Practical Dermoscopy

Jie Liu • Xian-biao Zou

Practical Dermoscopy

PEOPLE'S MEDICAL PUBLISHING HOUSE
PMPH

Springer

Jie Liu
Department of Dermatology
Peking Union Medical College Hospital
Beijing, China

Xian-biao Zou
Department of Dermatology
South China Hospital, Shenzhen University
Health Science Center
Shenzhen, China

ISBN 978-981-19-1459-1 ISBN 978-981-19-1460-7 (eBook)
https://doi.org/10.1007/978-981-19-1460-7
Jointly published with People's Medical Publishing House, PR of China

This Springer imprint is published by the registered company Springer Nature Singapore Pte Ltd.
The registered company address is: 152 Beach Road, #21-01/04 Gateway East, Singapore 189721, Singapore

Foreword 1

Dermoscopy is the most developed assisted diagnostic technique in skin imaging. In recent decades, dermoscopy has been widely accepted and used by dermatologists worldwide, with a large number of professional books and papers published. This technique was introduced to China late, but it developed rapidly. The Huaxia Skin Image and Artificial Intelligence Cooperation (HSIAIC) was established in May 2018 and it aims to cooperate with doctors and research teams from hospitals, universities, and research institutes all over China to promote the development of skin imaging and related artificial intelligence.

Practical Dermoscopy, written by the young dermatologist team from HSIAIC led by Prof. Jie Liu and Prof. Xian-biao Zou, provides a comprehensive introduction to the basic theories, devices, terminology, diagnostic strategies, and algorithms of dermoscopy, as well as the dermoscopic features of skin tumors, inflammatory skin diseases, infectious skin diseases, and hair and nail diseases, especially the correlation between dermoscopic findings and clinical characteristics and histopathology. It should be emphasized that all the images in this book are from Chinese patients, the most common Fitzpatrick skin types among whom are type III and type IV; therefore, some dermoscopic features may differ from those in other skin types. Finally, this book introduces the application of artificial-intelligence-assisted diagnosis in dermoscopy. This book is a monograph for doctors in relevant specialties to study dermoscopy, and it can be an important reference book for them.

The preparation of this book was supported by the Executive Committee of the International Dermoscopy Society. I would like to express my sincere thanks to Prof. H. Peter Soyer, Founding President of the International Dermoscopy Society; Prof. Aimilios Lallas, President of the International Dermoscopy Society; and other members of the International Dermoscopy Society.

I would also like to express my sincere congratulations to the writing team on their work, and I look forward to the further development of dermoscopy.

Hongzhong Jin

Director of Department of Dermatology
Peking Union Medical College Hospital
Beijing, China

Chairman of the Committee of the Dermatology Branch
of China International Exchange and Promotive Association
for Medical and Health Care
Beijing, China

Director of Huaxia Skin Image and Artificial Intelligence
Cooperation (HSIAIC)
Beijing, China

Director of the Rare Skin Disease Committee of the China Alliance
for Rare Disease
Beijing, China

Foreword 2

In my role as founding president of the International Dermoscopy Society, it is my honor and pleasure to write a foreword for the English translation of the first Chinese dermoscopy textbook, *Practical Dermoscopy*. While our own book, *Dermoscopy: The Essentials* has been translated into Chinese, the production of a Chinese text illustrates the keen interest of our Chinese colleagues in adapting dermoscopy to serve the needs of China's people. I have seen this interest for myself during my recent dermoscopy workshops at the Annual Meetings of the Chinese Dermatologist Association in Suzhou and Guangzhou, where I have participated as an invited international guest speaker over the last few years.

In addition, it is an excellent idea to have this book translated into English to provide better information for clinicians worldwide serving members of the Chinese diaspora, which extends to all inhabited continents and every major city worldwide. A weakness of many previous dermoscopy texts has been a lack of non-Caucasian skin representations, which is a problem due to the subtly different presentations of many diseases in skin with different levels of pigmentation. The wide variety of images in this book will be a useful educational tool in this respect.

The excellent and detailed photographs are supported by informative schematic drawings and histopathology images showing the correlation of dermoscopic and histopathologic structures. The authors should be commended for the uniformly high quality of these illustrations and their excellent instructional value.

I am very pleased to serve alongside this volume's author, Professor Jie Liu, on the executive board of the International Dermoscopy Society, and I have also been honored with an invitation to be a consultant for the Huaxia Skin Image and Artificial Intelligence Cooperation, as Chinese dermoscopists have expanded into the exciting new area of AI-assisted diagnosis and management.

Practical Dermoscopy follows the expanding role of dermoscopy, originally developed to examine melanocytic lesions and pigmented and non-pigmented skin lesions, to investigate uses in wider skin disease diagnosis, particularly inflammoscopy, entomodermoscopy, nail dermoscopy, and trichoscopy. This fully illustrated guide to dermoscopy should become essential for any clinician with an interest in dermatological diseases. In conclusion, I would like to compliment Professor Jie Liu and colleagues for authoring this very well illustrated and comprehensive textbook on dermoscopy.

H. Peter Soyer, MD FACD FAHMS

The University of Queensland
Dermatology Research Center
Brisbane, Queensland, Australia

Founding President
International Dermoscopy Society

Foreword 3

It is with great pleasure that I write the foreword to the new book of Prof. Jie Liu and Prof. Xian-biao Zou, *Practical Dermoscopy*. Including information on the history of the method, the instrument itself, criteria seen in tumors and inflammatory diseases, and diagnostic methods and algorithms, I strongly believe that it represents a complete guide that will be useful for all clinicians, irrespective of their level of experience. I am confident that this book will significantly enhance the dissemination of dermatoscopy and motivate numerous young researchers to generate ideas for future research in areas that are still much needed.

It is true that dermatoscopy radically changed not only our daily practice but also the field of dermatology itself. As a field dealing mainly with morphology, dermatology was literally redefined when the previously unexplored world of sub-macroscopical structures came to light. In addition, research in dermatoscopy generated novel ideas led to questions on previously established concepts and demolished pre-existing "dogmas." The most characteristic example is the radical change in the concepts of melanoma genesis and the biological significance of nevi. Our perception today is very much different from the "old-world" theory that melanoma represents a malignant transformation of nevi. Of course, this modification was not a result of dermatoscopy alone, but our ability to "see" melanoma in the early stages significantly contributed to the questioning of the previously predominant theory of "pre-melanomas."

While there is no doubt that our ability to diagnose skin cancer earlier is the most important impact of dermatoscopy, it is not the only one. Numerous cutaneous inflammations and infections have been dermatoscopically investigated, and their morphological characteristics need to be re-considered, re-established, and re-written in a combined macroscopic and submacroscopic context.

Finally, dermatoscopy continuously generates an increasing number of passionate teachers and researchers, exemplifying how clinicians continuously strive for self-improvement to provide better service to their patients.

Bright examples of passionate teachers and researchers are the editors of this book, which I invite to you to acquire and read in depth.

With my best wishes,

Aimilios Lallas

Department of Dermatology
Aristotle University of Thessaloniki
Thessaloniki, Greece

President of the International Dermoscopy Society
Graz, Austria

Preface

Dermoscopy is a convenient, noninvasive, real-time, and effective diagnostic tool that has been the most developed and studied in the field of skin imaging. It has been widely adopted around the world and is known as "the dermatologist's stethoscope." As the diagnostic strategies, patterns and terminology have been established, the application of dermoscopy has gradually expanded from pigmented and non-pigmented skin tumors to other skin conditions, including inflammatory, infectious and autoimmune skin diseases as well as hair and nail diseases. Apart from assisting in diagnosis, dermoscopy has also been used for monitoring responses of treatment. In recent years, with the development of image-based artificial intelligence (AI), the combination of AI and dermoscopy has become one of the research hotspots in dermatology, with increasing publications in prestigious journals.

Dermoscopy has not been introduced into China for long, but it is developing rapidly. Multiple skin imaging and AI cooperative groups have been established in China, including the Huaxia Skin Image and Artificial Intelligence Cooperation (HSIAIC), Chinese Skin Image Database (CSID), and Dermatology Artificial Intelligence Development Alliance of China (DAIDAC), all of which have made efforts to promote the education, application, and research on dermoscopy. For instance, the HSIAIC has held a national conference on dermoscopy for many years and has launched online courses to disseminate this technology in China.

In 2015, our team published the first textbook on dermoscopy in China, *Atlas of Dermoscopy of Xiehe (PUMCH)*, which comprehensively introduced the basic knowledge of dermoscopy and dermoscopic features of some diseases. It turned out to be very popular all over the country and nearly 10,000 copies have been sold. It has helped Chinese dermatologists in better using dermoscopy in their clinical practice, yet there is still much space for improvement. In the past five years, with the accumulation of practice and investigation, dermatologists have gained a deeper understanding of dermoscopy and the knowledge is in need of updating. That is why this book came about.

Practical Dermoscopy introduces the latest progresses in dermoscopy and shares with readers the clinical, dermoscopic, and histopathological images that are collected during our clinical practice. The first chapter describes the basic knowledge, history, and principles of dermoscopy. In Chapter 2, some of the current devices are introduced. In Chapters 3 and 4, terminology and analytical strategies are generally introduced. Chapters 5 to 11 focus on neoplastic dermatoses, consisting of benign melanocytic neoplasms, malignant melanomas, basal cell carcinomas, seborrheic keratosis and related diseases, vascular diseases, squamous cell neoplasms, and other neoplasms. The clinical characteristics are introduced briefly, while the dermoscopic features and their causes are highlighted with a large number of pictures. Chapters 12 to 14 introduce the dermoscopic manifestations of nonneoplastic dermatoses, including inflammatory skin diseases, infectious and parasitic skin diseases, hair and nail diseases. It should be noted that most dermoscopic features of these diseases are nonspecific, so a comprehensive analysis combined with medical history and clinical features is needed to avoid misdiagnosis. Chapter 15 introduces the history, present and future of computer-aided diagnosis based on dermoscopic images, since it has become a focus of attention these days.

We would like to express our gratitude to all the editors for their passion and dedication, to Prof. H. Peler Soyer and Prof. Aimilios Lallas for writing the foreword, to Prof. Hongzhong Jin for his full support over the course of writing this book and to all of our colleagues and friends for their appreciation of this book. We hope that *Practical Dermoscopy* will be a gift for the 100th anniversary of Peking Union Medical College Hospital! We hope that you will enjoy reading it!

Beijing, China

Jie Liu
Xian-biao Zou

Introduction of Editors

Chief Editors

Jie Liu
Xian-biao Zou

Deputy Editors

Chenyu Zhu
Chang Shu

Consultants

Hongzhong Jin
H. Peter Soyer
Aimilios Lallas

Contents

About the Editors and Contributors

About the Editors

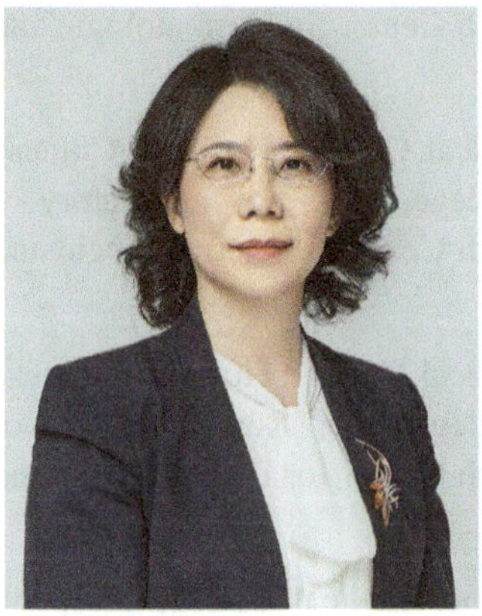

Jie Liu Deputy Director of Dermatology Department, Peking Union Medical College Hospital, professor/chief physician, doctoral supervisor. Her main research areas are skin imaging, artificial intelligence, and cutaneous lymphoma. In 2015, she was awarded the Outstanding Young Dermatologist by the Chinese Dermatologists Association. She is also an executive board of the International Dermoscopy Society (IDS) and a member of the International Society for Cutaneous Lymphoma (ISCL), the Deputy Director and Secretary-General of the Rare Skin Disease Committee of the China Alliance For Rare Disease, the Deputy Director and Secretary-General of the Huaxia Skin Image and Artificial Intelligence Cooperation (HSIAIC). She is also the reviewer of the Journal of Investigative Dermatology, Journal of the American Academy of Dermatology, British Journal of Dermatology, Journal of the European Academy of Dermatology and Venereology, and Chinese Journal of Dermatology, etc. She has taken charge of multiple national research projects and contributes to over 100 papers published by famous issues at home and abroad. She has led the publication of more than 10 consensuses in the skin imaging field. She is also the editor-in-chief of *Practical Dermoscopy*, *Atlas of Dermoscopy of Xiehe (PUMCH), Typical Cases and Analyses (PUMCH),* and is the main interpreter of the Chinese version of *Dermoscopy in General Dermatology*.

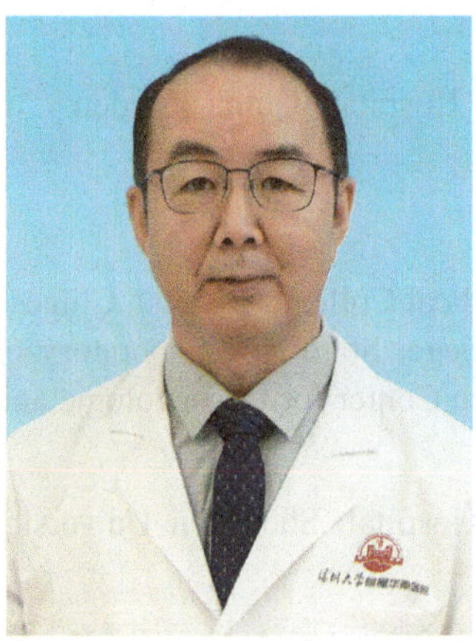

Xian-biao Zou Clinical Professor of Dermatology & Director of Department of Dermatology, South China Hospital, Health Science Center, Shenzhen University. He is the Deputy Secretary-General of the World Association of Chinese Dermatologists, the headman of the Skin Imaging Group, a member of the standing committee of Combination of Traditional and Western Medicine Dermatology, and a member of Chinese Science Writers Association. He has been engaged in dermatology for more than 30 years and has profound attainments in photodynamic therapy and skin imaging. He is also the main interpreter of the Chinese version of *Color Atlas of Differential Diagnosis in Dermatopathology*, *Diagnostic Dermoscopy*, *Dermatologic Ultrasound with Clinical and Histologic Correlations*, and *Identification of Pathogenic Fungi*, among others.

Contributors

Cheng Chi Department of Dermatology, Peking Union Medical College Hospital, Chinese Academy of Medical Science & Peking Union Medical College, State Key Laboratory of Complex Severe and Rare Diseases, National Clinical Research Center for Dermatologic and Immunologic Diseases, Beijing, China

Jie Liu Department of Dermatology, Peking Union Medical College Hospital, Chinese Academy of Medical Science & Peking Union Medical College, State Key Laboratory of Complex Severe and Rare Diseases, National Clinical Research Center for Dermatologic and Immunologic Diseases, Beijing, China

Zhaorui Liu Department of Dermatology, Peking Union Medical College Hospital, Chinese Academy of Medical Science & Peking Union Medical College, State Key Laboratory of Complex Severe and Rare Diseases, National Clinical Research Center for Dermatologic and Immunologic Diseases, Beijing, China

Yixin Luo Department of Dermatology, Peking Union Medical College Hospital, Chinese Academy of Medical Science & Peking Union Medical College, State Key Laboratory of Complex Severe and Rare Diseases, National Clinical Research Center for Dermatologic and Immunologic Diseases, Beijing, China

Chang Shu Department of Dermatology, Peking Union Medical College Hospital, Chinese Academy of Medical Science & Peking Union Medical College, State Key Laboratory of Complex Severe and Rare Diseases, National Clinical Research Center for Dermatologic and Immunologic Diseases, Beijing, China

Juncheng Wang Department of Dermatology, Peking Union Medical College Hospital, Chinese Academy of Medical Science & Peking Union Medical College, State Key Laboratory of Complex Severe and Rare Diseases, National Clinical Research Center for Dermatologic and Immunologic Diseases, Beijing, China

Shiqi Wang Department of Dermatology, Peking Union Medical College Hospital, Chinese Academy of Medical Science & Peking Union Medical College, State Key Laboratory of Complex Severe and Rare Diseases, National Clinical Research Center for Dermatologic and Immunologic Diseases, Beijing, China

Yukun Wang Department of Dermatology, Peking Union Medical College Hospital, Chinese Academy of Medical Science & Peking Union Medical College, State Key Laboratory of Complex Severe and Rare Diseases, National Clinical Research Center for Dermatologic and Immunologic Diseases, Beijing, China

Fengying Xie Beihang University, Beijing, China

Chenchen Xu Department of Dermatology, Guang'anmen Hospital, China Academy of Chinese Medical Sciences, Beijing, China

Yiguang Yang Beihang University, Beijing, China

Chenyu Zhu Department of Dermatology, Peking Union Medical College Hospital, Chinese Academy of Medical Science & Peking Union Medical College, State Key Laboratory of Complex Severe and Rare Diseases, National Clinical Research Center for Dermatologic and Immunologic Diseases, Beijing, China

Xian-biao Zou Department of Dermatology, South China Hospital, Shenzhen University Health Science Center, Shenzhen, China

Yue Zeng Department of Dermatology, South China Hospital, Shenzhen University Health Science Center, Shenzhen, China

Shan Zhang Department of Dermatology, Peking Union Medical College Hospital, Chinese Academy of Medical Science & Peking Union Medical College, State Key Laboratory of Complex Severe and Rare Diseases, National Clinical Research Center for Dermatologic and Immunologic Diseases, Beijing, China

Zhiyu Pang Department of Dermatology, Peking Union Medical College Hospital, Chinese Academy of Medical Science & Peking Union Medical College, State Key Laboratory of Complex Severe and Rare Diseases, National Clinical Research Center for Dermatologic and Immunologic Diseases, Beijing, China

Introduction

1

The diagnosis of skin diseases is highly based on morphology. With continuous development of technology, there are emerging skin imaging technologies available for clinicians to aid in diagnosis and evaluation of diseases as well as cosmetic assessment, including manual and computer graphics, photography and videography, Wood's lamp, reflective confocal microscopy (RCM), VISIA skin analysis system, high frequency skin ultrasound, optical coherence tomography (OCT), etc., all of which are in vivo, non-invasive, real-time, fast, and dynamic. Dermoscopy, as an important part of skin imaging, has attracted the attention of dermatologists and has shown increasing application in clinical practice due to its convenience and capability to assist in making a quick diagnosis.

1.1 History and Nomenclature of Dermoscopy

Dermatology is a discipline based on visual diagnosis. Previous examination and evaluation of skin lesions mainly relied on the naked eye before dermoscopy was introduced. As early as 1590, Dutch glass manufacturer H. Jansen and his son Z. Jansen invented microscope. In 1663, J.C. Kohlhaus first used skin surface microscopy to observe the capillaries of the nail fold. In 1893, G. Unna used the term "diaskopie" to describe how immersion oil was used together with a microscope. In 1923, J. Saphier used the German word "dermatoskopie" in his publications. In 1925, German scholar Hans Hinselman invented colposcopy, which was latterly used to diagnose skin ulcers and tumors in 1933. In 1951, L. Goldman investigated melanomas and melanocytic nevi with monocular epiluminescence tools and subsequently invented the first portable dermoscope in 1958 and named it "dermascopy". In 1971, Rona MacKie confirmed the practical value of dermoscopy in differential diagnosis of benign and malignant pigmented skin lesions. In 1981, P. Fritsch and R. Pechlaner observed pigment network in benign and malignant melanocytic lesions. In 1987, H. Pehamberger et al. used the term "epiluminescence microscopy (ELM)" to describe this technique and established pattern analysis, a dermoscopic diagnostic method for pigmented skin lesions. In 1989, H.P. Soyer et al. explained the correlation between dermoscopic features and histopathological structures. In the same year, the first Consensus Conference on dermoscopy was held in Hamburg, Germany, to develop a standardized terminology for this technique, and the website of the International Dermoscopy Society was also established. In 1991, J. Kreusch and G. Rassner published the first monograph, *Dermoscopy Atlas*. In 2001, the first polarized dermoscope was developed in the United States. In 2003, the International Dermoscopy Society published the first consensus on dermoscopic diagnosis of pigmented skin lesions. In 2007, a proposal for standardized dermoscopy reports was published. The recommendations include: clinical information of the patients; description of the lesion; using the two-step method; using standardized terms defined in the Dermoscopy Consensus Report published in 2003 to describe structures (for new terms, a definition should be given); imaging equipment and magnification; clinical and dermoscopic pictures of the lesion; diagnosis or differential diagnosis; suggested subsequent management. The optional points include the algorithm used and comments for the pathologists to guide the excision if necessary. In 2016, an international consensus on the standardized terminology of dermoscopy was published (see Chap. 3 for details). Over time, dermoscopic equipment has continuously been renovated, and dermoscopic diagnostic techniques and processes have also been improved.

Although clinical applications of dermoscopy started later in China than in European and American countries, the development of it is very encouraging. In recent years, a number of academic organizations have been established in China, including the Skin Imaging Group of the Combination of Traditional and Western Medicine Dermatology (Prof. Xianbiao Zou as the leader), the Skin Imaging Group of the Dermatology Branch of the China International Exchange and Promotive Association for Medical and Health Care (Prof. Jie Liu as the leader), etc.

J. Liu, X. Zou, *Practical Dermoscopy*, https://doi.org/10.1007/978-981-19-1460-7_1

Many skin imaging and artificial intelligence (AI) collaborative organizations, such as the Huaxia Skin Image and Artificial Intelligence Cooperation (HSIAIC), Chinese Skin Image Database (CSID) and Dermatology Artificial Intelligence Development Alliance of China (DAIDAC), have been set up following the lead of major skin imaging centers. Apart from the establishment of academic organizations, atlases, monographs and consensuses on dermoscopy have been published one after another by experts nationwide. In 2014, Prof. Xingqi Zhang from the Department of Dermatology of the First Affiliated Hospital of Sun Yat-sen University edited and published the *Atlas of Dermoscopy in Pigmented and Hair Diseases*. In 2015, Prof. Qiuning Sun and Prof. Jie Liu from the Dermatology Department of Peking Union Medical College Hospital coedited and published the *Atlas of Dermoscopy of Xiehe (PUMCH),* the first dermoscopic textbook in Chinese, which comprehensively introduced the clinical applications of dermoscopy. Subsequently, several national skin imaging groups published over ten expert consensuses on dermoscopic diagnoses, experts translated and published several foreign monographs on dermoscopy. In addition, online and offline courses have also been launched to promote education and dissemination of dermoscopy in China. A number of domestic leading skin imaging centers, including the Dermatology Department of Peking Union Medical College Hospital, the Dermatology Department of Peking University First Hospital, the Dermatology Department of Air Force General Hospital, and the Dermatology Department of the Fourth Affiliated Hospital of PLA General Hospital, have held dermoscopic training classes nationwide, many domestic manufacturers have also developed dermoscopic equipments in China. In 2018, Prof. Jie Liu from the Dermatology Department of Peking Union Medical College Hospital was elected as the Representative of the Board (Asia) of the Executive Board Committee of the International Dermoscopy Society. In May of the same year, HSIAIC was established, focusing on promoting the development of dermoscopy in China to be in line with international standards. In November 2018, Huaxia Skin Image Cloud-School went online, in which the Skin Imaging Course of Xiehe (PUMCH) introduced the basics and applications of dermoscopy. In recent years, special sessions on dermoscopy have been held at almost all domestic dermatology academic conferences. Dermoscopic diagnoses have also been included in the 2018 edition of the higher education textbook *Dermatovenereology*. A prototype of the AI diagnostic app for skin disease, which focuses on dermoscopic and clinical diagnoses, has also been launched. Thanks to the united efforts of experts and organizations, the clinical practice of dermoscopy in China is expected to be increasingly popular and widespread in the future.

Over the 100-year development of dermoscopy, many names have emerged for this technique, such as ELM, amplified surface microscopy, cutaneous microscopy, surface microscopy, dermascopy, dermoscopy, incident light microscopy, diascopy, dermatoscopy, and skin microscopy, among which "dermoscopy" and "dermatoscopy" are most commonly used in the published literature. The term "Dermoscopy" was first introduced by Friedman in 1991, and it was accepted by most dermatologists. Juliana Berk Krauss et al. searched "dermoscopy" and "dermatoscopy" on PubMed and found that 3900 papers used the former, while only 500 papers used the latter. However, experts did not reach an agreement on the standardized use of the two terms on the Third Consensus Conference of the International Dermoscopy Society in 2016, so they were both used in the consensuses on dermoscopy. In addition, many new terms have emerged due to the different application of dermoscopy, including inflammoscopy for dermoscopy used for the diagnosis of inflammatory skin diseases, entomodermoscopy for parasite examination, trichoscopy for scalp and hair, onychoscopy for nail examination, capillaroscopy for nail fold capillary examination (with the magnification from 50 times to more than 200 times), mucoscopy for oral or genital mucosa examination, and teledermoscopy for telemedicine diagnosis. Despite the numerous names, the most commonly used one is still "dermoscopy."

1.2 Principles and Classification of Dermoscopy

Dermoscopy, as a non-invasive, portable, and real-time diagnostic tool, is similar to otoscopy, ophthalmoscopy, and laryngoscopy, since all of them have the function of magnification. Dermoscopy is an extension of the naked eye, it can filter out reflected light and allows observation of deeper structures than a mere magnifying glass, assisting in observing pigmented changes in the epidermis and reticular dermis, and vascular changes in the superficial and middle layers of the dermis. Therefore, dermoscopy got the reputation of "dermatologist's stethoscope".

The latest research shows that the minimum unit of light that can be detected by human eyes is photon. Generally speaking, however, the smallest resolvable size of normal-vision eyes is 0.1 mm at a 25 cm distance of distinct vision, that is, the human eye can distinguish 10 pixels within a 1 mm unit. The resolution of human eyes is generally 0.25–0.30 mm, that is, the human eye can distinguish 3–4 pixels within a 1 mm distance. The width of the reticular lines of typical pigment network in a nevus and a capillary loop in the skin is less than 0.05 mm, which cannot be observed by the naked eye. But with the help of dermoscopy, these microstructures can be observed.

The stratum corneum of the skin has a certain degree of transmittance, with the cells closely arranged in a layered structure. The keratinocytes and oil film on the surface of skin have a specular reflection effect on illumination light. Since the refractive index of the stratum corneum (1.55) is higher than that of air (1.0), most of the incident light is reflected off the skin surface, therefore, it is impossible to observe the color and structural changes in the deep epidermis and dermis with the naked eye. Light can pass through the smooth and oily epidermis to reach the deeper dermis, based on this principle, early nonpolarized dermoscopy (NPD) required olive oil, mineral oil, couplant, ethanol, glycerin, or even water as mediators to eliminate the reflected light and improve the penetration of the light to a depth of 0.05–0.1 mm (Fig. 1.1). However, there was a possibility of cross-infection since it requires direct contact with the skin lesions and the glass plate. The advent of polarized dermoscopy (PD) solved this problem well.

As we know, light, like all the electromagnetic waves, is a transverse wave. The plane formed by the vibration direction and the propagation direction is known as the vibration plane. Light, whose vibration plane is limited to a fixed direction, is called plane-polarized light or linearly polarized light. While light, whose vibration plane is evenly distributed in all directions, is called natural light. PD achieves cross-polarization by two polarizers, which can turn the natural light into polarized light. The observation depth of PD can reach the deep layers of epidermis, dermal–epidermal junction, and the papillary dermis, while the area from the surface to 60–100 μm is the blind area. PD allows light to pass through the polarizer without contacting the skin lesions and therefore prevents cross-infection, but it has the disadvantage of low light intensity and poor resolution. Polarized dermoscopy can be further divided into polarized contact dermoscopy (PCD) and polarized noncontact dermoscopy (PNCD). Better image quality can be achieved when using PD with immersion liquid. Currently, most dermoscopes are available for multi-modal observation. NPD and PD have their own advantages, and they can display different dermoscopic features (Table 1.1). Due to the different observation depths and levels, more information can be obtained when using both non-polarized and polarized modes.

The advantage of dermoscopy is that it can improve the diagnostic accuracy of melanoma, with a sensitivity of 89.7% and specificity of 92.0%, reducing unnecessary biopsies or surgical resections of benign lesions. The biopsy rate of skin lesions by general practitioners in the United States is 30%, while 15% for dermatologists who do not use dermoscopy and 5% for dermatologists who use dermoscopy. In addition, the application of dermoscopy has gradually expanded to nonpigmented skin diseases, hair diseases, nail

Table 1.1 Comparison of the differences between nonpolarized and polarized dermoscopy

	NPD	PCD/PNCD
Observing depth	Superficial (the epidermis and the dermal–epidermal junction)	Deeper (the dermal–epidermal junction and superficial dermis)
Contact	Requires contact with the skin and liquid immersion	Does not require contact with the skin or liquid immersion
Colors	Better at observing blue-white veil	Better at observing pigmentation and red/pink
Structures	Better at observing peppering, milia-like cysts and comedo-like openings	Better at observing shiny-white streaks and blood vessels
patterns	Showing homogeneous blue in a blue nevus	Showing heterogeneous with different shades of blue

NPD nonpolarized dermoscopy, *PCD* polarized contact dermoscopy, *PNCD* polarized noncontact dermoscopy

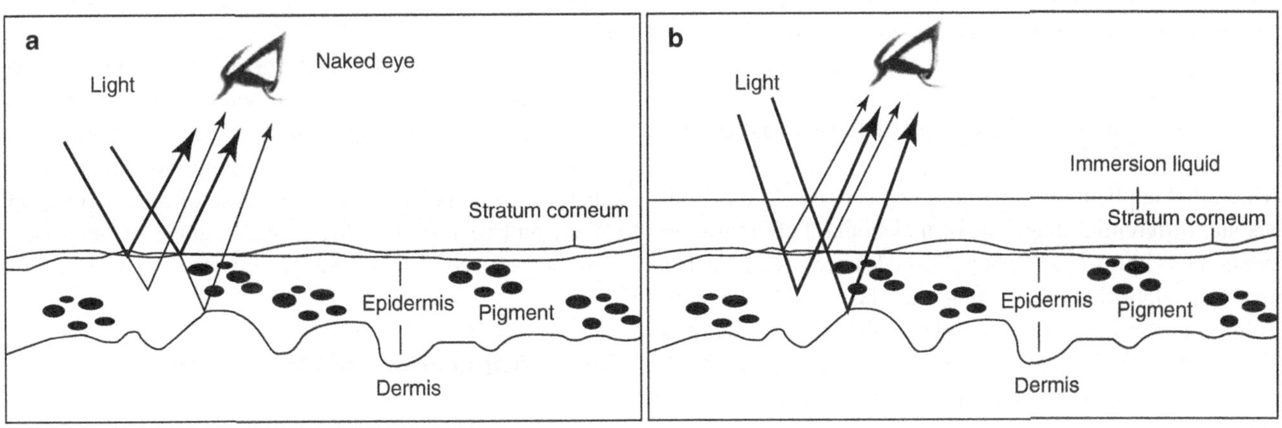

Fig. 1.1 Principle of dermoscopic imaging. (**a**) Observation with naked eye; (**b**) observation with nonpolarized dermoscopy

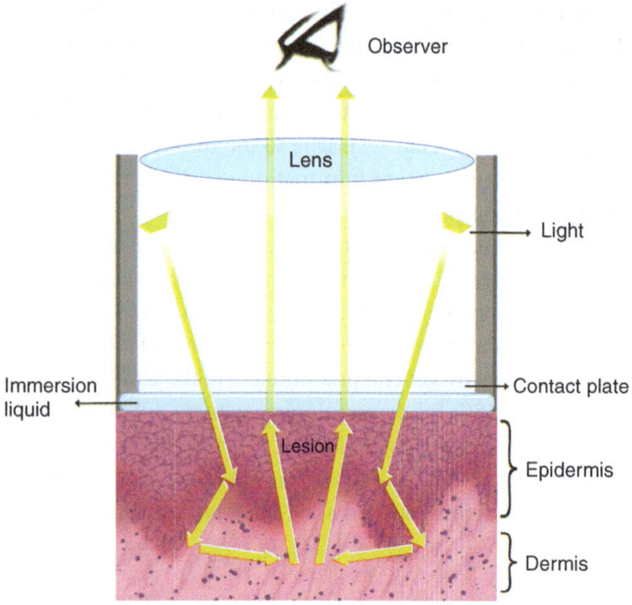

Fig. 1.2 Basic structure of a dermoscope

diseases, autoimmune diseases and other fields, increasing the clinical diagnostic rate by 5–30%.

Currently, there is no international standard for the classification of dermoscopy equipment. Depending on their structures, dermoscopes can be divided into six categories: classic handheld dermoscopes, handheld dermoscopes that attach to digital cameras, dermoscopes with image acquisition accessories, dermoscopes that attach to smartphones, desktop dermoscopic systems, and polarized total body photographic systems (see Chap. 2 for details) that can be generally divided into portable and desktop dermoscopes. A portable dermoscope is composed of an eyepiece, contact plate, light source (halogen lamp or LED lamp), battery, camera clasp, and so on (Fig. 1.2). The contact plate is mostly made of polysilicon-coated glass with built-in scale marks to measure the size of the lesions. The small contact plate makes it easy to observe finger web, skin folds, and nail bed capillaries. A desktop dermoscope is connected to a workstation and the image data storage and analysis system.

1.3 Diagnostic Algorithms of Dermoscopy

The initial application of dermoscopy is to assist in diagnosis and differential diagnosis of melanoma. Different diagnostic algorithms have been published successively, such as two-step algorithms (including the classic two-step algorithm and top-down two-step algorithm), pattern analysis, the ABCD rule, the Menzies method, the seven-point checklist, the three-point checklist, the CASH algorithm, the revised version of pattern analysis, the Chaos and Clues, the Triage Amalgamated Dermoscopic Algorithm, the Prediction without Pigment and the color wheel approach.

Table 1.2 Color and location of melanin under dermoscopy

Color	Representation
Black	Stratum spinosum
Light or dark brown	Dermal–epidermal junction
Gray-bluish	Papillary dermis
Blue	Reticular dermis
White	Fibrosis or regression (the white color must be lighter than that of the periphery skin)
Red	Hemoglobin inside vessels

The Chaos and Clues is a simple process to analyze the characteristics of lesion under dermoscopy step by step, which is practicable and easy to operate, with great potential for development. The above methods are all based on colors, structures or blood vessels viewed under dermoscopy. Colors presented under dermoscopy include black, red, white and brown (Table 1.2, Fig. 1.3). Features of the structures include global and local features (Table 1.3). Vascular morphology includes dots, clods, linear, coiled, looped, serpentine, helical, curved, monomorphous and polymorphous, while the vascular arrangement is classified into crown vessels, string of pearls, arborizing vessels, and targetoid vessels (see Chap. 3 for details). Dermoscopic features combined with clinical manifestations and medical history enable dermatologists to quickly make a clinical diagnosis.

1.4 Correlation and Differences Between Dermoscopy and Histopathology

Dermoscopy and histopathology are two different diagnostic methods. As a convenient, easy-to-learn, non-invasive, real-time diagnostic tool, dermoscopy can be widely used in the diagnosis of pigmented and nonpigmented skin tumors and non-neoplastic dermatoses. Since histopathology is the "gold standard" in the diagnosis of skin tumors, the diagnostic criteria of dermoscopy is derived from comparative analysis of dermoscopic features and their correlated histopathologic structures. These two methods have certain differences in application, which are listed in detail in Table 1.4. Dermoscopy can improve the accuracy of skin lesion screening, guide clinical decision and help to optimize the treatment. However, the observing depth of dermoscopy is limited to epidermis and superficial or papillary dermis. Because of that, dermoscopy cannot replace histopathology, whose scope of observation can reach as deep as the subcutaneous tissue and adipose layer.

1.5 Applications of Dermoscopy

1. Early detection of melanoma and differentiate it from pigmented nevus.
2. Monitoring lesions been suspicious of melanoma.

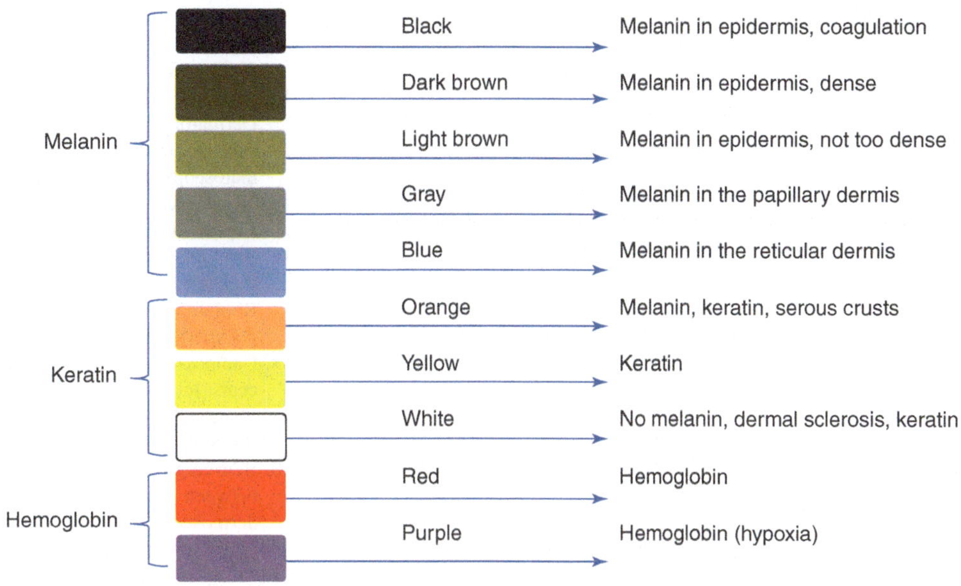

Fig. 1.3 The color under dermoscopy is formed by different combinations of keratin, melanin, hemoglobin, collagen and foreign bodies and is related to the depth of the pigment. (Copyright © 2012 From An Atlas of Dermoscopy by Ashfaq A Marghoob, Josep Malvehy, and Ralph P. Braun. Reproduced by permission of Taylor and Francis Group, LLC, a division of Informa plc.)

Table 1.3 Structures under dermoscopy

Global patterns	Local features of melanocytic lesions	Local features of nonmelanocytic lesions
Reticular pattern	Pigment network	Milia-like cysts
Globular pattern	Dots and globules	Comedo-like openings
Cobblestone pattern	Streaks	Exophytic papillary structures
Homogeneous pattern	Pigmentation	Red lacunas
Parallel pattern	Hypopigmentation	Leaf-like areas
Starburst pattern	Regression structures	Central white area
Multicomponent pattern	Vascular structures	
Unspecific pattern	Blue-white veil	

Table 1.4 Differences between dermoscopy and histopathology

Characteristics	Dermoscopy	Histopathology
Invasiveness	Non-invasive	Invasive
Real-time and dynamic	Yes	No
Operating equipment	Simple	Difficult
Operator	Single	Multiplayer
Number of tests	Dozens or more	Generally no more than 3
Degree of difficulty	Simple	Difficult
Diagnostic time	1–5 min	Hours to days
Convenience	Convenient, suitable for follow-up	Inconvenient
Direction of the epidermis	Horizontal	Vertical
Depth of observation	Superficial or papillary dermis	Adipose layer
Display accuracy	Nests of melanocytes, vessels	Cell level
Diagnostic value	Screening	Gold standard

3. Assist in the diagnosis of nonmelanocytic benign and malignant tumors, such as basal cell carcinoma, actinic keratosis, squamous cell carcinoma, adnexal tumor, hemangioma, and seborrheic keratosis.
4. Assist in the diagnosis of inflammatory diseases, such as lichen planus, psoriasis, Darier's disease, and urticarial vasculitis.
5. Assist in the diagnosis of parasitic and infectious diseases, such as pediculosis pubis, scabies, insect bite dermatitis, molluscum contagiosum, skin warts, and condyloma acuminatum.
6. Assist in the diagnosis and differential diagnosis of hair diseases such as alopecia areata, syphilitic alopecia, tinea capitis, trichotillomania, and androgenic alopecia. Hair follicle density and hair texture can be observed, and the curative effect can be evaluated.
7. Assist in the diagnosis and differential diagnosis of nail lesions, such as subungual hemorrhage, nail melanoma, nail lichen planus, periungual wart, and onychomycosis. The capillaries of the nail fold can be examined for early diagnosis and differential diagnosis of rheumatic diseases and predict their prognosis.
8. Determine the surgical margin of skin tumor and dynamically monitor postoperative recurrence.
9. Monitor the adverse effect caused by long-term topical corticosteroid preparations in the treatment of dermatitis, eczema, or psoriasis.
10. Establish AI-aided diagnosis and telemedicine system for skin diseases, which is helpful to improve the diagnosis of skin diseases in remote areas or primary medical institutions.

Further Reading

1. Braun RP, Rabinovitz HS, Oliviero M, et al. Dermoscopy of pigmented skin lesions. J Am Acad Dermatol. 2005;52(1):109–21.
2. Kittler H, Marghoob AA, Argenzianor G, et al. Standardization of terminology in dermoscopy/dermatoscopy: results of the third consensus conference of the International Society of Dermoscopy. J Am Acad Dermatol. 2016;74(6):1093–106.
3. Bahmer FA, Fritsch P, Kreusch J, et al. Terminology in surface microscopy. Consensus meeting of the Committee on Analytical Morphology of the Arbeitsgemeinschaft Dermatologische Forschung, Hamburg, Federal Republic of Germany, Nov. 17, 1989. J Am Acad Dermatol. 1990;23(6 Pt 1):1159–62.
4. Massie D, De Giorgi V, Soyer HP. Histopathologic correlates of dermoscopic criteria. Dermatol Clin. 2001;19(2):259–68.
5. Argenziano G, Soyer HP, Chimenti S, et al. Dermoscopy of pigmented skin lesions: results of a consensus meeting via the Internet. J Am Acad Dermatol. 2003;48(5):679–93.
6. Malvehy J, Puig S, Argenzianor G, et al. Dermoscopy report: proposal for standardization. Results of a consensus meeting of the International Dermoscopy Society. J Am Acad Dermatol. 2007;57(1):84–95.
7. Coelho De Sousa V, Oliverira A. Inflammoscopy in the diagnosis of hypertrophic lichen planus. J Am Acad Dermatol. 2015;73(5):e171–3.
8. Torres F, Tosti A. Trichoscopy: an update. G Ital Dermatol Venereol. 2014;149(1):83–91.
9. Sheu SL, Cho HG, Nord KM. Videodermoscopy as a novel tool for dermatologic education. Cutis. 2017;100(2):E25–7.
10. Zalaudek I, Giacomel J, Cabo H, et al. Entodermoscopy: a new tool for diagnosing skin infections and infestations. Dermatology. 2008;216(1):14–23.
11. Cutolo M, Melsens K, Wijnant S, et al. Nailfold capillaroscopy in systemic lupus erythematosus: a systematic review and critical appraisal. Autoimmun Rev. 2018;17(4):344–52.
12. Kadurina M, Dimitrov B. Dermoscopy—a new diagnostic approach of pigmented skin lesions. Biotechnol Biotechnol Equip. 2005;19(2):23–7.
13. Grover C, Jakhar D. Onychoscopy: a practical guide. Indian J Dermatol Venereol Leprol. 2017;83(5):536–49.
14. Berk-Krauss J, Laird ME. What's in a name—dermoscopy vs dermatoscopy. JAMA Dermatol. 2017;153(12):1235.
15. Nischal KC, Khopkar U. Dermoscope. Indian J Dermatol Venereol Leprol. 2005;71(4):300–3.
16. Sun QN, Liu J. Atlas of dermoscopy of Xiehe (PUMCH). Beijing: People's Medical Publishing House; 2015.
17. Roldan-Marin R, Puig S, Malvehy J. Dermoscopic criteria and melanocytic lesions. G Ital Dermatol Venereol. 2012;147(2):149–59.
18. Campos-Do-Carmo G, Ramos-E-Silva M. Dermoscopy: basic concepts. Int J Dermatol. 2008;47(7):712–9.
19. Zhang QN. Principle and application of polarized light. Info Teach Res Wkly. 2010;14:26–7.
20. Benvenuto-Andrade C, Dusza SW, Agero AL, et al. Differences between polarized light dermoscopy and immersion contact dermoscopy for the evaluation of skin lesions. Arch Dermatol. 2007;143(3):329–38.
21. Liu Y, Xin R, Sun XM. Applicability analysis of eye resolution, satellite resolution and mapping scale. Heilongjiang Agric Sci. 2012;9:126–9.
22. Braun RP, Rabinovitz HS, Oliviero M, et al. Pattern analysis: a two-step procedure for the dermoscopic diagnosis of melanoma. Clin Dermatol. 2002;20(3):236–9.
23. Marghoob AA, Braun R. Proposal for a revised 2-step algorithm for the classification of lesions of the skin using dermoscopy. Arch Dermatol. 2010;146(4):426–8.
24. Rosendahl C, Cameron A, Mccoll I, et al. Dermatoscopy in routine practice—'chaos and clues'. Aust Fam Physician. 2012;41(7):482–7.
25. Soyer HP, Argenziano G, Chimenti S, et al. Dermoscopy of pigmented skin lesions. Eur J Dermatol. 2001;11(3):270–6.
26. Zou XB, Liu HX, Lu M, Wen H. Clinical application of skin imaging. Chin J Dermatol. 2017;50(7):467–71.

2 Dermoscopic Devices

The dermoscopic devices on the market at present are mainly divided into six categories: classic handheld dermoscopes, handheld dermoscopes that attach to digital cameras, dermoscopes with image acquisition accessories, dermoscopes that attach to smartphones, desktop dermoscopic systems, and polarized total body photographic systems, which will be briefly introduced in this chapter. Since most of these devices are easy to obtain at various international conferences and in online channels, also the agents change frequently, device acquisition approaches will not be mentioned in this book. We hereby certify that there is no conflict of interest between the authors of this book and the dermoscope manufacturers mentioned.

2.1 Classic Handheld Dermoscopes

Classic handheld dermoscopes are mainly used for direct examination of skin lesions with the naked eye, and most are equipped with an internal standard illumination source. Classic handheld dermoscopes have the advantages of easy portability, direct in vivo observation of skin lesions, more realistic and abundant information on skin lesions, and a low price relative to other types of dermoscopes. However, handheld dermoscopes cannot record and save images and are more suitable for rapid outpatient screening.

Handheld dermoscopes are divided into polarized and nonpolarized (immersion) types depending on how epidermal reflections are eliminated. Nonpolarized (immersion) dermoscopes are older and more classic in design than polarized dermoscopes, and some dermoscope manufacturers are still producing similar devices. Immersion dermoscopes eliminate surface reflections through liquid infiltration of the lens and skin lesions, and they can obtain clear image of the epidermis and the dermal–epidermal junction. However, it is necessary to disinfect the lens, select the infiltrating solution, coat and wipe the lens each time, which is inconvenient. Moreover, the lens contacting the skin may compress blood vessels and thereby affect observations. Therefore, there are few scenarios where immersion dermoscopes must be used at present.

Immersion dermoscope requires an infiltrating solution. Generally, liquids with a refractive index exceeding that of air can be used as infiltrating solutions, such as alcohol gel, water, paraffin oil, and ultrasonic coupling agents. For skin lesions without rupture, alcohol gel (such as hand sanitizer) can be used for disinfection. For broken skin, paraffin oil or other anhydrous infiltrating solutions can be used. After use, the lens should be disinfected with alcohol-soaked cotton or gauze.

Polarized dermoscopes are easier to use, have no contact with lesions, avoid the compression of blood vessels, allow the observation of certain manifestations that can be viewed uniquely by polarized dermoscopy (e.g., shiny white streaks, rosettes, and rainbow patterns), and are ready to use without consumables or preparation. They could obtain deeper structures than immersion dermoscopes. However, polarized dermoscopy may miss some lesion features, such as milia-like cysts in seborrheic keratoses and nail fold capillaries. Therefore, dermoscopes on the market in recent years have both polarized and nonpolarized lenses (or light sources) for observation. This type of equipment includes DermLite DL100 and Carbon from 3Gen, VISIOMED Luminis from Canfield (United States), and mini3000 and NC1 from Heine (Germany).

2.2 Handheld Dermoscopes That Attach to Digital Cameras

Since dermoscopic images, similar to photographs, serve as objective evidence of lesions, they are often retained for observation and research, which play a significant role in dermatology; hence, dermoscopes that attach to digital cameras have gradually emerged on the market. Initially, these devices were only adapter kits for connecting body scopes and digital cameras; later, dermoscopes specifically for digital cameras were developed. This kind of dermo-

J. Liu, X. Zou, *Practical Dermoscopy*, https://doi.org/10.1007/978-981-19-1460-7_2

scope, with a high-resolution single lens reflex (SLR) digital camera, can provide a wide field of view and obtain high-quality photos. However, these dermoscopes are typically used only by professional medical institutions and dermoscopy specialists because of the tedious process of photographing target lesions and the need for a trained photographer. Such equipment includes Delta 20T from Heine and DermoGenius II from DermoScan (Germany), the DermLite Foto series from 3Gen, and VEOS SLR from Canfield (United States).

2.3 Dermoscopes with Image Acquisition Accessories

Dermoscopes with image acquisition accessories are all-in-one dermoscopes, integrating a lens and an image collector (such as a CCD camera) in the same device. Preset by the manufacturer, the lens and image collector can match better in an integrated device, and users can obtain very high magnification without adjusting the focal length and setting the image acquisition area. Since the body of the device is integrated with a screen, users can instantly view the image, and images can be transmitted to a computer screen or smart device for viewing and processing via wireless signals. However, integrated devices are often slow in image acquisition; sometimes, the restoration of the color is low, while the price is high, and the image collector is not easily upgraded. These devices are more suitable for hair observations, dermoscopy reports, and medical aesthetic institutions. This type of equipment includes VISIOMED D200EVO and E50+ from Canfield, DermLite Cam from 3Gen (United States), Dynamify from DermoScan (Germany), CH-DS50 from Chuang Hon (Guangzhou, China), and so on.

2.4 Dermoscopes That Attach to Smartphones

With the progress in smartphones, many cell phones are comparable to professional digital cameras in terms of image capture and quick photography; therefore, dermoscopes that attach to smartphones are unique in the current skin market. The advantages of these dermoscopes are that they can be easily attached to a smartphone by a snap, magnet, or clip, and the dermoscope can be removed and sterilized separately, making use and cleaning easy, and the image quality is high (depending on the imaging quality of the smartphone used), allowing direct observation of the details of lesions on some large-screen devices. These devices combine usability with storage, preservation, and analysis functions, and some apps can be used directly to analyze images (e.g., the risk level of pigmented nevi) and are popular with dermatologists as a compromise between high-quality images and usability. However, this type of dermoscope is affected by both the dermoscope itself and the cleanliness of the phone lens, as dust and grease on the lens can easily lead to problems in imaging quality. Phones are easy to drop and lose; therefore, data security must receive special attention in the design and use of these devices. This type of equipment includes DermLite DL1, DL200, DL3N, DL4, and HÜD from 3Gen United States); Handyscope from Fotofinder; iC1 and NC2 from Heine (Germany); MoleScope II from MetaOptima (Canada); VEOS HD1, HD2, and DS3 from Canfield United States); IDS-1100 from Illuco (South Korea); DMT-100 and DMT-200 from Dermat; and BN-FDJ-I from Bening (Beijing, China).

2.5 Desktop Dermoscopic Systems

Desktop dermoscopic systems are mostly used in medical institutions for patient documentation and management, data storage and analysis, and the monitoring of skin lesions (including information analysis and hair processing). Desktop dermoscopic systems can be integrated into skin image management systems for medical, educational, and research applications. Desktop dermoscopic systems can be used for batch examinations and the integration and comprehensive application of multiple skin examinations (polarized, nonpolarized, UV, and hair dermoscopy; also polarized total body photography and 3D photography). The advantages of desktop devices are that they are similar to SLR digital cameras in terms of imaging quality and field of view, and they are similar to all-in-one dermoscopes in terms of lenses and image collectors. Moreover, desktop devices are easier to use and more functional than smartphone devices, they have safe storage and backup of data. However, these devices are large and not portable, and some institutions with large examination volumes may need specialized technicians for their operation. Desktop devices are suitable for the issuing of examination reports by medical institutions, patient management, and secondary development of data. This type of equipment includes MoleMax HD from Derma Medical Systems (Austria); C-Cube 2 from Pixience (UK); VISIOMED from Canfield (United States); Dermoscope from FotoFinder; DermoGenius ultra from DermoScan (Germany); HS500 from Horus (Italy); Dermoscopy-II from Dermat (Beijing, China); CH-DSIS-2000 and 2000 Plus from Chuang Hong (Guangzhou, China); BN-PFMF-8001 from Benning (Nanjing, China); DDC/DSC-100 from Jinhong; HXSK-III from Honskin (Beijing, China); and CBS-907/908, CBS 4K ultra HD from CBS (Taiwan, China).

2.6 Polarized Total Body Photographic Systems

Polarized total body photographic systems are independent of dermoscopic systems but are often used together with desktop dermoscopic systems. These systems capture macroscopic and fine images of the entire skin surface and information on almost all lesions on the skin surface. The devices are equipped with image analysis software that facilitates clinician mapping, measuring, and tracking of skin lesions such as pigmented lesions and the recording and monitoring of changes in skin lesions throughout the body, greatly reducing the time required for patient evaluation. With the help of a given digital dermoscopic system, quick location of lesions can be accomplished, and dermoscopic images can be categorized, thus providing an objective record of and simple access to the follow-up images of skin tumors.

Polarized 3D total body photographic systems provide additional information on the texture and volume of the skin surface for the follow-up of pigmented lesions and lesions of systemic distribution, including malignant melanomas, dysplastic nevus syndrome lesions, nonmelanotic skin tumors, psoriatic lesions, cutaneous T-cell lymphoma lesions, drug rashes, pre- and postoperative plastic surgery, breast surgery, burn, lymphedema, vitiligo, neurofibromatosis, and management for documentation as well as analysis. Devices in this category include Bodystudio ATBM from FotoFinder (Germany), Derma Medical Systems from MoleMax (Austria), Vectra 3D from Canfield (United States), and DermoScan X2 from DermoScan (Germany).

2.7 Conclusion

A variety of dermoscopic devices are available depending on the users' specific requirements. The cost, imaging quality, and usability of these devices are often considered. For the purpose of a dermatologist's "stethoscope," classic handheld dermoscopes or dermoscopes that attach to smartphones are recommended due to their good portability, fast start-up, and convenience. For photoarchiving, analysis, and report issuance by institutional users, desktop devices are most suitable. A rating of these devices by convenience is as follows: classic handheld dermoscopes > dermoscopes that attach to smartphones > handheld dermoscopes that attach to digital cameras > desktop dermoscopic systems. A rating of these devices by image quality is as follows: dermoscopes that attach to SLR digital cameras ≈ desktop dermoscopic systems > classic handheld dermoscopes > integrated dermoscopic devices.

Further Reading

1. Massone C, Di-Sterfani A, Soyer HP. Dermoscopy for skin cancer detection. Curr Opin Oncol. 2005;17(2):147–53.
2. Dermoscopic equipment. In: Dermoscopedia. https://dermoscopedia.org/Overview_dermoscopic_equipment(Jul 13, 2018). Accessed 30 Oct 2019.

3 Terminology in Dermoscopy

Dermoscopy, as a widely used noninvasive diagnostic tool, has gradually developed its unique language in clinical practice and research. Due to the application of dermoscopy in new fields and the introduction of polarized dermoscopy, the terms of dermoscopy proliferated rapidly, including many features that are difficult to observe with nonpolarized dermoscopy. There are two types of terminology: the metaphoric terminology and the descriptive terminology.

Metaphoric terminology refers to a class of terms that vividly compare features seen under dermoscopy to real-life objects, such as "starburst pattern," "leaflike areas," and "strawberry pattern," which are easy to learn and grasp for beginners. However, due to the large amount of terms and the fact that some metaphors are ambiguous or inappropriate, it can be difficult to memorize and communicate to some extent.

Descriptive terminology consists of five basic elements: "lines," "dots," "clods," "circles," and "pseudopods" (Fig. 3.1). It is called "structureless" if none of these five elements is present. The five building blocks, together with color and, if necessary, distribution, like the letters of the alphabet, are sufficient to describe all kinds of dermoscopic features, whether simple or complex, so that metaphorical terms can be translated as descriptive terms accurately when needed. Descriptive terminology is relatively new, but it has become popular with clinicians because of its simplicity and logic. Its major disadvantage is that some complex features, which can be vividly described by metaphorical terms, would be verbose and cumbersome in descriptive expression.

In recent years, experts have made efforts to standardize dermoscopic terminology and established a dictionary of standardized dermoscopic terms for skin tumors that contains both metaphoric and descriptive terms, as shown in Tables 3.1 and 3.2. The correspondence between descriptive and metaphoric terms as well as their definitions and related diseases are shown in Table 3.1. The vascular structures with their definitions in skin tumors are described in Table 3.2.

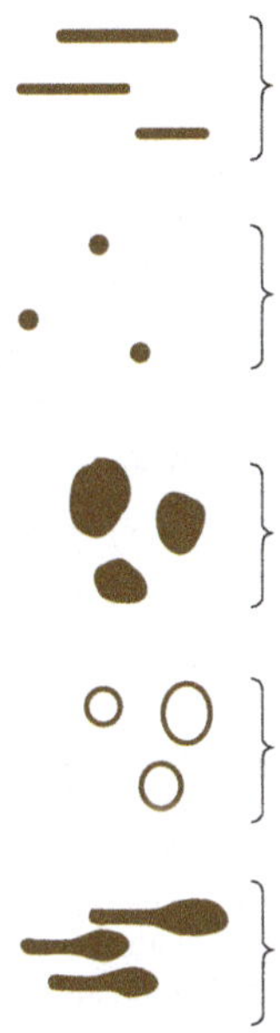

Fig. 3.1 Schematic diagram of descriptive terminology

Both metaphoric and descriptive terminology have pros and cons. The current consensus includes: (1) Dermoscopic features can be appropriately described by both metaphoric and descriptive terms; (2) Metaphoric terms should have definitions; (3) When describing new dermoscopic features, a pre-existed metaphoric or descriptive term should be preferred rather than a newly invented one; (4) Discard the inappropriate metaphoric terms and keep the most appropriate and easy-to-understand ones. Be aware of standardization and consistency when using terminology during the daily work, research, and training.

With the accumulation of clinical practice and the deepening of research, dermoscopy has been applied to non-neoplastic skin diseases, such as inflammatory and infectious skin diseases. The 2020 Consensus of the International Dermoscopy Society was aimed to standardize the terminology and basic parameters of dermoscopy for non-neoplastic skin diseases and identified 5 standardized basic parameters

J. Liu, X. Zou, *Practical Dermoscopy*, https://doi.org/10.1007/978-981-19-1460-7_3

Table 3.1 Descriptive terms, corresponding metaphoric terms, and their definitions

Descriptive terminology	Metaphoric terminology	Definitions	Main dermatoses[a]
1. Lines			
Lines, reticular	Pigment network	Grid-like pattern formed by interconnecting pigmented lines surrounding hypopigmented holes; typical pigment network with minimal variability in the color, thickness, and spacing of the lines which distributing symmetrically	Melanocytic nevus, solar lentigo, dermatofibroma
Lines, reticular, and thick	Broadened network	Widening of the network lines	Melanoma
Lines, reticular, and thin	Delicate network	Light-brown, thin network lines	Melanocytic nevus
Lines, reticular, and thick or reticular lines that vary in color	Atypical pigment network	Network with increased variability in the color, thickness, and spacing of the lines of the network; asymmetrically distributed; gray color	Melanoma
Lines, reticular, white			Melanoma, Spitz nevus, dermatofibroma
Lines, reticular, hypopigmented, around brown clods	Negative pigment network (former synonyms: inverse network, reticular depigmentation)	Serpiginous interconnecting broadened hypopigmented lines that surround elongated and curvilinear globules	Melanoma, Spitz nevus
Lines, white, perpendicular[b]	Shiny white streaks (former synonyms: chrysalis, chrysalids, crystalline)	Short discrete white lines oriented parallel and orthogonal (perpendicular) to each other seen only under polarized dermoscopy	Melanoma, BCC, Spitz nevus, dermatofibroma
Lines, branched	Branched streaks	Broadened or widened network with broken lines and incomplete connections	Melanocytic lesion
Lines, radial (always at periphery)	Streaks		Reed nevus, melanoma, recurrent nevus
Lines, radial and segmental	Radial streaming	Radial linear extensions at the lesion edge	Melanoma, recurrent nevus
Lines, radial, connected to a central common base	Leaflike areas (sometimes variously shaped large clods have also been termed leaflike areas)	Brown to gray-blue discrete linear or bulbous structures coalescing at a common off-center base creating structures that resemble a leaflike pattern	BCC
Lines, radial, converging to a central dot or clod	Spoke wheel area (sometimes a clod within a clod has also been termed spoke wheel area/concentric structure)	Well-circumscribed radial projections, usually light-brown but sometimes blue or gray in color meeting at a central darker clod that has a dark brown, black, or blue color	BCC
Lines, curved, and thick	Cerebriform pattern (former synonyms: brainlike appearance) to describe the pattern and fissures and ridges (former synonyms: gyri and sulci and fat fingers) to describe the structural components of the pattern	Thick curved lines created by gyri and keratin-filled sulci; these gyri and sulci coalesce forming a brainlike appearance pattern	SK
Lines, brown, curved, parallel, thin	Fingerprinting	Light-brown thin curved lines that do not interconnect to form a network; these tend to be linear to curvilinear; corresponding to small and thin gyri	Solar lentigo
Lines, curved, and thick, in combination with clods	Crypts	Keratin-filled invaginations that are larger than comedo-like openings	SK
Lines, parallel, short, crossing ridges (volar skin)	Fibrillar pattern	Linear pigmented filamentous lines of similar length with one end at the furrows and crossing the ridges at a certain angle	Acral nevus
Lines, parallel, thick, on the ridges (volar skin)	Parallel ridge pattern	Volar pigmentation forming lines, parallel, diffuse, and irregular, along the ridges or cristae superficiales (raised portion of the dermatoglyphics)	Acral lentiginous melanoma

Table 3.1 (continued)

Descriptive terminology	Metaphoric terminology	Definitions	Main dermatoses[a]
Lines, parallel, thin, in the furrows and crossing the ridges (volar shin)	Lattice like pattern	Volar pigmentation forming thin lines, parallel on the furrow or sulci superficialis (invaginations in dermatoglyphics) and crossing perpendicular on the ridges	Acral nevus
Lines, parallel, thin, in the furrows (volar shin)	Parallel furrows pattern	Volar pigmentation forming solid or dotted lines, parallel, thin, on the furrows (sulci superficiales or invaginations in dermatoglyphics); the lines are occasionally doubled, each line is beside the furrows	Acral nevus
Lines, angulated, or polygonal (facial skin)	Rhomboids/zig-zag pattern	Gray-brown angulated lines forming a polygonal shape around adnexal ostial openings	Lentigo maligna melanoma
Lines, angulated, or polygonal (nonfacial skin)	Angulated lines/polygons	Gray-brown lines that are connected at an angle or coalescing to form polygons	Lentiginous melanoma (nonfacial, nonacral)
2. Clods			
Clods, small, round, or oval	Globules	Regular globules with minimal variability in their color, size, and shape; irregular globules with variability in color, size, shape, or spacing and distributed in an asymmetric fashion	Various diagnoses
Clods, brown, circumferential	Rim of brown globules	Globules distributed at the periphery of lesion	Growing nevi
Clods, brown, yellow, or orange (rarely black)	Comedo-like openings	Round to oval keratin-filled clefts	SK
Clods, brown, or blue, concentric (clod within a clod)	Concentric globules		BCC
Clods, brown or skin colored, large and polygonal	Cobblestone pattern	Polygonal globules symmetrically distributed throughout lesion	Intradermal nevus
Clods, blue, large, clustered	Blue-gray ovoid nests	Well-circumscribed ovoid structures with confluent or near confluent blue-gray pigmentation	BCC
Clods, blue, small	Blue globules		BCC
Clod within a clod (concentric clods)	Variant of spoke wheel area		BCC
Clods, white, shiny[b]	Shiny white blotches and strands	White structures in the form of circles, oval structures, or large structureless areas that are bright-white longer and less well-defined lines oriented parallel or distributed haphazardly, or forming blotches (shiny white clods); seen only under polarized dermoscopy	BCC
Clods, pink and small	Milky-red globules		Melanoma
Clods, red or purple	Red lacunas		Hemangioma
3. Dots[c]		Regular dots clustered at the center of the lesion, or located on the network lines (also called target network); irregular dots display any distribution other than that is described above	
Dots, any color	Granularity or granules	Consists of fine dots with a blue-gray color	Various diagnoses
Dots, gray	Peppering	Consists of fine dots with a blue-gray color	Melanoma, LPLK
Dots, gray and circles, gray	Annular-granular pattern	Dots and structureless areas arranged around follicle openings (and involving adnexal opening)	Lentigo maligna melanoma

(continued)

Table 3.1 (continued)

Descriptive terminology	Metaphoric terminology	Definitions	Main dermatoses[a]
Dots or clods, white, clustered, or disseminated	Milia-like cysts, cloudy or starry	White to yellowish round opalescent structures corresponding to intraepidermal cysts; when they are small and bright they are called starry; when they are larger and less bright, they are called cloudy	SK
Dots, white, four arranged in a square[b]	Rosettes	Four bright-white dots or clods arranged together as a square (or a 4-leaf clover)	AK, SCC
Dots, peripheral, four arranged in lines	Linear dots		Pigmented Bowen's disease
Dots, brown, central (in the center of hypopigmented spaces between reticular lines)	Targetoid dots		Congenital melanocytic nevus
4. Circles			
Circles, white			SCC
Circles, concentric	Circle within a circle		Lentigo maligna melanoma
Circles, incomplete	Asymmetric pigmented follicular openings	Pigment associated with adnexal opening that does not uniformly surround the entire opening or curved (or crescent-shaped) pigment lines partially surrounding adnexal openings	Lentigo maligna melanoma
5. Pseudopods		Bulbous and often kinked projections seen at the lesion edge, either directly associated with a network or solid tumor border	
Pseudopods, circumferential or lines, radial, circumferential	Starburst pattern	This pattern consists of peripheral globules, pseudopods, or streaks (or a combination of them), located around the entire perimeter of the lesion	Reed nevus
6. Structureless			
Structureless zone, brown or black	Blotch	Dark structureless areas; regular blotch is defined as one blotch located in the center of the skin lesion and surrounded by pigmented network; irregular blotch is defined as more than one blotch or a blotch that is located off-center	Atypical nevus (centric structureless zone), melanoma(eccentric structureless zone)
Structureless zone, blue	Blue-whitish veil	An irregular shaped blotch of blue hue with an overlying whitish ground-glass haze	Melanoma
Structureless zone, pink	Milky-red areas	Milky-white appearance or pinkish structureless areas (strawberry and ice cream-like), formed by a red vascular blush with no specific distinguishable vessels	Melanoma
Structureless zone, white	Scar-like depigmentation	Area that is whiter than surrounding normal-appearing skin (true scarring); it should not be confused with hypopigmentation or depigmentation caused by simple loss of melanin; shiny white structures and blood vessels are not seen in areas of regression	Melanoma
Structureless zone, white, central	Central white patch	Central white structureless area	Dermatofibroma
Structureless zone, polychromatic	Rainbow pattern	Circumscribed structureless areas displaying colors of the whole spectrum of visible light	Various diagnoses
Structureless, red, interrupted by follicular openings	Strawberry pattern	Reddish pseudonetwork (erythema and wavy fine vessels) around hair follicle openings that are accentuated with a white halo appearance	AK
Structureless, brown (tan), eccentric			Melanoma

Table 3.1 (continued)

Descriptive terminology	Metaphoric terminology	Definitions	Main dermatoses[a]
Structureless, any color	Homogenous pattern	A pattern lacking any definable pigment structures, structureless pattern	Various diagnoses
Structureless zone, brown, interrupted by follicular openings (facial skin)	Pseudonetwork	A structureless pigmented area interrupted by nonpigmented adnexal openings	Facial pigmented lesions
7. Else			
Sharply demarcated, scalloped border	Moth-eaten border	Border with concave or sharp punched-out invaginations	Solar lentigo, SK

AK actinic keratosis, *BCC* basal cell carcinoma, *LPLK* lichen planus-like keratosis, *SCC* squamous cell carcinoma, *SK* seborrheic keratosis
[a] Varies depending on context
[b] Only visible under polarized dermoscopy
[c] Dots are all small and round in the same size and shape but not larger than the terminal hair generally, while the clods vary in size and shape

Table 3.2 Suitable terms and definitions for vessel morphology and distribution of skin tumors

Descriptive term	Metaphoric term	Definition	Main dermatoses[a]
1. Vessels morphology			
Dots		Tiny pinpoint vessels	Melanocytic lesions, Bowen's disease
Clods	Red-purple lacunas	More or less sharply demarcated, roundish, or oval areas with a reddish, red-bluish, maroon, or dark-red to black coloration, separated from each other by intervening stroma, without vessels inside the lacunae	Hemangioma
Linear		Linear, mildly curved vessels, considered irregular when different sizes, shapes, and curves with a haphazard, or random, distribution are presented and considered regular when short and fine (thin) linear vessels prevail	Various diagnoses
Coiled	Glomerular	Tightly coiled vessels resembling the glomerular apparatus of the kidney	Bowen's disease
Looped	Hairpin	Two parallel linear vessels forming a half looped or hairpin-like structure	SK, warts
Serpentine	Linear irregular	Linear vessels with multiple bends	Flat BCC, melanoma
Helical	Corkscrew	Twisted looped vessels with bends twisted along a central axis	Melanoma, cutaneous metastasis
Curved	Comma	Linear, curved, short vessels	Intradermal nevus
Monomorphous		One type of vessel dominates	Various skin tumors
Polymorphous		Multiple types of vessels are present	May indicate malignancy in appropriate context, for example, in flat melanocytic lesions
2. Vessels distribution			
Radial	Crown vessels	Radial, serpentine, or arborizing vessels at the periphery of the lesion that radiate toward the center but do not cross the midline of the lesion	Sebaceous hyperplasia
Serpiginous	String of pearls	Coiled or dotted vessels arranged in lines	Clear cell acanthoma
Branched	Arborizing vessels	Bright-red, sharply in focus, large or thick-diameter vessels dividing into smaller vessels	BCC
Clustered		Coiled or glomerular vessels arranged in groups	Bowen's disease
Centered dots	Targetoid vessels	Red dots (vessels) in the center of hypopigmented space between reticular lines	Congenital melanocytic nevus

BCC basal cell carcinoma, *SK* seborrheic keratosis
[a] Significance of vascular structures depends on the context and is generally weaker than that of pigmented structures

and 31 subitems. The five standardized parameters to be assessed include: (1) vessels (including morphology and distribution); (2) scales (including color and distribution); (3) follicular findings; (4) other structures (including color and morphology); (5) specific clues. Table 3.3 describes all the terms and basic parameters included in the consensus, as well as their previous nomenclature, corresponding histopathological findings, and related dermatoses. It should be emphasized that the distribution of each parameter in the lesion determines its disease relevance, thus predominant structures which are visible in the larger part of the lesion have a higher disease relevance. In general, there are usually one or two predominant criteria for non-neoplastic skin diseases, whose diagnostic accuracy needs to be verified by controlled studies. Moreover, similar subitems need to be specified if they are relevant to unique or differential features of some diseases because of the presence of corresponding specific histological findings. For example, linear vessels may occur in both rosacea and discoid lupus erythematosus, but in rosacea vessels are denser and larger and form a polygonal network due to dermal capillaries significantly dilated and connected into a network. However, it should be noted that the standardized terminology for non-neoplastic skin diseases has some limitations, as the level of evidence is only V in most of studies on dermoscopy of non-neoplastic dermatosis (based on the 2011 Oxford level of evidence).

This chapter introduces the newly published standardized dermoscopic terms of neoplastic and non-neoplastic dermatoses, in order to lay a solid theoretical foundation for the education and research on dermoscopy.

Table 3.3 Standardized terms and basic parameters in non-neoplastic dermatoses

Terms and parameters	Previous nomenclature/included findings	Corresponding histological findings	Main dermatoses
1. Vessels			
1.1. Vessels morphology			
Dotted	Dotted, pinpoint, glomerular and globular	Dilated vessels in elongated dermal papillae	Psoriasis, dermatitis, lichen planus, pityriasis rosea, lichen sclerosus, porokeratosis, lichen simplex chronicus, secondary lichenification, tinea corporis, mycosis fungoides, impetigo, and plane warts
Linear (without bends or branches)	Linear	Dilated dermal vessels located in parallel to the skin surface	Mycosis fungoides, rosacea, lichen planus, discoid lupus erythematosus, granulomatous dermatoses, and atrophic diseases
Linear with branches	Arborizing, branched and crown-like	Branching dermal vessels	Discoid lupus erythematosus, granulomatous dermatoses, seborrheic dermatitis, molluscum contagiosum, and pityriasis lichenoides chronica
Linear curved	Comma-shaped, chalice-shaped, hairpin-like, linear irregular, tortuous, corkscrew-like, spermatozoa-like and linear-helical	Convoluted dermal vessels	Zoon's balanitis, lichen sclerosus, pityriasis lichenoides chronica, granulomatous dermatoses, discoid lupus erythematosus, and telangiectasia macularis eruptive perstans
1.2. Vessels distribution			
Uniform	Regular, homogeneous and diffuse	–	Psoriasis, lichen simplex chronicus, secondary lichenification, mycosis fungoides, and plane warts
Clustered	Clustered and "in cluster"	–	Dermatitis, common warts, and pityriasis rosea
Peripheral	Peripheral	–	Lichen planus, discoid lupus erythematosus, pityriasis rosea, molluscum contagiosum
Reticular	Regular, "in plexus," net-like and network-like	–	Rosacea, psoriasis, urticaria, necrobiosis lipoidica and telangiectasia macularis eruptive perstans
Unspecific	Patchy, asymmetric, irregular, scattered, sparse and unspecific	–	Dermatitis, pityriasis rosea, pityriasis lichenoides chronica
2. Scales			
2.1. Scales color			
White	White and gray	Hyperkeratosis (especially parakeratosis)	Psoriasis (all variants, except pustular, genital, and inverse psoriasis), hypertrophic lichen planus, discoid lupus erythematosus, subacute lupus erythematosus, pityriasis rosea, mycosis fungoides, pityriasis lichenoides chronica and tinea corposis
Yellow (scales and crusts)	Yellow	Serum ± hyperkeratosis	Dermatitis, pemphigus vulgaris, rosacea, and Darier's disease

Table 3.3 (continued)

Terms and parameters	Previous nomenclature/included findings	Corresponding histological findings	Main dermatoses
Brown	Brown	Keratin + melanin or exogenous pigment (e.g., dirt)	Terra firma-forme dermatosis and dermatosis neglecta
2.2. Scales distribution			
Diffuse	Diffuse, regular and homogeneous	–	Psoriasis and lichen simplex chronicus
Central	Central	–	Hypertrophic lichen planus, discoid lupus erythematosus, leishmaniasis and pityriasis lichenoides chronica
Peripheral	Peripheral, collarette scaling and squamous collarette	–	Pityriasis rosea, tinea corporis and erythema annulare centrifugum and subacute lupus erythematosus
Patchy	Patchy, irregular, sparse, and scattered	–	Dermatitis, mycosis fungoides, pityriasis rubra pilaris, lichen simplex chronicus, lichen planus and pityriasis lichenoides chronica
3. Follicular findings			
Follicular plugs	Follicular plugs, yellow "tears," "Demodex tails," "Demodex follicular openings," comedo-like openings and rosettes	Follicular hyperkeratosis alone (white plugs) or combined with serum (yellow plugs) or melanin (brown plugs)	Hypertrophic lichen planus, discoid lupus erythematosus, leishmaniasis, demodicosis, and lichen sclerosus
Follicular red dots	Follicular red dots	Perifollicular inflammation	Early discoid lupus erythematosus, follicular mycosis fungoides, and follicular mucinosis
Perifollicular white color	Perifollicular white halo and perifollicular depigmentation	Perifollicular fibrosis or epidermal hyperplasia and perifollicular depigmentation	Discoid lupus erythematosus, rosacea, hypertrophic lichen planus, and vitiligo
Perifollicular pigmentation	Perifollicular pigmentation or hyperpigmentation	Perifollicular pigment deposits	Vitiligo
4. Other structures			
4.1. Color			
White	White and chalk-white	Fibrosis, reduction of melanocytes or melanin, epidermal hyperplasia (acanthosis or hypergranulosis), or calcium deposits	Lichen sclerosus, morphoea, necrobiosis lipoidica, primary cutaneous B-cell lymphoma, vitiligo, idiopathic guttate hypomelanosis, achromic pityriasis versicolor, lichen nitidus, molluscum contagiosum, prurigo nodularis, xanthogranuloma, calcifications, and gouty tophi
Brown	Brown	Melanin in the basal layer of the epidermis or superficial dermis	Melasma, tinea nigra, friction melanosis, morphea, urticaria pigmentosa, pityriasis versicolor, lichen amyloidosis, and macular amyloidosis
Gray	Gray	Melanin or ochronotic pigment in the papillary dermis	Lichen pigmentosus, lichen planus, melasma, and exogenous ochronosis
Blue	Blue	Melanin or ochronotic pigment in reticular dermis	Ashy dermatosis and exogenous ochronosis
Orange	Orange and salmon	Dermal granulomas and other dense cellular infiltrations, or hemosiderin deposits in the dermis	Granulomatous dermatoses, xanthogranuloma, primary cutaneous B-cell lymphomas, Zoon's balanitis, pityriasis lichenoides chronica, pityriasis rubra pilaris, papular syphiloderm, and pigmented purpuric dermatosis
Yellow	Yellow	Lipid deposits in the dermis and pustules	Necrobiosis lipoidica, xanthelasma, pustular psoriasis, and xanthogranuloma
Purple	Purple, violet, hemorrhagic areas, and petechiae	Extravasation of erythrocytes (purpura) or thrombosed vessels	Pigmented purpuric dermatosis, vasculitis, lichen sclerosus, and common and plantar warts

(continued)

Table 3.3 (continued)

Terms and parameters	Previous nomenclature/included findings	Corresponding histological findings	Main dermatoses
4.2. Morphology			
Structureless (diffuse—as a background—or focal)	Structureless (diffuse or focal), background, amorphous, blots, blotches and irregular	–	Granulomatous dermatoses, primary cutaneous B-cell lymphomas, lichen sclerosus, pityriasis lichenoides chronica, Zoon's balanitis, xanthogranuloma, friction melanosis, urticaria pigmentosa, xanthelasma, pityriasis versicolor, pigmented purpuric dermatosis, and solitary mastocytoma
Dots/globules	Dots/globules, confetti-like, clouds, cloud-like, petaloid-like, milium-like cysts, corn pearls, hubs and globular	–	Lichen planus, lichen pigmentosus, ashy dermatosis, lichen sclerosus, molluscum contagiosum, morphoea, lichen amyloidosus, macular amyloidosis, and pigmented purpuric dermatosis
Lines (parallel, reticular, perpendicular, angulated or unspecifically arranged)	Streaks, crystalline-like/chrysalis, crystalline leaf venation, reticular, network-like, streaming lines, projections, radiant strips, spicules, and bulb-like projections	–	Tinea nigra, friction melanosis, morphoea, lichen sclerosus, urticaria pigmentosa, prurigo nodularis, lichen amyloidosus, macular amyloidosis, xanthogranuloma, and common warts
Circles	Circles, annular, arciform, and curvilinear-worm like	–	Melasma, exogenous ochronosis, and primary cutaneous B-cell lymphomas
5. Specific clues	Wickham striae, peripheral keratotic structure with two free edges, spongiotic vesicles, "jet with contrail," nits and lice, dilated follicular openings, etc.	Variable but highly specific and sensitive	Lichen planus, porokeratosis, chronic hand eczema, scabies, pediculosis, granuloma faciale, etc.

Further Reading

1. Benvenuto-Andrade C, Dusza SW, Agero AL, et al. Differences between polarized light dermoscopy and immersion contact dermoscopy for the evaluation of skin lesions. Arch Dermatol. 2007;143(3):329–38.
2. Pan Y, Gareau DS, Scope A, et al. Polarized and nonpolarized dermoscopy: the explanation for the observed differences. Arch Dermatol. 2008;144(6):828–9.
3. Pellacani G, Seidenari S. Comparison between morphological parameters in pigmented skin lesion images acquired by means of epiluminescence surface microscopy and polarized-light videomicroscopy. Clin Dermatol. 2002;20(3):222–7.
4. Agero AL, Taliercio S, Dusza SW, et al. Conventional and polarized dermoscopy features of dermatofibroma. Arch Dermatol. 2006;142(11):1431–7.
5. Wang SQ, Dusza SW, Scope A, et al. Differences in dermoscopic images from nonpolarized dermoscope and polarized dermoscope influence the diagnostic accuracy and confidence level: a pilot study. Dermatol Surg. 2008;34(10):1389–95.
6. Argenziano G, Soyer HP, Chimenti S, et al. Dermoscopy of pigmented skin lesions: results of a consensus meeting via the Internet. J Am Acad Dermatol. 2003;48(5):679–93.
7. Zalaudek I, Giacomel J, Argenziano G, et al. Dermoscopy of facial nonpigmented actinic keratosis. Br J Dermatol. 2006;155(5):951–6.
8. Kittler H, Marghoob AA, Argenziano G, et al. Standardization of terminology in dermoscopy/dermatoscopy: results of the third consensus conference of the International Society of Dermoscopy. J Am Acad Dermatol. 2016;74(6):1093–106.
9. Ran ML, Liu J, Zou XB, Luo YX, Cui Y. Standardization of terminology and device parameters in dermoscopy for diagnosis: an expert consensus statement. Chin J Dermatol. 2017;50(7):472–7.
10. Liu J. Explanation and elaboration for the standardization of terminology in dermoscopy/dermatoscopy: results of the Third Consensus Conference of the International Society of Dermoscopy. Chin J Dermatol. 2017;50(4):299–304.
11. Errichetti E, Stinco G. Dermoscopy in general dermatology: a practical overview. Dermatol Ther (Heidelb). 2016;6(4):471–507.
12. Errichetti E, Stinco G. The practical usefulness of dermoscopy in general dermatology. G Ital Dermatol Venereol. 2015;150(5):533–46.
13. Lallas A, Giacomel J, Argenziano G, et al. Dermoscopy in general dermatology: practical tips for the clinician. Br J Dermatol. 2014;170(3):514–26.
14. Lallas A, Zalaudek I, Argenziano G, et al. Dermoscopy in general dermatology. Dermatol Clin. 2013;31(4):679–94.
15. Errichetti E, Zalaudek I, Kittler H, et al. Standardization of dermoscopic terminology and basic dermoscopic parameters to evaluate in general dermatology (non-neoplastic dermatoses) :an expert consensus on behalf of the International Dermoscopy Society. Br J Dermatol. 2020;182(2):454–67.
16. Liu J, Zou XB. Explanation and elaboration for "standardization of dermoscopic terminology and basic dermoscopic parameters to evaluate in general dermatology (non-neoplastic dermatoses): an expert consensus on behalf of the International Dermoscopy Society". Chin J Dermatol. 2020;53(6):409–14.

4 Diagnostic Strategies and Algorithms of Dermoscopy

The initial application of dermoscopy was the diagnosis of skin tumors, with the particular aim to enhance clinicians' ability to diagnose malignant melanoma (MM). Various diagnostic strategies and approaches were created in succession, such as the two-step algorithm (including the classic two-step algorithm, the revised two-step algorithm and the top-down two-step algorithm), pattern analysis, the ABCD rule, the Menzies method, the seven-point checklist, the three-point checklist, the CASH algorithm, the triage amalgamated dermoscopy algorithm (TADA), prediction without pigment, and the color wheel. This chapter mainly introduces the methods mentioned above to help readers construct their preferred and applicable diagnostic approaches. Of note, in clinical practice, clinicians should apply appropriate strategies according to their own experience in dermoscopy, the specific circumstances, and the features of particular cases. Terminology is based on the consensus of the International Society of Dermoscopy (IDS).

4.1 The Two-Step Algorithm

4.1.1 The Revised Two-Step Algorithm

In 2001, the Board of the Consensus Net Meeting agreed on a two-step algorithm for the classification of pigmented skin lesions (the classic two-step algorithm), mainly to improve MM diagnostic sensitivity. The algorithm is designed to evaluate lesions on glabrous and nonglabrous skin but not those on skin appendages such as nails or mucous membranes or hair disorders. The first step of this algorithm requires the clinician to distinguish whether the lesion is melanocytic or not. If the lesion is of melanocytic origin, the clinician moves on to the second step of the algorithm to decide whether the lesion is benign or malignant. However, the classic two-step algorithm cannot be used to adequately describe vascular patterns; therefore, clinicians have difficulty in evaluating hypomelanotic or amelanotic neoplasms with this algorithm. Subsequently, the revised two-step algorithm was proposed, which has become one of the most important and commonly used diagnostic strategies.

Step 1: Determine Whether the Lesion Is Melanocytic or Nonmelanocytic

The first step of the algorithm has seven different diagnostic levels. The observer should analyze the lesion according to these levels in succession.

Level 1: Search for Criteria Associated with Melanocytic Lesions

A lesion presenting the dermoscopic patterns shown below should be considered melanocytic; therefore, the clinician can move to the second step.

1. Pigment network: a reticular pattern consisting of intersecting pigmented lines and hypopigmented holes. The network usually thins at the peripheral.
2. Pseudonetwork: in facial area, a diffuse homogeneous pigmented area interrupted by nonpigmented adnexal openings resulting in a network appearance.
3. Negative network: a grid-like pattern consisting of intersecting serpiginous and hypopigmented lines surrounding elongated and curvilinear globules.
4. Streaks: including radial streaming (radially arranged lines extending at the lesion edge), pseudopods (thick and bulbous projections at the lesion edge, usually radiate from a tumor border), and branched streaks (broadened or widened network with broken lines and incomplete connections).
5. Aggregated globules: multiple globules with variability in color (brown, gray, or dark) and size and clustered in distribution.
6. Homogenous blue pigmentation: a blue-colored structureless pattern.
7. Parallel furrow pattern: on palms and soles, pigmented solid or dotted lines, parallelly arranged, on the skin furrows; the lines are sometimes doubled with each line beside the furrows.

J. Liu, X. Zou, *Practical Dermoscopy*, https://doi.org/10.1007/978-981-19-1460-7_4

8. Parallel ridge pattern: on palms and soles, pigmented lines, parallelly, diffusely or irregularly arranged along the skin ridges.

In addition, ulceration can be observed in invasive MM.

Importantly, we also stress that there are exceptions to the two-step algorithm. Here, the presence of the above features does not mean that the lesion must be melanocytic. For example, pigment networks and similar structures are also commonly present in dermatofibroma (DF), seborrheic keratosis (SK), solar lentigo (SL), etc., and streaks as long as similar structures can be seen in SK, basal cell carcinoma (BCC), pigmented Bowen's disease, etc. However, other accompanying dermoscopic characteristics can help to differentiate these diseases from melanocytic lesions, such as typical central scar-like depigmentation with a peripheral reticular pattern in DF lesions. Detailed dermoscopic features of abovementioned dermatoses with such exceptions will be discussed in the following chapters.

Level 2: Search for Criteria Associated with Pigmented BCC

The classic diagnostic pattern for pigmented BCC includes the following:

One negative criterion: the absence of a pigment network.

Six positive criteria include the following:

1. Large blue-gray ovoid nests: well-circumscribed ovoid structures with confluent or near confluent blue-gray pigmentation.
2. Multiple blue-gray nonaggregated globules: well-circumscribed roundish to ovoid structures, blue-gray or brown, larger than dots and smaller than ovoid nests, multiple but not aggregated.
3. Leaflike areas: brown to gray/blue discrete linear or bulbous structures coalescing at a common off-center base, creating structures that resemble a leaflike pattern.
4. Spoke wheel areas: well-circumscribed radial projections, usually light brown but sometimes blue or gray in color, meeting at a central darker clod that has a dark brown, black, or blue color.
5. Ulcerations: a loss of the epidermis and superficial dermis, usually located in the center, and sometimes covered by crusts.
6. Branched/arborizing blood vessels: large, thick and focused bright-red vessels gradually divided into smaller branches.

If a lesion fulfils the negative criterion and one or more positive criteria, the diagnosis of pigmented BCC can be primarily made.

Level 3: Search for Criteria Associated with SK

Common dermoscopic features of SK include the following:

1. Sharply demarcated borders.
2. Moth-eaten border: a clearly defined border of which some portions are scalloped, giving a moth-eaten appearance.
3. Milia-like cysts: white-to-yellow round structures; when they are small and bright (contrasted with darker surroundings), they are called "starry" and sometimes appear in melanocytic lesions; when they are larger in size and blurred in appearance, they are called "cloudy," usually seen in SK and the number of such milia-like cysts is mostly more than 3.
4. Comedo-like opening: round to oval craters with central dark keratin plugs.
5. Crypts: larger and longer depressions filled with keratins.
6. Fissures and ridges pattern: fissures are linear comedo-like openings that present as brown or dark curved linear structures, and the elevated parts are called ridges.
7. Cerebriform pattern: a combination of multiple fissures (sulci) and ridges (gyri), giving a brain-like appearance.
8. Hairpin blood vessels: blood vessels that are twisted upon themselves and appear as "U"-shaped and hairpin-like.

Level 4: Search for Criteria Associated with Vascular Diseases

The most typical dermoscopic feature of common vascular diseases such as hemangioma, angiokeratoma and port-wine stains is red-purple lacunae (more or less sharply demarcated, roundish, or oval areas with a reddish, red-bluish, maroon, or dark-red to black coloration, separated from each other by intervening stroma, without vessels inside the lacunae). If such red-purple lacunae exist, the lesion is considered to be of vascular origin.

Level 5: Search for Specific Vascular Patterns Associated with Nonmelanocytic Lesions

At this diagnostic level, the remaining lesions are usually nonpigmented or hypopigmented. The clinician should examine specific vascular patterns (including the morphology and arrangement), other nonvascular features (including scales, background color and hair follicle findings), and the medical history to make a comprehensive diagnosis.

For example, the presence of crown vessels (radial, serpentine, or arborizing vessels at the periphery of a lesion that radiate towards the center but do not cross the midline of the lesion) indicates the possibility of sebaceous hyperplasia and molluscum contagiosum. Since the clinical manifestations of these two conditions are quite different, the diagnosis would not be difficult. Another example is the presence of glomerular vessels, which should remind observers of the possibility of squamous cell carcinoma (SCC) and related entities.

Level 6: Search for Specific Vascular Patterns Associated with Melanocytic Lesions

Specific vascular patterns also exist in melanocytic lesions, especially in malignant conditions. Under dermoscopy, the blood vessels of MM are often polymorphous, including dotted, linear irregular (serpentine), atypical hairpin, and corkscrew vessels. Furthermore, milky-red areas (milky-white to pinkish structureless areas) can also be seen in MM. The comma vessel is a classic vascular finding in intradermal nevi.

Level 7: Structureless Lesions
Lesions in level 7 fail to be identified through levels 1–6 and are usually regarded as "structureless." However, these lesions are sometimes not completely unable to provide a clue for the diagnosis. For instance, a lesion with blue-white veils and crystalline structures is still suspicious for MM. Therefore, this level is also considered the default level, and lesions should be further evaluated during the second step because these lesions often need histopathological investigations or close monitoring of their changes.

Step 2: Determine Whether the Melanocytic Lesion Is Benign or Malignant
After the primary evaluation in the first step, lesions meeting diagnostic levels 1, 6, and 7 are evaluated in the second step to further investigate whether they are benign nevi, suspicious nevi, or MM. Various approaches have been created to help in this step, including pattern analysis, the ABCD rule, the Menzies method, the seven-point checklist, the three-point checklist, the revised version of pattern analysis, and chaos and clues, and are discussed below.

4.1.2 The Top-Down Two-Step Approach

In 2018, Ralph P. Braun, Ashfaq A. Marghoob and Aimilios Lallas proposed a new approach building upon the classic and revised two-step algorithm, named the top-down two-step approach on the official website of the IDS—https://dermoscopedia.org. In this new approach, the first step requires the clinician to establish a specific diagnosis if possible, and the second step further requires the clinician to distinguish between a benign nevus and MM.

Step 1: Establish a Specific Diagnosis If Possible
The first step includes the nine diagnostic levels listed below. The observer should make a definitive diagnosis upon the recognition of related dermoscopic patterns. The detailed dermoscopic characteristics of these nine diseases can be found in their corresponding chapter.

Level 1: benign nevus (excluding intradermal nevus)
Level 2: DF
Level 3: intradermal nevus
Level 4: BCC
Level 5: SCC
Level 6: SK and lentigo
Level 7: angioma/angiokeratoma/hemangioma
Level 8: sebaceous hyperplasia
Level 9: clear cell acanthoma

Step 2: Rule Out MM
If none of the nine categories of diagnoses can be made, the lesions in the second step are usually suspicious for MM or cannot be safely diagnosed. The latter group mainly includes nevi that demand further evaluation and MM lesions that lack the usual disorganized distribution of structures and colors. It is of vital importance to understand that the second step mainly aims at improving the detection of MM, so each lesion included should undergo careful assessment of any possible signs of MM. In addition, the clinical background of each lesion should be provided and considered on a whole scale, such as the patient's age when the lesion appears and the history of rapid enlargement and symptoms, since the differential diagnosis of MM must depend on comprehensive information as much as possible.

1. **Nevi Demanding Special Attention**
   (a) The two-component pattern and the multicomponent symmetric pattern are common in patients with atypical mole syndrome, but biopsy or close monitoring is advised when the lesion appears significantly different compared to other nevi in the same patient.
   (b) Homogeneous tan to pink areas are common in nevi in patients with Fitzpatrick skin type I-II but can also be present in amelanotic and hypomelanotic melanomas. Therefore, a biopsy is recommended if the lesion with such a pattern is an outlier.
   (c) The tiered peripheral globular pattern is usually associated with spitzoid nevi. If such a pattern appears in an elderly patient, the lesion should be biopsied.
   (d) The typical starburst pattern is usually associated with Reed's nevi. A lesion with such a pattern can be closely monitored (patient age younger than 12) or biopsied (older patients).
2. **MM Patterns and Specific Structures**
   The detailed dermoscopic features and patterns of various types of MM will be discussed in the related chapter. In summary, MM usually manifests as a disorganized and asymmetric distribution of various structures and colors, of which many features are quite specific, especially when appearing in groups. Under very rare circumstances, atypical MM lesions tend to be regular and symmetric in shape, yet they almost always reveal one of the following features: a starburst pattern, negative network, blue-black or gray color, shiny white streaks, vessels, or ulceration. In addition, if a lesion is considered structureless (with no dermoscopic structures or with only nonspecific structures), a biopsy is needed when it is palpable.

4.2 Pattern Analysis

Unlike other structured analytic approaches, pattern analysis requires clinicians to accurately recognize certain dermoscopic patterns that imply whether the melanocytic lesions are benign, suspicious, or malignant in the second step of the two-step algorithm. Compared with other algorithms, pattern analysis is often faster to make a decision and better in terms of diagnostic accuracy. However, clinicians must have enough experience in dermoscopy to correctly distinguish a vast variety of dermoscopic patterns. Therefore, this is not an appropriate choice for beginners since it needs a long period of training and practice.

The ten most common dermoscopic patterns in benign nevi include reticular diffuse, reticular patchy, peripheral reticular with central hypopigmentation, peripheral reticular with central hyperpigmentation, homogenous areas, peripheral reticular with central globules, peripheral globules with a central network or homogenous area/the starburst pattern, globular, two components and multicomponent. The definitions and diagrams of these patterns are described in Chap. 5. MM lesions usually manifest multiple colors (more than 2), irregularity in shape and asymmetry in distribution. Therefore, the ten most common dermoscopic patterns of MM include an atypical pigment network, irregular streaks, a negative pigment network, chrysalis/crystalline, atypical dots and globules, irregular blotches, blue-white structures over raised areas, blue-white structures over flat areas, atypical vascular structures, and peripheral brown structureless areas. Please refer to Chap. 6, where the above patterns are elaborated in detail.

Obtaining familiarity with these patterns and sufficient dermoscopic practice gradually lead to a strong instinct in experts to make rapid and accurate diagnoses.

4.3 The ABCD Rule of Dermoscopy

The ABCD rule of dermoscopy was first described by Nachbar and Stolz et al. in 1994, and the efficacy of this rule was demonstrated afterwards by Binder et al. and Dolianitis et al. The ABCD rule was the first algorithm based on dermoscopy to help clinicians decide whether a melanocytic lesion is benign, suspicious or MM. The ABCD rule is very easy to learn and practice and is especially suited for novices. The classic ABCD rule is explained below.

A: Asymmetry

A lesion is bisected by two mutually perpendicular lines. The first line should be placed so that the lesion is bisected with the "most symmetry," and the second line is then placed 90° to the first line through the center. Then, the symmetry of the lesion contour, colors, and structures is assessed. Lesions that are symmetric in both axes are given 0 points, those asymmetric in one axis are given 1 point, and those asymmetric in two axes are given 2 points. The points of A range from 0 to 2.

B: Border

A lesion is divided equally into eight pie-shaped segments. Then, the number of segments with abrupt perimeter cut-off is counted. When the entire border of the lesion reveals a sharp cut-off, then the maximum score of eight is given. The minimum score of zero is given when all the borders tend to be blurry in the peripheries. The points of B range from 0 to 8.

C: Color

The presence of white, red, light brown, dark brown, blue-gray and black colors is of diagnostic value. White areas usually correspond with regression structures. Red indicates vascularity or inflammatory infiltration. The other four colors are related to melanin at different depths in the involved skin. The number of presented colors mentioned above is counted. The points of C range from 1 to 6.

D: Dermoscopic Structures

The presence of the following dermoscopic structures is considered meaningful: pigment networks, structureless areas (hypo- or hyperpigmented), branched streaks (including streaks, pseudopods, radial streaming and branched streaks), dots, and globules. Of note, structureless areas can be hypo- or hyperpigmented but must encompass at least 10% of the lesion area. Dots and branched streaks are counted when there are at least two of each in number. The categories of the above dermoscopic structures are counted. The points of D range from 1 to 5.

TDS: Total Dermoscopy Score

After evaluating the four dimensions of the lesion features, the TDS is calculated so that a final decision can be made.

$$\text{TDS} = (A \times 1.3) + (B \times 0.1) + (C \times 0.5) + (D \times 0.5)$$

The lesion is considered benign with a TDS < 4.75 and highly suspected as malignant with a TDS > 5.45. Suspicious lesions with a TDS between 4.75 and 5.45 should be biopsied or closely monitored with a low threshold for excision to maximize MM diagnostic sensitivity.

In addition, Kittler et al. proposed an extension to the classic ABCD rule by including a new scale of morphological change (E) since both subjective information offered by the patient's medical history and objective information provided by comparison with baseline lesion morphology are important to improve the detection of MM. This modification results in a slight but significant increase in diagnostic accuracy when applying the ABCD rule.

However, there are many exceptions to the ABCD rule. For instance, nevi with dermoscopic globular patterns and papillomatous surfaces can have a high TDS. Amelanotic, hypomelanotic and deep nodular MM can commonly score a TDS < 5.45. Under these circumstances, some dermoscopic features that are not contained in the ABCD rule, such as regression structures, milky-red areas and atypical vessels, can be extra diagnostic clues.

4.4 The Menzies Method

To simplify the diagnostic approach of MM under dermoscopy, Menzies et al. created the Menzies method to allow dermoscopists with limited experience to learn and apply this method in daily practice. The diagnostic sensitivity of the Menzies method is 92%, and the specificity is 71%. The Menzies method requires a clinician to observe the presence or absence of only the following dermoscopic features. An MM lesion must have neither of the two negative features but at least one of the nine positive features.

Negative Features

1. Symmetry of the pigmentation pattern: the method does not require the shape of the lesion to be symmetric, but all the patterns in the lesion should be symmetrically distributed, including colors.
2. Single color: this feature includes black, gray, blue, red, dark brown, and tan colors. White color is not scored.

Positive Features

1. Blue-white veil: This feature is found in 51% of invasive MM lesions, with a specificity of 97%, and is histopathologically correlated with melanin in the middle dermis, with compact orthokeratosis of the overlying epidermis.
2. Multiple brown dots, focally distributed: this feature is found in 30% of MM lesions, with a specificity of 97%, and is histopathologically associated with intraepidermal melanoma cells.
3. Radial streaming: This feature is found in 18% of MM lesions, with a specificity of 96%, and histopathologically results from confluent radial nests of melanoma cells at the intraepidermal areas or the dermal–epidermal junction.
4. Pseudopods: This feature is found in 23% of invasive MM lesions, with a specificity of 97%, and shares the same histopathological background as radial streaming.
5. Scar-like depigmentation: This feature is found in 36% of invasive MM lesions, with a specificity of 93%, and is considered the final phase of regression.
6. Peripheral black dots/globules: This feature is found in 42% of invasive MM lesions, with a specificity of 92%, and is histopathologically related to melanin accumulation in the stratum corneum arising from pagetoid spread of malignant melanocytes.
7. Multiple colors: This feature is scored when at least five types of colors are present in the lesion, including red, tan, dark brown, black, gray, and blue. Multiple colors are found in 53% of invasive melanoma lesions, with a specificity of 92%, and are histopathologically correlated with increased vasculature (red) or melanin in different skin layers (others).
8. Multiple blue-gray dots: This feature is found in 45% of invasive melanoma lesions, with a specificity of 91%, and is histopathologically correlated with melanophages in the acute phase of the regression process.
9. Broadened network: A broadened network is present in 35% of invasive melanoma lesions, with a specificity of 86%, and histopathologically corresponds to the expansion of melanocytic nests at the dermal–epidermal junction.

4.5 The Seven-Point Checklist

The seven-point checklist, published in 1998, allows clinicians to quantitively score melanocytic lesions by recognizing several dermoscopic features. Specifically, the major criteria consist of an atypical pigment network, blue-white veil, and atypical vascular pattern (linear irregular or dotted vessels that cannot be present within areas revealing regression structures). The presence of each major criterion is assigned 2 points. The minor criteria include irregular streaks, irregular dots/globules, irregular blotches, and regression structures. The presence of each minor criterion is assigned 1 point. The diagnosis of MM requires a lesion to obtain a minimum total score of 3, while a lesion with a total score < 3 is considered a benign nevus. The overall sensitivity of the seven-point checklist is 95%, and the specificity is 75%.

4.6 The Three-Point Checklist

The three-point checklist is a simple and effective diagnostic algorithm especially suited for novices. The overall sensitivity was 86.7%, and the overall specificity was 71.9% in a study for validation by Zalaudek et al. The three criteria are as follows:

1. Asymmetry: This is defined as asymmetry in the distribution of dermoscopic colors and/or structures in one or two perpendicular axes, regardless of the lesion shape or contour.

2. Atypical pigment network.
3. Blue-white structures: these include blue-white veil and regression structures (i.e., any blue and/or white color visible within the lesion).

The presence of two or three criteria favors the diagnosis of a malignancy (MM or BCC), and the lesion should be excised.

4.7 The CASH Algorithm

The CASH (color, architecture, symmetry, homogeneity) algorithm is a newly developed dermoscopic method based on pattern analysis for better adaption by clinicians with limited experience in dermoscopy. A study showed that the CASH algorithm had a comparable sensitivity and specificity to other methods, including the ABCD rule, Menzies method and seven-point checklist.

When applying the CASH algorithm, a clinician assesses the lesion in four aspects and assigns each criterion a number of points, including its number of colors (range 1–6), architectural disorder (range 0–2), symmetry (range 0–2) and level of homo-/heterogeneity (range 0–7). Then, the given points for each criterion are summed. A lesion is suspicious for MM if the total score is 8 or higher, whereas it is considered a probably benign nevus if the total score is less than 8.

Color

Colors scored in the CASH algorithm consist of light brown, dark brown, black, red, white and blue. The presence of each category is assigned one point.

Architecture

Architecture, or architectural disorder, represents the overall orderliness of the lesion contour and/or content based on "the global perception of the order *vs.* the disorder of the lesion." This criterion is scored from zero to two points. A lesion presenting no or merely mild disorder is assigned zero points, while a lesion with moderate or marked disorder is assigned one or two points, respectively.

Symmetry

Similar to the ABCD rule, a lesion is bisected by two perpendicular lines (the first line across the diameter that has the greatest symmetry). If the lesion is biaxially symmetric, it is assigned a score of zero. If the lesion is monoaxially or biaxially asymmetric, it is assigned a score of one or two points, respectively.

Homo-/Heterogeneity

This criterion is based on how many specific dermoscopic structures are present. The categories are counted, and the number equals the points that the lesion is assigned (zero to seven). Dermoscopic structures that are scored include pigment networks (typical or atypical), dots/globules, blotches (>10% of the lesion area), regression structures, streaks (radial streaks and pseudopods), blue-white veils and polymorphous vessels (vessels of various shapes and sizes).

4.8 The Revised Version of Pattern Analysis

The revised version of pattern analysis is a new modification of pattern analysis in which the unclear terminology is replaced with standardized descriptive terminology to facilitate beginner learning and application of such a dermoscopic method.

The basic geometric elements of all the dermoscopic patterns are lines, pseudopods, circles, clods and dots. If none of the elements are seen, a lesion is defined as structureless. The combinations of those elements and the repetitions of the same single element contribute to the formation of various dermoscopic patterns. However, one or two repetitions of a basic element are usually not sufficient to form a pattern, and a pattern has to cover a significant part of the lesion (at least 25% of the lesion surface). Patterns formed by lines can be reticular, branched, parallel, radial or curved. Exceptions are as follows: (1) any pseudopods or two or more radial lines are sufficient to form a pattern, and (2) any reticular lines not due to collision with another lesion are sufficient to form a pattern. Consequently, any unclear metaphorical term can be transformed into a simple and logical descriptive term. For instance, the classic dermoscopic pattern "blue ovoid nests" in BCC can be simply transformed into blue clods.

Colors under dermoscopy usually relate to different chromogenic materials in the skin. The most important is melanin, and others include keratin, hemoglobin, collagen, etc. In the revised version of pattern analysis, the shades of brown, gray and other colors are not differentiated. The number of colors present is classified as only one or more. Moreover, if relevant, colors can be classified as predominantly melanin-related or not.

Based on the combination of basic elements and colors, every dermoscopic pattern can be described in a simple and logical way that even beginners can easily understand and use. However, the precise description of the dermoscopic appearance is of even more vital importance with the revised version of pattern analysis.

The description starts with pigmentation structures. First, the clinician decides whether a lesion has one or more than one pattern. If the lesion has only one pattern, the present color(s) are further assessed. Lesions with only one pattern and one color must be symmetric. If a lesion with one pattern has various colors, clinicians must further decide whether the lesion is symmetric in the context of the combination of its pattern and colors. Lesions with multiple patterns can be analyzed in a similar way. First, a clinician decides whether the combination of these patterns is symmetric or not, following the order from the most specific patterns to the least specific patterns. For the five basic elements, lines and pseudopods are prioritized, followed by circles, clods, and dots. Structureless is the last to be considered because it has the least specificity.

4.9 Chaos and Clues

"Chaos and clues" is an analytic method assisting clinicians in deciding whether a pigmented lesion should be biopsied. In daily practice, it is unnecessary to analyze every dermoscopic feature very closely in detail because most lesions are benign and can be easily diagnosed by specific dermoscopic patterns. A clinician can quickly recognize most benign lesions through adequate experience since benign lesions seldom manifest suspicious patterns under dermoscopy. The overall diagnostic sensitivity of chaos and clues is 90.6% (MM 79.3%, BCC 98.5%, and SCC 86.5%), with a specificity of 62.7% for MM of any subtype.

The decision-making process includes two steps. The first step starts with the clinician looking for "chaos" along with "red flags" in the pigmented lesion. If a lesion is suspicious, then the clinician decides whether it is likely to be malignant by assessing the presence of "clues" in the second step (Fig. 4.1).

Chaos

"Chaos" is defined as the presence of any asymmetry in the pattern, color and border abruptness under dermoscopy. Chaos in dermoscopic patterns requires a lesion to have two or more patterns (each covering at least 20% of the lesion surface, except for peripheral black dots/clods, radial or segmental lines and pseudopods). Chaos in color requires a lesion to consist of more than one type of color with asymmetric distributions. Chaos in border abruptness is defined as definite and asymmetric variability in the abruptness of the demarcation of the border of a lesion.

Red Flags

"Red flags" are conditions that should raise the clinician's alertness of malignancy. They mainly include the following:

1. Patient's concern or clinical evidence of changes.
2. A lesion developing disordered dermoscopic features that break the benign patterns.
3. Dermoscopic clues of changes, including peripheral clods, radial lines and pseudopods, present in elderly patients.
4. Dermoscopic uniqueness, or the dermoscopic ugly duckling sign, defined as a lesion with dermoscopic patterns distinct from other lesions in the same patient.

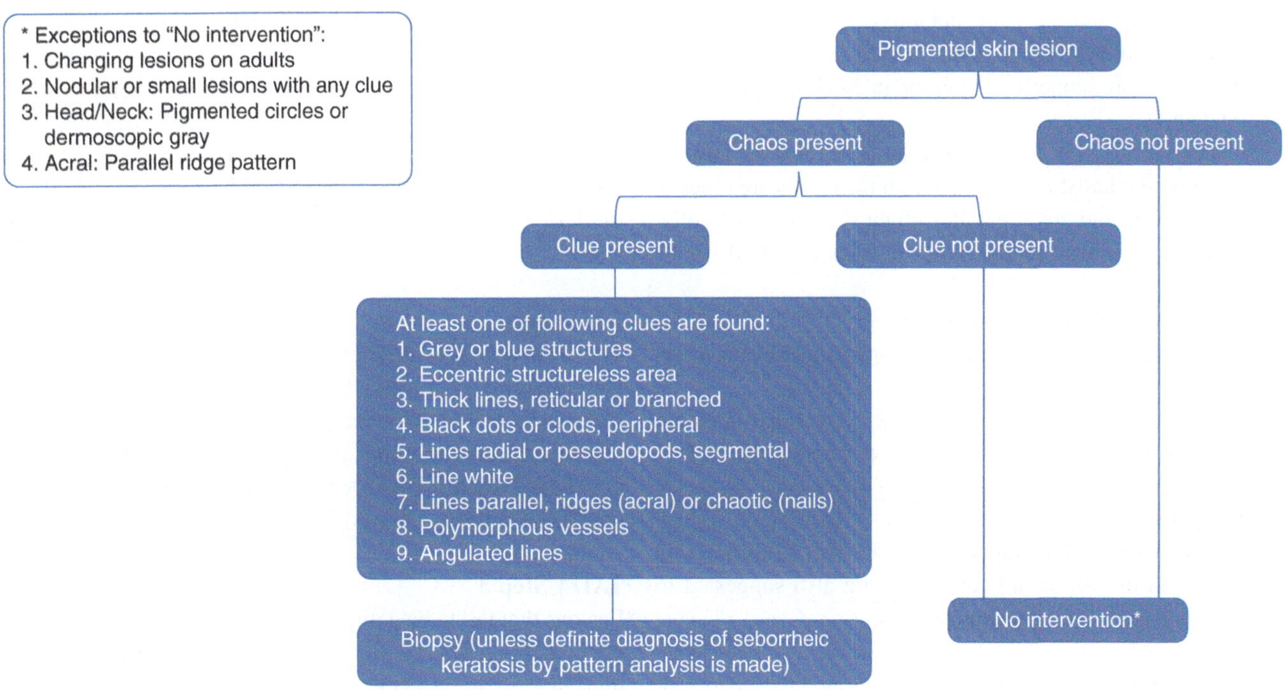

Fig. 4.1 Flowchart of chaos and clues (original design by Harald Kittler, Cliff Rosendahl, Aksana Marozava via https://dermoscopedia.org/Chaos_and_Clues)

Clues

"Clues" are features that further favor a diagnosis of the malignancy of a pigmented lesion and are described as follows:

1. Gray or blue structures (including gray or blue structureless areas): Gray color correlates with melanin located in the superficial dermis, commonly seen in MM in situ, pigmented BCC and pigmented SCC, while blue color indicates melanin in the deep dermis, most frequently seen in pigmented BCC and MM.
2. Eccentric structureless areas: An eccentric structureless area covers a sufficient portion of a lesion, is eccentrically located, and has colors different from those of the surrounding normal skin. Melanin-related colors favor the diagnosis of MM. Structureless areas with pink colors indicate increased vascularity, while white colors indicate fibrosis.
3. Thick lines reticular: This clue specifically indicates MM and is related to predominantly MM tumor cells in the widened rete ridges.
4. Black dots and clods, peripheral: Black dots and clods that are peripherally located are correlated with pigmented pagetoid melanocytes or nests of melanocytes in MM. However, they can also be found in pigmented BCC and pigmented SCC.
5. Lines radial or pseudopods, segmental: Lines radial can be seen in MM, pigmented BCC and pigmented SCC, while pseudopods specifically indicate MM. These clues are related to the peripheral nests of tumor cells.
6. White lines: White lines must be clearly lighter than the surrounding normal skin and might merely be seen in polarized mode. White lines are commonly present in BCC and are sometimes present in MM and pigmented SCC in situ.
7. Lines parallel on the ridges (acral) or chaotic parallel lines on the nails: Lines parallel on the ridges are clues to acral MM, and lines parallel chaotic (various in color, interval, or width) on the nails are related to MM on the nail matrix.
8. Polymorphous vessels: Vascular structures of various morphologies usually indicate malignancy (MM and pigmented BCC, but not pigmented SCC in situ).
9. Angulated lines: On chaotic lesions, angulated lines are clues to MM and are rarely seen in pigmented BCC.

Exceptions

To further improve the diagnostic sensitivity of this method, lesions with the following conditions are also suggested to be biopsied even if no chaos is present.

1. Any changing lesion (reported in the medical history or during clinical and dermoscopic monitoring) in an adult.
2. A nodular or small lesion (<6 mm in diameter) that has any of clues of malignancy.
3. Any lesion on the head or neck with pigmented circles and/or any dermoscopic gray.
4. Any lesion on acral skin with a parallel ridge pattern.

4.10 The TADA

The TADA is a method designed for the triage of cutaneous malignancies, with a sensitivity of 94% and a specificity of 72%. The TADA includes three steps. A clinician attempting to use the TADA needs to determine whether the lesion has the following patterns:

1. Unequivocal clinical and dermoscopic features of SK, DF, or angioma.
2. Disorder of color and structure distribution: Lesions with disordered (asymmetric, chaotic, or random) distributions of colors and structures are considered disorganized.
3. Starburst pattern.
4. Blue-black or gray color.
5. Shiny white structures under polarized dermoscopy.
6. Negative network.
7. Any vascular structure or ulceration.

The following is a simplified flowchart of the TADA (Fig. 4.2).

TADA Step 1

The first step requires a clinician to determine whether this lesion can be diagnosed as SK, DF or angioma through unequivocal clinical and dermoscopic criteria. Experienced dermoscopists can further recognize other benign lesions, such as sebaceous hyperplasia, clear cell acanthoma and intradermal nevus. If a definitive diagnosis of a benign lesion can be made, no further evaluation is required; if not, the lesion should be included in the assessment of the next steps.

TADA Step 2

The second step is to determine whether the lesion displays an organized or disorganized pattern under dermoscopy. Lesions revealing disorganized patterns (asymmetric or chaotic distribution of colors and structures) should be biopsied or referred to an expert for reassessment, while lesions with organized patterns fall into the last step of the TADA.

TADA Step 3

Lesions that fail to be definitively diagnosed as benign lesions but reveal organized dermoscopic patterns are included in the third step of the TADA. The last step is designed to detect cutaneous malignancies mimicking benign lesions as much as possible. If the lesion displays any of the following dermoscopic patterns, a biopsy is suggested:

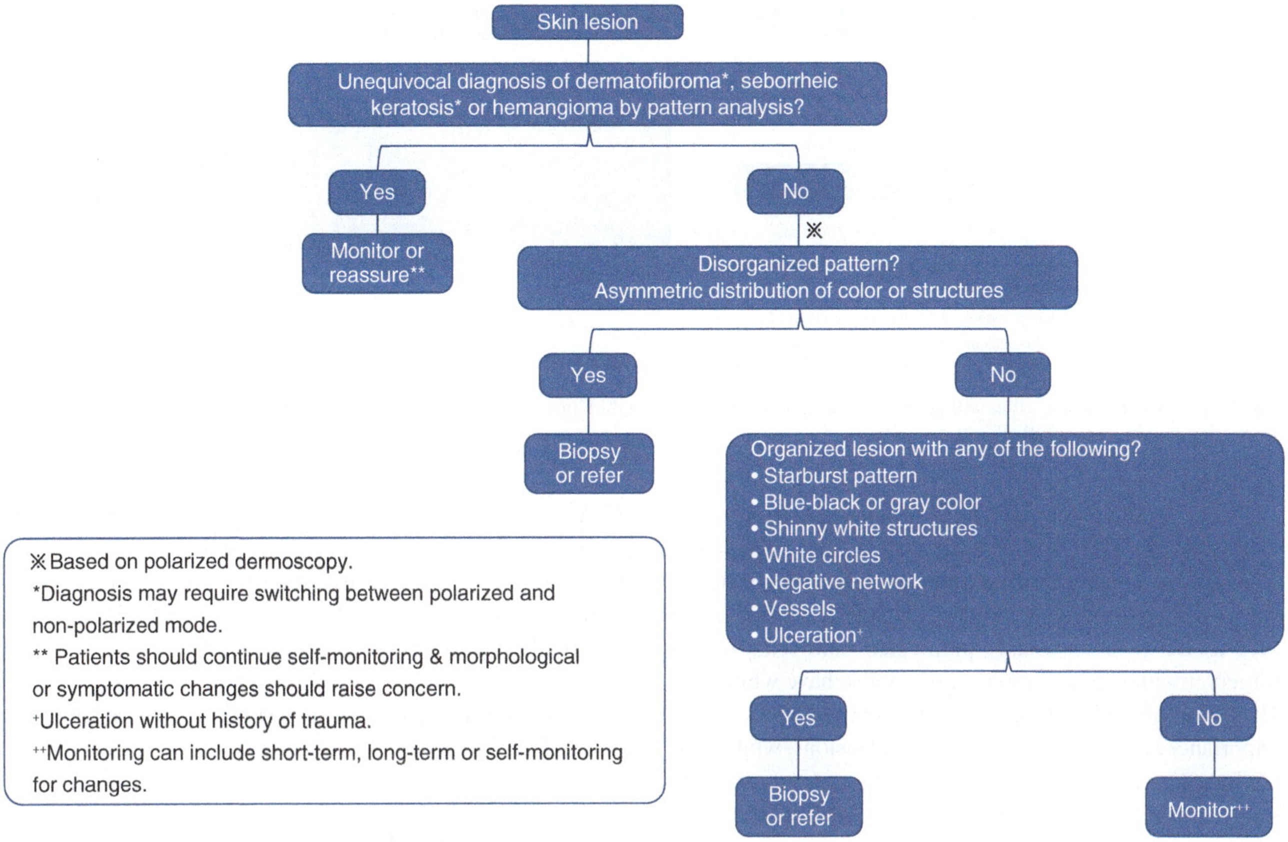

Fig. 4.2 Flowchart of the TADA (original design by Ashfaq A. Marghoob, Natalia Jaimes via https://dermoscopedia.org/TADA)

1. Starburst pattern, especially in elderly patients
2. Blue-black or gray colors
3. Shiny white structures or negative network
4. Vascular structures or ulceration

In addition, any volar lesion with a parallel ridge pattern should also be considered.

4.11 Prediction Without Pigment

Prediction without pigment is an algorithm based on pattern analysis designed for the evaluation of lesions without evidence of melanin pigmentation. In other words, there must be an absence of brown and gray color, and the presence of black, purple or blue color must result from blood rather than melanin.

As mentioned in Sect. 4.9, benign nonpigmented lesions such as nonpigmented nevi, benign keratinocytic lesions (including viral warts), DF, hemangiomas, sebaceous hyperplasia and benign cystic diseases are commonly encountered in daily practice and easily recognized by experienced clinicians. In addition, nonpigmented lesions are also simple to detect.

"Red flags" also exist in nonpigmented lesions. Specifically, a patient's concern or evidence of changes clinically or dermoscopically, as well as lesions developing disordered dermoscopic features that break the benign patterns, should raise the attention of clinicians.

Ulcerations are very common in BCC; therefore, the presence or absence of ulcerations is the first criterion to evaluate. Additionally, white lines under polarized and/or nonpolarized dermoscopy are clues to the nonpigmented variants of cutaneous malignancies. Subsequently, other white clues (white structureless areas and white circles in the raised lesions) and vascular patterns are also important in the evaluation of nonpigmented lesions. The flowchart of prediction without pigment is shown below (Fig. 4.3).

Step 1: Is There Ulceration?
Of note, ulcerations due to significant trauma should be excluded, and dermoscopy can help to detect small ulcerations that are difficult to recognize with the naked eye (micro-ulceration). Other features secondary to ulcerations, such as increased vascular structures and white circles, can be found near the ulcerated areas.

Step 2: Are There White Clues?
White clues are defined as

1. White lines in any nonpigmented lesion.
2. White structureless areas or white circles under dermoscopy or clinical evidence of keratin in any raised nonpigmented lesion.

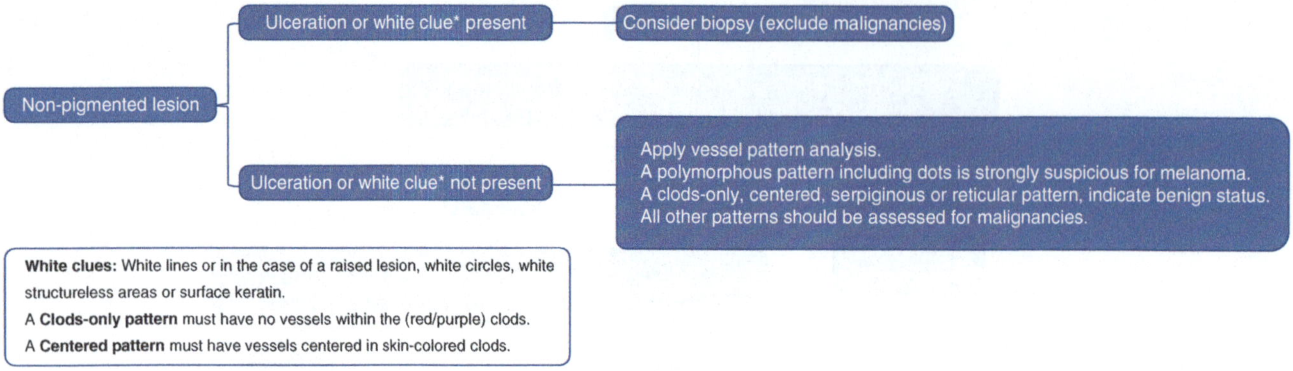

Fig. 4.3 Flowchart of prediction without pigment (original design by Harald Kittler, Cliff Rosendahl, Aksana Marozava via https://dermoscopedia.org/Prediction_without_Pigment)

White lines in nonpigmented lesions can be found in malignancies such as BCC, SCC, and amelanotic MM. Vascular patterns are usually necessary to consider at the same time to make a prediction. However, benign lesions such as DF (lesions usually pigmented) and scars (due to surgery, trauma, cryotherapy, etc.) can also have white lines. Therefore, obtaining an accurate medical history is of vital importance in these conditions. In raised lesions, white structureless areas, white circles and prominent keratins on the lesion surface usually indicate SCC or keratoacanthoma (KA), especially the white circles.

Step 3: Are the Vascular Patterns Consistent with Malignancy?

It is only necessary to analyze vascular patterns when the nonpigmented lesions reveal no ulcerations and white clues. If any ulcerations or white clues are present, vascular patterns can be supplementary to make a prediction but not to impede the decision of biopsy.

Eight categories of vascular structures, including dots, clods, linear straight, linear looped, linear curved, linear serpentine, linear helical and linear coiled, and eight types of vascular arrangements, including random, clustered, serpiginous, linear, centered, radial, reticular and branched, are identified in the revised pattern analysis.

Vascular patterns consistent with a benign diagnosis are as follows:

1. A pattern of (red, purple and/or blue) clods-only: This pattern is consistent with the diagnosis of hemangioma in a stable lesion. However, any evidence of changes, the presence of linear vessels, or any vessels seen within the red or purple clods of a hemangioma are suspicious.
2. A pattern of centered vessels only: This pattern is consistent with the diagnosis of a viral wart, congenital nevus, or SK in a stable lesion. Of note, the background color should not be dark-pink or red (seen in some nodular MM).
3. A pattern of serpiginous vessels only: This pattern is consistent with the diagnosis of clear cell acanthoma.
4. A pattern of reticular vessels only: This pattern is associated with chronic sun-damaged skin and telangiectasia macularis perstans.

All other vascular patterns in lesions of concern should be assessed for biopsy.

4.12 The Color Wheel Approach

Orit Markowitz proposed a practical dermoscopic algorithm named "the color wheel approach" that serves as a complement to the two-step algorithm and traditional pattern analysis. This approach is designed to help clinicians decide whether to perform a biopsy of the assessed lesion rather than differentiating melanocytic or nonmelanocytic origin or stressing the final diagnosis.

The color wheel approach is mainly based on four aspects of the lesion: the clinical history, clinical and dermoscopic colors, morphology and supplementary pattern analysis. After the assessment of patient risk factors and the gross features of the lesion, the four steps of the color wheel can be used to create a list of possible diagnoses (Fig. 4.4).

Step 1: Is the Lesion Flat or Raised (Based on Inspection and Palpation)?

Step 2: What Color Is the Lesion on Clinical Assessment?

The clinical color wheel spectrum includes pink-clear, pale brown, brown-black, and others (yellow, purple, red). Combined with the information that the lesion is raised or flat, the clinician can subsequently narrow down the differential diagnosis.

Step 3: What Color Is the Lesion Under Dermoscopic Examination?

The clinician can cross-reference the list of possible diagnoses that remain after step 2 using the respective color

Fig. 4.4 Clinical and dermoscopic color wheel indicating differential diagnosis (original design by Orit Markowitz in the book A Practical Guide to Dermoscopy, Wolters Kluwer)

Color	Clinical Color Wheel Diagnosis
Brown/Black	Melanoma, Ink-jet Lentigo/Seborrheic Keratosis, Pigmented Bowen's Disease, Dermatofibroma, Benign Nevus
Pale Brown	Melanoma, Lentigo/Seborrheic Keratosis, Pigmented Bowen's Disease, Dermatofibroma, Benign Nevus
Purple	Angiokeratoma, Lichen Planus-Like Keratosis
Red	Angioma
Pink/Clear	Amelanotic Melanoma, Squamous Cell Carcinoma, Basal Cell Carcinoma, Porokeratosis, Cyst/Milia, Dermatofibroma, Benign Nevus, Clear Cell Acanthoma, Sebaceous Hyperplasia, Spitz Nevus
Color	**Dermoscopic Color Wheel Diagnosis**
Blue/Gray/Black	Lichen Planus-Like Keratosis, Melanoma, Basal Cell Carcinoma, Congenital Nevus/Blue Nevus, Ink-jet Lentigo/Seborrheic Keratosis, Hemorrhage/Angiokeratoma
Brown	Dermatofibroma, Benign Nevus, Lentigo/Seborrheic Keratosis, Melanoma, Pigmented Bowen's Disease
Yellow	Seborrheic Keratosis, Cyst/Milia, Sebaceous Hyperplasia, Malignant Erosion, Squamous Cell Carcinoma/Basal Cell Carcinoma
Red	Angioma/Angiokeratoma, Vascular Patterns of Melanoma, Squamous Cell Carcinoma, Clear Cell Acanthoma, Basal Cell Carcinoma, Dermatofibroma, Benign Nevus, Seborrheic Keratosis, Spitz Nevus

wheel corresponding to the relevant dermoscopic color (red, multicolored, brown and yellow).

Step 4: Is Further Pattern Analysis Needed to Decide Whether To Perform a Biopsy?

If the final list of differential diagnoses includes malignancies, the lesion should be further analyzed for limited benign or malignant patterns to rule out related diagnoses.

Further Reading

1. Argenziano G, Soyer H, Chimenti S, et al. Dermoscopy of pigmented skin lesions: results of a consensus meeting via the Internet. J Am Acad Dermatol. 2003;48(5):679–93.
2. Scope A, Benvenuto-Andrade C, Agero AL, et al. Nonmelanocytic lesions defying the two-step dermoscopy algorithm. Dermatol Surg. 2006;32(11):1398–406.
3. Marghoob AA, Braun R. Proposal for a revised 2-step algorithm for the classification of lesions of the skin using dermoscopy. Arch Dermatol. 2010;146(4):426–8.
4. Agero A, Taliercio S, Dusza S, et al. Conventional and polarized dermoscopy features of dermatofibroma. Arch Dermatol. 2006;142(11):1431–7.
5. Menzies S, Westerhoff K, Rabinovitz H, et al. Surface microscopy of pigmented basal cell carcinoma. Arch Dermatol. 2000;136(8):1012–6.
6. Ahlgrimm-Siess V, Cao T, Oliviero M, et al. Seborrheic keratosis: reflectance confocal microscopy features and correlation with dermoscopy. J Am Acad Dermatol. 2013;69(1):120–6.
7. Braun R, Rabinovitz H, Krischer J, et al. Dermoscopy of pigmented seborrheic keratosis: a morphological study. Arch Dermatol. 2002;138(12):1556–60.
8. Stricklin S, Stoecker W, Oliviero M, et al. Cloudy and starry milia-like cysts: how well do they distinguish seborrheic keratoses from malignant melanomas? J Eur Acad Dermatol Venereol. 2011;25(10):1222–4.
9. Zalaudek I, Argenziano G. Dermoscopy of actinic keratosis, intraepidermal carcinoma and squamous cell carcinoma. Curr Probl Dermatol. 2015;46:70–6.
10. Morales A, Puig S, Malvehy J, et al. Dermoscopy of molluscum contagiosum. Arch Dermatol. 2005;141(12):1644.
11. Zaballos P, Ara M, Puig S, et al. Dermoscopy of sebaceous hyperplasia. Arch Dermatol. 2005;141(6):808.
12. Menzies SW, Kreusch J, Byth K, et al. Dermoscopic evaluation of amelanotic and hypomelanotic melanoma. Arch Dermatol. 2008;144(9):1120–7.
13. Braun RP, Rabinovitz H, Oliviero M, et al. Dermoscopic diagnosis of seborrheic keratosis. Clin Dermatol. 2002;20(3):270–2.
14. Argenziano G, Zalaudek I, Ferrara G, et al. Dermoscopy features of melanoma incognito: indications for biopsy. J Am Acad Dermatol. 2007;56(3):508–13.
15. Puig S, Argenziano G, Zalaudek I, et al. Melanomas that failed dermoscopic detection: a combined clinicodermoscopic approach for not missing melanoma. Dermatol Surg. 2007;33(10):1262–73.
16. Annessi G, Bono R, Sampogna F, et al. Sensitivity, specificity, and diagnostic accuracy of three dermoscopic algorithmic methods in the diagnosis of doubtful melanocytic lesions: the importance of light brown structureless areas in differentiating atypical melanocytic nevi from thin melanomas. J Am Acad Dermatol. 2007;56(5):759–67.
17. Carli P, Quercioli E, Sestini S, et al. Pattern analysis, not simplified algorithms, is the most reliable method for teaching dermoscopy

for melanoma diagnosis to residents in dermatology. Br J Dermatol. 2003;151(2):981–4.
18. Nachbar F, Stolz W, Merkle T, et al. The ABCD rule of dermatoscopy. J Am Acad Dermatol. 1994;30(4):551–9.
19. Binder M, Kittler H, Steiner A, et al. Reevaluation of the ABCD rule for epiluminescence microscopy. J Am Acad Dermatol. 1999;40(2):171–6.
20. Dolianitis C, Kelly J, Wolfe R, et al. Comparative performance of 4 dermoscopic algorithms by nonexperts for the diagnosis of melanocytic lesions. Arch Dermatol. 2005;141(8):1008–14.
21. Kittler H, Seltenheim M, Dawid M, et al. Morphologic changes of pigmented skin lesions: a useful extension of the ABCD rule for dermatoscopy. J Am Acad Dermatol. 1999;40(4):558–62.
22. Menzies SW, Ingvar C, Crotty KA, et al. Frequency and morphologic characteristics of invasive melanomas lacking specific surface microscopic features. Arch Dermatol. 1996;132(10):1178–82.
23. Argenziano G, Fabbrocini G, Carli P, et al. Epiluminescence microscopy for the diagnosis of doubtful melanocytic skin lesions: comparison of the ABCD rule of dermatoscopy and a new 7-point checklist based on pattern analysis. Arch Dermatol. 1998;134(12):1563–70.
24. Soyer HP, Argenziano G, Zalaudek I, et al. Three-point checklist of dermoscopy. A new screening method for early detection of melanoma. Dermatology. 2004;208(1):27–31.
25. Henning J, Stein JA, Yeung J, et al. Cash algorithm for dermoscopy revisited. Arch Dermatol. 2008;144(4):554–5.
26. Rosendahl C, Cameron A, Mccoll I, et al. Dermatoscopy in routine practice—'chaos and clues'. Austr Family Phys. 2012;41(7):482–7.
27. Tschandl P, Rosendahl C, Kittler H. Dermatoscopy of flat pigmented facial lesions. J Eur Acad Dermatol Venereol. 2015;29(1):120–7.
28. Rogers T, Marino ML, Dusza SW, et al. A clinical aid for detecting skin cancer: the triage amalgamated dermoscopic algorithm (TADA). J Am Board Family Med. 2016;29(6):694–701.
29. Rogers T, Marino M, Dusza SW, et al. Triage amalgamated dermoscopic algorithm (TADA) for skin cancer screening. Dermatol Pract Concep. 2017;7(2):39–46.
30. Carrera C, Marchetti MA, Dusza SW, et al. Validity and reliability of dermoscopic criteria used to differentiate nevi from melanoma: a web-based international dermoscopy society study. JAMA Dermatol. 2016;152(7):798–806.
31. Argenziano G, Longo C, Cameron A, et al. Blue-black rule: a simple dermoscopic clue to recognize pigmented nodular melanoma. Br J Dermatol. 2011;165(6):1251–5.
32. Braun RP, Gaide O, Oliviero M, et al. The significance of multiple blue-grey dots (granularity) for the dermoscopic diagnosis of melanoma. Br J Dermatol. 2007;157(5):907–13.
33. Balagula Y, Braun RP, Rabinovitz HS, et al. The significance of crystalline/chrysalis structures in the diagnosis of melanocytic and nonmelanocytic lesions. J Am Acad Dermatol. 2012;67(2):194.e1–8.
34. Pizzichetta MA, Talamini R, Marghoob AA, et al. Negative pigment network: an additional dermoscopic feature for the diagnosis of melanoma. J Am Acad Dermatol. 2013;68(4):552–9.
35. Rosendahl C, Cameron A, Tschandl P, et al. Prediction without Pigment: a decision algorithm for non-pigmented skin malignancy. Dermatol Pract Concept. 2014;4(1):59–66.
36. Rosendahl C, Cameron A, Argenziano G, et al. Dermoscopy of squamous cell carcinoma and keratoacanthoma. Arch Dermatol. 2012;148(12):1386–92.
37. Markowitz O. Practical guide to dermoscopy. Philadelphia: Wolters Kluwer; 2017. p. 120–50.

Benign Melanocytic Tumors

5

Benign melanocytic tumors are a group of skin tumors derived from melanocytes and are the most common skin tumors in humans. The initial purpose of dermoscopy is to distinguish malignant melanoma lesions from benign melanocytic tumors (such as nevi). Compared with macroscopic observation, dermoscopy can improve the diagnostic accuracy by 20–30%, thus reducing the number of unnecessary skin biopsies and surgeries performed.

5.1 Common Dermoscopic Patterns of Pigmented Nevi

The two-step algorithm, established in 2001, is the most commonly used method for dermoscopic diagnosis of pigmented lesions. For lesions identified as being of melanocytic origins in the first step, the second step is to determine whether these melanocytic lesions are benign, suspicious, or malignant. Pattern analysis is the most commonly used dermoscopic diagnostic method for nevi. Based on the evaluation of a large number of nevi, most nevi were found to show the following ten dermoscopic patterns. These patterns of benign nevi all demonstrate symmetry in terms of color, structures, and patterns, among which the homogeneous pattern and the peripheral globule/starburst pattern have three variants. Color variation is responsible for the homogenous pattern, including homogenous tan, brown and blue pigmentation. The peripheral globule/starburst pattern includes a single layer of globules at the periphery, peripheral tiering, and the typical starburst pattern.

The ten dermoscopic patterns of benign nevi are as follows, and schematic diagrams are shown in Fig. 5.1:

(i) **Reticular Diffuse** (Fig. 5.2). Diffuse homogenous network with a relatively uniform thickness and color of the network lines. The holes of the network are of relatively uniform size. The network tends to fade at the periphery. This pattern is frequently seen in acquired nevi (especially those developing in individuals with a darker skin phenotype) and is commonly seen in congenital nevi, especially those located on the lower extremities.

(ii) **Reticular Patchy** (Fig. 5.3). Homogenous network with a relatively uniform thickness and color of the network lines. The network is present in focal patches that are separated by homogenous structureless areas that are lighter in color than the network lines. The structureless areas have the same color as the background skin or are slightly darker than the background skin. This pattern is commonly seen in acquired nevi located on the trunk and in superficial congenital nevi, especially those located on the lower extremities.

(iii) **Peripheral Reticular with Central Hypopigmentation** (Fig. 5.4). A relatively uniform network at the periphery of the lesion with a central homogenous and hypopigmented (relative to the color of the network) structureless area. The structureless area has the same color as the background skin or is slightly darker (but lighter in color than the network lines). This pattern is commonly seen in acquired nevi, especially those found in individuals with a fair skin phenotype.

(iv) **Peripheral Reticular with Central Hyperpigmentation** (Fig. 5.5). A relatively uniform network at the periphery of the lesion with a central homogenous, hyperpigmented structureless area or blotch. The blotch has a darker color than the network lines. This type of acquired nevus is more common in individuals with a darker skin phenotype.

(v) **Homogenous** (Fig. 5.6). A tan, brown, and blue (may be pink occasionally) color may be present. Primarily consists of a diffuse homogenous structureless pattern. On occasion, a few globules and/or small focal network fragments may be evident. The homogenous tan pattern is usually found in acquired nevi in individuals with fair skin phenotypes, while the brown pattern is found in congenital nevi, and the blue pattern is found in blue nevi. Nevi in very fair-skinned individuals (including redheads) can manifest a homogenous pink pattern (N.B.: amelanotic and hypomelanotic melanomas can

J. Liu, X. Zou, *Practical Dermoscopy*, https://doi.org/10.1007/978-981-19-1460-7_5

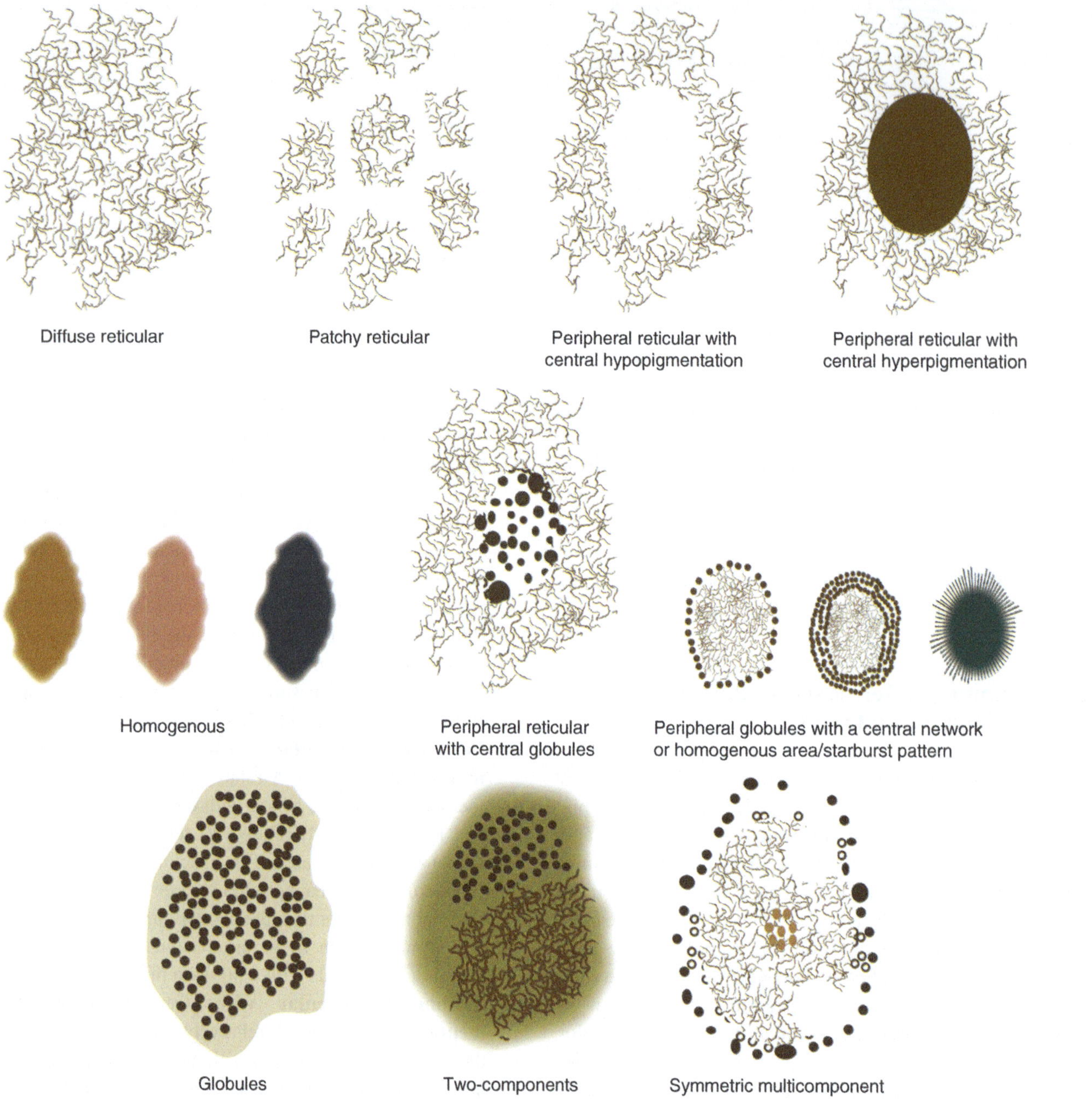

Fig. 5.1 Schematic diagrams of the ten benign nevus patterns

manifest in a similar manner; however, most melanomas will also reveal atypical blood vessels and/or crystalline structures).

(vi) **Peripheral Reticular with Central Globules** (Fig. 5.7). A relatively uniform network at the periphery of the lesion with central globules. The histopathological features of these nevi are often the same as those in congenital nevi.

(vii) **Peripheral Globules with a Central Network or Homogenous Area/Starburst Pattern** (Figs. 5.8 and 5.9). The central component of this type of nevus is either reticular or homogenous. The presence of one row of relatively uniform brown globules surrounding the entire perimeter of the lesion is indicative of an actively growing nevus (i.e., not yet undergoing senescence). When the globules at the perimeter are tiered (more than one row of globules), then it is considered to be a starburst pattern, which is commonly seen in Spitz nevi. The classic starburst pattern consists of streaks, radial streaming, or pseudopods present around the entire perimeter of the lesion, giving the appearance of an exploding star.

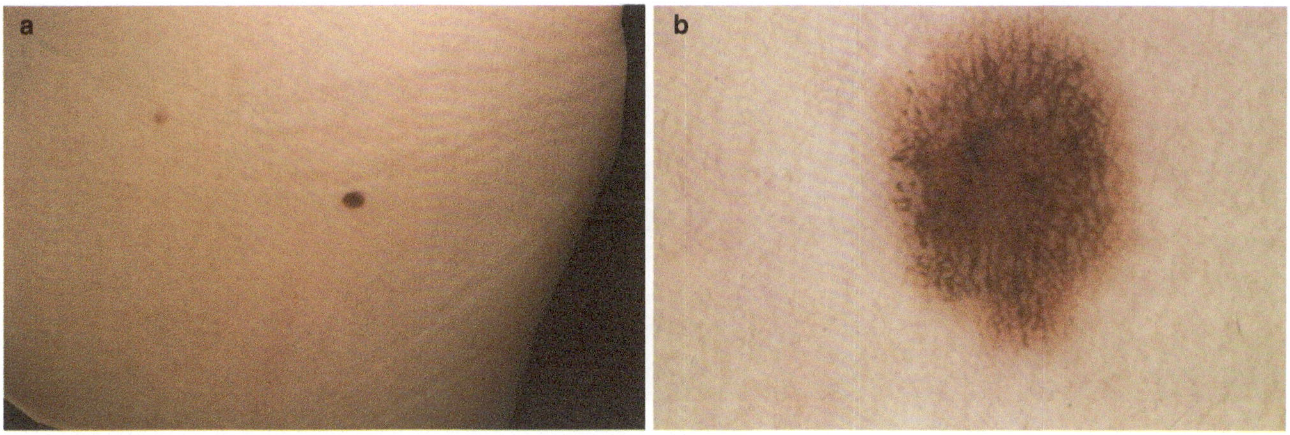

Fig. 5.2 Clinical and dermoscopic images of the diffuse reticular pattern. (**a**) A brown patch on the trunk. (**b**) Dermoscopy shows a diffuse reticular pattern (×30)

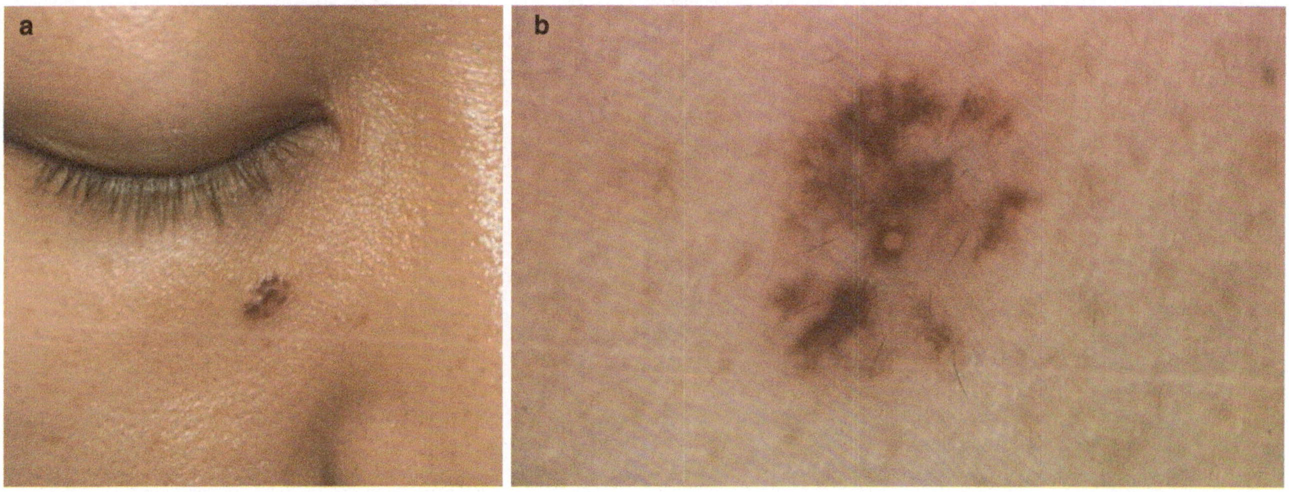

Fig. 5.3 Clinical and dermoscopic images of the patchy reticular pattern. (**a**) A brown patch on the right face. (**b**) Dermoscopy shows a patchy reticular pattern, which is characterized by a homogenous network with a relatively uniform thickness and color of the network lines, which are separated by homogenous structureless areas that are lighter in color than the network lines (×30)

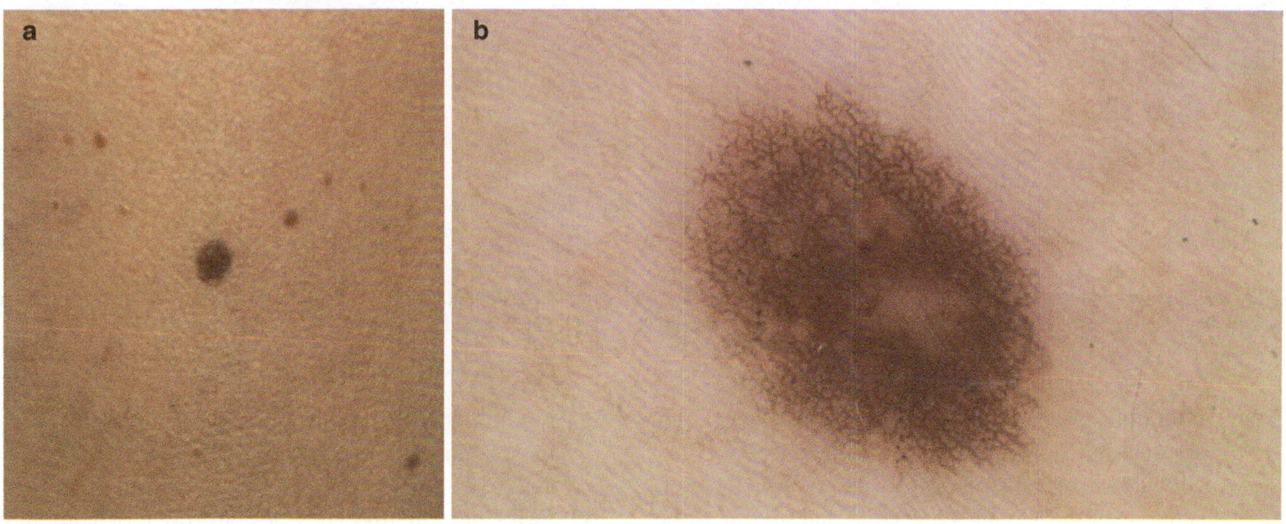

Fig. 5.4 Clinical and dermoscopic images of the peripheral reticular with central hypopigmentation pattern. (**a**) A brown patch on the trunk, slightly raised in the center. (**b**) Dermoscopy shows a peripheral reticular with central hypopigmentation pattern (×30)

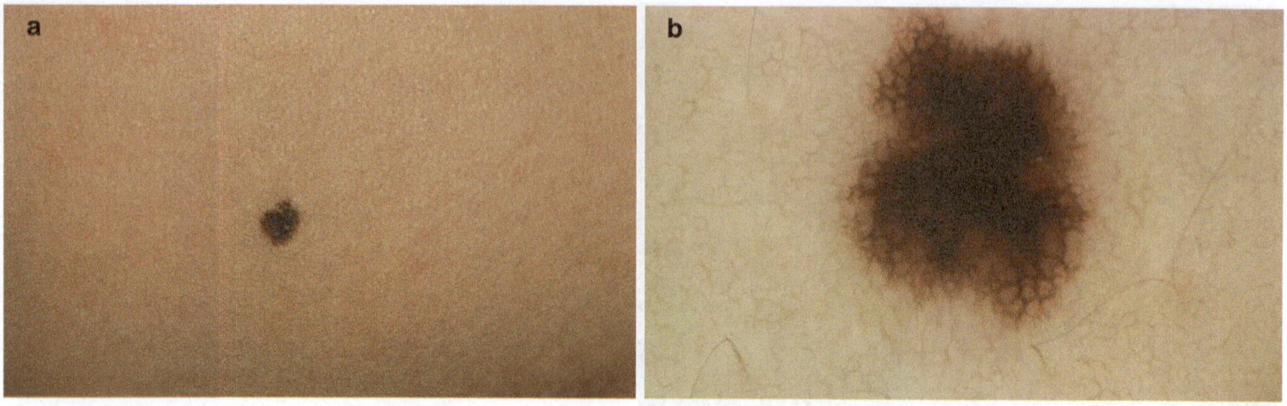

Fig. 5.5 Clinical and dermoscopic images of the peripheral reticular with central hyperpigmentation pattern. (**a**) A dark-brown patch on the left chest wall. (**b**) Dermoscopy shows a peripheral reticular with central hyperpigmentation pattern (×30)

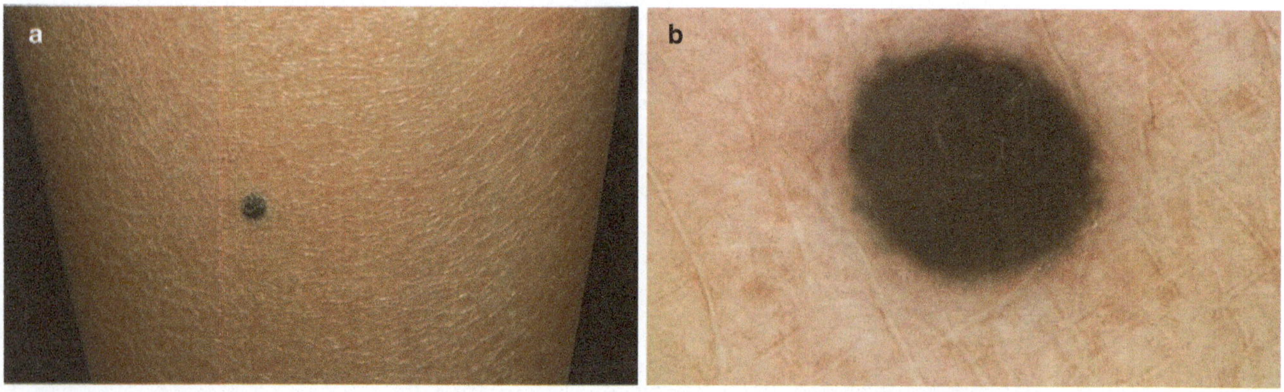

Fig. 5.6 Clinical and dermoscopic images of the homogenous pattern. (**a**) A blue-black papule on the lower limb. (**b**) Dermoscopy shows a blue-black homogeneous structureless area (×30)

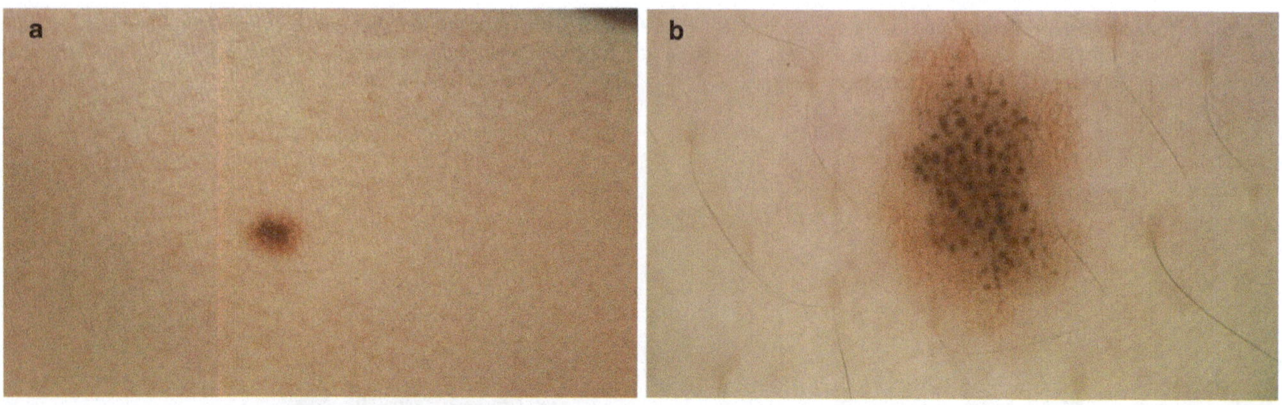

Fig. 5.7 Clinical and dermoscopic images of the peripheral reticular with central globule pattern. (**a**) A brown papule on a yellow-brown patch located on the back. (**b**) Dermoscopy shows a peripheral reticular with central globule pattern (×30)

(viii) **Globular**. Globules of similar shape, size, and color are distributed symmetrically throughout the lesion. Globules are usually round to oval in shape. However, sometimes the globules are large and appear to be compressing each other, creating angulated shapes reminiscent of cobblestones. This pattern is seen most commonly in congenital nevi (Figs. 5.10, 5.11, and 5.12).

(ix) **Two Components.** These lesions reveal two different patterns (reticular-globular, reticular-homogenous, or

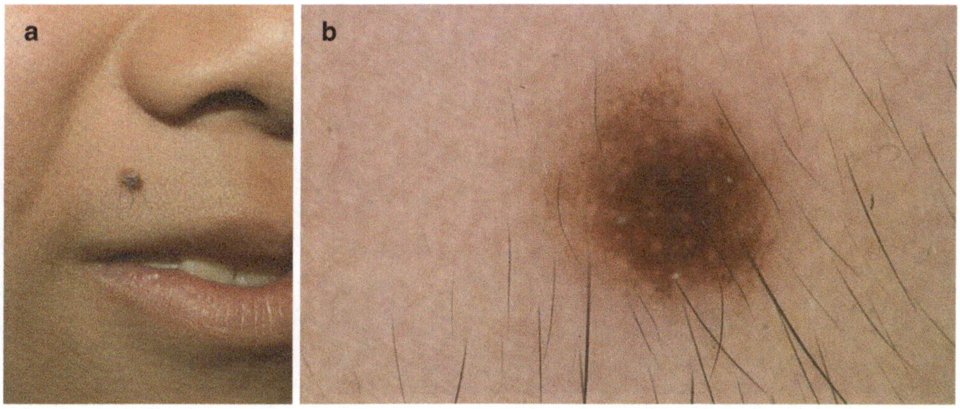

Fig. 5.8 Clinical and dermoscopic images of the peripheral globule pattern. (**a**) A brown patch on the face. (**b**) Dermoscopy shows a pattern of peripheral globules with a central pseudonetwork, indicating that the lesion is an actively growing nevus (×30)

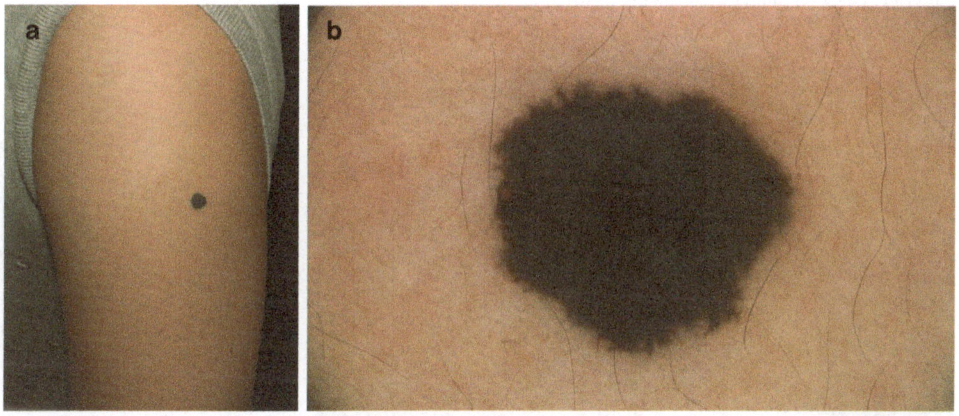

Fig. 5.9 Clinical and dermoscopic images of the starburst pattern. (**a**) A blue-black plaque on the upper arm. (**b**) Dermoscopy shows a blue-black homogeneous pattern in the center and a starburst pattern with radial lines at the periphery (×20)

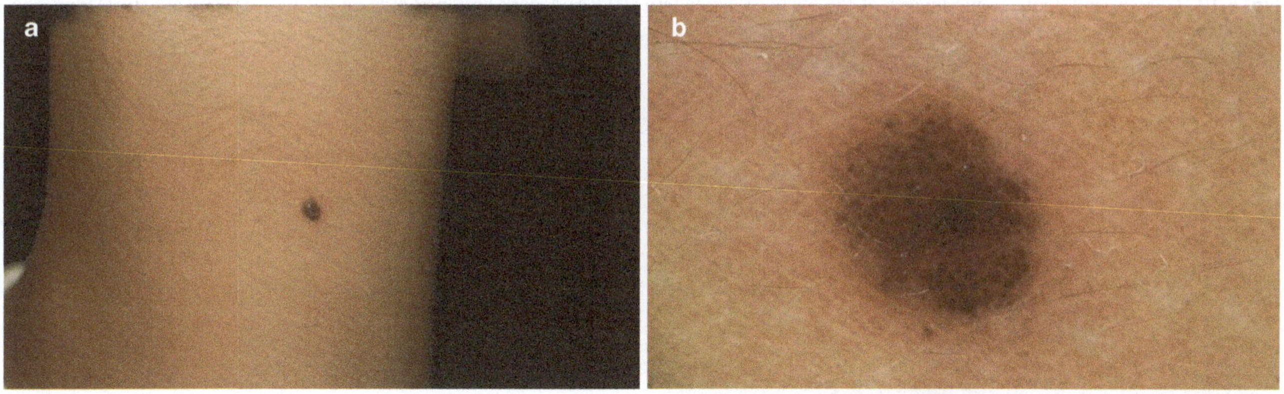

Fig. 5.10 Clinical and dermoscopic images of the globular pattern. (**a**) A brown papule on the neck. (**b**) Dermoscopy presents a globular pattern (×30)

globular-homogenous). Half of the lesion manifests one pattern, while the other half of the lesion manifests a different pattern.

(x) **Multicomponent** (Fig. 5.13). Two definitions exist for the multicomponent pattern (N.B.: only the first definition applies to benign nevi). In one definition, a lesion with a multicomponent pattern presents organized and/or symmetrically distributed typical dots/globules, typical networks, and homogenous areas. This pattern is associated with benign nevi. In the second definition, a lesion with a multicomponent pattern needs to have an axis of symmetry only in one axis, with symmetrically distributed globules, network, blotches, dots, veil, regression structures, and/or structureless areas. Here, three or more structures are required to classify the lesion as having a multicomponent pattern (N.B.: although a symmetric multicomponent pattern favors a benign nevus, any lesion displaying a multicomponent pattern other than that described in the first definition should be viewed with caution).

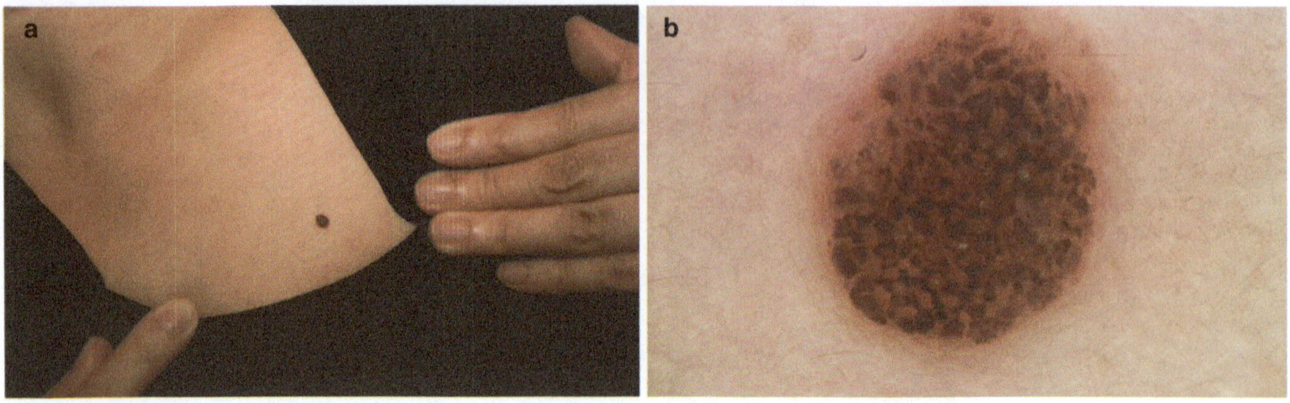

Fig. 5.11 Clinical and dermoscopic images of the cobblestone pattern (I). (**a**) A dark-brown papule on the upper chest wall. (**b**) A cobblestone pattern is observed under dermoscopy (×40)

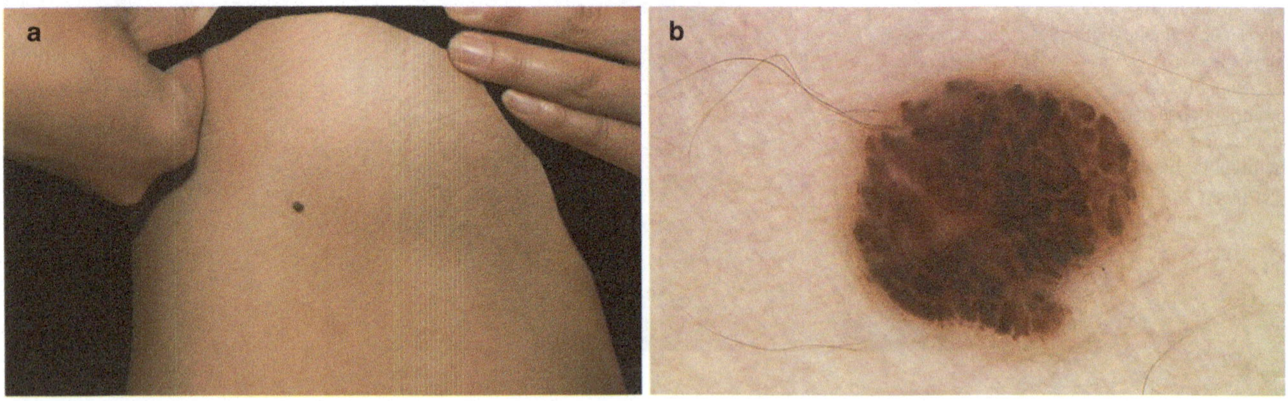

Fig. 5.12 Clinical and dermoscopic images of the cobblestone pattern (II). (**a**) A dark-brown papule on the right chest wall. (**b**) Dermoscopy presents a cobblestone pattern, on which a hair can be seen (×40)

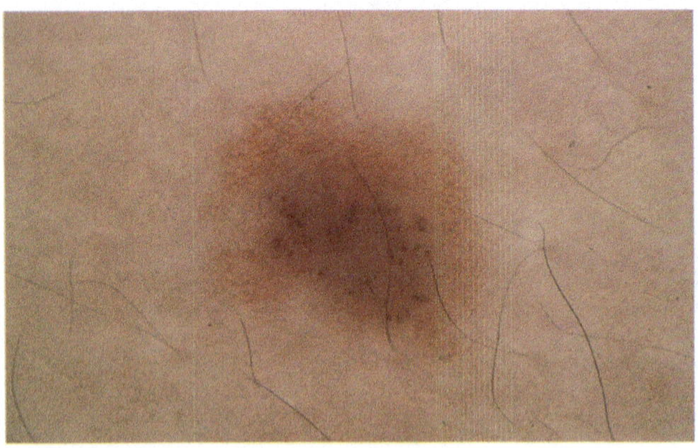

Fig. 5.13 Clinical and dermoscopic images of the multicomponent pattern. Dermoscopy shows a combination of homogeneous, globular and reticular patterns (×30)

> **Tip**
> The central pigmentation of a benign nevus, corresponding to pigmented parakeratosis histologically, may be mistaken for a blotch. Tape can peel off the stratum corneum and easily remove or dilute the central pigmentation of a nevus, while a blotch is not affected by tape.

5.2 Dermoscopic Features of Common Pigmented Nevi

5.2.1 Junctional Nevi

Pigmented nevi can be divided into three types according to the distribution of nevus cells on skin histology: junctional nevi, intradermal nevi, and compound nevi. The color of a junctional nevus is dark, varying from light brown and dark-brown to black. A junctional nevus has a smooth and hairless surface. Junctional nevi can occur on any part of the skin or mucosa. The palm, plantar area, vulva, nail bed, and other special locations are often the location of junctional nevi.

Pathologically, nevus cells containing a large amount of melanin are found in the lower part of the epidermis or in the epidermis near the dermis.

The dermoscopic manifestations of junctional nevi are as follows:

(i) Reticular pattern. The reticular pattern is usually brown in color, with dots and globules (indicating a period of growth), and the pigment network is denser in the center of the skin lesion than in the surrounding areas (Figs. 5.14 and 5.15).
(ii) Due to the different anatomical structures of special locations of junctional nevi, the lesions show the corresponding characteristics under dermoscopy. Please refer to Sect. 5.3 below.

Tip
If there is no typical benign pattern, when the lesion diameter is less than 7 mm, regular follow-up can be performed. If the diameter ≥7 mm, the lesion should be excised for biopsy.

5.2.2 Compound Nevi

A compound nevus is similar to a junctional nevus in appearance but is slightly raised and may be accompanied by hair. The nests of nevus cells are located not only at the dermal–epidermal junction but also in the dermis.

The dermoscopic manifestations of compound nevi are as follows:

(i) Globular pattern. The size of the globules is similar (Fig. 5.16)
(ii) Cobblestone pattern
(iii) The common vascular pattern is linear regular or comma shaped

5.2.3 Intradermal Nevi

Intradermal nevi are most common in adults. Intradermal nevi can occur on the head, face, and neck. This type of nevus manifests as a hemispheric or papillomatous protru-

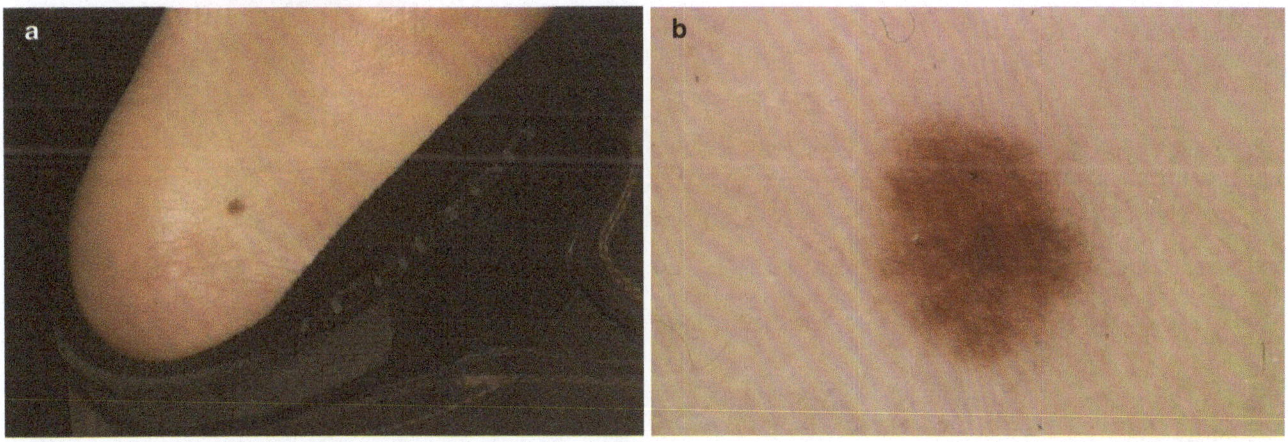

Fig. 5.14 Clinical and dermoscopic images of a junctional nevus (1). (**a**) A black patch on the skin above the heel. (**b**) Dermoscopy shows a reticular pattern (×30)

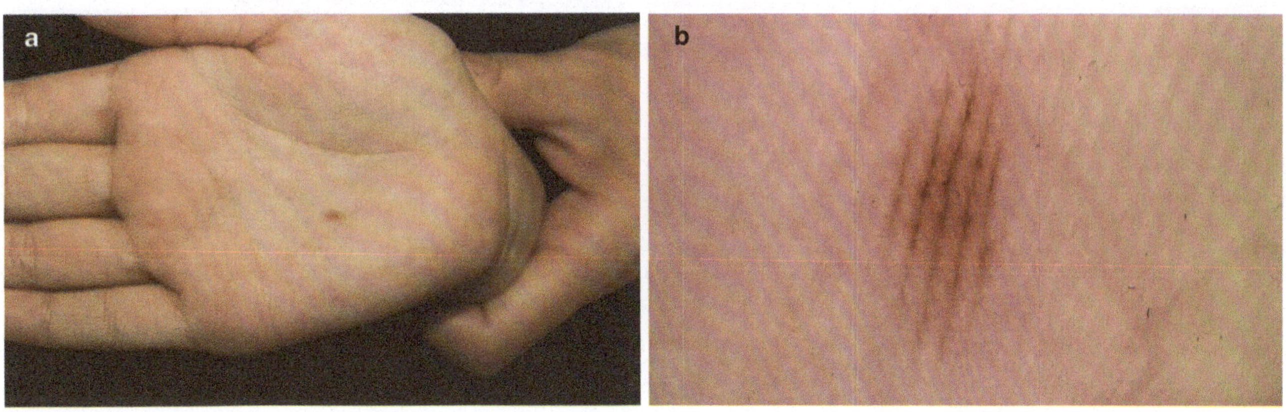

Fig. 5.15 Clinical and dermoscopic images of a junctional nevus (2). (**a**) A black patch on the right palm. (**b**) Dermoscopy shows a typical parallel furrow pattern (×30)

sion, may have a pedicle, and often has hair on the surface. Pathologically, nevus cells may be arranged in nests or cords in the dermis. The nests in the superficial dermis often contain a moderate amount of melanin, while the cells in the deep dermis are spindle-like and arranged in bundles but lack melanin.

> **Tip**
> Sometimes an intradermal nevus is difficult to distinguish from seborrheic keratosis, and the wobble test can be performed. The ability to compress the lesion and sway it back and forth under dermoscopy is indicative of an intradermal nevus.

The dermoscopic manifestations of intradermal nevi are as follows:

(i) A pale brown homogeneous pattern, occasionally as a globular pattern (Figs. 5.17 and 5.18).
(ii) Hypopigmented or nonpigmented nevi are characterized by a vascular structure, with the comma-shaped vessels being the most common type (Fig. 5.19).

5.2.4 Congenital Melanocytic Nevi

Congenital melanocytic nevi (CMN) are found at birth and vary in size, ranging from a few millimeters to larger, with some CMN affecting the entire back, neck, scalp, or even an entire limb. A CMN can gradually grow with age. CMN with

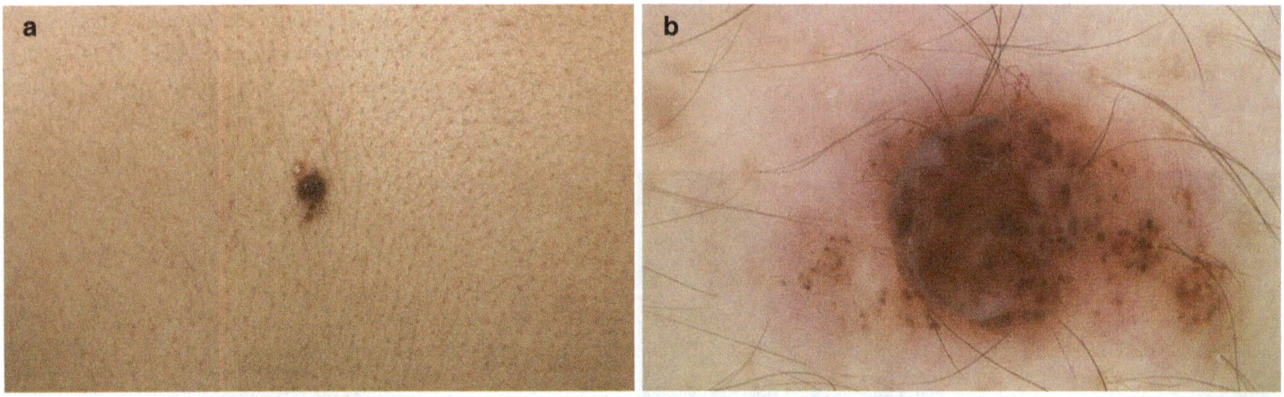

Fig. 5.16 Clinical and dermoscopic images of a compound nevus. (**a**) A dark patch on the back, with a papule in the center. (**b**) Dermoscopy shows a globular pattern on a brown background, with scattered globules and brown spots at the periphery. This is one of the typical patterns of benign nevi, with hairs in the center (×30)

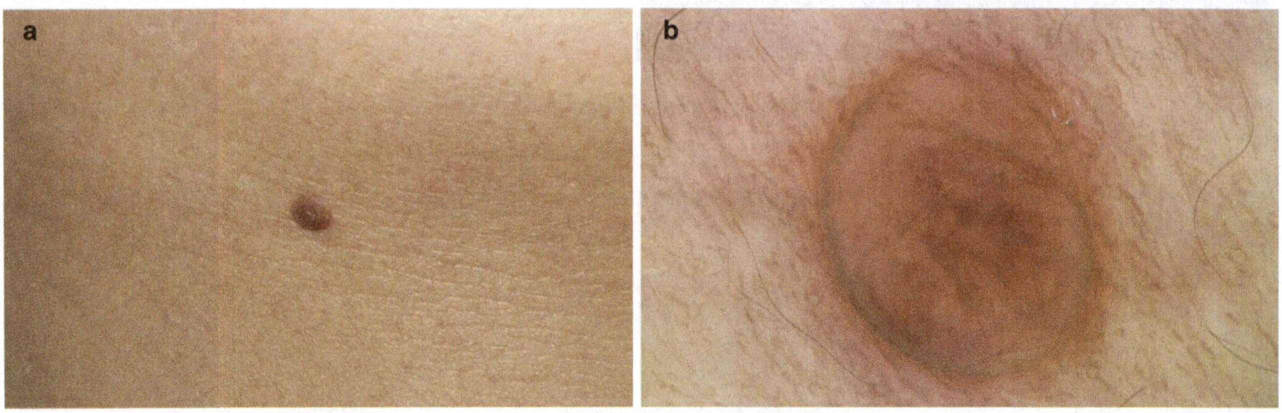

Fig. 5.17 Clinical and dermoscopic images of an intradermal nevus (1). (**a**) A brown papule with a broad base on the abdomen. (**b**) Dermoscopy shows a pale brown homogeneous pattern, and the lesion can be compressed and swayed, suggesting an intradermal nevus (×30)

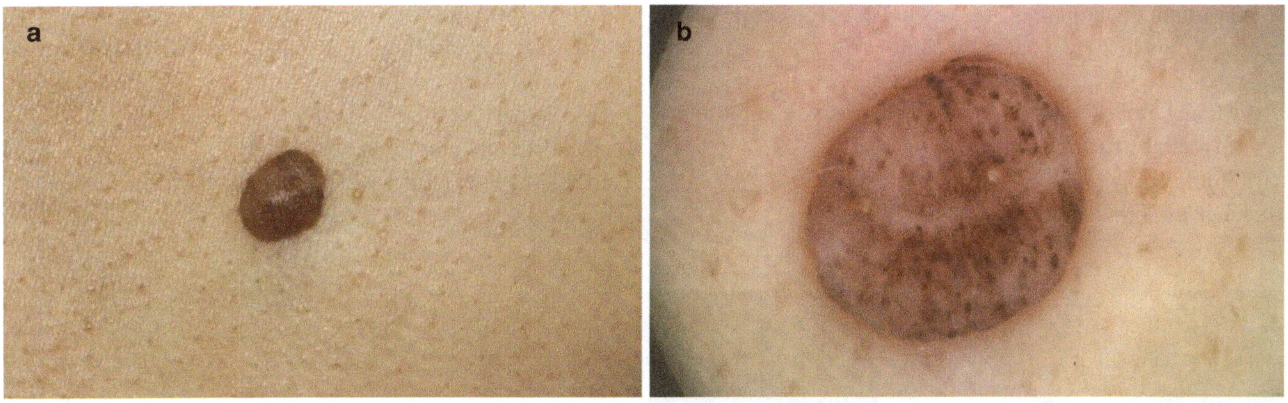

Fig. 5.18 Clinical and dermoscopic images of an intradermal nevus (2). (**a**) A brown papule on the chest. (**b**) A globular pattern on a pale brown background is seen under dermoscopy (×20)

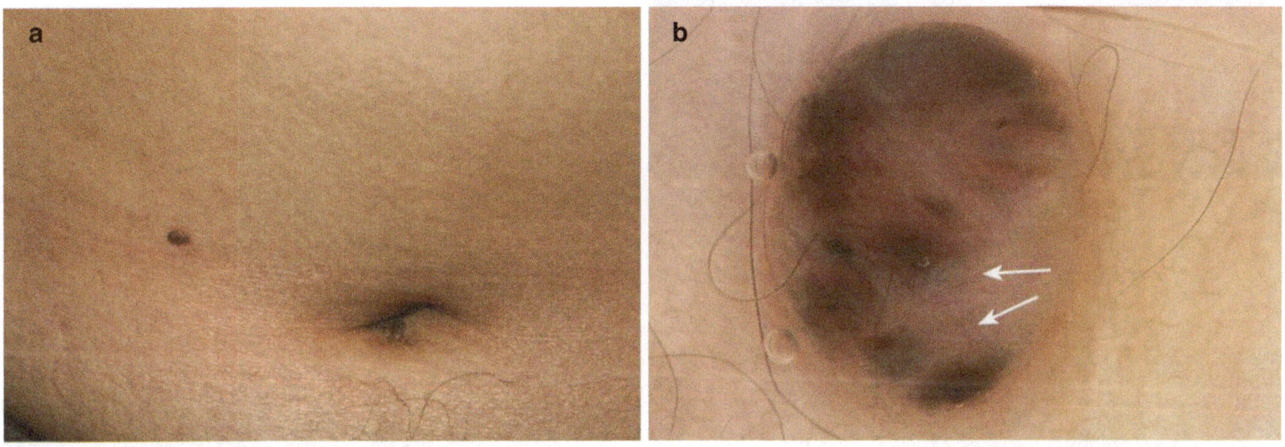

Fig. 5.19 Clinical and dermoscopic images of an intradermal nevus (3). (**a**) A brown papule on the abdomen. (**b**) Dermoscopy shows pale brown and dark-brown homogeneous patterns, with scattered comma-shaped vessels (white arrow, ×30)

folds and a verrucous appearance on the surface are called verrucous melanocytic nevi, those with hypertrichosis are called furred nevi, and those with a diameter of 20 cm or larger in adulthood are called congenital giant nevi and have a higher risk of malignancy. Pathologically, a CMN may involve the lower part of the dermal reticular layer, subcutaneous fat, fascia, or deeper tissue. The characteristic pathological manifestations of a CMN are single-celled nevus cells distributed diffusely in the middle and lower parts of the dermal reticular layer and even the subcutaneous interlobular septa, which can invade blood vessel walls, cutaneous appendages (such as hair follicles and sweat glands) and nerves. The common dermoscopic structures and patterns of CMN are described below.

Tip

Malignant melanoma developing in smaller CMN tends to appear after puberty and is more likely to originate at the dermal–epidermal junction and at the peripheral edge of a CMN. Thus, dermoscopy is an ideal instrument to evaluate smaller CMN for melanoma. In contrast, malignant melanoma occurring in large CMN develops earlier in life and frequently originates below the dermal–epidermal junction. Thus, dermoscopy has a limited role in evaluating large CMN, especially those are thick and rugous.

The common structures of CMN under dermoscopy are as follows (Figs. 5.20 and 5.21):

(i) Honeycomb-like networks, sometimes exhibiting a mycelial structure
(ii) Globules
(iii) Diffuse brown structureless areas
(iv) Milia cysts
(v) Target network with vessels located in the holes of the target network
(vi) Hypertrichosis
(vii) Perifollicular pigment changes
(viii) Blood vessels of varying morphologies

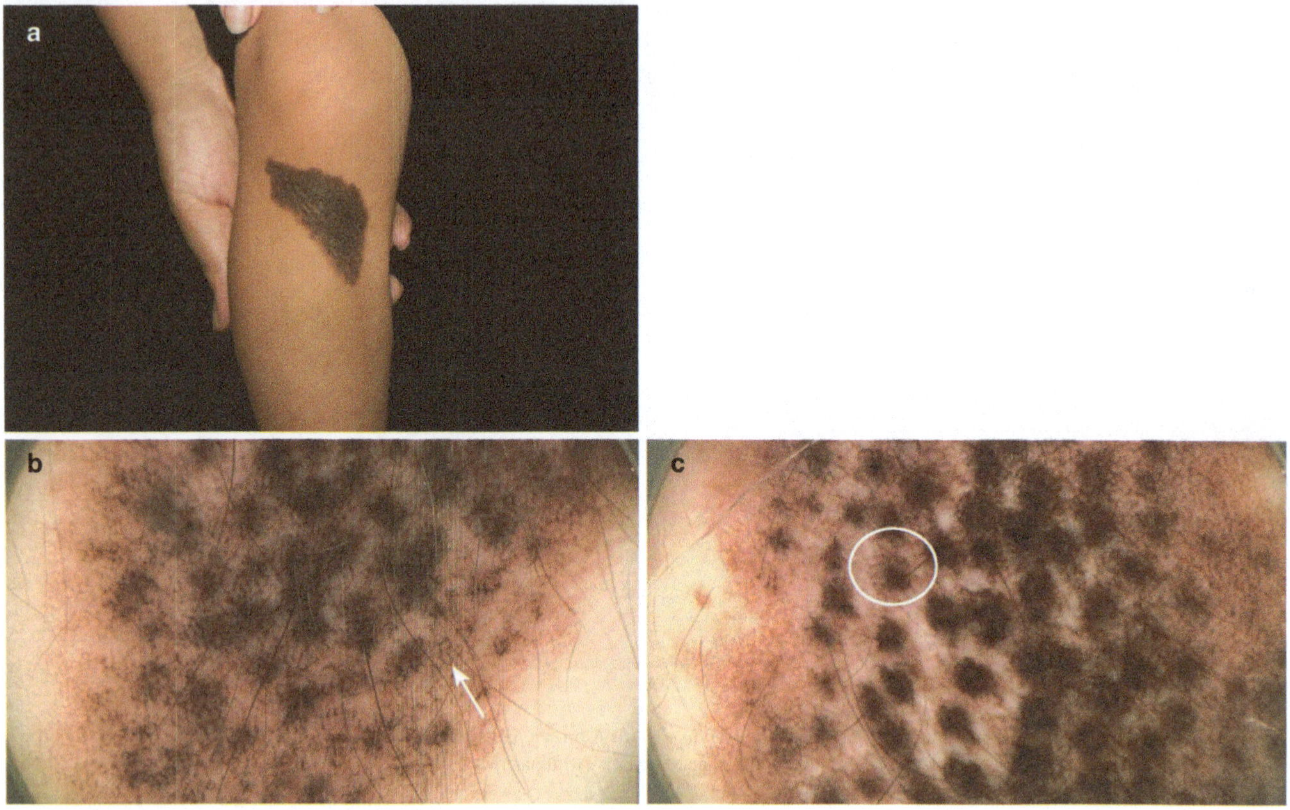

Fig. 5.20 Clinical and dermoscopic images of a congenital melanocytic nevus (1). (**a**) A brown and black patch occurring since birth on the right lower limb with hypertrichosis. (**b**) Under dermoscopy, a light brown background with brown honeycomb-like networks, mycelial structures (white arrows), brown to black globules of different sizes, and hypertrichosis can be seen (×20). (**c**) Dermoscopy shows the pigment around hair follicles (white circle) (×20)

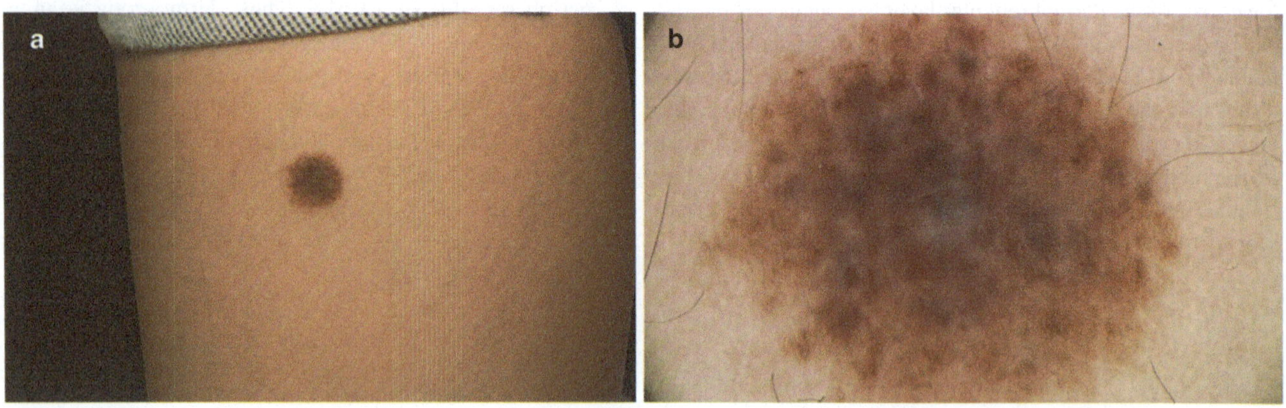

Fig. 5.21 Clinical and dermoscopic images of a congenital melanocytic nevus (2). (**a**) A brown patch on the lower limb, which was present since birth. (**b**) Dermoscopy shows a light brown background with brown honeycomb-like networks, a mycelial structure, a blue-gray structureless area and a blotch, showing a multicomponent pattern (×20)

The common dermoscopic patterns of CMN are as follows:

(i) Globular. This pattern often occurs in CMN on the head, neck, and trunk, especially in patients aged less than 12 years.
(ii) Reticular. This pattern is common in the CMN on the extremities, especially in patients aged more than 12 years.
(iii) Peripheral reticular with central globules (Fig. 5.22).
(iv) Homogeneous brown pattern (Fig. 5.23).
(v) Multicomponent pattern (Fig. 5.24).

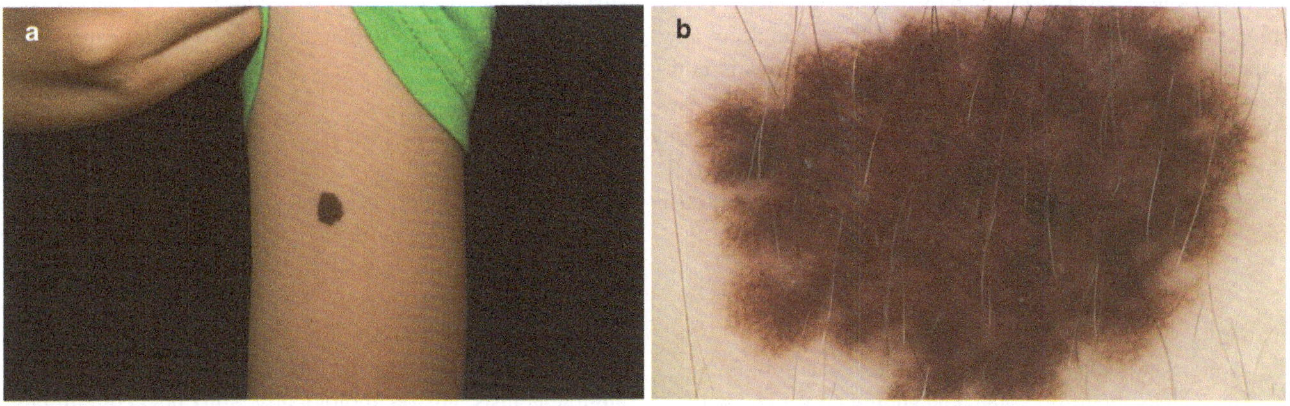

Fig. 5.22 Clinical and dermoscopic manifestations of a congenital melanocytic nevus (3). (**a**) A brown patch on the upper limb since birth. (**b**) Dermoscopy shows a brown background with scattered globules in the center and peripheral networks (×30)

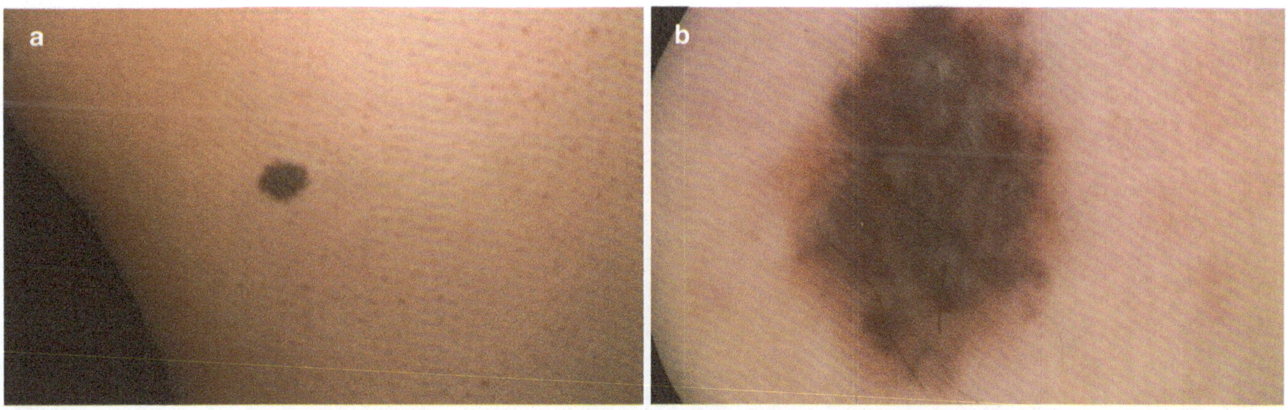

Fig. 5.23 Clinical and dermoscopic manifestations of the homogeneous brown pattern of a congenital melanocytic nevus. (**a**) A brown patch on the lower limb since birth. (**b**) Dermoscopy shows diffuse brown structureless areas and blue-gray structureless areas (×20)

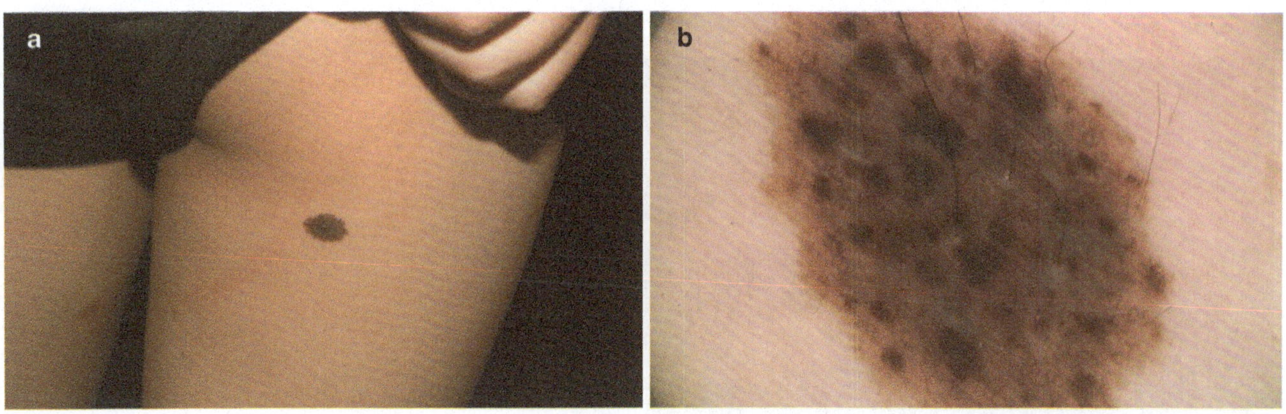

Fig. 5.24 Clinical and dermoscopic manifestations of the multicomponent pattern of a congenital melanocytic nevus. (**a**) Yellow-brown plaques on the flexural aspect of the right thigh since birth. (**b**) Dermoscopy shows dots/globules and homogeneous dark-brown pigmentation on a tan reticular background (×20)

5.2.5 Blue Nevi

A blue nevus is a benign tumor originating from melanocytes in the dermis. A blue nevus is often acquired and usually occurs in children or adolescents. Blue nevi can be divided into common blue nevi, cellular blue nevi, and malignant blue nevi (which can originate from cellular blue nevi, Ota's nevi, Ito's nevi, etc.). A blue nevus is a well-defined, blue or blue-gray, blue-black hemispheric papule that can occur anywhere. Histopathologically, a common blue nevus is composed of elongated, dendritic melanocytes with long axes parallel to the epidermis, mostly located in the upper and middle dermis. Cellular blue nevi are hypertrophic spindle melanocytes that lack melanin granules and are distributed in nests or bundles.

Tip
A metastatic malignant melanoma lesion can mimic a blue nevus; therefore, blue nevi should be viewed with caution.

The common dermoscopic manifestations of blue nevi are as follows (Figs. 5.25 and 5.26):

(i) Homogeneous. Blue nevi can be blue, blue-gray, blue-brown or blue-black.
(ii) Clear boundary. The pigment can fade at the peripheral area.
(iii) White cicatricial hypopigmentation, dots/globules, vessels, streaks, or reticular structures may appear locally.

5.2.6 Spitz Nevi

A Spitz nevus (spindle cell and epithelioid cell nevus), also known as a benign juvenile melanoma, usually occurs on the cheek or ear in children and on the trunk or limbs in adults. Spitz nevi often present as isolated, pink, brown, or dark-brown papules or nodules. Spitz nevi often have a uniform color and a smooth and verrucous surface, accompanied by angiotelectasis. Histopathologically, Spitz nevi contain large epithelioid nevus cells and spindle nevus cells, often extending from the epidermis to the reticular layer of the dermis,

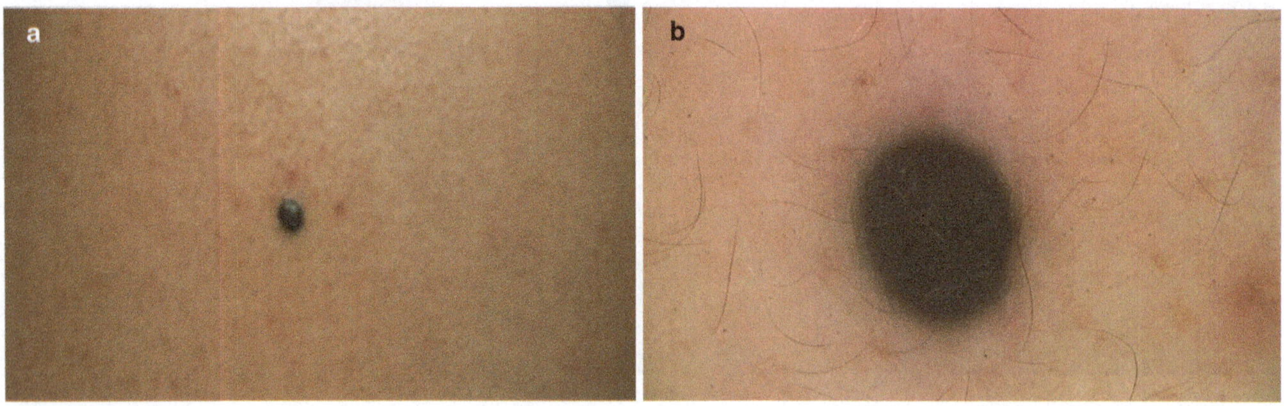

Fig. 5.25 Clinical and dermoscopic manifestations of a blue nevus (1). (**a**) A well-defined blue papule on the upper arm. (**b**) Under dermoscopy, the lesion shows a blue-black homogeneous pattern (×30)

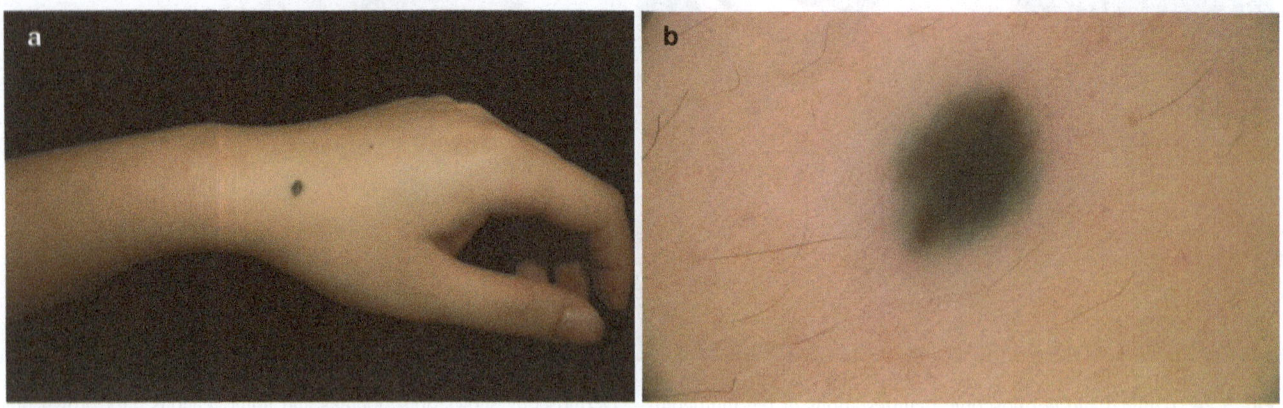

Fig. 5.26 Clinical and dermoscopic manifestations of a blue nevus (2). (**a**) An oval-shaped blue patch with a sharp boundary. (**b**) Dermoscopy shows a blue-brown homogeneous structure (×20)

with a single cell, nest or cluster distribution. Nevus cells have large nuclei, obvious nucleoli, and abundant cytoplasm. Nevus cells are long elliptical cells, with their long axis perpendicular to the epidermis. The Kamino body and maturation of the nevus cells can be seen. Sometimes there are obvious fissures between the tumor and the surrounding tissues.

The common dermoscopic manifestations of Spitz nevi are as follows (Fig. 5.27):

(i) A Spitz nevus should be considered when the following three dermoscopic patterns are present: the starburst pattern (51%), a pattern of regularly distributed dotted vessels (19%), and the globular pattern with reticular depigmentation (17%) (Fig. 5.28).
(ii) Raised or nodular Spitz nevi may present curled, hairpin or irregular linear blood vessels, which are often symmetrically distributed and surrounded by white halos or lines.
(iii) Other patterns include reticular, homogeneous, atypical/multicomponent, etc.
(iv) Other features include reticular depigmentation, superficial black networks, blue-white veils, etc.
(v) Asymmetric lesions with spitzoid features (both flat/raised and nodular) under dermoscopy should be excised to rule out melanoma.
(vi) Symmetric spitzoid nodules under dermoscopy should also be excised or closely monitored, irrespective of age, to rule out atypical Spitz tumors.
(vii) Symmetric flat spitzoid lesions under dermoscopy should be managed according to the age of the patient.

Tip
A Spitz nevus with a dermoscopic atypical/multicomponent pattern is highly suspicious for malignant melanoma, and biopsy is recommended.

5.2.7 Halo Nevi

A halo nevus, which is a nevus with a hypopigmented halo around it, most commonly occurs in children or adolescents with multiple nevi. Halo nevi can occur in patients with vitiligo. Histopathologically, halo nevi can be a junctional, compound or intradermal nevus, and fully developed halo nevi present lymphocytes infiltrating the central area.

The dermoscopic manifestations of halo nevi are as follows:

(i) More than 80% of halo nevi have the globular or homogeneous pattern in the center and a hypopigmented halo (Fig. 5.29).
(ii) The center of a halo nevus presents a pale brown or pink homogeneous area with dotted vessels after complete regression.
(iii) The dermoscopic structure of a halo nevus is stable and does not change with the reduction of the nevus and halo.

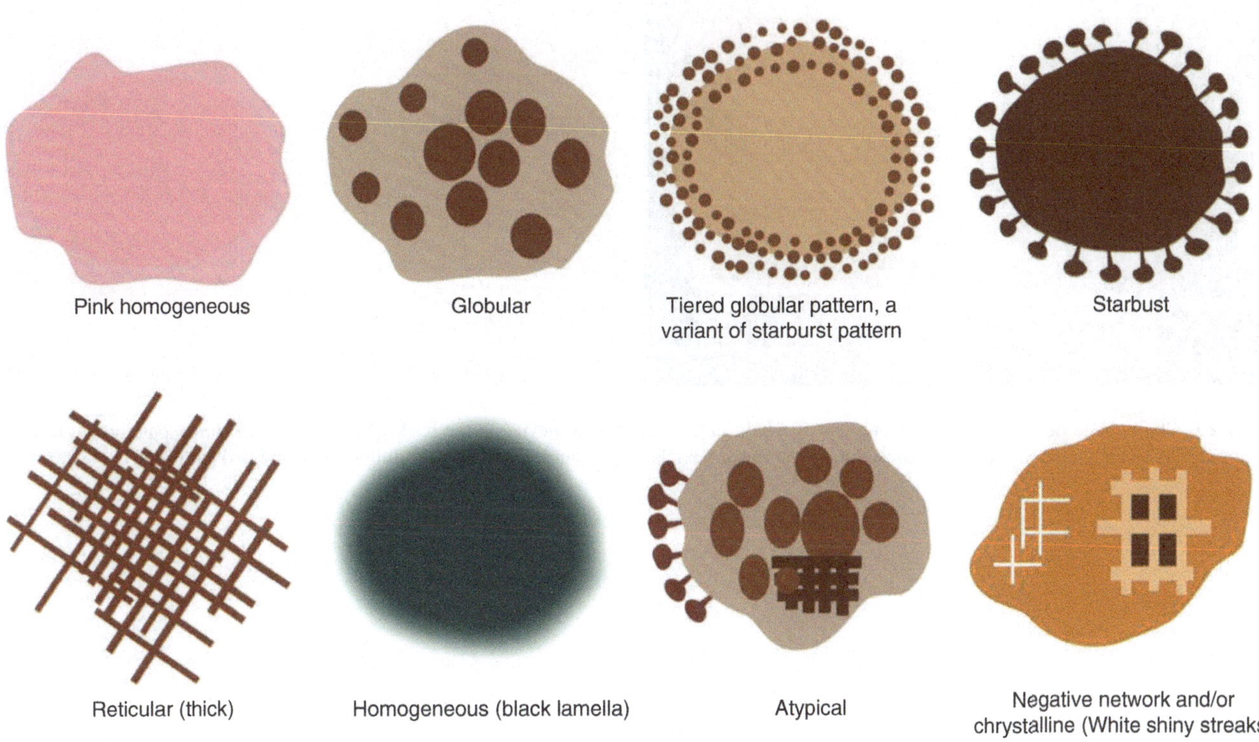

Fig. 5.27 Schematic diagrams of common dermoscopic manifestations of Spitz nevi

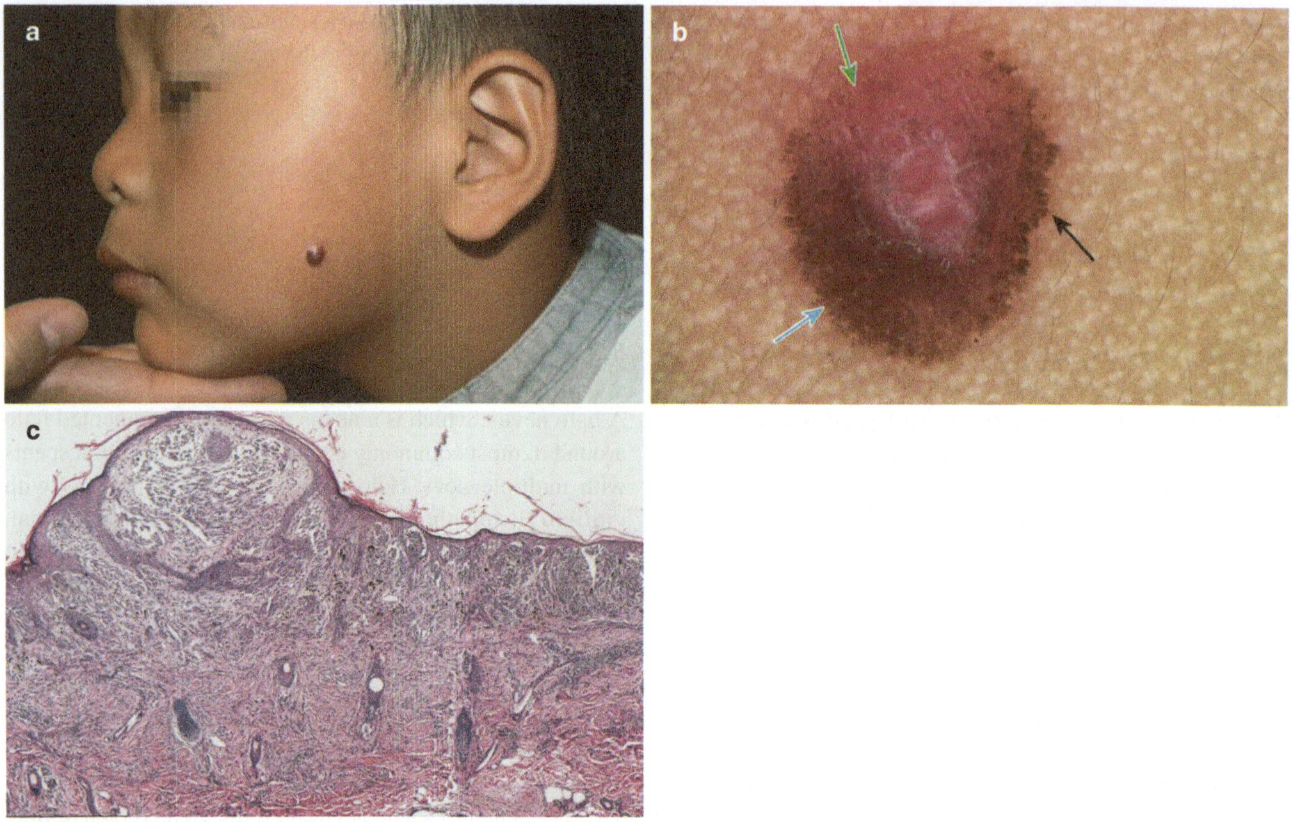

Fig. 5.28 Clinical, dermoscopic and histopathological findings of a Spitz nevus. (**a**) A reddish-brown hemispheric papule on the left cheek. (**b**) Under dermoscopy, the starburst pattern (black arrow), globular pattern (blue arrow), milk-pink homogeneous pattern (green arrow), shiny white streaks and reticular depigmentation are observed (×20). (**c**) Histopathology shows hyperkeratosis with focal parakeratosis, and nests of cells composed of spindle cells and epithelioid cells are found at the dermal–epidermal junction and in the superficial dermis. Fissures can be seen, and lymphocytes infiltrate the dermal papillary layer, which is consistent with a Spitz nevus (hematoxylin and eosin ×100)

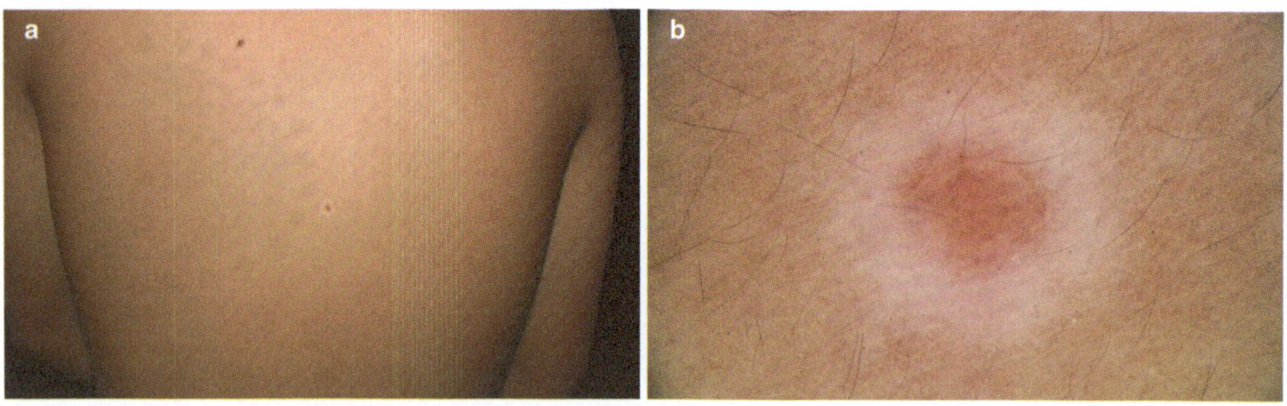

Fig. 5.29 Clinical and dermoscopic manifestations of a halo nevus . (**a**) A halo nevus on the back. (**b**) Dermoscopy shows pale brown to pink homogeneous areas, scattered brown globules, dotted and linear vessels in the center, and a surrounding hypopigmented halo (×20)

5.2.8 Nevus Spilus

Nevus spilus clinically presents as a macula or papule, with a size ranging from a needle to a rice grain, on a lighter brown patch. Various melanocyte proliferative diseases can occur on a nevus spilus, including junctional nevi, compound nevi, intradermal nevi, blue nevi, and even malignant melanoma. Nevus spilus can be unilateral, localized or distributed along Blaschko's lines.

The dermoscopic manifestations of nevus spilus are as follows (Fig. 5.30):

(i) The brown patch presents homogeneous, light brown networks.
(ii) The most common patterns for the macula or papule under dermoscopy are the reticular pattern or the reticular pattern coexisting with the homogeneous/globular pattern.

5.2.9 Dysplastic Nevi

A dysplastic/hyperalgesia nevus (DN) is a special type of nevus with a phenotype between that of a benign nevus and a malignant melanoma. Whether a DN can be an independent subtype of nevi is still a controversy. DN clinically resemble melanomas since they frequently share some or all of the clinical ABCDE morphological features of malignant melanomas (A, asymmetry; B, border irregularity; C, color variability; D, diameter >6 mm; E, evolving). The differentiation of DN from malignant melanomas is difficult. Compared with other methods, pattern analysis can better distinguish DN and malignant melanomas.

The common dermoscopic patterns of DN are as follows:

A DN may have the reticular, globular, or homogeneous pattern or a combination of these patterns.

Dermoscopic differentiation between DN and malignant melanomas can be performed as follows:

(i) Identify the overall structural pattern and whether it is a common dermoscopic pattern of a typical benign nevus.
(ii) Determine whether there are specific local features of a malignant melanoma.
(iii) Determine whether the patterns are arranged in an orderly manner.
(iv) Be highly suspicious of a malignant melanoma when a lesion has more than five colors.

5.2.10 Recurrent Melanocytic Nevi

A recurrent melanocytic nevus is also known as a pseudomelanoma due to recurrence after curetting, excision or laser treatment. A recurrent melanocytic nevus is usually confined to the scarred area of a surgically excised nevus and appears within 6 months after surgery without special histological changes. A recurrent melanocytic nevus should be distinguished from a recurrent atypical nevus, which has significant cellular atypia.

> **Tip**
> In cases with lesions beyond the surgical scar, surgical excision is recommended. Otherwise, the resection of the recurrent nevus is not necessary.

Reactive pigmentation may occur after the removal of a pigmented nevus. Dermoscopy is of great significance in distinguishing a recurrent nevus from a recurrent malignant melanoma and reactive pigmentation.

The dermoscopic manifestations of recurrent melanocytic nevi are as follows (Fig. 5.31):

(i) Globular pattern and nonhomogeneous pigmentation appearing on a scar.
(ii) Radial lines, symmetry, and an eccentric growth pattern.

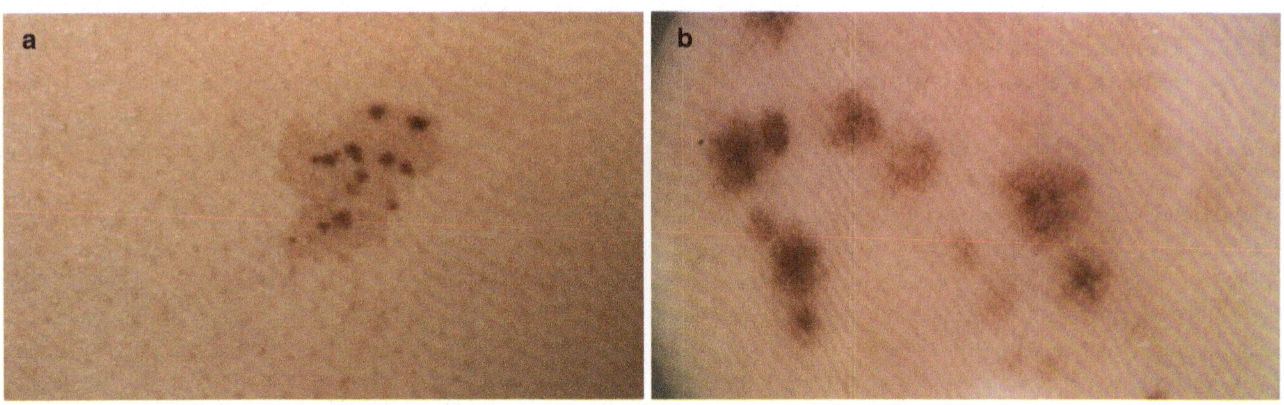

Fig. 5.30 Clinical and dermoscopic manifestations of nevus spilus. (**a**) Nevus spilus on the left lower limb. (**b**) Dermoscopy shows multiple dark-brown networks with central dark pigmentation on a light brown pigmentated patch (×20)

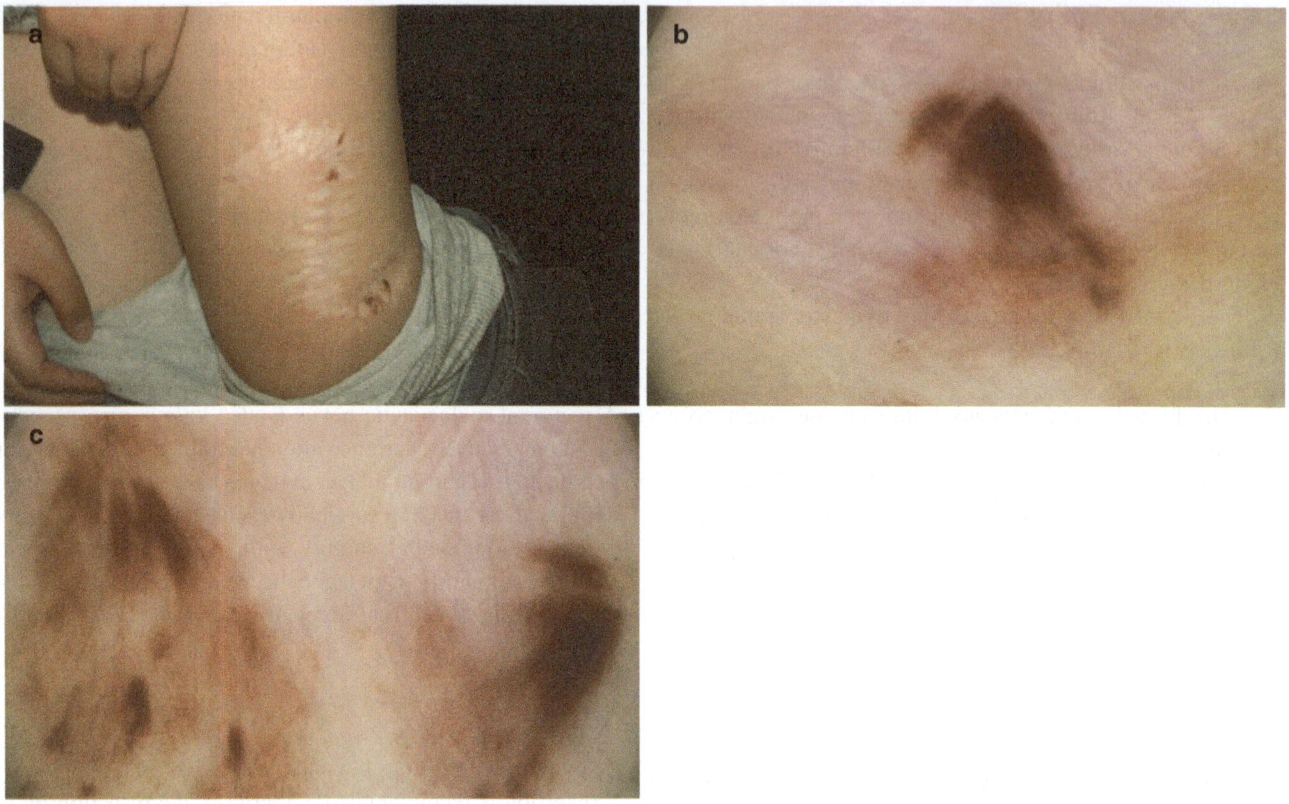

Fig. 5.31 Clinical and dermoscopic manifestations of a recurrent nevus. (**a**) Multiple brown patches on the surgical scar on the left thigh. (**b**) Dermoscopy shows light brown to dark-brown nonhomogeneous pigmentation area with radial streaks on a pink homogeneous background (×20). (**c**) The reticular pattern, homogeneous pattern and radial streaming on the white scar area (×20)

The dermoscopic manifestations of recurrent malignant melanomas are as follows:

Circles (especially on the face and neck); eccentric pigmentation at the edges of the lesion; a chaotic, discontinuous growth pattern; and pigmentation beyond the scar boundaries.

The dermoscopic manifestations of reactive pigmentation are as follows:

A regular pigment network with fine continuous streaks or wide homogeneous streaks.

5.3 Dermoscopic Features of Pigmented Nevi in Special Locations

5.3.1 Facial Melanocytic Nevi

Due to epidermal thinning on the facial skin and the presence of adnexal openings, facial melanocytic nevi often show the pseudonetwork pattern under dermoscopy, which presents as pigmentation around the adnexal openings that are devoid of any pigment (Fig. 5.32).

The common dermoscopic patterns of facial nevi are as follows:

(i) Junctional nevi often show a pseudonetwork pattern.
(ii) Compound nevi and intradermal nevi on the face share the same dermoscopic characteristics as those on the trunk and limbs (Fig. 5.32).

5.3.2 Acral Melanocytic Nevi

Because of the unique anatomical characteristics of palmar and plantar skin, pigmented lesions often appear in a parallel pattern. The anatomical characteristics of palmar and plantar skin are as follows:

(i) Thick stratum corneum: melanin in the superficial dermis appears bluish rather than brown in color in palmar and plantar skin owing to the physical property of light, namely, the Tyndall effect.
(ii) Furrows (sulcus superficialis) and ridges (crista superficialis) (Fig. 5.33): these two structures are distinguished by the observations that ridges are wider than furrows and eccrine ducts open on the surface of ridges. Benign nevi often present the parallel furrow pattern, while malignant melanoma shows the parallel ridge pattern.

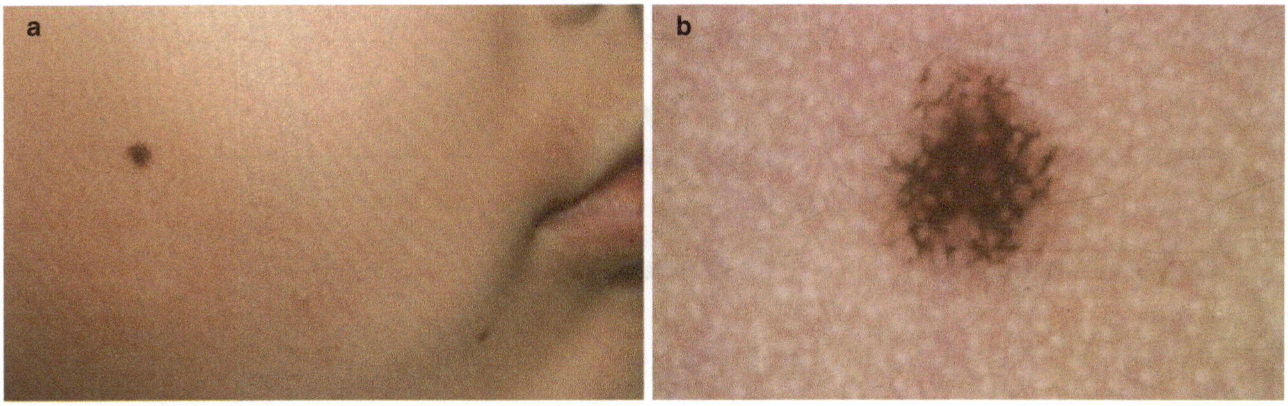

Fig. 5.32 Clinical and dermoscopic manifestations of the pseudonetwork pattern of a facial lesion. (**a**) A facial melanocytic nevus in a child. (**b**) Dermoscopy shows brown pigmentation around the nonpigmented follicular openings, resulting in a pseudonetwork pattern (×30)

Fig. 5.33 Schematic diagram of the anatomy of volar skin. (Copyright © 2012 From An Atlas of Dermoscopy by Ashfaq A Marghoob, Josep Malvehy, and Ralph P. Braun. Reproduced by permission of Taylor and Francis Group, LLC, a division of Informa plc.)

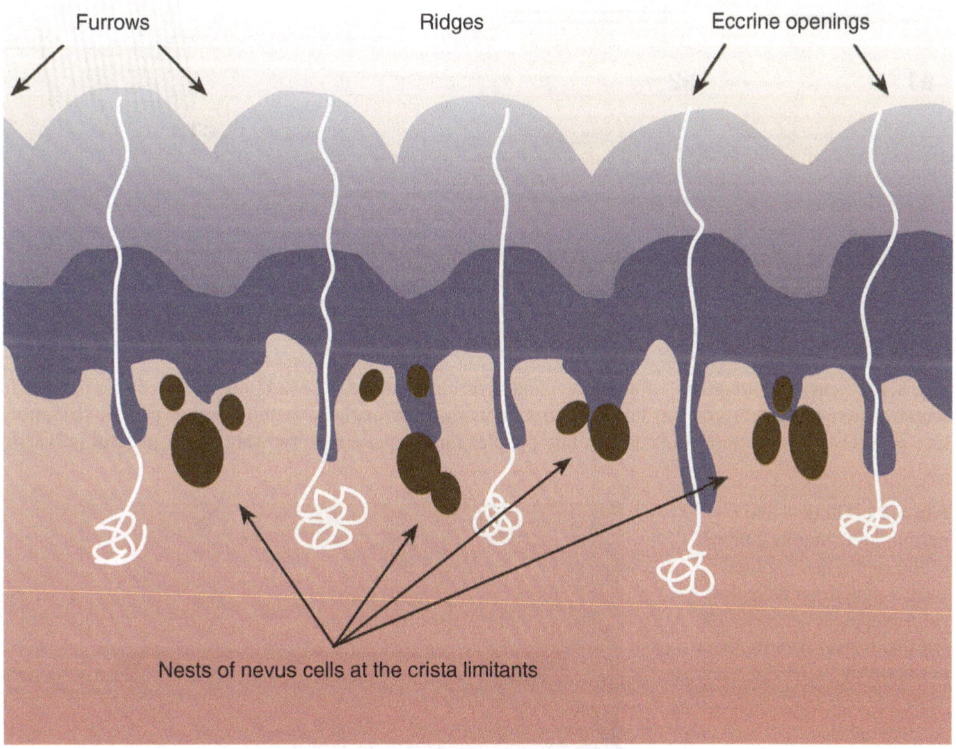

(iii) Absence of follicular openings: eccrine openings, located in the center of ridges, appear as regularly spaced small white dots on ridges under dermoscopy.

The classic dermoscopic patterns of acral melanocytic nevi (schematic diagram of the classic dermoscopic mode and its subtypes are shown in Fig. 5.34):

(i) Parallel furrow pattern: This pattern is common on the weight-bearing parts of the palms and soles. There are four parallel furrow pattern subtypes, consisting of the single-line variant (Fig. 5.35), the double-line variant (Fig. 5.36), the single-dotted-line variant (Fig. 5.37), and the double-dotted-line variant (Fig. 5.38).

(ii) Lattice-like pattern (Fig. 5.39): This pattern is the most common pattern on the arch area of the sole and can also be seen on the palms. The lattice-like pattern presents the parallel furrow pattern with the addition of parallel pigmented bands that crossover the ridges from one furrow to the next, similar to the rungs of a ladder.

(iii) Fibrillar pattern: This pattern consists of dense fibrillar pigmentation composed of multiple thin parallel lines that cross both furrows and ridges. This pattern results from the effects of intermittent/constant horizontal

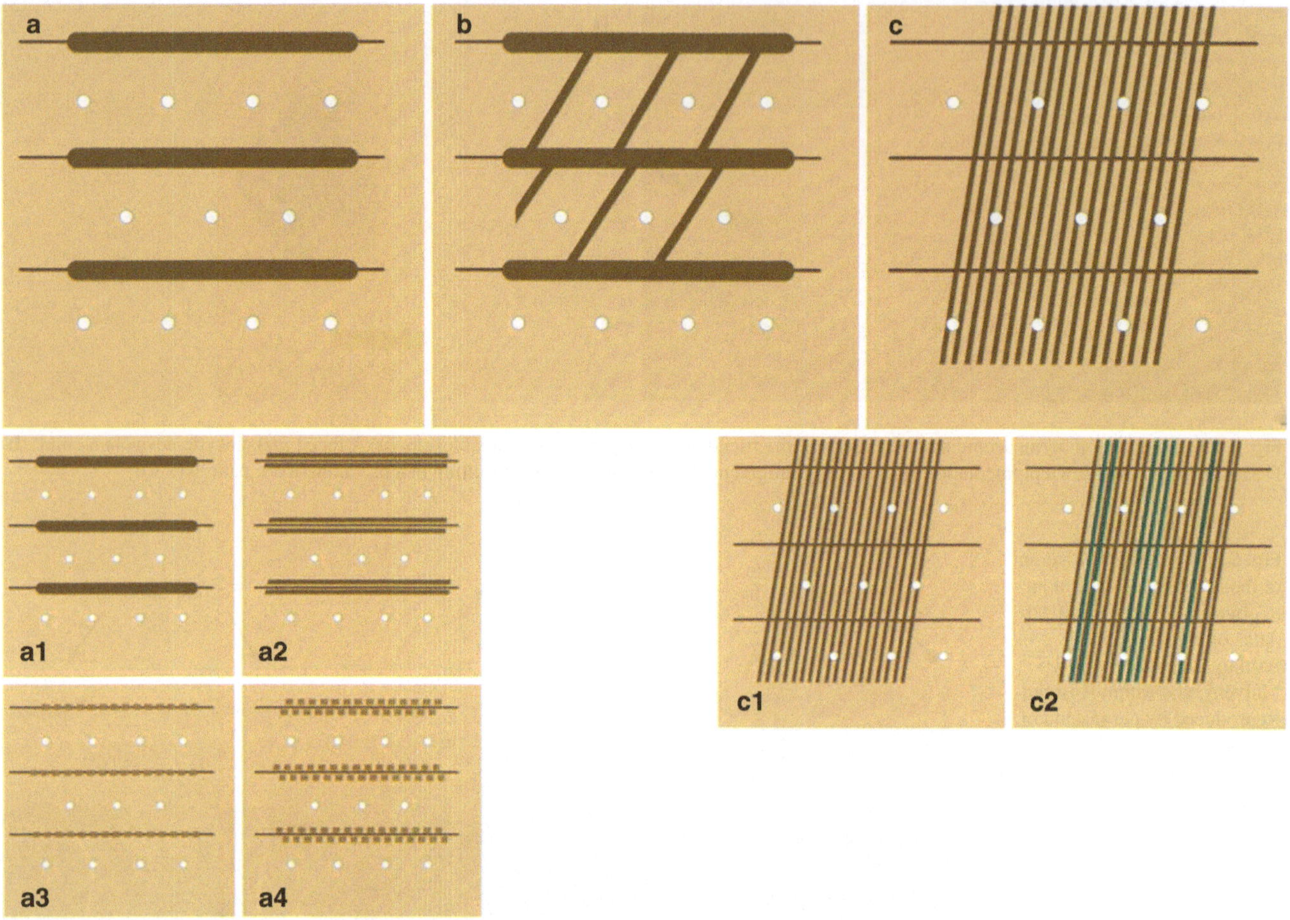

Fig. 5.34 Schematic diagrams of acral nevi and their classic dermoscopic patterns and subtypes. (**a**) Parallel furrow pattern: (**a1**) single-line parallel furrow pattern; (**a2**) double-line parallel furrow pattern; (**a3**) single-dotted-line parallel furrow pattern; (**a4**) double-dotted-line parallel furrow pattern. (**b**) Lattice pattern. (**c**) Fibrillar pattern: (**c1**) fine typical fibrillar pattern; (**c2**) atypical fibrillar pattern

Fig. 5.35 Clinical and dermoscopic manifestations of the single-line parallel furrow pattern on the palm. (**a**) A benign acral nevus. (**b**) Parallel furrow pattern under dermoscopy (×30)

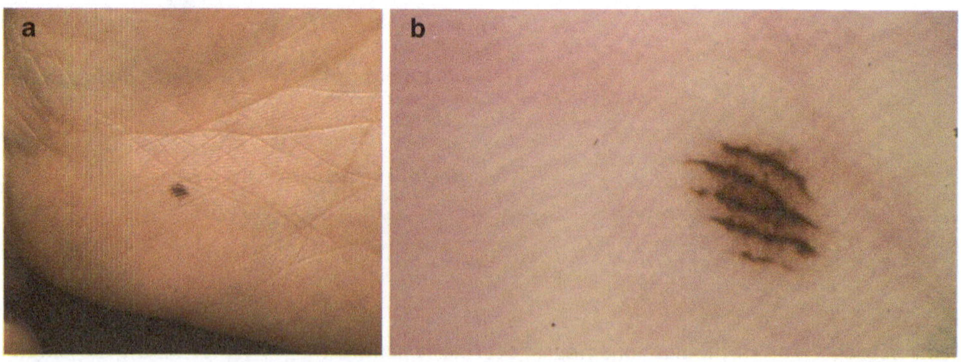

Fig. 5.36 Clinical and dermoscopic manifestations of the double-line-furrow pattern. (**a**) A benign acral nevus on the sole. (**b**) Dermoscopy shows a double-line parallel furrow pattern (×30)

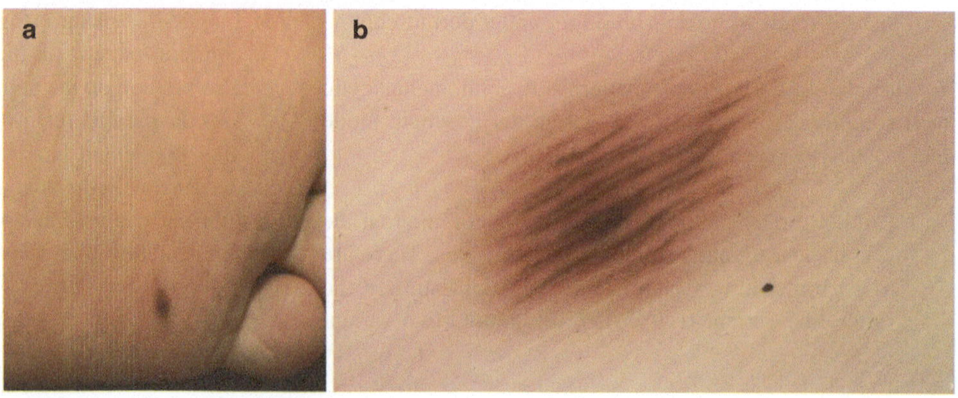

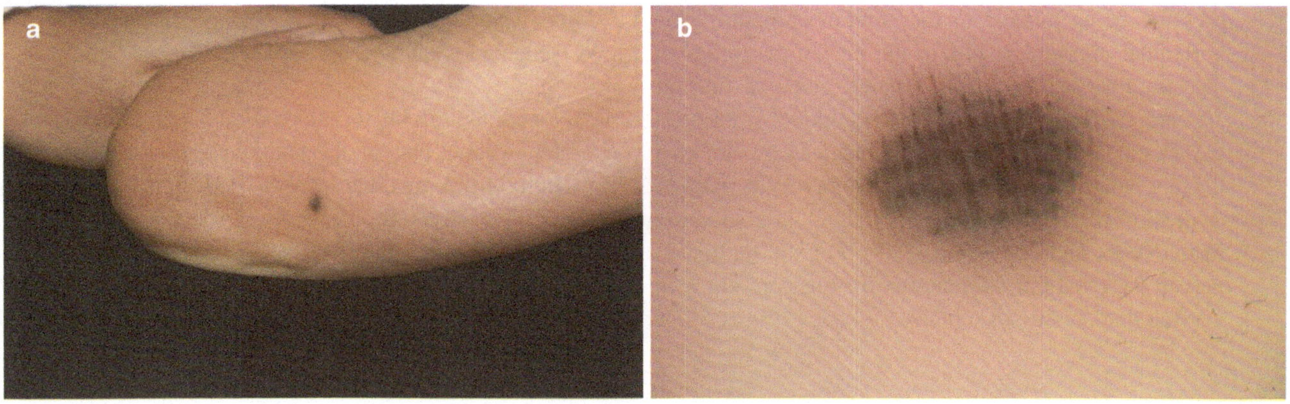

Fig. 5.37 Clinical and dermoscopic manifestations of the single-dotted-line parallel furrow pattern. (**a**) A benign acral nevus on the sole. (**b**) Dermoscopy shows a single-dotted-line parallel furrow pattern (×30)

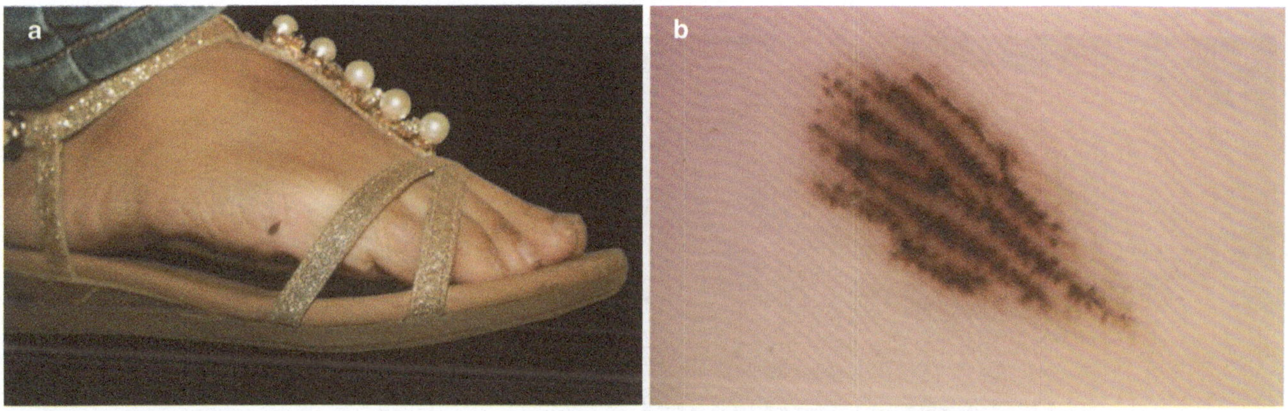

Fig. 5.38 Clinical and dermoscopic manifestations of the double-dotted-line parallel furrow pattern. (**a**) A benign acral nevus on the lateral margin of the sole. (**b**) Dermoscopy shows a double-dotted-line parallel furrow pattern (×30)

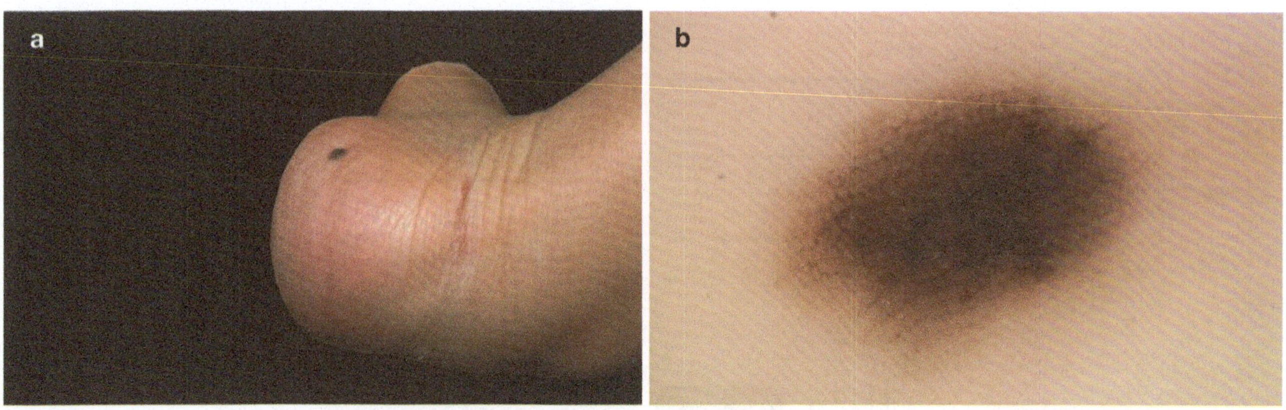

Fig. 5.39 Clinical and dermoscopic manifestations of the lattice-like pattern. (**a**) A benign acral nevus on the heel. (**b**) Dermoscopy shows a lattice-like pattern (×30)

pressure being applied to the stratum corneum. This horizontal pressure results in the melanin columns in the stratum corneum being slanted, giving a fibrillar appearance. The fibrillar pattern is commonly seen on the weight-bearing parts of the sole. There are two fibrillar pattern subtypes. For the benign fibrillar pattern (typical fibrillar pattern), the lines show little variation in thickness and color (Fig. 5.40). For the malignant variant (atypical fibrillar pattern), the lines present with varying thicknesses and colors.

Tip
In fact, an acral nevus on the palms with the atypical fibrillar pattern should be viewed with suspicion.

Other benign patterns of acral melanocytic nevi are as follows (schematic diagrams are shown in Fig. 5.41):

(i) Nonparallel-globular pattern (Fig. 5.42).
(ii) Homogenous pattern: this pattern consists of a uniformly tan-to-brown area that involves both furrows and ridges and is devoid of any other structures or patterns (Fig. 5.43).
(iii) Reticular pattern without association with the furrows and ridges (Fig. 5.44).
(iv) Peas in a pod pattern: this pattern refers to the parallel furrow pattern together with dots/globules on the ridges (Fig. 5.45).
(v) Nontypical patterns (Fig. 5.46): these patterns do not have any features of the benign patterns and do not have any acro-lentiginous-melanoma-specific patterns.

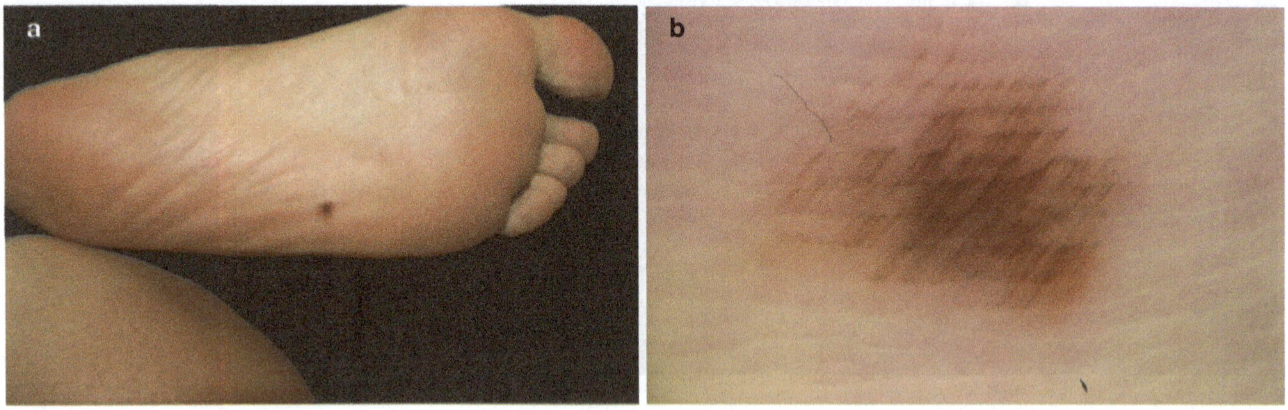

Fig. 5.40 Clinical and dermoscopic manifestations of the fibrillar pattern. (**a**) A benign acral nevus on the sole. (**b**) Dermoscopy shows the fibrillar pattern (×30)

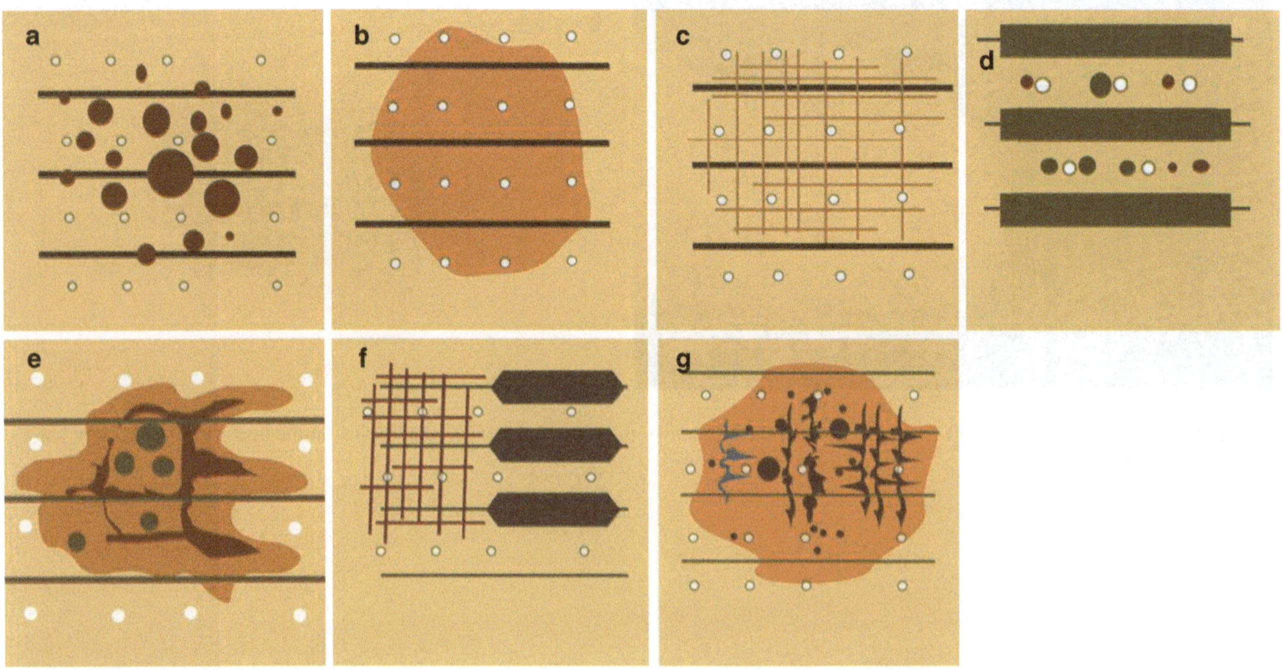

Fig. 5.41 Schematic diagrams of other benign patterns of acral melanocytic nevi under dermoscopy. (**a**) Globular pattern that is not associated with the parallel pattern. (**b**) The homogenous pattern. (**c**) The reticular pattern that is not associated with skin markings. (**d**) The peas in a pod pattern. (**e, g**) Atypical patterns. (**f**) The transition pattern

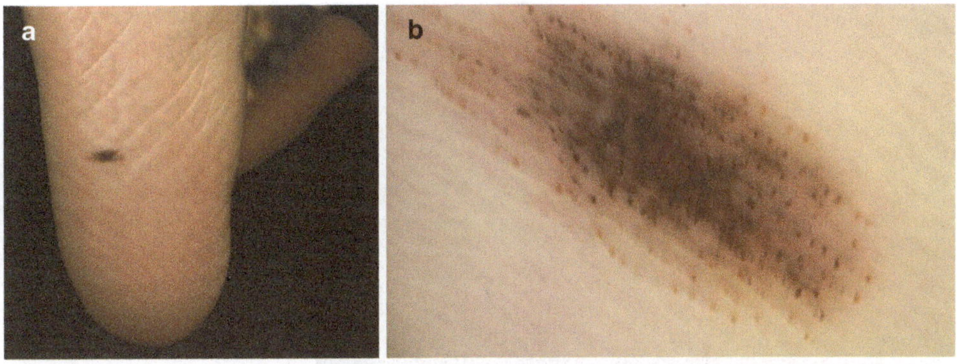

Fig. 5.42 Clinical and dermoscopic manifestations of the globular pattern in an acral nevus. (**a**) A benign acral nevus on the sole. (**b**) Dermoscopy shows the globular pattern without associations with the parallel pattern (×50)

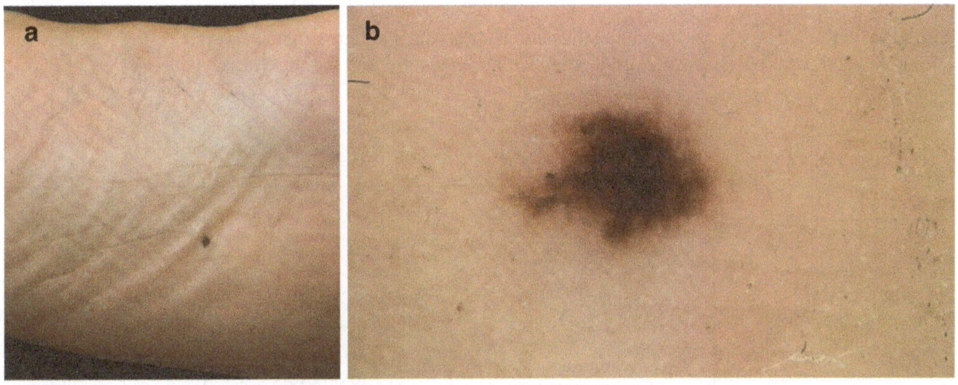

Fig. 5.43 Clinical and dermoscopic manifestations of the homogenous pattern in an acral nevus. (**a**) A benign acral nevus on the sole. (**b**) Dermoscopy shows a homogenous pattern, and uninvolved eccrine openings on the ridges can be seen (×30)

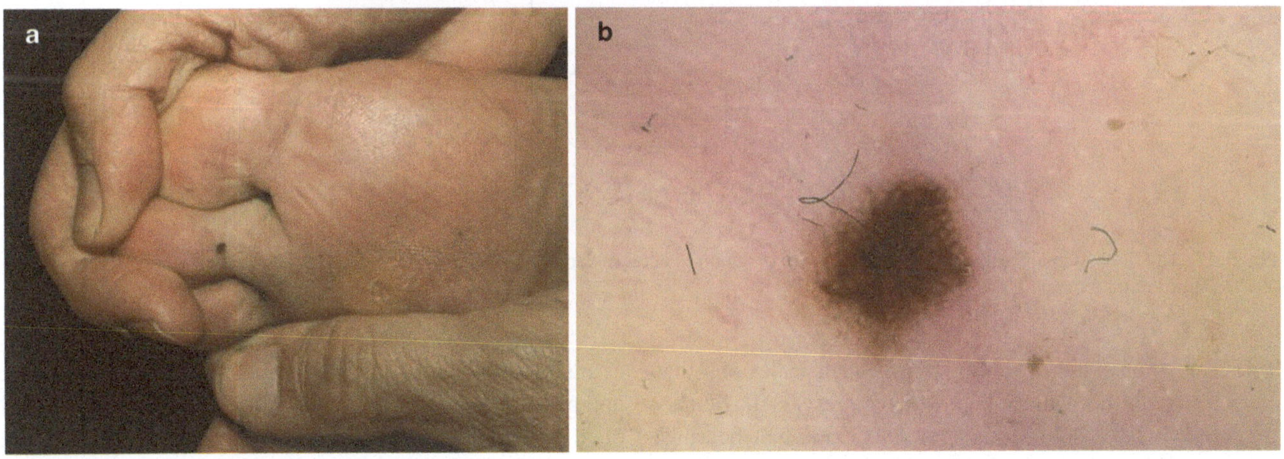

Fig. 5.44 Clinical and dermoscopic manifestations of the reticular pattern in an acral nevus. (**a**) A benign acral nevus on the sole. (**b**) Dermoscopy shows the reticular pattern that is not associated with skin markings (×30)

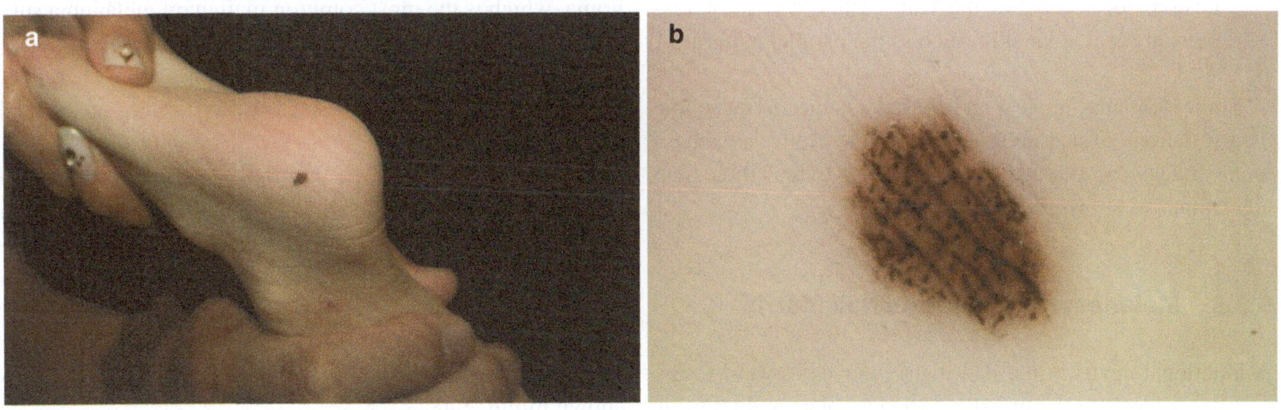

Fig. 5.45 Clinical and dermoscopic manifestations of the "peas in a pod" pattern in an acral nevus. (**a**) A benign acral nevus on the heel. (**b**) Dermoscopy shows the peas in a pod pattern (×30)

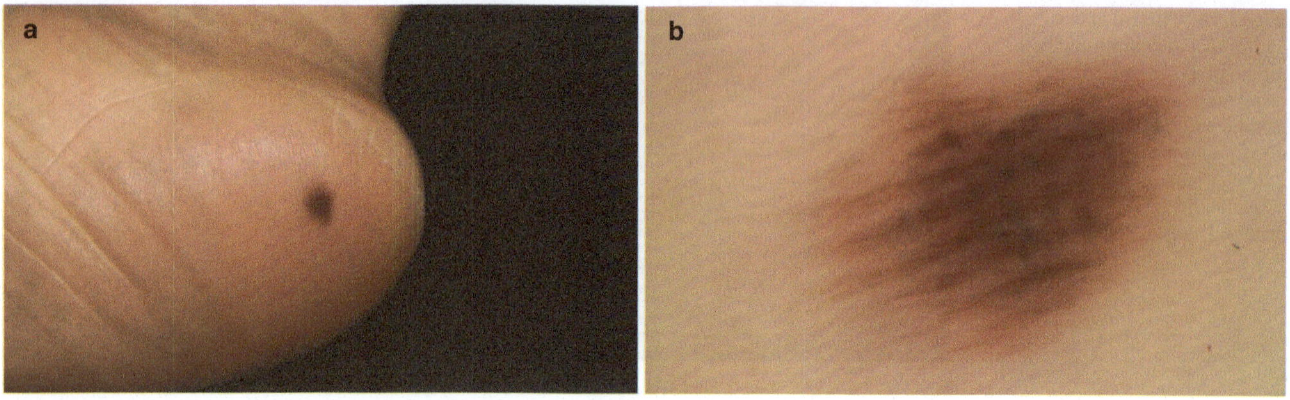

Fig. 5.46 Clinical and dermoscopic manifestations of atypical patterns in an acral nevus. (**a**) A benign acral nevus on the heel. (**b**) Dermoscopy shows atypical patterns, consisting of the globular, homogenous, and parallel furrow patterns (×30)

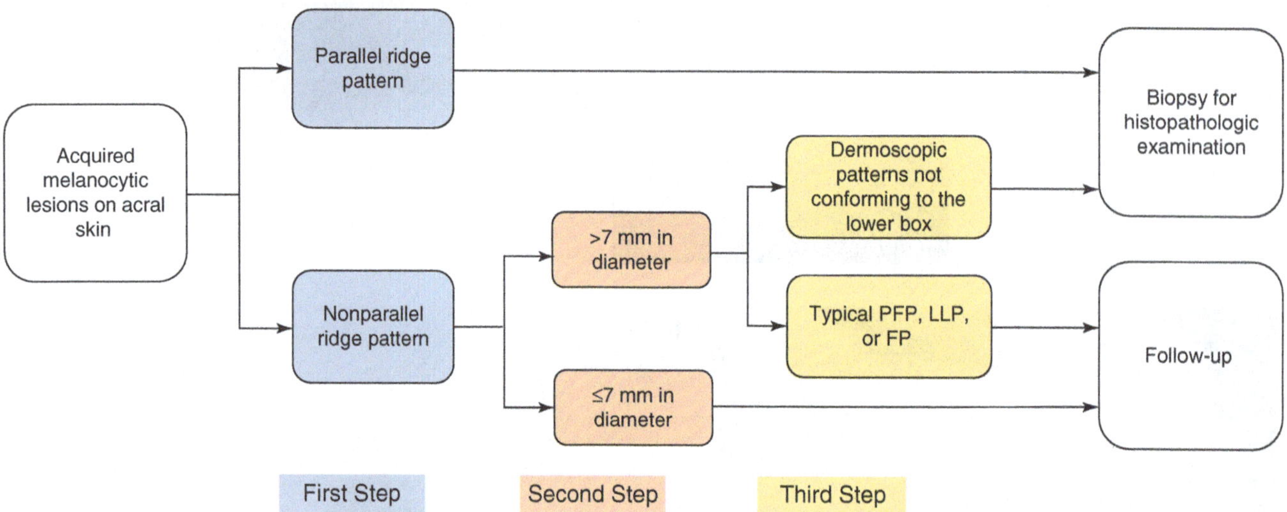

Fig. 5.47 The three-step algorithm for the management of acquired acral melanocytic lesions. *PFP* parallel furrow pattern, *LLP* lattice-like pattern, *FP* fibrillar pattern

(vi) Transition pattern: this pattern is seen in lesions that crossover the Wallace line, which represents the demarcation line delineating glabrous (non-hair-bearing) from nonglabrous (hair-bearing) skin. Lesions located above the Wallace line will show dermoscopic features of nonglabrous skin, such as the reticular pattern. Lesions located below the Wallace line will show features of acral volar skin, such as the parallel pattern.

Some scholars suggest that based on the dermoscopic manifestations of acquired acral nevi, the clinical management strategy can be carried out according to the "three-step algorithm," as shown in Fig. 5.47.

5.3.3 Melanocytic Nevi of the Nail Matrix

A junctional nevus in the nail matrix moves forward to the nail free edge with the growth of the nail plate and presents as a slightly elevated longitudinal dark-brown band on the nail plate. A few nail nevi may have malignant changes. Nail plate pigmentation is relatively common in black people and can be caused by minor trauma, where pigmentation is caused by the activation of melanocytes. A nail matrix nevus needs to be differentiated from an acral malignant melanoma, which is the most common malignant melanoma subtype in the Asian population and is most commonly found in the nails of the thumbs, index fingers, or big toes. Therefore, pigment bands should be closely observed if they are located in those areas.

For nail dermoscopy, an infiltration mode, which can fill the cavities, is recommended. Of note, not all nail pigmentations originate from melanocytes, such as exogenous pigmentation and subnail hemorrhage. If small pigment particles <0.1 mm in diameter are observed under dermoscopy, the lesion can be considered to be of melanocyte origin. The diagnostic procedure for melanocytic nail pigmentation is shown in Fig. 5.48.

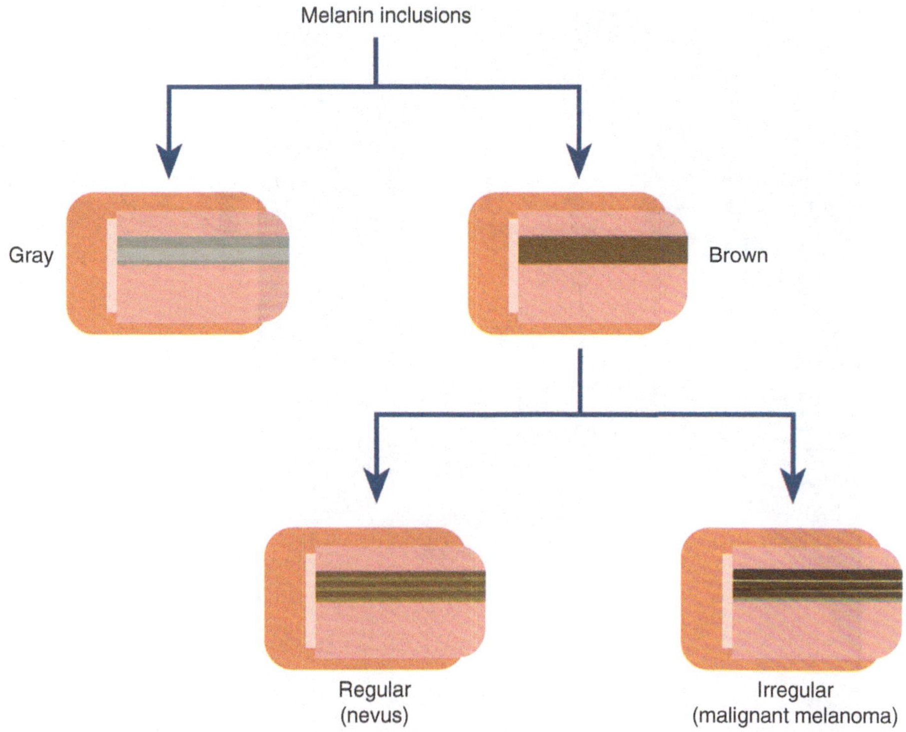

Fig. 5.48 Diagnostic procedure for melanocytic nail pigmentations. In the first step, a clinician has to determine whether the nail pigmentation has a gray or brown color. For lesions with gray color, lentigo, drug-induced pigmentation, and ethnic nail pigmentation should be considered. For lesions with brown color, clinicians need to move to the second step to determine whether the brown bands are regular (nevus) or irregular (malignant melanoma)

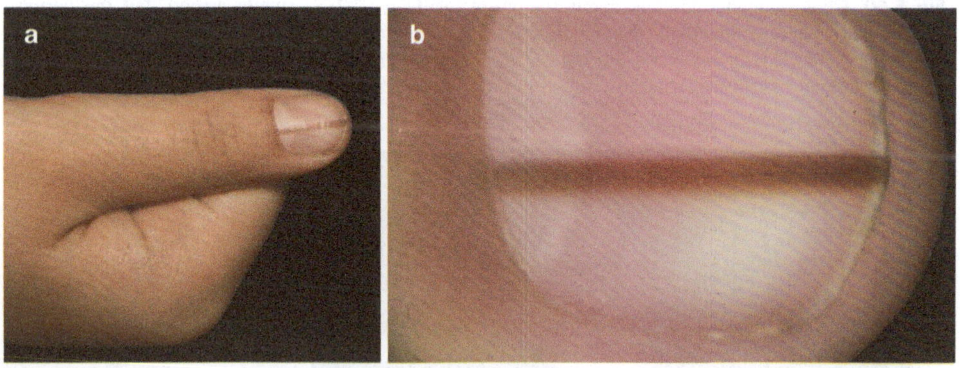

Fig. 5.49 Clinical and dermoscopic manifestations of a melanocytic nevus of the nail matrix (1). (**a**) Brown bands of a thumbnail. (**b**) Dermoscopy shows longitudinal brown parallel lines of the same width. Hutchinson's sign is negative (×20)

The dermoscopic manifestations of melanocytic nevi of the nail matrix are as follows (Figs. 5.49 and 5.50):

(i) Regular pattern: longitudinal brown or light brown parallel lines with regular gaps and width, with a uniform color.
(ii) Pseudo-Hutchinson's sign: this sign shows that the pigment of the nail matrix is visible through the translucent cuticula.
(iii) More than half of patients have pigmentation bands with the width less than 1/3 of the nail plate.

The dermoscopic features of nail malignant melanomas are as follows (Fig. 5.51):

(i) Irregular pattern: the band comprises multiple longitudinal brown to black lines with irregular and nonparallel spacing and thickness.
(ii) A rapidly growing nail matrix melanoma presents as nonparallel bands, and the band on the proximal side is wider.
(iii) In the advanced stage, nail plate atrophy or onychomadesis can be seen, which is directly caused by damage to the nail matrix due to tumor growth.
(iv) Pigmentation of the nailfold cuticle and the surrounding skin can be seen, which is known as Hutchinson's sign. If pigmentation is invisible to the naked eye but visible under dermoscopy, it is called micro-Hutchinson's sign.
(v) Pigmented bands often involve more than 2/3 of the width of the nail plate.

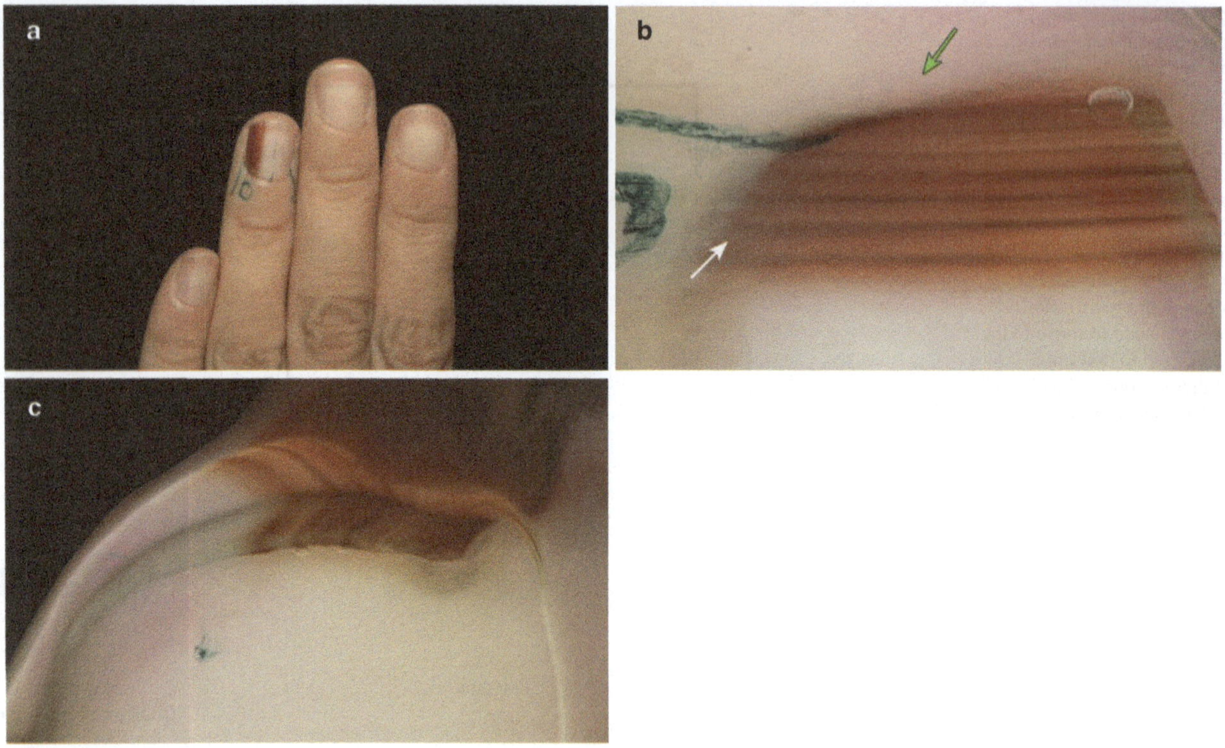

Fig. 5.50 Clinical and dermoscopic manifestations of a nail nevus (2). (**a**) Brown bands of a fingernail. (**b**) Under dermoscopy, longitudinal brown parallel lines with uniform width and gap are observed. The pigment of the nail matrix can be seen through the translucent cuticula (white arrow), but the peripheral skin has no pigmentation (green arrow), namely, pseudo-Hutchinson's sign (×30). (**c**) No pigmentation in the hyponychium under dermoscopy (×30)

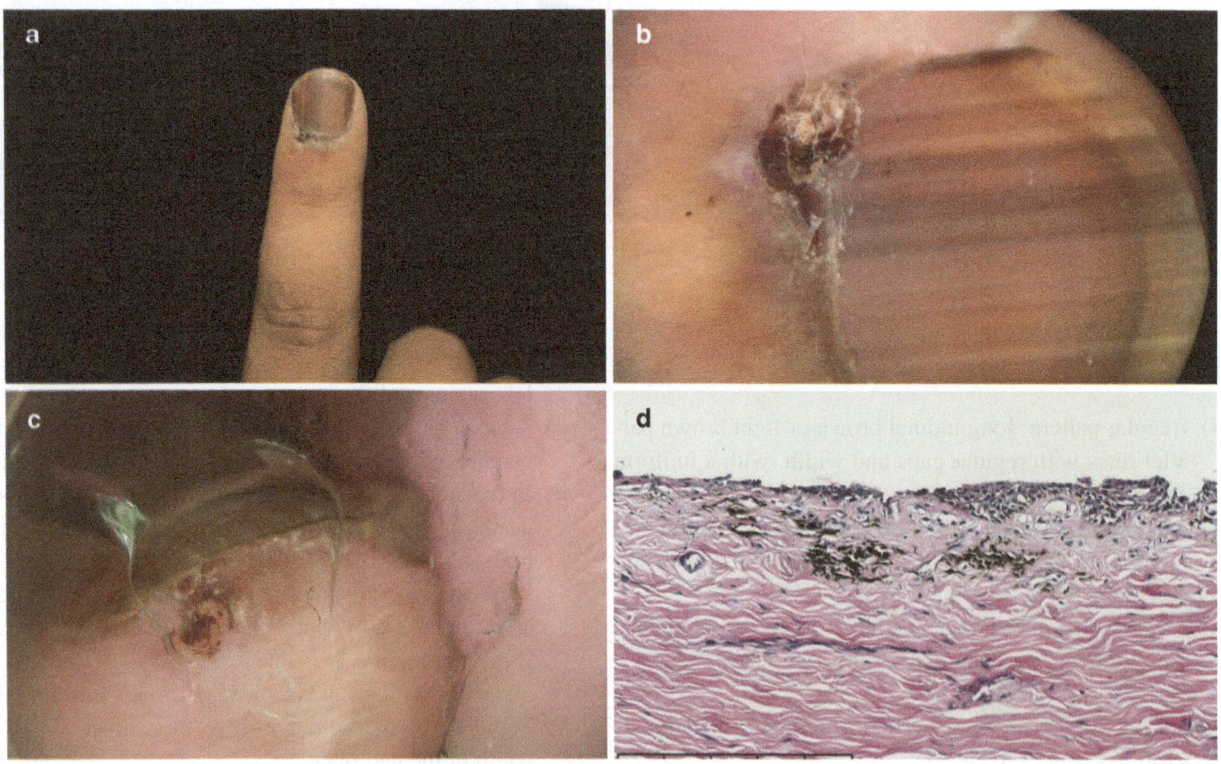

Fig. 5.51 Clinical and dermoscopic manifestations of a nail melanoma. (**a**) A black to brown pigmentation on a fingernail, with nailfold cuticle ulceration. (**b**) Dermoscopy shows ulcers; brown to black bands of the nail plate, with irregular color, spacing and width; and the pigmentation of the surrounding skin (×20). (**c**) Dermoscopy shows Hutchinson's sign (×20). (**d**) Histological examination showed small nests of cells with hyperchromatic pleomorphic nuclei consistent with a malignant melanoma (hematoxylin and eosin, ×200)

5.3.4 Benign Melanocytic Tumors of the Mucosa

Benign melanocytic tumors of the mucosa (oral cavity, vulva, etc.) are usually brown to gray. Multiple melanin spots on the lips may be associated with some systemic diseases, requiring vigilance for Peutz–Jeghers syndrome.

The dermoscopic features of benign melanocytic tumors of the mucosa are as follows (Figs. 5.52 and 5.53):

(i) The pattern is relatively symmetrical and regular.
(ii) The parallel pattern is common in small lesions.
(iii) The homogeneous pattern (structureless areas) can be seen in large lesions.
(iv) The reticular pattern and ring-like structures (including their variant types of a fish-scale-like pattern and hyphal pattern) are found.
(v) The most common color is brown or gray.

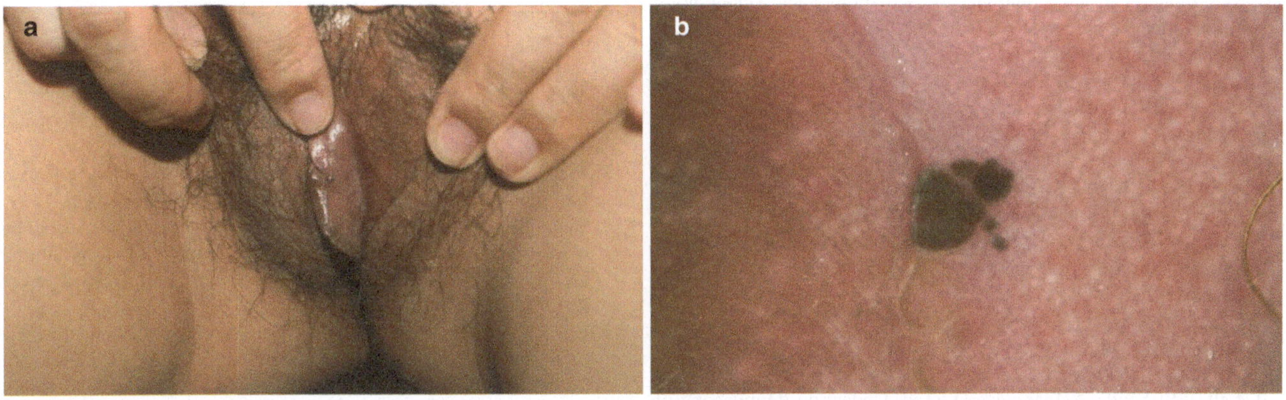

Fig. 5.52 Clinical and dermoscopic manifestations of a benign melanocytic tumor of the vulva. (**a**) Dark-brown papules of the vulva. (**b**) The dark-brown homogeneous pattern is seen under dermoscopy (×30)

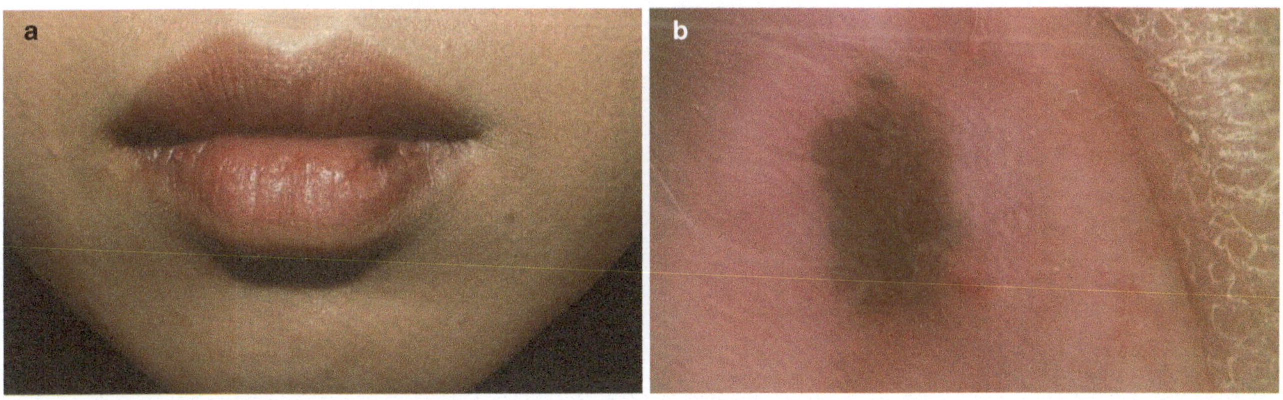

Fig. 5.53 Clinical and dermoscopic manifestations of a benign melanocytic tumor of the lower lip. (**a**) A dark-brown patch on the lower lip. (**b**) Dermoscopy shows a symmetrical and regular grayish-brown fish-scale-like pattern (×30)

Further Reading

1. Piccolo D, Smolle J, Argrnziano G, et al. Teledermoscopy—results of a multicenter study on 43 pigmented skin lesions. J Telemed Telecare. 2000;6(3):132–7.
2. Argenziano G, Soyer HP, Chimenti S, et al. Dermoscopy of pigmented skin lesions: Results of a consensus meeting via the Internet. J Am Acad Dermatol. 2003;48(5):679–93.
3. Carli P, Qrercioli E, Sestini S, et al. Pattern analysis, not simplified algorithms, is the most reliable method for teaching dermoscopy for melanoma diagnosis to residents in dermatology. Br J Dermatol. 2003;148(5):981–4.
4. Skin Imaging Group, Committee on Dermatology and Venereology Association of Integrative Medicine. Dermoscopic diagnosis of nevus. Chin J Lepr Skin Dis. 2017;33(2):65–9.
5. Blum A, Simionescu O, Argenziano G, et al. Dermoscopy of pigmented lesions of the mucosa and the mucocutaneous junction: results of a multicenter study by the International Dermoscopy Society (IDS). Arch Dermatol. 2011;147(10):1181–7.
6. Kim JK, Nelson KC. Dermoscopic features of common nevi: a review. G Ital Dermatol Venereol. 2012;147(2):141–8.
7. Cengiz FP, Emiroglu N, Ozkaya DB, et al. Dermoscopic features of small, medium, and large-sized congenital melanocytic nevi. Ann Dermatol. 2017;29(1):26–32.
8. Antonella DC, Francesco S, Andrea G, et al. The spectrum of dermatoscopic patterns in blue nevi. J Am Acad Dermatol. 2012;67(2):199–205.
9. Lallas A, Apalla Z, Ioannides D, et al. Update on dermoscopy of Spitz/Reed naevi and management guidelines by the International Dermoscopy Society. Br J Dermatol. 2017;177(3):645–55.
10. Kolm I, Di Stefani A, Hofmann-Wellenhof R, et al. Dermoscopy patterns of halo nevi. Arch Dermatol. 2006;142(12):1627–32.
11. Kamińska-Winciorek G. Dermoscopy of nevus spilus. Dermatol Surg. 2013;39(10):1550–4.
12. Suh KS, Park JB, Kim JH, et al. Dysplastic nevus : Clinical features and usefulness of dermoscopy. J Dermatol. 2019;46(2):e76–7.
13. Blum A, Hofmann-Wellenhof R, Marghoob AA, et al. Recurrent melanocytic nevi and melanomas in dermoscopy: results of a multicenter study of the International Dermoscopy Society. JAMA Dermatol. 2014;150(2):138–45.
14. Botella-Estrada R, Nagore E, Sopena J, et al. Clinical, dermoscopy and histological correlation study of melanotic pigmentations in excision scars of melanocytic tumors. Br J Dermatol. 2006;154(3):478–84.
15. Thomas L, Phan A, Pralong P, et al. Special locations dermoscopy: facial, acral, and nail. Dermatol Clin. 2013;31(4):615–24.
16. Toshiaki S, Hiroshi K. Dermoscopic patterns of acral melanocytic nevi: their variations, changes, and significance. Arch Dermatol. 2007;143(11):1423–6.
17. French LE, Laugier P, Saurat JH. Diagnosis and management of nail pigmentations. J Am Acad Dermatol. 2007;56(5):835–47.
18. Benati E, Ribero S, Longo C, et al. Clinical and dermoscopic clues to differentiate pigmented nail bands: an International Dermoscopy Society study. J Eur Acad Dermatol Venereol. 2017;31(4):732–6.
19. Lin J, Koga H, Takata M, et al. Dermoscopy of pigmented lesions on mucocutaneous junction and mucous membrane. Br J Dermatol. 2009;161(6):1255–61.
20. Marghoob AA, Malvehy J, Braun RP. Atlas of dermoscopy. 2nd ed. CRC Press; 2012;98–275.

6 Melanoma

Melanoma, also known as malignant melanoma, is a type of malignant tumor that arises from melanocytes with a high degree of malignancy, fast progression, and poor prognosis. Dermoscopy serves as a valuable aid in diagnosing melanoma. It is also the earliest indication of dermoscopy.

6.1 Dermoscopic Analysis of Melanocytic Neoplasms

The earliest application of dermoscopy is to identify benign and malignant melanocytic neoplasms. Studies have shown that dermoscopy is an effective diagnostic tool in recognizing early melanoma, which can greatly improve diagnostic accuracy. Common diagnostic algorithms include pattern analysis, the ABCD rule, the Menzies method, the seven-point checklist, the three-point checklist, and the CASH algorithm.

Pattern analysis, among all the methods, requires the most knowledge and recognition of patterns of nevi and melanoma, with the highest diagnostic accuracy if used by experienced clinicians. The dermoscopic patterns of melanocytic nevi include reticular pattern, globular pattern, homogeneous pattern, starburst pattern, etc. The specific patterns of melanoma include atypical pigment network, irregular streaks, irregular dots and globules, irregular blotches, and blue-white veil, etc. (see Table 6.1). In addition, there are some site-specific patterns, such as pseudonetwork, asymmetric pigmented follicular openings, annular-granular patterns, and rhomboidal structures on facial skin and parallel ridge patterns, irregular diffuse pigmentation, and multicomponent pattern on palms and soles.

6.2 Types of Cutaneous Melanoma

The four main types of primary cutaneous melanoma, according to histopathological findings, are as follows:

1. Lentigo maligna melanoma (LMM)
2. Superficial spreading melanoma (SSM)
3. Acral lentiginous melanoma (ALM)
4. Nodular melanoma (NM)
5. Other rare and specific types, such as amelanotic melanoma and connective tissue hyperplastic melanoma

According to the 2017 National Comprehensive Cancer Network (NCCN) guidelines, melanoma can be classified into another four types based on a new standard:

1. Chronic sun damage (CSD): melanomas induced by long-term exposure to sun, with significant solar elastosis
2. Nonchronic sun damage (non-CSD): melanomas that are not induced by long-term exposure to sun
3. Acral: melanomas located on soles, palms, or subungual sites
4. Mucosal melanoma: melanomas located on mucosal membranes

6.3 Dermoscopic Manifestations of Various Melanomas

6.3.1 Chronic Sun-Damage Melanoma

CSD-melanomas are commonly seen in the elderly on exposed sites, most often on the face, especially the cheeks, nose, neck, or lips. They are induced by long-term chronic sun exposure and manifest as asymmetric macules with irregular borders, which can be yellowish-brown, brown, or black. CSD-melanomas are usually flat and gradually expand into the surrounding areas up to several centimeters. They can become nodules due to aggressive growth. This type includes lentigo maligna (LM) and LMM, with LM referring to melanoma in situ and LMM referring to invasive melanoma.

J. Liu, X. Zou, *Practical Dermoscopy*, https://doi.org/10.1007/978-981-19-1460-7_6

Table 6.1 Dermoscopic patterns of melanoma

Common characteristic patterns	Schematic	Definition
Atypical pigment networks	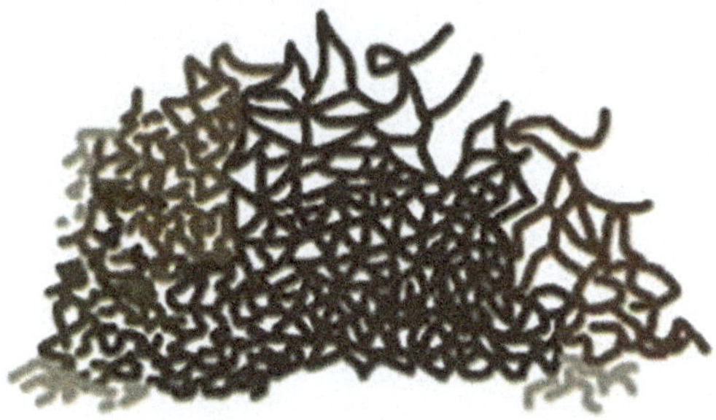	Pigmented lines varying in size, color, thickness, or distribution
Irregular streaks (pseudopods and radial streaming)	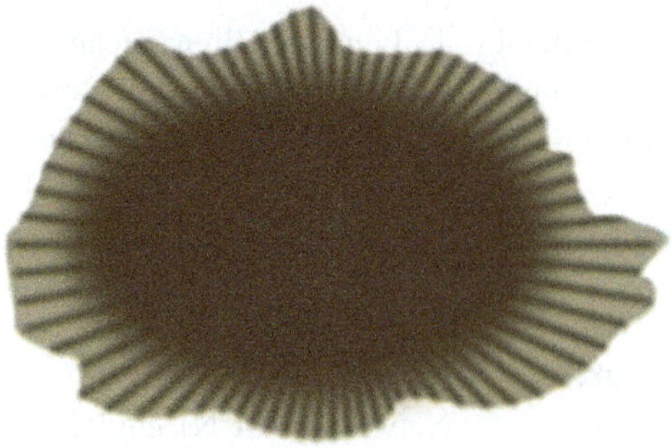	Pseudopods: distorted bulbous projections at the margin and directly connected to the main tumor mass Radial streaming: radial linear extensions of the lesion margin Irregularly distributed peripheral streaks at the lesion margins are highly suggestive of melanoma
Negative pigment network	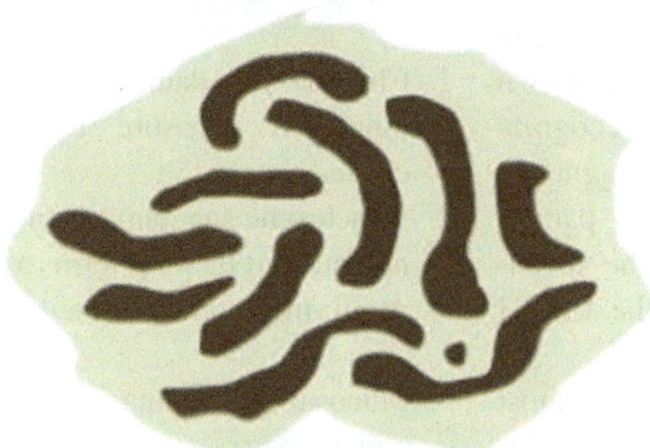	Serpiginous hypopigmented thick lines interconnected with each other and surrounded by long, curved globules, whose distribution is generally asymmetric and focal in melanoma
Shiny white streaks (crystalline structures)	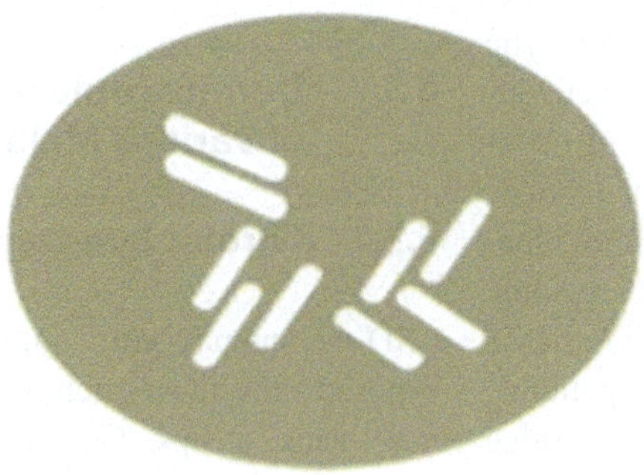	Discrete short white lines parallel or perpendicular to each other, seen only under polarized dermoscopy; also seen in nonmelanocytic lesions, including basal cell carcinoma, dermatofibroma and lichen planus-like keratosis

Table 6.1 (continued)

Common characteristic patterns	Schematic	Definition
Irregular dots and globules	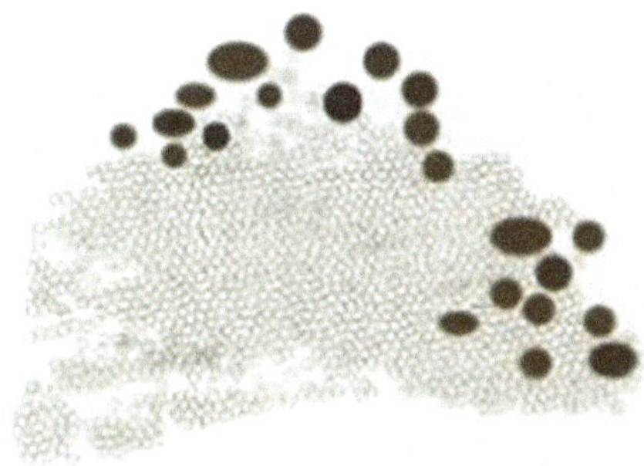	Irregular dots vary in color, size, shape, and interval or asymmetrically distributed, mostly found at the periphery of the lesion, usually not on gridlines; globules are larger than dots
Irregular blotches	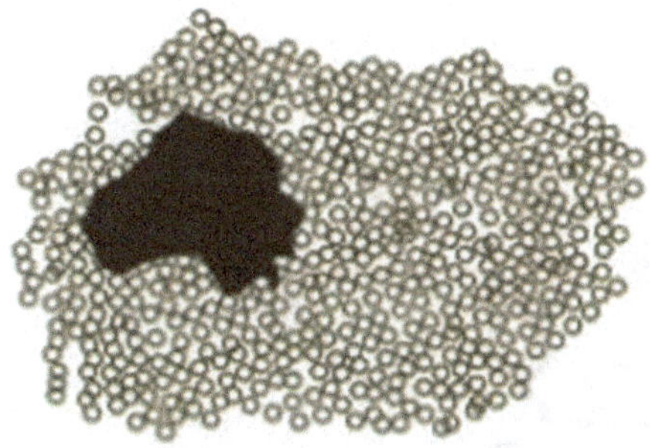	Blotches that are heterogeneous in shade and deviate from the center of the lesion (asymmetric)
Peripheral brown structureless zone	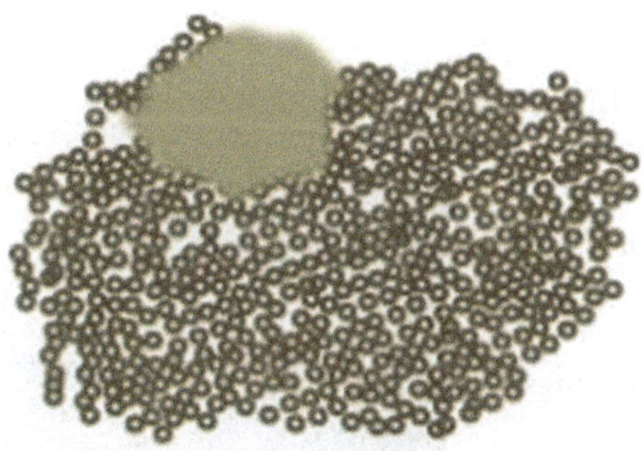	Light brown or yellow-brown structureless areas appear at the edge of the lesion and are not encircled by grids or globules
Blue-white veil	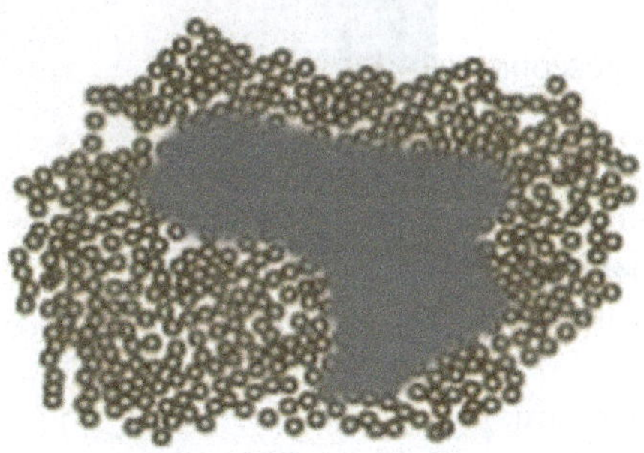	Irregularly shaped blue blotches covered with white ground-glass-like haze

(continued)

Table 6.1 (continued)

Common characteristic patterns	Schematic	Definition
Regression structures (scar-like depigmentation and/or peppering/granularity)	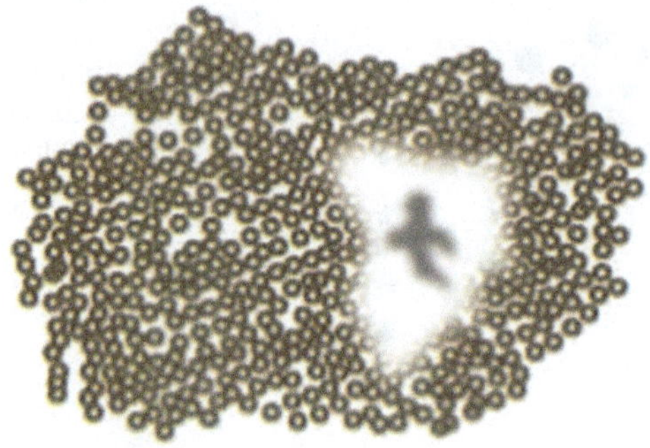	Scar-like depigmentation: areas that are whiter than the surrounding normal skin (true scar) without shiny white structures or vessels, must be distinguished from hypopigmentation or depigmentation due to simple pigment loss Peppering/granularity: accumulation of blue-gray dots
Atypical vascular structures	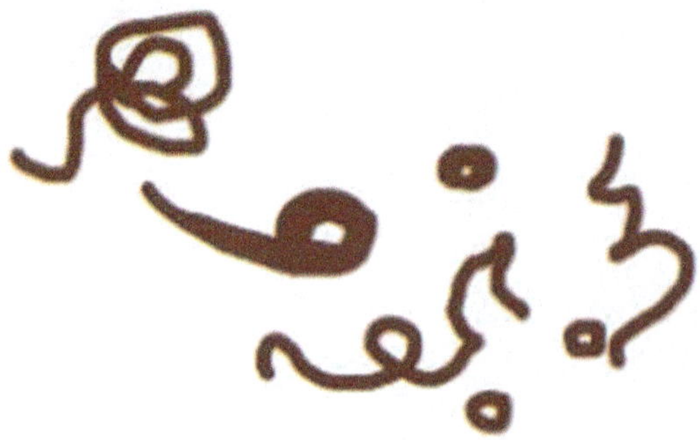	Milky-red areas with dots, linear, serpiginous or twisted vessels. Melanoma should be considered when more than one vascular pattern is present within a lesion, which is the typical feature of hypomelanotic and amelanotic melanoma

The common dermoscopic manifestations of LM and LMM are as follows (Figs. 6.1, 6.2, 6.3, 6.4, and 6.5):

1. Asymmetric pigmentation of follicular openings
2. Annular-granular pattern
3. Dots aggregated around the adnexal openings
4. Short and polygonal lines around the adnexal openings
5. Rhomboidal structures
6. Dark blotches (also called homogeneous patterns)

In addition, Pralong et al. proposed four rare dermoscopic manifestations:

1. Darkening at dermoscopic examination: brown or gray patches under dermoscopy, but invisible to the naked eye.
2. Target-like pattern: a dark dot in the center of the dark circle of a hyperpigmented follicular opening.
3. Red rhomboidal structure: a rhomboidal vascular structure that separates follicular openings from each other.
4. Increased density of the vascular network: a vascular network that is denser than that of the surrounding normal skin.

6.3.2 Nonchronic Sun-Damage Melanoma

6.3.2.1 Superficial Spreading Melanoma

SSM is the most common type in fair-skinned people and occurs primarily on the trunk in males and the legs in females. Approximately half of all SSMs develop on pre-existing nevi.

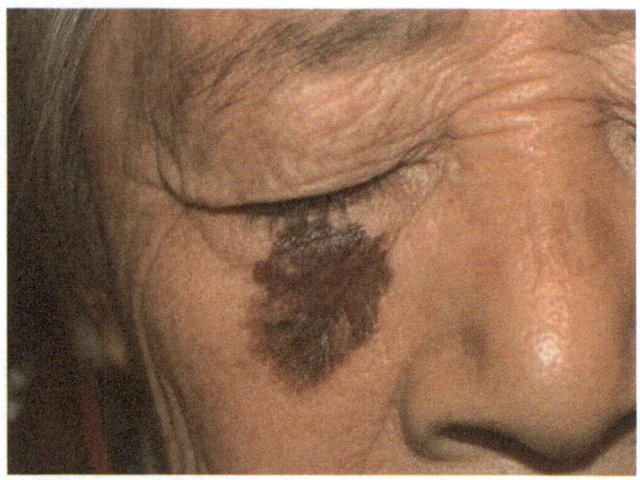

Fig. 6.1 Clinical picture of LMM: an approximately 4 cm brownish-black patch on the right cheek with irregular shape and uneven color

Initially, SSM is an asymptomatic tan to black macule with variable pigmentation and irregular edges when in situ. SSM typically begins with a slow and horizontal growth (radial growth) pattern confined to the epidermis or dermal papillae, and then followed by a more rapid vertical growth pattern.

The common dermoscopic characteristics of SSM are as follows (Figs. 6.6, 6.7, 6.8, 6.9, 6.10, 6.11, 6.12, 6.13, and 6.14):

1. Various colors
2. Atypical pigment network

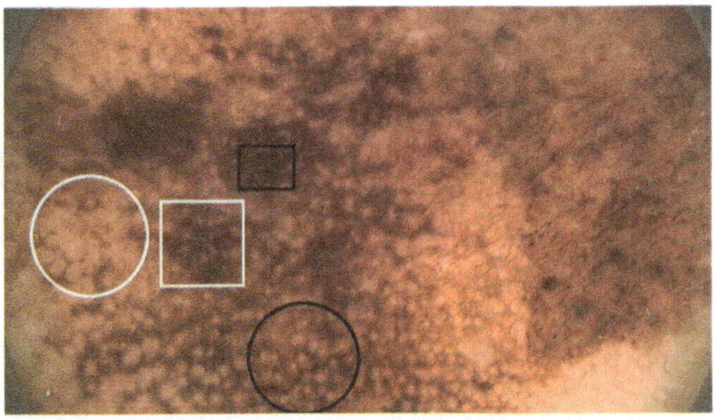

Fig. 6.2 Dermoscopic picture of LMM: asymmetric pigmentation of follicular openings (white circles); rhomboidal structures (black circles); dark blotches with follicular openings still visible (white rectangles); dark blotches with follicular openings invisible (black rectangles) (×30)

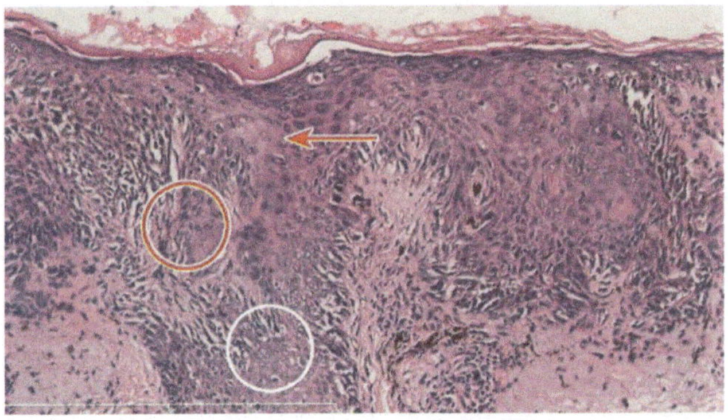

Fig. 6.3 Histopathology of LMM: pigment granules can be seen in the stratum corneum; Paget-like atypical cells can be seen in the stratum granulosum and stratum spinosum; nested and scattered atypical cells are in the basal layer; atypical cells and pigment granules can be seen in the hair follicles and superficial dermis (HE ×100)

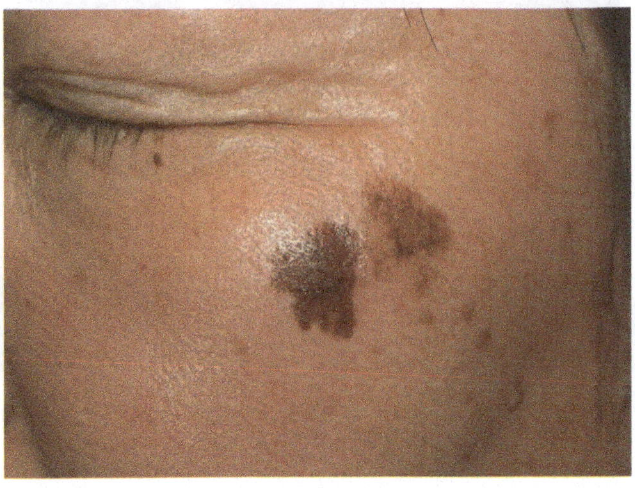

Fig. 6.4 Clinical picture of LM: an approximately 3 × 6 cm brownish-black patch on the left cheek with irregular, dumbbell shape, and uneven color

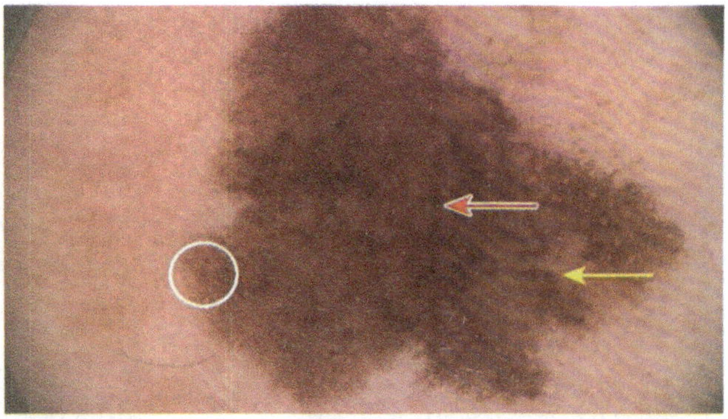

Fig. 6.5 Dermoscopic picture of LM: lesions with uneven color and irregularly shaped border. The red arrow refers to asymmetric pigmentation of the follicular openings, the yellow arrow refers to dots aggregated around the adnexal openings and the white circle refers to concentric structures (×30)

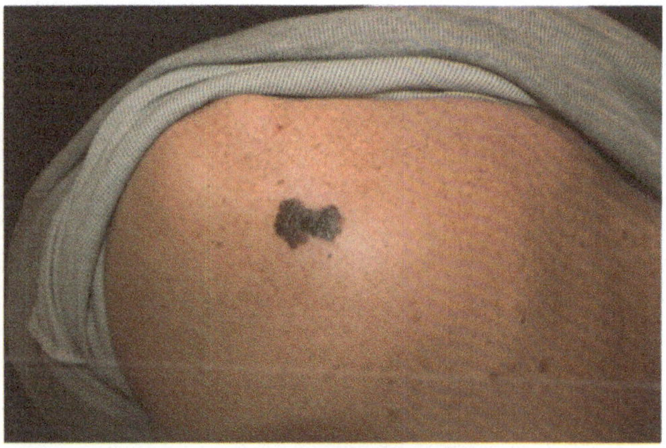

Fig. 6.6 Clinical picture of SSM: an approximately 3 × 5 cm brownish-black plaque on the back with irregular shape and unclear border

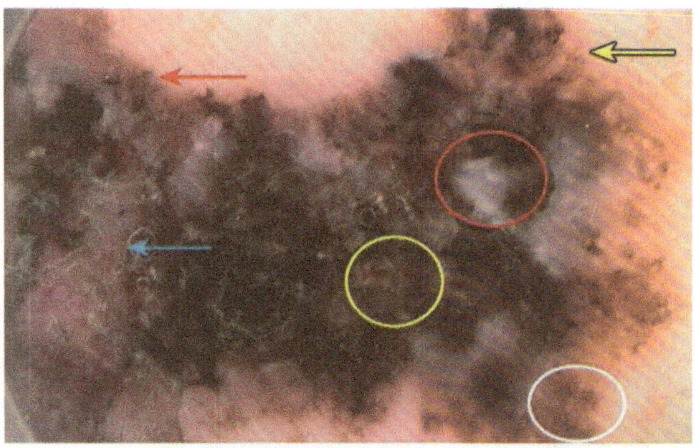

Fig. 6.7 Dermoscopic picture of SSM: asymmetric multi-pigmented structures. The red arrow refers to peripheral irregular dots and globules, yellow arrow refers to irregular streaks, blue arrow refers to multiple vascular structures, red circle refers to scar-like depigmentation, white circle refers to atypical widened pigment network, and yellow circle refers to blotches (×30)

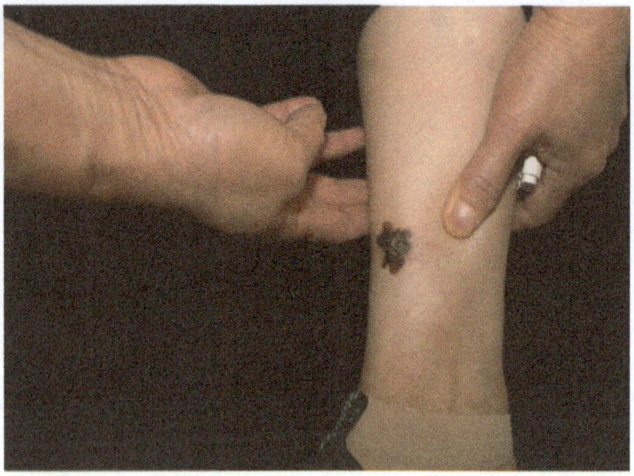

Fig. 6.8 Clinical picture of SSM: an approximately 3 × 3 cm brownish-black plaque on the right calf with irregular shape and unclear border

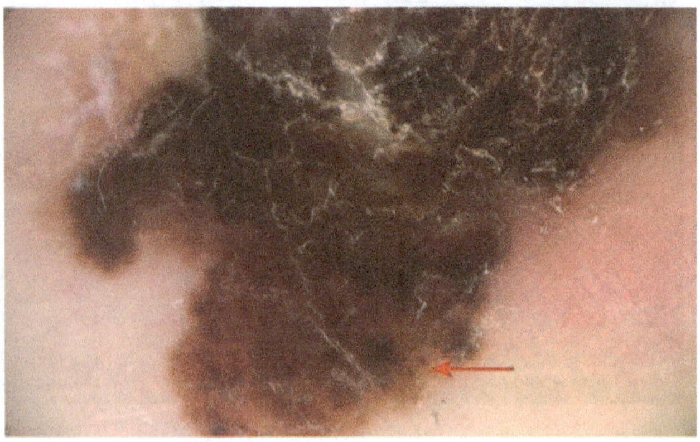

Fig. 6.9 Dermoscopic picture of SSM: asymmetric multi-pigmented structures and irregular blotches. The red arrow refers to peripheral irregular dots and globules (×30)

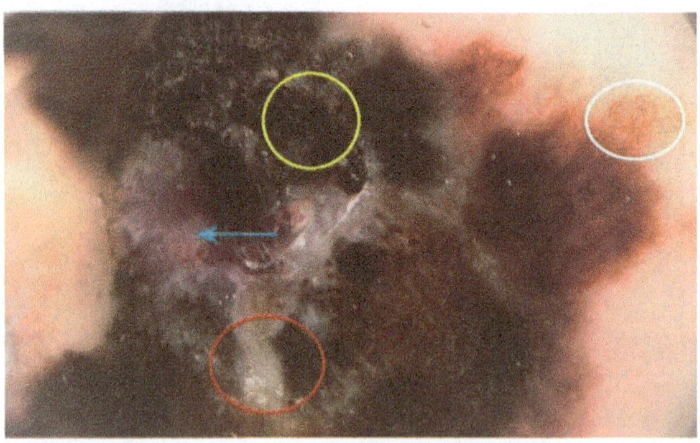

Fig. 6.10 Dermoscopic picture of SSM: asymmetric multi-pigmented structures. The blue arrow refers to multiple vascular structures, red circle refers to scar-like depigmentation, white circle refers to atypical pigment network, and yellow circle refers to blotches (×30)

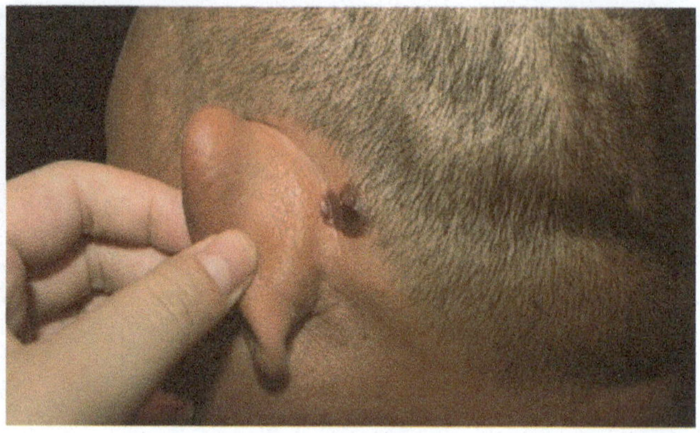

Fig. 6.11 Clinical picture of SSM: an approximately 2 × 2 cm brownish-black plaque behind the left ear with irregular shape, unclear border, and an elevated black nodule in the center

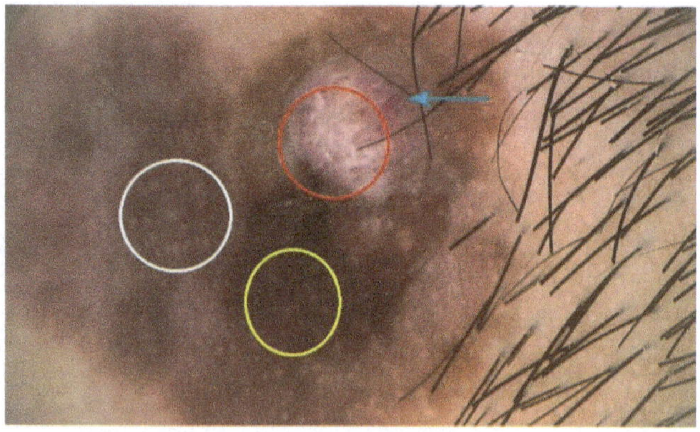

Fig. 6.12 Dermoscopic picture of SSM: asymmetric multi-pigmented structures. The blue arrow refers to multiple vascular structures, red circle refers to scar-like depigmentation and shiny white streaks, white circle refers to atypical widened pigment network, and yellow circle refers to blotches (×30)

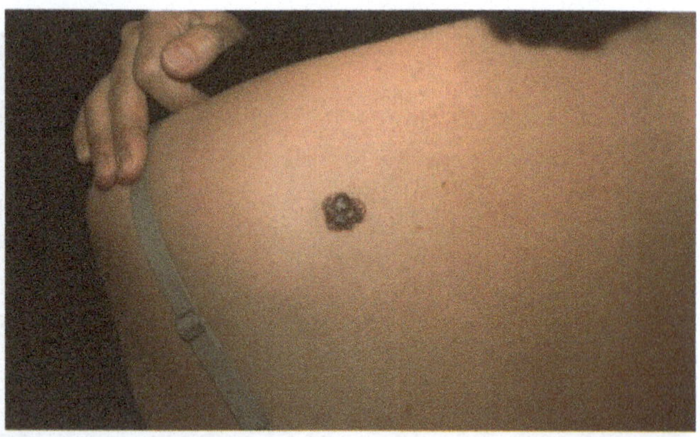

Fig. 6.13 Clinical picture of SSM: an approximately 2 × 2 cm brownish-black plaque on the back with irregular shape, unclear border, and an elevated black nodule in the center

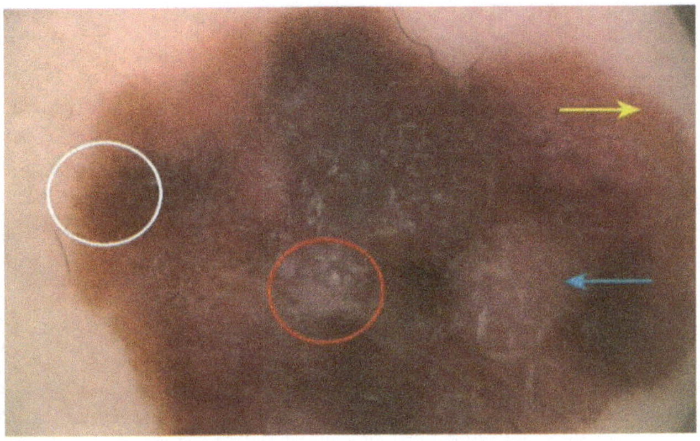

Fig. 6.14 Dermoscopic picture of SSM: asymmetric multi-pigmented structures. The blue arrow refers to multiple vascular structures, red circle refers to scar-like depigmentation and shiny white streaks, white circle refers to an atypical pigment network, and yellow arrow refers to radial streaming (×30)

3. Irregular streaks (pseudopods and radial streaming)
4. Negative network
5. Shiny white streaks (crystalline structure)
6. Irregular dots and globules (peripheral)
7. Irregular blotches
8. Peripheral brown structureless zone
9. Blue-white veil
10. Regression structures (scar-like depigmentation and/or peppering/granularity)
11. Atypical vascular structures

Atypical pigment network is one of the earliest manifestations of SSM. Irregular streaks in SSM suggest radial growth, and shiny white streaks, which are visible only under polarized dermoscopy, suggest aggressive growth. The presence of both dots and linear vessels in the same lesion is highly suggestive of melanoma. Melanoma with a depth <0.76 mm is more likely to show atypical pigmentation network than a thicker one, while melanoma with a depth >0.76 mm is more likely to show atypical vascular structures and blue-white veil. Je-Ho Mun et al. found that in the Asian population, the most common dermoscopic manifestations of melanoma on the trunk included asymmetric and multiple colors, followed by irregular dots, blue-white veil, atypical pigment network, and atypical vascular structures, with an occurrence of more than 50% for each of them, which is statistically different from that of benign nevi.

6.3.2.2 Nodular Melanoma

NM is the second most common type of melanoma in fair-skinned people. NM can occur anywhere on the body, especially on the trunk, head, and neck. NM is usually a blue to black nodule, but sometimes pink to red, which may be ulcerated or bleeding with rapid growth, and an elevated nodule can be formed within a few months. NM lacks the ABCD features since NM arises as rapid invasive vertical growth instead of radial growth. NM is more likely to develop into amelanotic and hypomelanotic melanoma (AHM) than other subtypes.

The common dermoscopic features of NM are as follows:

1. Various colors
2. Blue-white veil
3. Shiny white streaks
4. Atypical vascular structures
5. Structureless areas

The common dermoscopic features of AHM are as follows (Figs. 6.15, 6.16, and 6.17):

1. Negative network
2. Shiny white streaks
3. Milky-red areas
4. Polymorphous atypical vascular structures

Nodular amelanotic melanomas are easily misdiagnosed and need to be differentiated from intradermal nevi, pyogenic granulomas, and skin adnexal tumors, and polymorphous vascular patterns are often suggestive of a diagnosis of nodular amelanotic melanoma. In terms of vascular, the most suggestive features of nodular amelanotic melanoma are

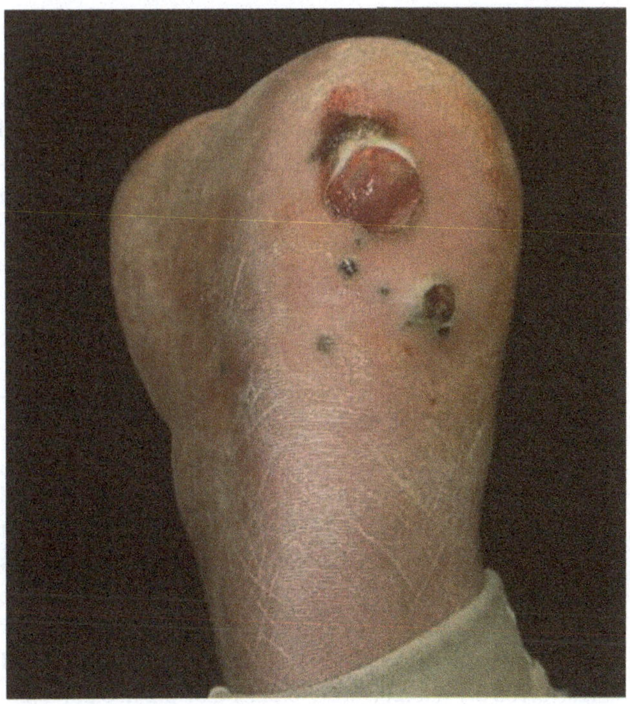

Fig. 6.15 Clinical picture of AHM on the heel: red, brown, and blue-black papules, patches, nodules of varying sizes on the sole with surface ulceration and exudation

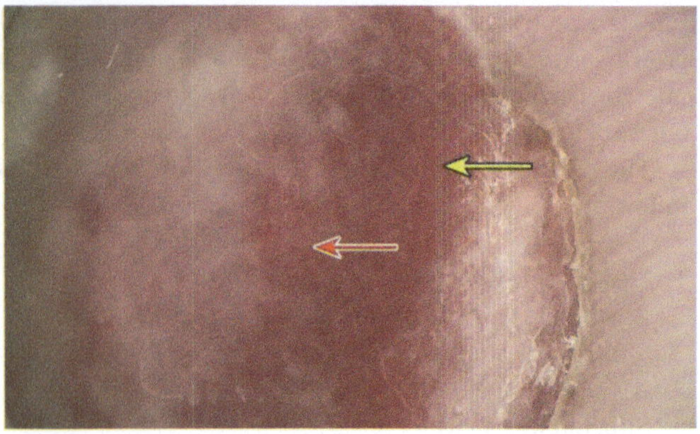

Fig. 6.16 Dermoscopic picture of AHM on the heel. The yellow arrow refers to milky-red areas, and red arrow refers to polymorphous atypical vascular structures (×30)

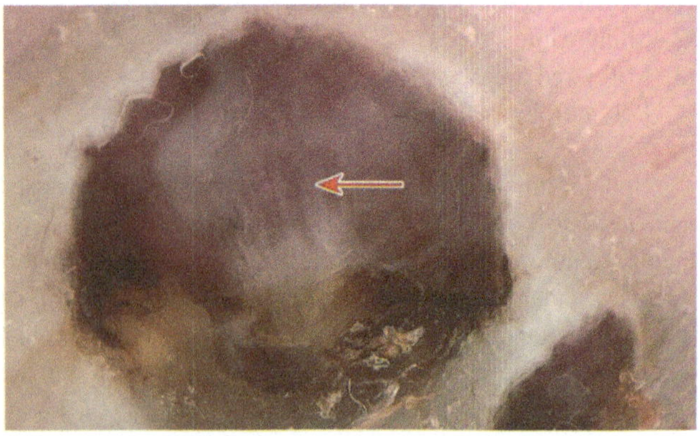

Fig. 6.17 Dermoscopic picture of AHM on the heel. The red arrow refers to polymorphous atypical vascular structures (×30)

prominent central vessels, hairpin-like vessels, milky-red areas, variable shades of pink, a combination of dots and linear vessels, and linear irregular vessels as the predominant vascular type.

6.3.3 Acral Melanoma

AM is the most common type of melanoma in Asian individuals. Therefore, the early diagnosis of it is very valuable in China. AM can occur on hairless areas like palms, soles, fingernails, and toenails. In the past, AM is also called acral lentiginous melanoma (ALM), but since the realization of the fact that the growth pattern and histopathologic findings of AM are different from those of lentiginous melanoma, the term AM is now preferred.

Common dermoscopic features of non-subungual AM (Figs. 6.18, 6.19, 6.20, 6.21, 6.22, 6.23, 6.24, 6.25, 6.26, 6.27, 6.28, 6.29, 6.30, and 6.31):

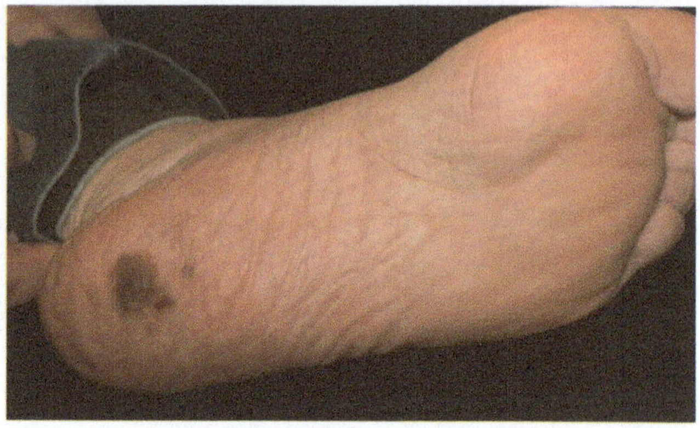

Fig. 6.18 Clinical picture of AM: approximately 5 × 7 cm irregular patches on the sole with asymmetric distribution and multiple colors (brown, black, light red)

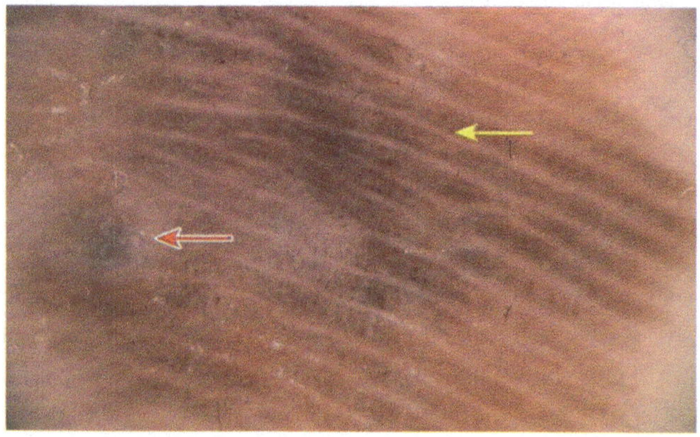

Fig. 6.19 Dermoscopic picture of AM: irregular lesions with multiple colors, typical parallel ridge pattern (yellow arrows) and multicomponent pattern. The red arrow refers to blue-white veil (×30)

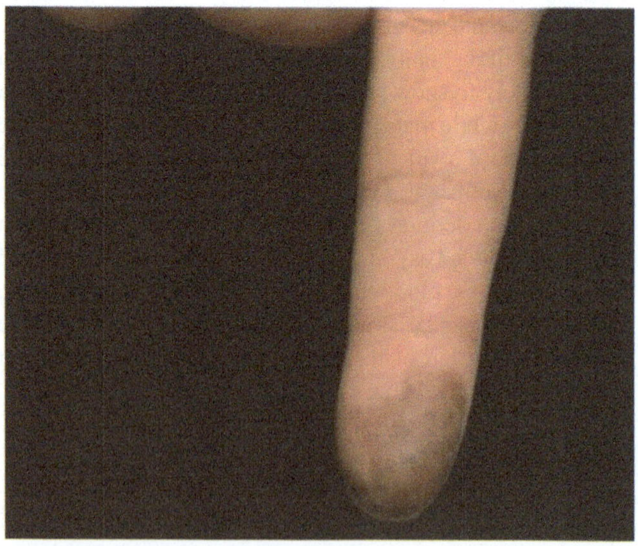

Fig. 6.20 Clinical picture of AM: brown patches with uneven color on the distal phalanx of the left index finger

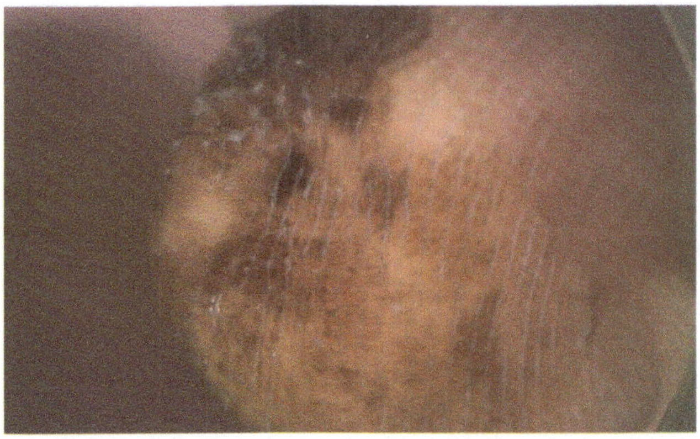

Fig. 6.21 Dermoscopic picture of AM: irregular lesions with multiple colors (white, light brown, dark brown, black), uneven distribution of pigmentation, parallel ridge pattern, and atypical fibrillar pattern (×30)

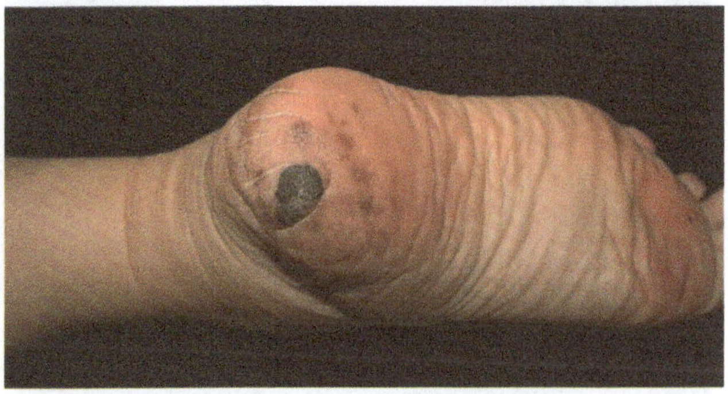

Fig. 6.22 Clinical picture of AM: 2 × 2 cm irregular black patch on the sole of the right foot, surrounded by light to dark brown patches of varying sizes

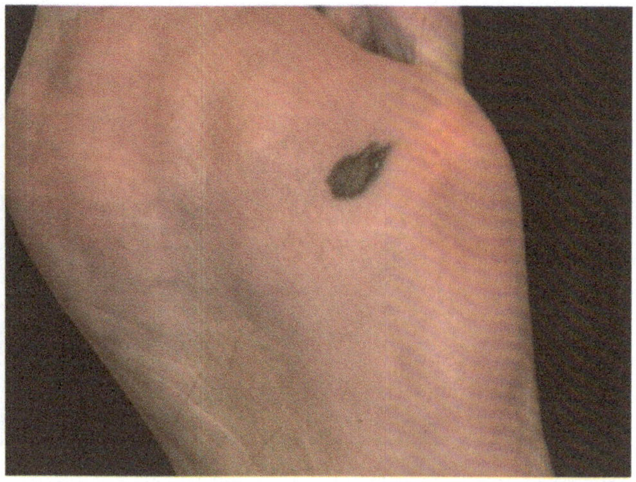

Fig. 6.24 Clinical picture of AM: an irregular brownish-black approximately 1 × 2 cm flamelike patch on the sole of the left foot

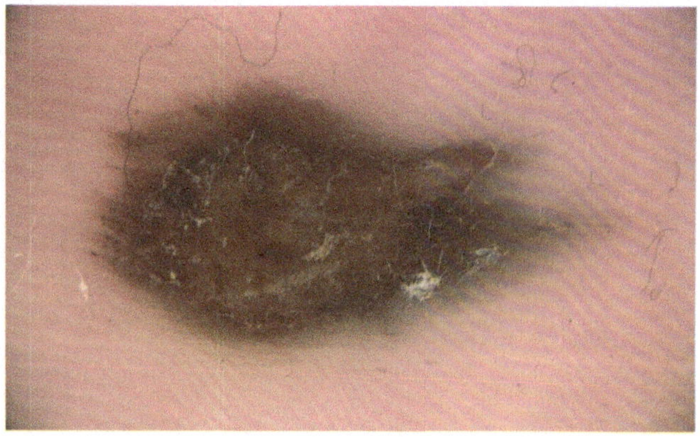

Fig. 6.25 Dermoscopic picture of AM: irregular lesion with various colors (white, light brown, dark brown, blue-gray, black), irregular diffuse pigmentation, blue-white veil, pigmented dots with pod-like distribution on the left edge (×30)

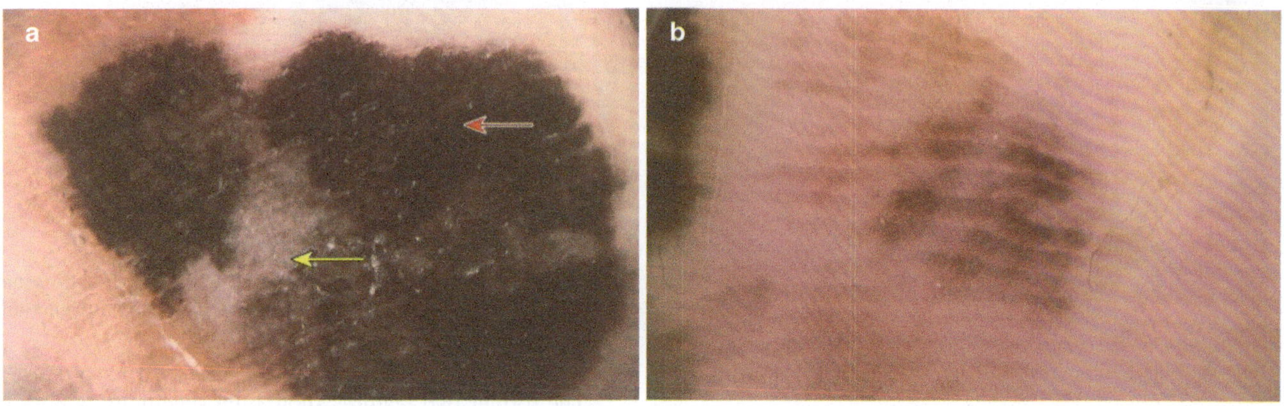

Fig. 6.23 (**a**) Dermoscopic picture of AM: irregular lesions with multiple colors (white, dark brown, black). The red arrow indicates irregular diffuse pigmentation, and yellow arrow indicates white regression structures (×30). (**b**) Dermoscopic picture of AM (satellite lesion): irregular lesion with typical parallel ridge pattern and atypical fibrillar pattern (×30)

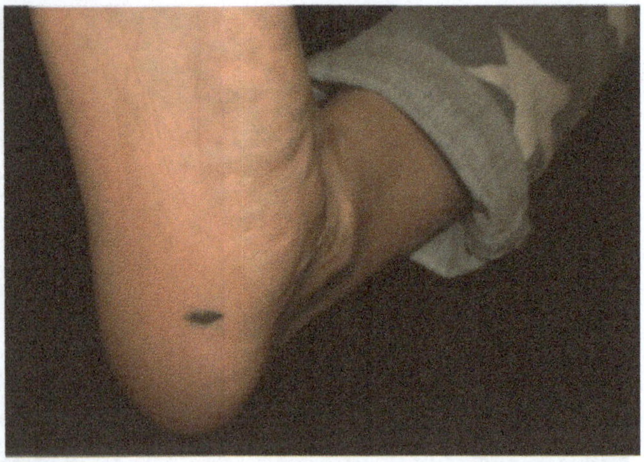

Fig. 6.26 Clinical picture of AM: fusiform black patch approximately 0.5 × 1.5 cm in size on the sole of the left foot

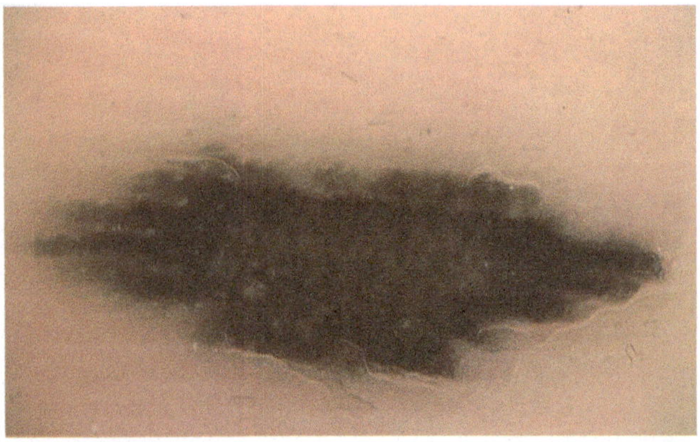

Fig. 6.27 Dermoscopic picture of AM: irregular lesions with various colors (white, brown, gray, black), irregular diffuse pigmentation surrounded by parallel ridge pattern (×30)

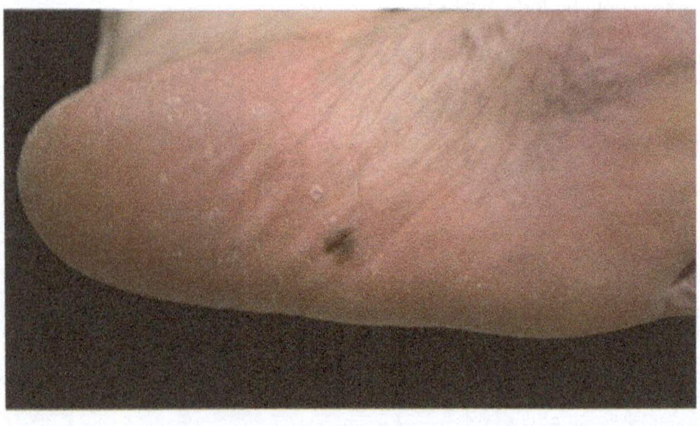

Fig. 6.28 Clinical picture of AM: light brown patch approximately 1 cm in diameter with irregular shape on the sole of the left foot

1. Parallel ridge pattern
2. Irregular diffuse pigmentation
3. Multicomponent pattern

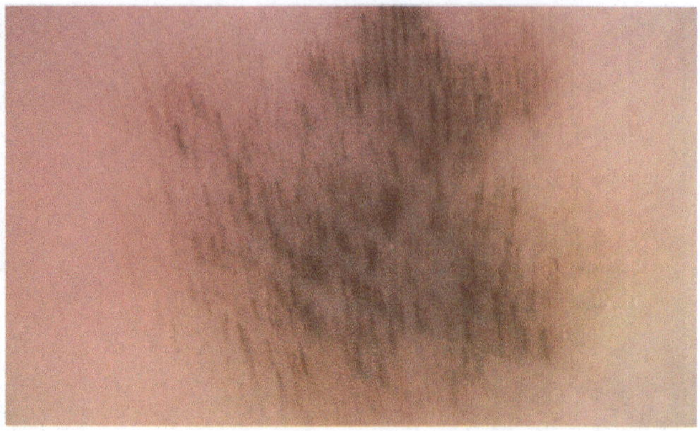

Fig. 6.29 Dermoscopic picture of AM: irregular lesions with atypical fibrillar pattern (×30)

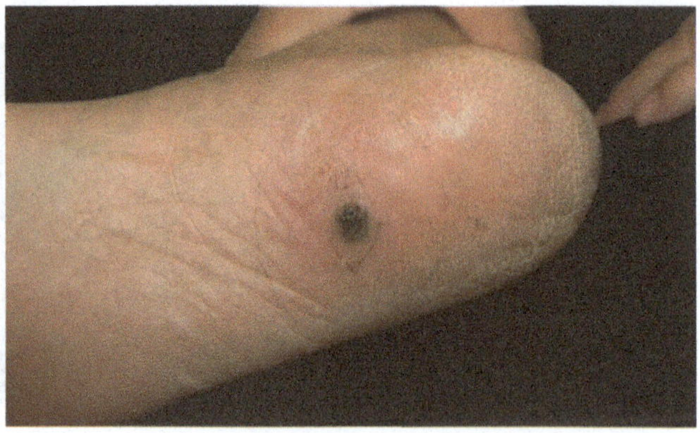

Fig. 6.30 Clinical picture of AM: brownish-black patch approximately 1.5 cm in size with irregular shape on the sole of the right foot

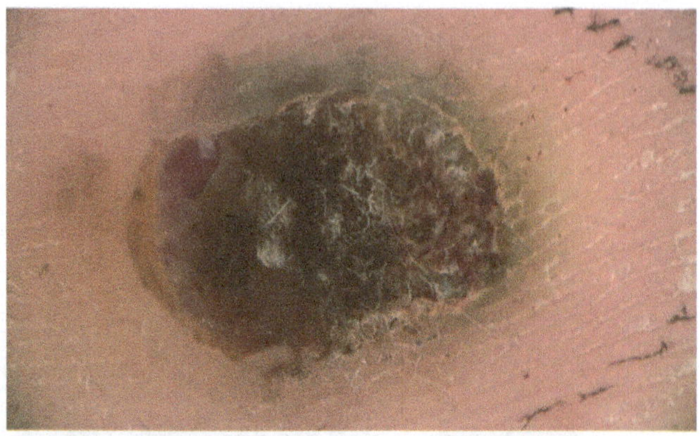

Fig. 6.31 Dermoscopic picture of AM: irregular lesion with various colors (white, milky-red areas, brown, black, blue-gray), irregular diffuse hyperpigmentation and ulceration (×30)

The former two features show high specificity in both in situ and invasive melanomas. The pigmentation of the parallel ridge pattern is distributed along the cristae cutis in parallel lines, contrast to the parallel furrow pattern, where pigmentation is distributed along the sulci cutis. Irregular diffuse pigmentation appears as irregular structureless pigmentation of different colors, such as brown, black, or gray, and is more often seen in highly aggressive and advanced lesions as opposed to the parallel ridge pattern. Advanced AMs show dermoscopic multicomponent patterns as other types of melanoma, such as multiple colors, irregular dots and globules, irregular streaks, atypical vascular structures, and blue-white veil. Some advanced AMs show atypical parallel furrow pattern, fibrillar pattern, and lattice-like pattern. In addition, ulceration is not used as a diagnostic criterion, but the presence of ulceration, especially non-trauma-induced ulceration, often indicates melanoma.

It is worth noting that the parallel ridge pattern can also occur in benign lesions such as pigmentation caused by para-phenylenediamine or antineoplastic drugs, pigmented macules on the extremities in Peutz–Jeghers syndrome, subcuticular hemorrhages on the extremities, and pigmented warts.

In addition, any fibrillar pattern in the palmar region and atypical fibrillar patterns on the soles (thicker lines, darker or grayish in color, with irregular shape) also need to be noted.

To better diagnose AM by dermoscopy, Lallas et al. conducted a multicenter study and proposed a new dermoscopic rule for the diagnosis of AM, i.e., the **BRAAFF scale:**

- **B**: Irregular **B**lotches (+1)
- **R**: Parallel **R**idge Pattern (+3)
- **A**: **A**symmetry of Structures (+1)
- **A**: **A**symmetry of Colors (+1)
- **F**: Parallel **F**urrow Pattern (−1)
- **F**: **F**ibrillar Pattern (−1)

Lesions with a total score of ≥1 are suspicious for AM.

Subungual melanoma can occur on both fingernails and toenails, mostly on the thumb and hallux.

The common dermoscopic features of subungual melanoma are as follows (Figs. 6.32, 6.33, 6.34, and 6.35):

1. Irregular bands on a brown background (most common), which may appear broader at the proximal end than the distal end
2. Hutchinson's sign (pigmentation of the nail folds and periungual skin)
3. Micro-Hutchinson's sign (only visible with dermoscopy, but not with the naked eye)
4. Nail plate destruction and distal fissuring

One study revealed that irregular bands on a brown background were the most common feature of melanoma (90.3%) among Ronger's seven features, followed by Hutchinson's sign (83.9%). While there was no significant difference between in situ and invasive melanoma in hemorrhagic spots and irregular dots/globules.

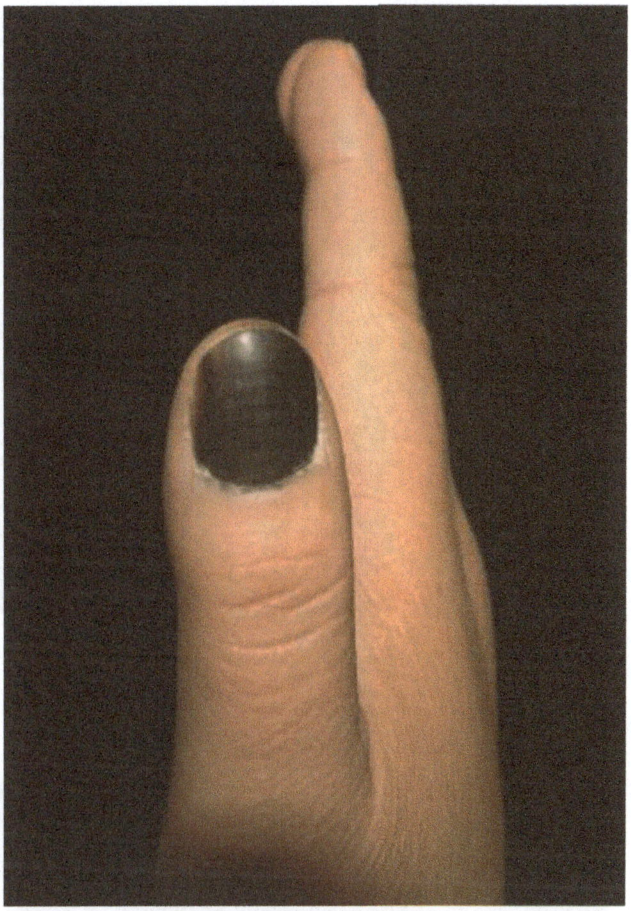

Fig. 6.32 Clinical picture of subungual melanoma: a diffuse brownish-black patch on the right thumbnail with irregular brownish-black pigmentation of the nail folds

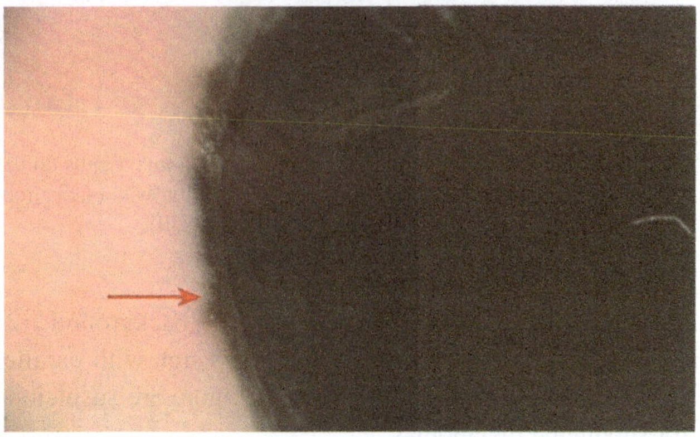

Fig. 6.33 Dermoscopic picture of subungual melanoma: diffuse brown-black uneven bands on a brown-black background. The red arrow refers to Hutchinson's sign (×30)

Currently, the Japanese 6-point measurement of longitudinal melanonychia is mostly used: Clinical assessment (one score for each positive item): (1) age > 30 years old; (2) course of disease < 5 years; and (3) significant changes within 3 months. Dermoscopic evaluation (2 points for each

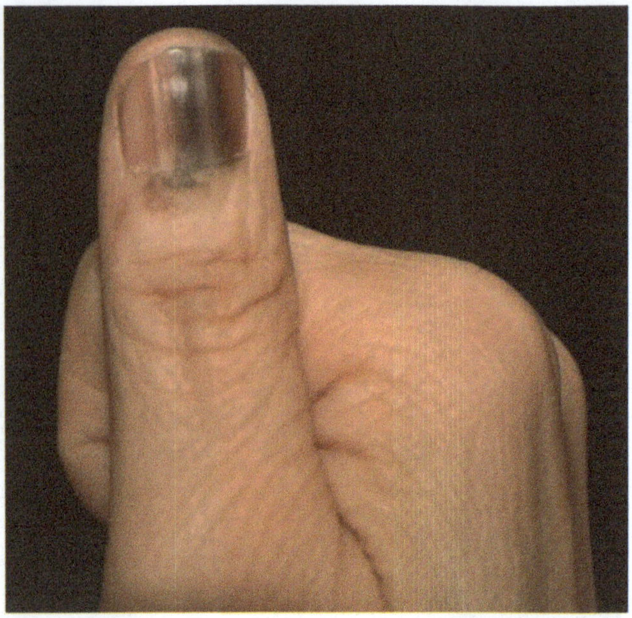

Fig. 6.34 Clinical picture of subungual melanoma: irregular brownish-black bands on the right thumbnail with irregular pigmentation of the nail folds and periungual skin

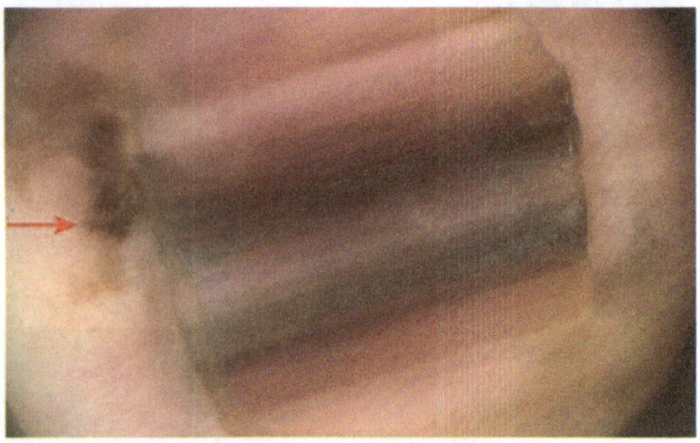

Fig. 6.35 Dermoscopic picture of subungual melanoma: bands on the nail plate with uneven width and uneven color (brown, black, red, white). The red arrow refers to Hutchinson's sign (×30)

positive item): (1) multiple colors in the background; (2) irregular lines or bands; (3) Hutchinson's sign with parallel ridge pattern. Lesions with 3 points or more are suspicious for subungual melanomas.

6.3.4 Mucosal Melanoma

Mucosal melanoma can occur at many sites, such as the lips, vulva, eyelids, oral cavity, and intestinal mucosa.

1. Early dermoscopic features include structureless areas and gray areas.
2. Advanced dermoscopic features show multicomponent pattern, i.e., asymmetric structure, multiple colors (white, red, light brown, dark brown, blue-gray), blue-white veil, irregular blotches, irregular streaks, and regression structures.

This chapter introduced the dermoscopic features of different types of melanoma. Understanding these manifestations can help us improve the diagnostic accuracy of melanoma and reduce misdiagnosis. However, there are still many diseases that are difficult to distinguish from melanoma clinically, such as pigmented basal cell carcinoma, special types of pigmented nevi, seborrheic keratosis, actinic keratosis, and lichen planus-like keratosis, etc. Therefore, when using dermoscopy in the diagnosis, clinicians should be familiar with the dermoscopic features of not only melanoma but also similar diseases. The final diagnosis requires a combination of clinical presentation, history, histopathologic and immunohistochemistric examination, as well as genetic testing if necessary.

Further Reading

1. Skin Imaging Group, Dermatology Branch, China Healthcare International Exchange and Promotion Association; Digital Diagnosis of Dermatological Diseases Subgroup of the Chinese Medical Association, Dermatology and Venereology Branch; Subspecialty Committee of Dermatologic Surgery, Dermatologists Branch, Chinese Medical Association; Skin Imaging Group, Skin Venereology Committee, Chinese Society of Integrative Medicine; China Medical Equipment Association Dermatology and Dermatological Aesthetics Branch Skin Imaging Equipment Group. Interpretation of *Codes for Terminology of Dermoscopy: Consensus on the Third Conference of International Society of Dermoscopy*. Chin J Dermatol. 2017;50(4):299–304.
2. Pralong P, Bathelier E, Dalle S, et al. Dermoscopy of lentigo maligna melanoma: report of 125 cases. Br J Dermatol. 2012;167(2):280–7.
3. Stante M, De Giorgi V, Capppugi P, et al. Non-invasive analysis of melanoma thickness by means of dermoscopy: a retrospective study. Melanoma Res. 2001;11(2):147–52.
4. Argenziano G, Fabbrocini G, Carli P, et al. Epiluminescence microscopy: criteria of cutaneous melanoma progression. J Am Acad Dermatol. 1997;37(1):68–74.
5. Mun JH, Ohn J, Kim WI, et al. Dermoscopy of Melanomas on the Trunk and Extremities in Asians. PLoS One. 2016;11(7):e0158374.
6. Menzies SW, Kreusch J, Byth K, et al. Dermoscopic evaluation of amelanotic and hypomelanotic melanoma. Arch Dermatol. 2008;144(9):1120–7.
7. Phan A, Dalle S, Touzet S, et al. Dermoscopic features of acral lentiginous melanoma in a large series of 110 cases in a white population. Br J Dermatol. 2010;162(4):765–71.
8. Saida T, Koga H, Uhara H. Key points in dermoscopic differentiation between early acral melanoma and acral nevus. J Dermatol. 2011;38(1):25–34.
9. Tanioka M. Benign acral lesions showing parallel ridge pattern on dermoscopy. J Dermatol. 2011;38(1):41–4.
10. Lallas A, Kyrgidis A, Koga H, et al. The BRAAFF checklist: a new dermoscopic algorithm for diagnosing acral melanoma. Br J Dermatol. 2015;173(4):1041–9.

11. Inoue Y, Menzies SW, Fukushima S, et al. Dots/globules on dermoscopy in nail-apparatus melanoma. Int J Dermatol. 2014;53(1):88–92.
12. Mun JH, Kim GW, Jwa SW, et al. Dermoscopy of subungual haemorrhage: its usefulness in differential diagnosis from nail-unit melanoma. Br J Dermatol. 2013;168(6):1224–9.
13. Lin J, Koga H, Takata M, et al. Dermoscopy of pigmented lesions on mucocutaneous junction and mucous membrane. Br J Dermatol. 2009;161(6):1255–61.
14. Li K, Xin L. Palpebral conjunctiva melanoma with dermoscopic and clinicopathological characteristics. J Am Acad Dermatol. 2014;71(2):e35–7.

Basal Cell Carcinoma

7

A basal cell carcinoma (BCC) is the most common malignant tumor of the skin, and its incidence has been rising steadily in recent decades. Although a BCC is usually slow-growing and rarely metastasizes, it can cause localized destruction and cosmetic disfigurement. Therefore, early diagnosis and treatment are of great importance. Dermoscopy has been shown to improve the diagnostic accuracy of BCCs and is a standard component of dermatologist office visits.

Dermoscopy can be helpful to differentiate BCC subtypes, which may have significant consequences for treatment. Pigmented BCCs (PBCCs) respond poorly to photodynamic therapy. Topical imiquimod is more effective for the treatment of BCCs with multiple small erosions. Furthermore, surgical excision is considered a standard treatment for nodular BCCs. In addition, dermoscopy can aid in determining the surgical margins of BCC lesions, evaluating the effectiveness of treatment, and following up after treatment.

The dermoscopic features of BCCs were first described more than a decade ago, and the list of BCC-related criteria has been updated and expanded several times. The dermoscopic features of BCCs can be classified into vascular structures, pigment-related structures, and other structures. The dermoscopic features of different BCC subtypes have already been described. Moreover, Menzies et al. proposed a simple dermoscopic model for diagnosing PBCCs based on the degree of pigmentation in BCCs.

PBCC is the most common nonmelanoma skin cancer in Chinese individuals. Clinically, PBCC should be differentiated from other pigmented diseases, such as malignant melanoma (MM) and benign melanocytic. On the other hand, non-PBCC should be differentiated from other nonpigmented diseases and inflammatory skin diseases.

The classification of the degree of pigmentation of a lesion is conducive to the differential diagnosis of BCCs. The screening out of superficial BCCs by classifying the types of pathology is helpful for the determination of treatment options and follow-ups. This book presents both classifications (Table 7.1).

Table 7.1 The common dermoscopic features of basal cell carcinomas

Vascular structures	Pigmentation structures	Other structures
Arborizing vessels	Leaflike structures	Ulcerations
Fine telangiectasias	Spoke-wheel areas	Multiple small erosions
Other morphological vessels	Blue-gray ovoid nests	Shiny white-red structureless areas
	Multiple blue-gray globules	White streaks
		Blue-white veil

7.1 Pigmented Basal Cell Carcinomas and Nonpigmented Basal Cell Carcinomas (Based on the Degree of Pigmentation)

BCC lesions can be classified according to the degree of pigmentation as follows: nonpigmented, mildly pigmented (<30%), pigmented (30–70%), and heavily pigmented (>70%). PBCCs occur more frequently in the Asian population than in the Caucasian population. Approximately 30% of BCCs that are clinically classified as nonpigmented manifest pigmented structures under dermoscopy.

7.1.1 Pigmented Basal Cell Carcinomas in Dermoscopy

7.1.1.1 Classic Features

1. One negative feature. No pigment network or streaks.
2. Six positive features:
   (a) Blue-gray ovoid nests/large blue clustered clods (Fig. 7.1).
   (b) Multiple blue-gray globules/small blue clods (Fig. 7.2).
   (c) Leaflike structures (Fig. 7.3).
   (d) Spoke-wheel-like structures (Fig. 7.4).

J. Liu, X. Zou, *Practical Dermoscopy*, https://doi.org/10.1007/978-981-19-1460-7_7

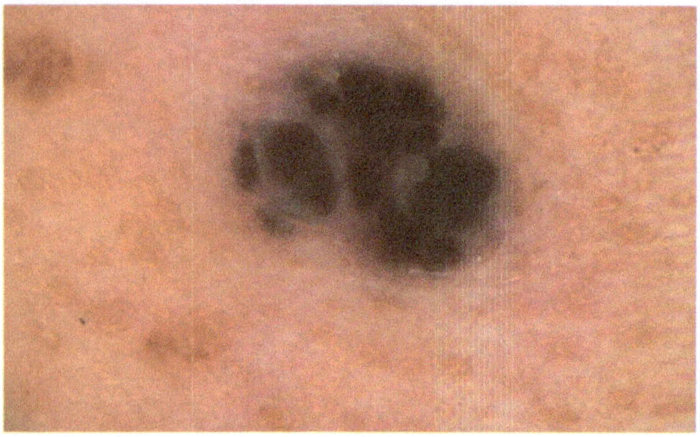

Fig. 7.1 Blue-gray ovoid nests. Well-circumscribed ovoid areas with confluent or nearly confluent pigmentation (×20)

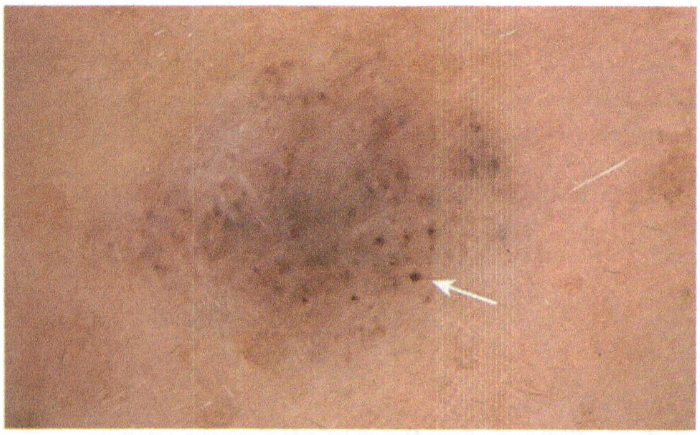

Fig. 7.2 Multiple blue-gray globules. Well-circumscribed globule, diameter >0.1 mm, larger than dots but smaller than ovoids, scattered (white arrow) (×20)

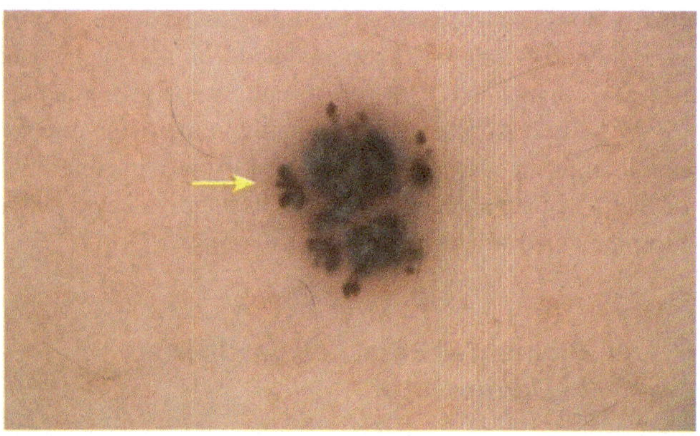

Fig. 7.3 Leaflike structures. Brown or blue-gray bulbous structures and extensions with a leaflike pattern (yellow arrow) (×20)

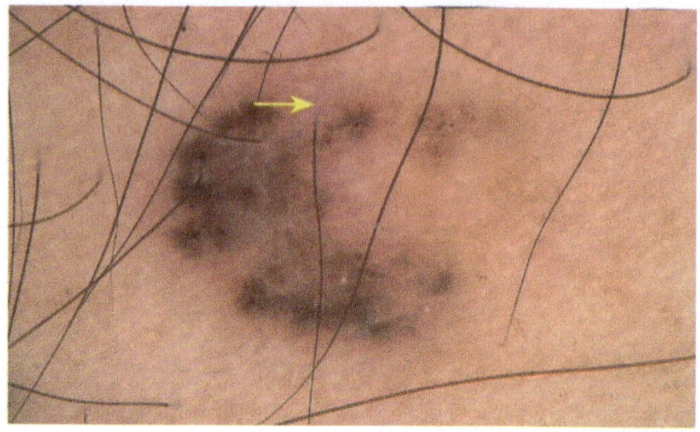

Fig. 7.4 Spoke-wheel-like structures. Well-defined radial projections, light brown or blue to gray. The central point is dark brown (yellow arrow) (×20)

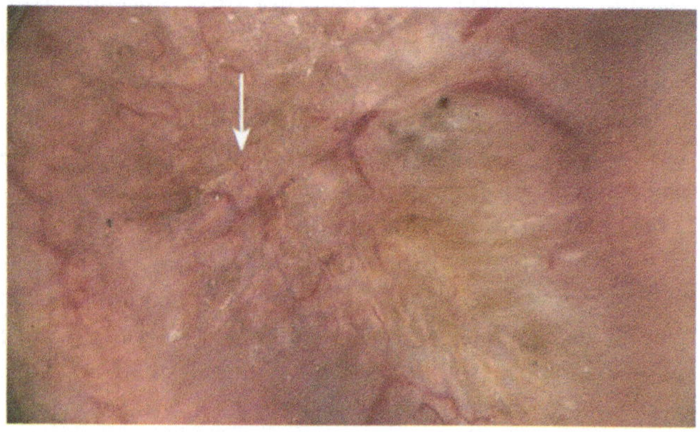

Fig. 7.5 Arborizing vessels. Thick multiple branching blood vessels in a tree-like pattern (white arrow) (×20)

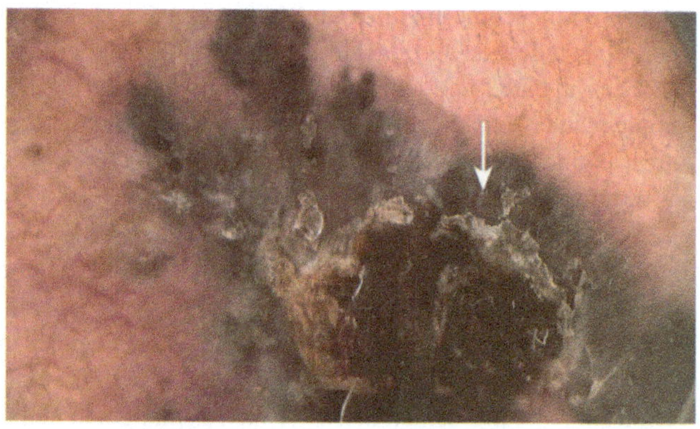

Fig. 7.6 Ulcerations. Shallow ulcerations that might be covered with congealed blood. No history of trauma (white arrow) (×20)

(e) Arborizing vessels (Fig. 7.5).
(f) Ulcerations (Fig. 7.6).

A diagnosis of PBCC based on the absence of a pigment network and the presence of at least one of six positive features in dermoscopy has been described.

7.1.1.2 Nonclassic Features

1. Concentric structures/globules; possibly the early stage of spoke-wheel-like structures (Fig. 7.7)
2. Multiple in-focus blue/gray dots; possibly the early stage of multiple blue/gray globules (Fig. 7.8)

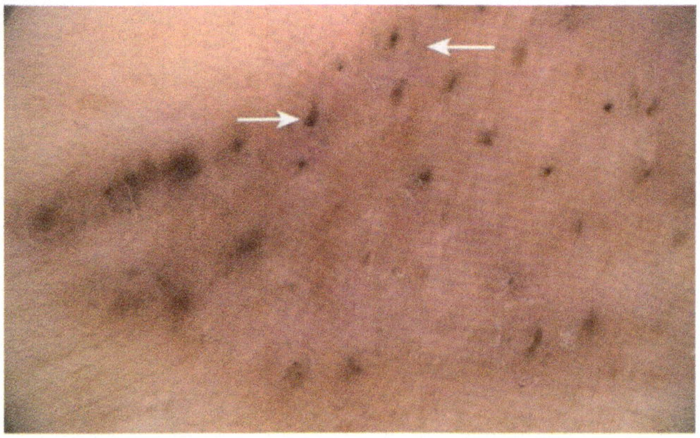

Fig. 7.7 Concentric structures/globules (white arrow) (×20)

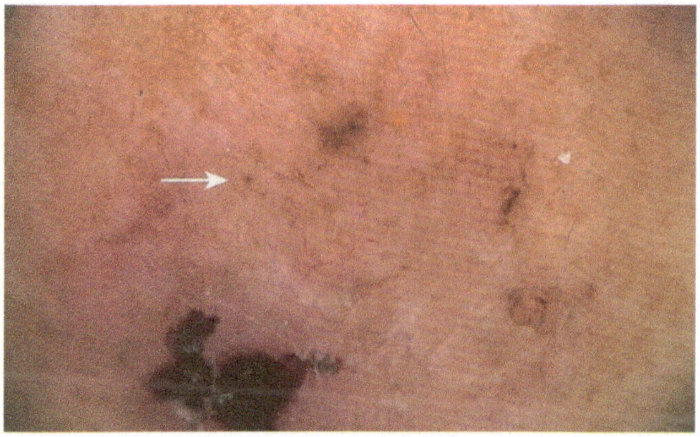

Fig. 7.8 Multiple in-focus blue/gray dots (white arrow) (×20)

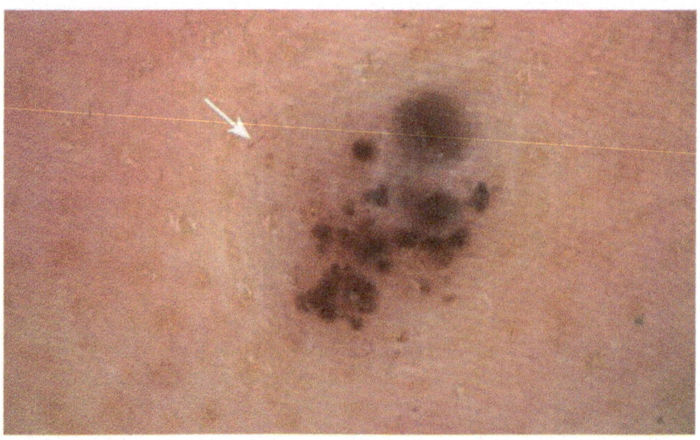

Fig. 7.9 Small fine telangiectasias (white arrow) (×40)

3. Small fine telangiectasias. Less than 1 mm in length, twisted and no obvious dendritic branches, distributed within a white or red background; possibly the early stage of arborizing telangiectasias (Fig. 7.9)
4. Multiple small and shallow erosions. More than 5 with a maximum diameter ≤1 mm; possibly the early stage of ulcerations

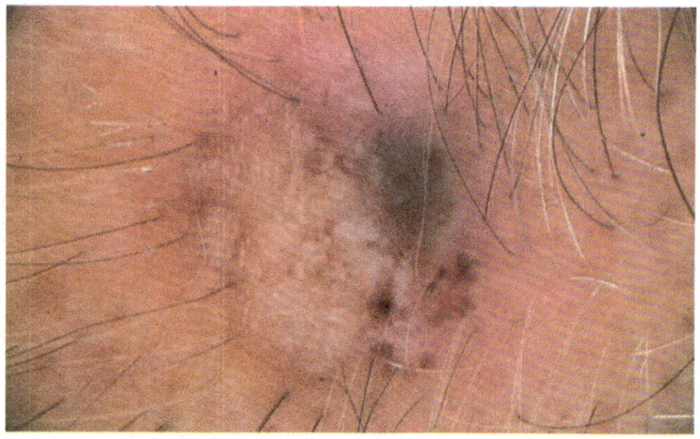

Fig. 7.10 Shiny white areas (×20)

5. Shiny white areas/crystalline structures (Fig. 7.10)
6. Blue-white veil/blue-white veil variant (Fig. 7.11)
7. Yellow-white structures

The blue-white veil variant is a bluish-white structure that appears diffusely throughout the lesion and may be surrounded by ulcerative foci and dendritic vessels. The blue-white veil variant is less common than the typical blue-white veil and histopathologically corresponds to anisotropic basal cell aggregates in the inner dermal nucleus accompanied by more diffusely distributed melanophages with fibrous hyperplasia between nests of atypical cells. In addition, the hyperkeratosis and thickening of the granular layer observed in typical blue-white veil structures are not observed in the blue-white veil variant (Figs. 7.12, 7.13, 7.14, 7.15, and 7.16).

Some of the nonclassic features might be the early stages of relative classic features. Arborizing vessels may look like small fine telangiectasias with pressure under contact dermoscopy. The use of noncontact dermoscopy is highly recommended in lesions with vascular structures.

In BCC, the dermoscopic features of melanocyte-derived lesions, such as MMs and benign melanocytic tumors, can also be observed (Table 7.2).

7.1.2 Nonpigmented Basal Cell Carcinomas in Dermoscopy

A clear diagnosis is often difficult to make in non-PBCCs. The differential diagnosis includes squamous cell carcinoma, Bowen's disease, skin appendage tumors, and inflammatory skin diseases. The dermoscopic features of non-PBCCs have been well established in recent years as dermoscopy has been developed. Dermoscopy can be an effective auxiliary diagnostic tool in non-PBCCs.

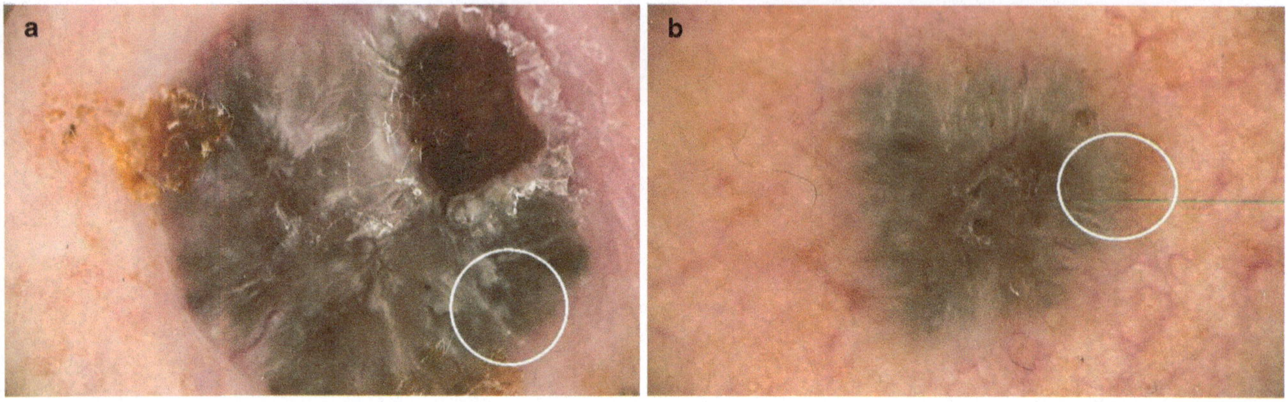

Fig. 7.11 Blue-white veil (white circle) (×20)

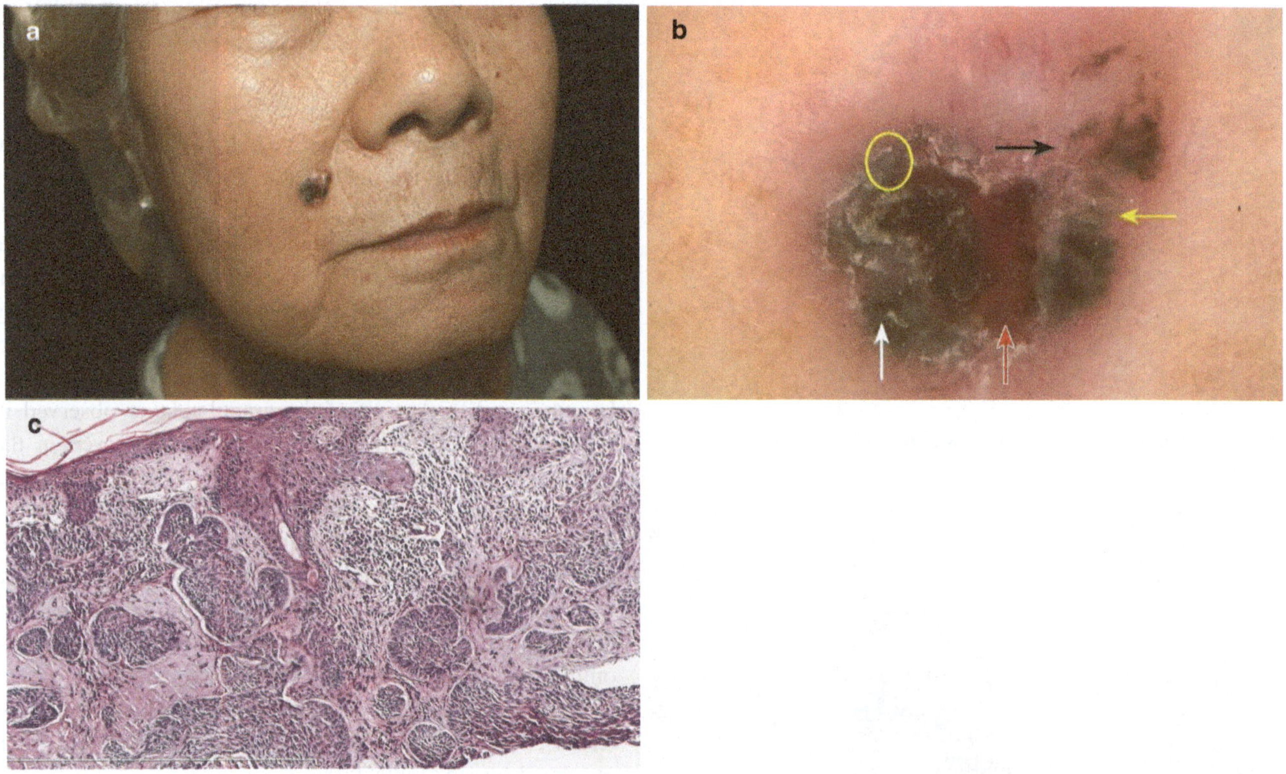

Fig. 7.12 Pigmented basal cell carcinoma. (**a**) Clinical image of a pigmented basal cell carcinoma. (**b**) Dermoscopic image: Large blue-gray ovoid nests (white arrow), leaflike areas (yellow arrow), arborizing vessels (black arrow), ulceration (red arrow), blue-white veil (yellow circle) (×20). (**c**) Histopathological image of a pigmented basal cell carcinoma (hematoxylin and eosin, ×40)

7.1.2.1 The Dermoscopic Features of Nonpigmented Basal Cell Carcinomas

1. Small fine telangiectasias. Less than 1 mm in length, twisted and no evident dendritic branches, distributed within a white or red background; possibly the early stage of arborizing vessels.
2. Multiple vascular structures. Including hairpin vessels, corkscrew vessels, and comma vessels.
3. Multiple small and shallow erosions. More than 5 with a maximum diameter ≤1 mm; possibly the early stage of ulcerations.
4. Shiny white areas/crystalline structures (can be visualized only with polarized dermoscopy).
5. Rosette sign (can be visualized only with polarized dermoscopy).
6. Milky-pink areas/shiny white-red structureless areas.

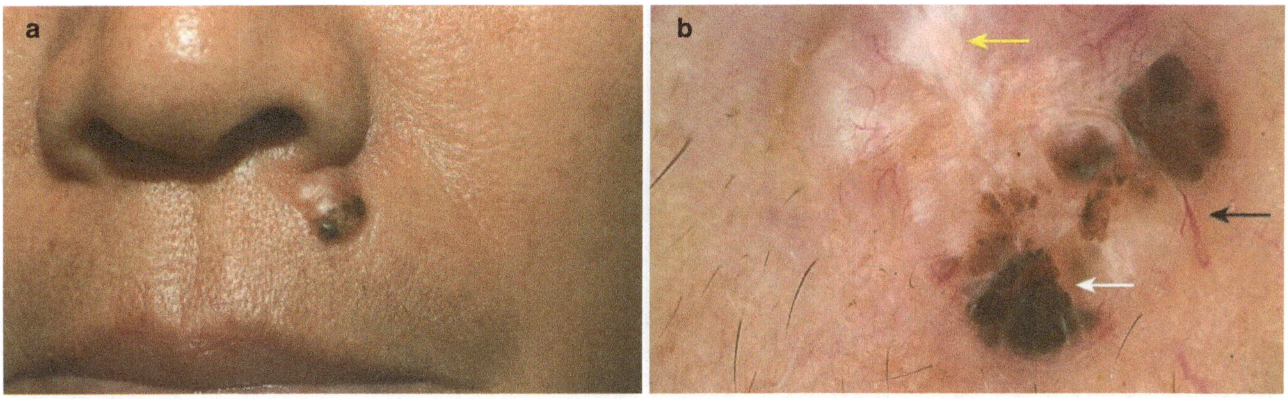

Fig. 7.13 Pigmented basal cell carcinoma. (**a**) Clinical image of a pigmented basal cell carcinoma. (**b**) Dermoscopic image: Large blue-gray ovoid nests (white arrow), arborizing vessels (black arrow), shiny white areas (yellow arrow) (×40)

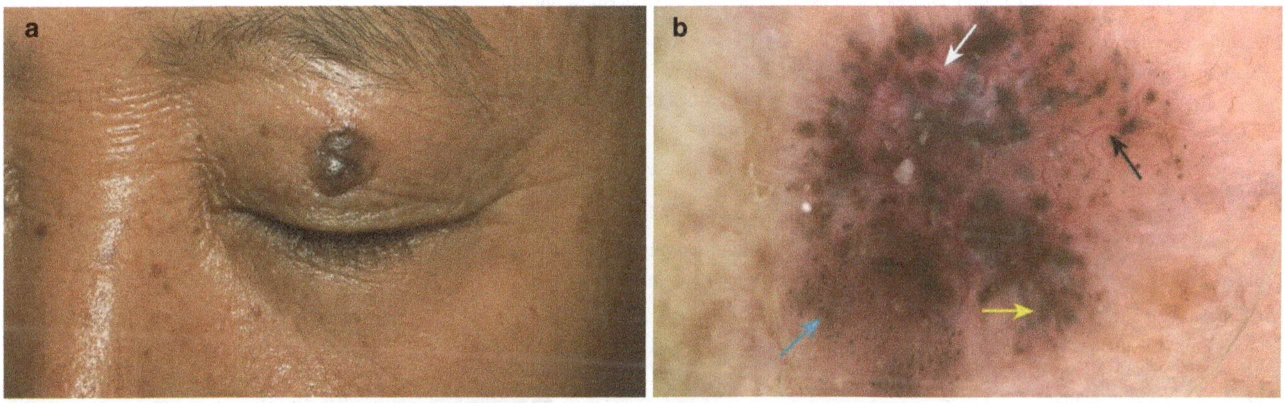

Fig. 7.14 Pigmented basal cell carcinoma. (**a**) Clinical image of a pigmented basal cell carcinoma. (**b**) Dermoscopic image: Large blue-gray ovoid nests (white arrow), multiple in-focus blue/gray dots (blue arrow), leaflike areas (yellow arrow), arborizing vessels (black arrow) (×20)

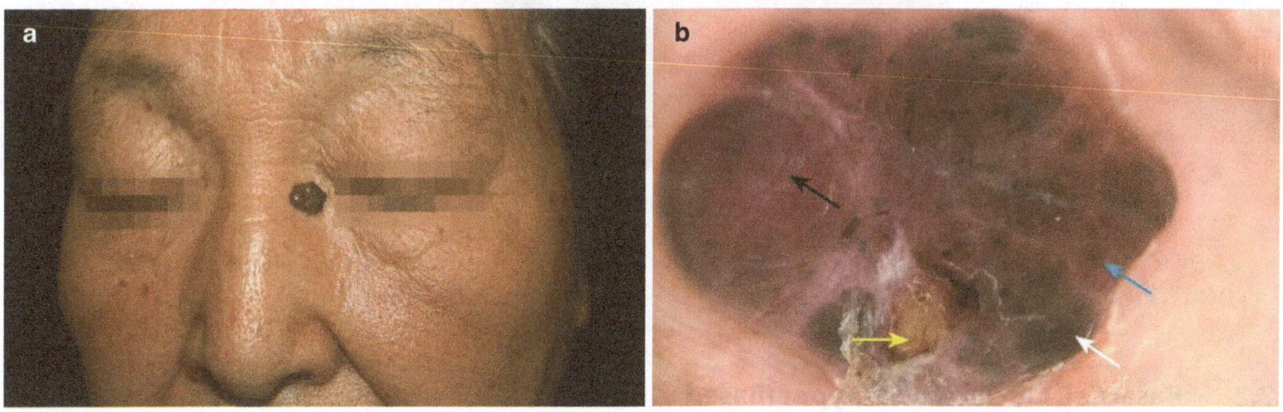

Fig. 7.15 Pigmented basal cell carcinoma. (**a**) Clinical image of a pigmented basal cell carcinoma. (**b**) Dermoscopic image: Large blue-gray ovoid nests (white arrow), multiple in-focus blue/gray dots (blue arrow), arborizing vessels (black arrow), ulcerations (yellow arrow) (×20)

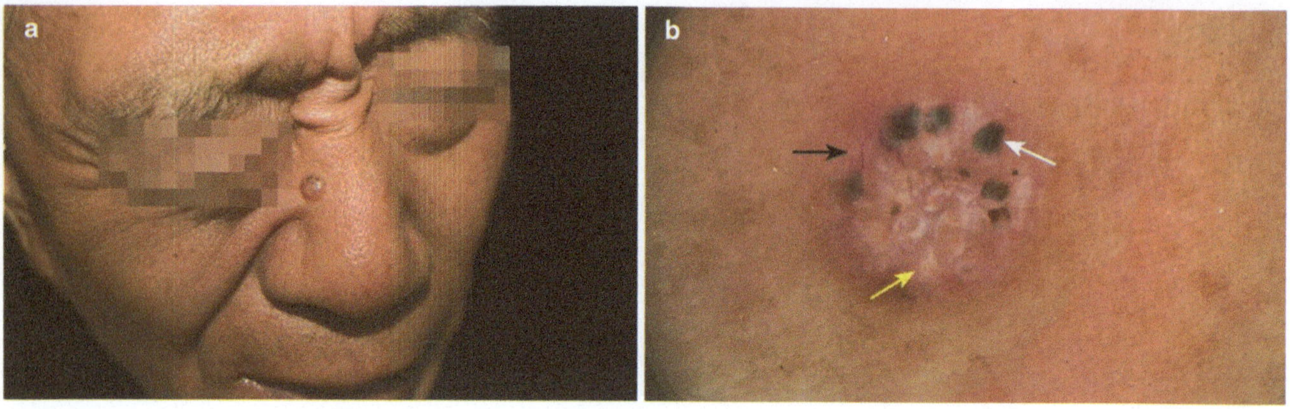

Fig. 7.16 Pigmented basal cell carcinoma. (**a**) Clinical image of a pigmented basal cell carcinoma. (**b**) Dermoscopic image: Large blue-gray ovoid nests (white arrow), arborizing vessels (black arrow), shiny white areas (yellow arrow) (×20)

Table 7.2 The features of BCC and MM/benign melanocytic tumors in dermoscopy

Dermoscopic features		BCC	MM/benign melanocytic tumors
Pigmented globules	Color	Blue-gray (sometimes brown)	Brown/black (sometimes blue)
	Location	Irregular	Aggregated
	Backgrounds	–	Brown
Streaks	Feature	Fuzzy	Clear
	Distribution	Some radiate	Always radiate
Hubs		White/hypopigmented/structureless	Pigmented/blue-white veil
Others		Other BCC features	Other melanocytic features

BCC basal cell carcinoma, *MM* malignant melanoma

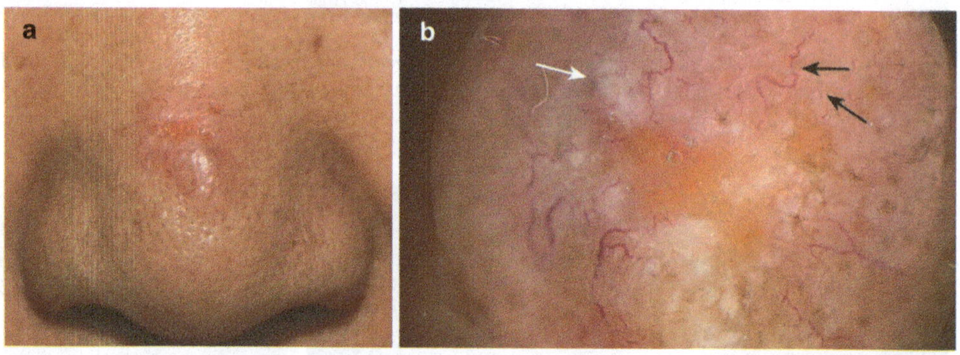

Fig. 7.17 Nonpigmented basal cell carcinoma. (**a**) Clinical image of a nonpigmented basal cell carcinoma. (**b**) Dermoscopic image: Shiny white areas (white arrow), corkscrew and arborizing vessels (black arrow) (×20)

Vascular structures are more common in non-PBCCs than in PBCCs (Figs. 7.17 and 7.18).

7.2 Basal Cell Carcinoma Subtypes (Based on the Pathological Classification Type)

The classification of BCC pathological types can help to guide the selection of treatment plans and posttreatment follow-up (Fig. 7.19).

7.2.1 Superficial Basal Cell Carcinomas in Dermoscopy

7.2.1.1 The Dermoscopic Features of Superficial Basal Cell Carcinomas

1. Leaflike structures
2. Small fine telangiectasias
3. Multiple small erosions
4. Milky-pink areas/shiny white-red background structureless areas
5. No arborizing vessels and no ulcerations (Fig. 7.20)

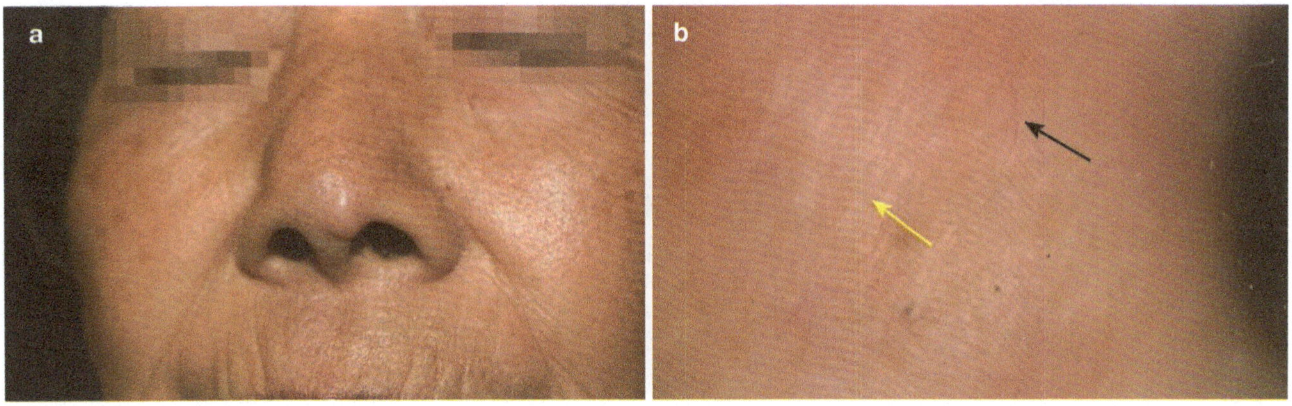

Fig. 7.18 Nonpigmented basal cell carcinoma. (**a**) Clinical image of a nonpigmented basal cell carcinoma. (**b**) Dermoscopic image: Shiny white areas (yellow arrow), arborizing vessels (black arrow) (×20)

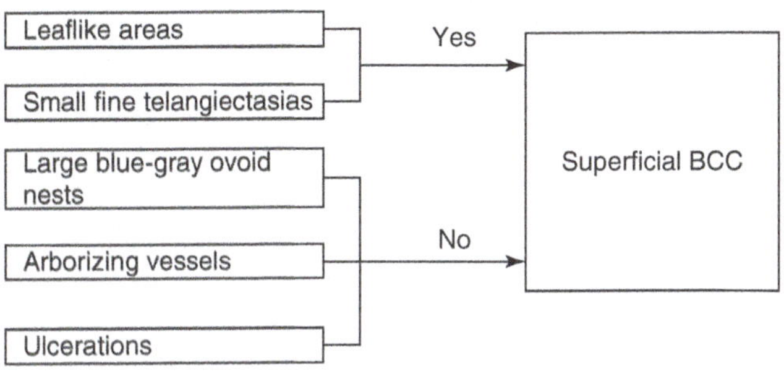

Fig. 7.19 Flowchart for the diagnosis of a superficial basal cell carcinoma (BCC)

Dermoscopy can assist in the differential diagnosis of superficial BBC and Bowen's disease (Table 7.3).

7.2.2 Nonsuperficial Basal Cell Carcinomas in Dermoscopy

7.2.2.1 The Dermoscopic Features of Nodular Basal Cell Carcinomas

1. Arborizing vessels
2. Large blue-gray ovoid nests
3. Multiple in-focus blue/gray dots
4. Ulcerations

> **Tip**
> Nodular BCC is the most common subtype of BCC.
> Large blue/gray ovoid nests are the most common pigmented structures in nonsuperficial BCCs.
> The presence of both branched vessels and ulcerations suggests a high likelihood of skin recurrence.

7.2.2.2 The Dermoscopic Features of Infiltrating Basal Cell Carcinomas

1. Arborizing vessels (smaller and with fewer branches)
2. Milky-pink areas
3. Large blue-gray ovoid nests and/or multiple in-focus blue/gray dots
4. Stellate pattern. A star-like appearance can be created by blood-filled vessels, surface morphology folds, or white linear mstructures

The stellate pattern has a higher incidence in infiltrating BCCs than in other BCC subtypes (Figs. 7.21, 7.22, and 7.23).

The concept of the "signature pattern" of BCCs has been recently introduced, referring to the observation that multiple BCCs in an individual usually display a repetitive dermoscopic pattern (Figs. 7.24 and 7.25).

Approximately 30% of PBCCs are misdiagnosed as non-PBCCs.

Pigmented structures can be found in all BCC types, corresponding to histopathological pigmentary incontinence or increased melanophagocytes located at the dermal–epidermal junction or in the dermis.

If the pathological changes are located at the dermal–epidermal junction, brownish features such as leaflike structures, spoke-wheel-like structures, and concentric structures can be observed. The probability that these lesions are superficial or infiltrating basal cell carcinomas is high.

If the pathological changes are located in the deep dermis areas, blue/gray features, such as blue/gray ovoid nests, multiple blue/gray globules, and multiple in-focus blue/gray dots, can be observed. The probability that these lesions are nodular basal cell carcinomas is high.

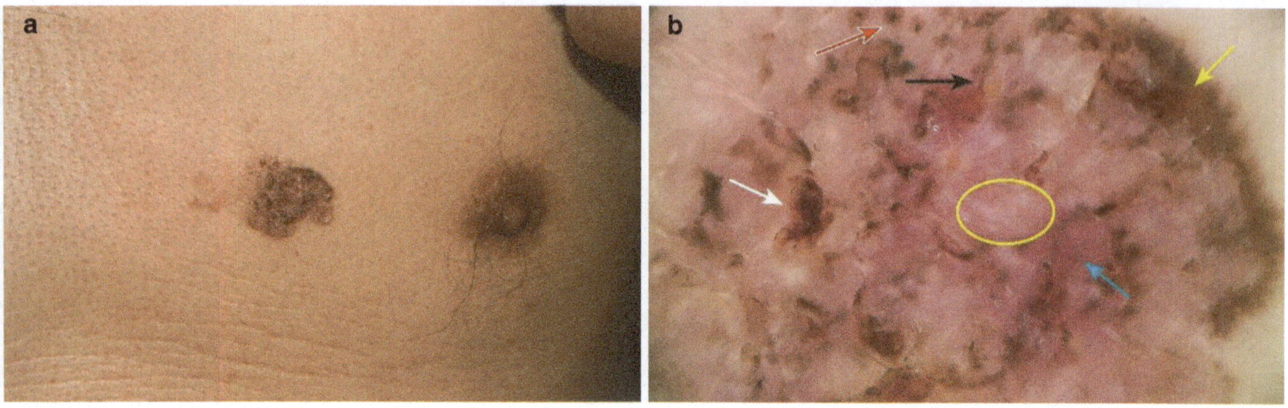

Fig. 7.20 Superficial BCC. (**a**) Clinical image of a superficial basal cell carcinoma. (**b**) Dermoscopic image: Leaflike areas (yellow arrow), concentric structures (red arrow), follicular plugs (black arrow), shiny white areas (yellow circle), multiple small erosions (white arrow), milky-pink areas (blue arrow) (×40)

Table 7.3 Superficial BCC and Bowen's disease in dermoscopy

Dermoscopic features	Superficial BCC	Bowen's disease
Pigmented structures	+++	+
Vascular structures		
Arborizing vessels/small fine telangiectasias	+++	+
Dots/globules	+, most on legs	+++
Shiny white streaks	+++	+
Ulcerations/erosions	+	+
Scales	White	White/yellow

BCC basal cell carcinoma

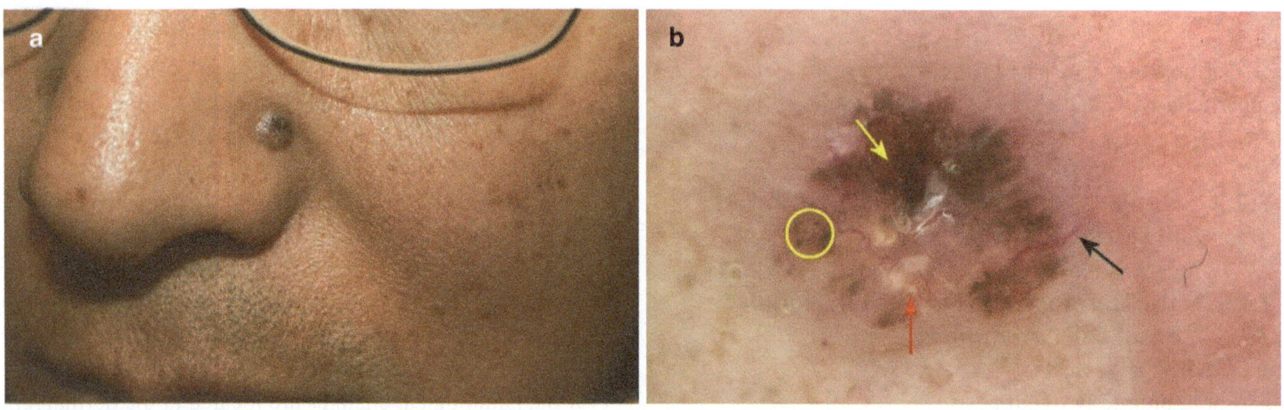

Fig. 7.21 Nodular basal cell carcinoma. (**a**) Clinical image of a nodular basal cell carcinoma. (**b**) Dermoscopic image: Arborizing vessels (black arrow), large blue-gray ovoid nests (yellow arrow), multiple in-focus blue/gray dots (yellow circle), milia-like cysts (red arrow) (×20)

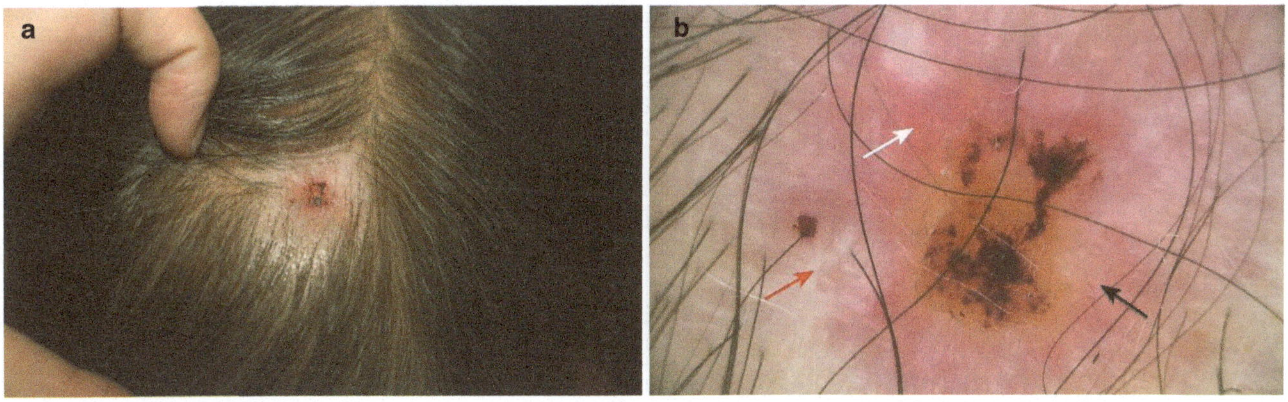

Fig. 7.22 Infiltrating basal cell carcinoma. (**a**) Clinical image of an infiltrating basal cell carcinoma. (**b**) Dermoscopic image: Arborizing vessels (black arrow), milky-pink areas (white arrow), shiny white streaks (red arrow), ulcerations in the center of the lesion, with the stellate pattern (×20)

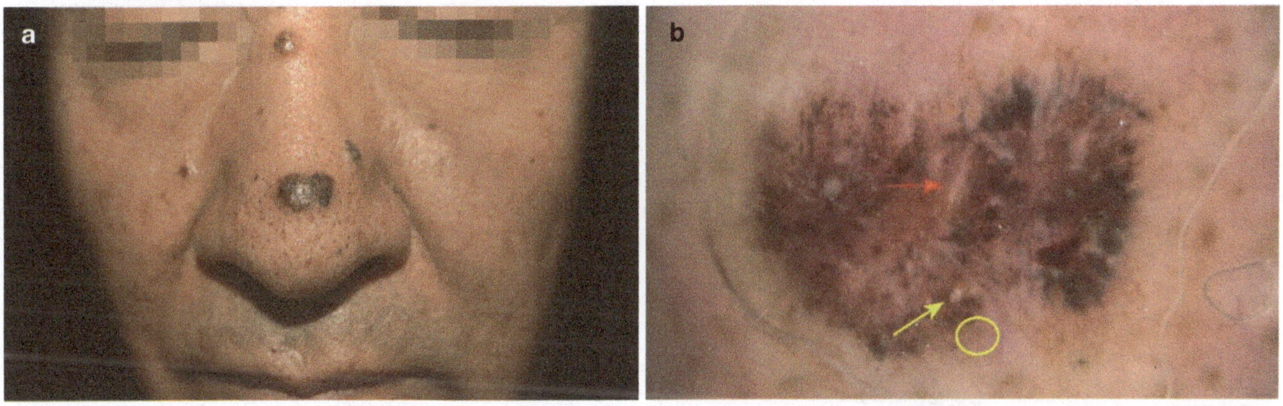

Fig. 7.23 Mixed basal cell carcinoma (nodular basal cell carcinoma and micronodular basal cell carcinoma). (**a**) Clinical image of a mixed basal cell carcinoma. (**b**) Dermoscopic image: Large blue-gray ovoid nests (yellow arrow), multiple in-focus blue/gray dots (yellow circle), ulcerations, shiny white streaks (red arrow), milia-like cysts and arborizing vessels (×40)

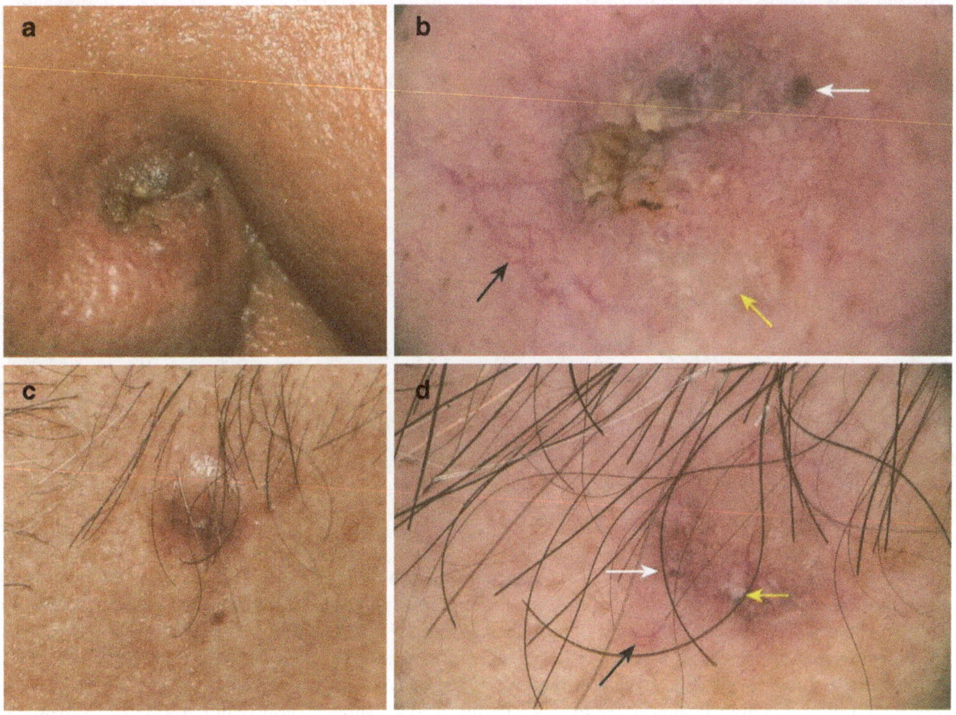

Fig. 7.24 Multiple basal cell carcinoma. (**a**) Clinical image of lesion a. (**b**) Dermoscopic image of lesion a: Arborizing vessels (black arrow), large blue-gray ovoid nests (white arrow), shiny white streaks (yellow arrow) (×20). (**c**) Clinical image of lesion b. (**d**) Dermoscopic image of lesion b: Arborizing vessels (black arrow), multiple in-focus blue/gray dots (white arrow), shiny white streaks (yellow arrow) (×20)

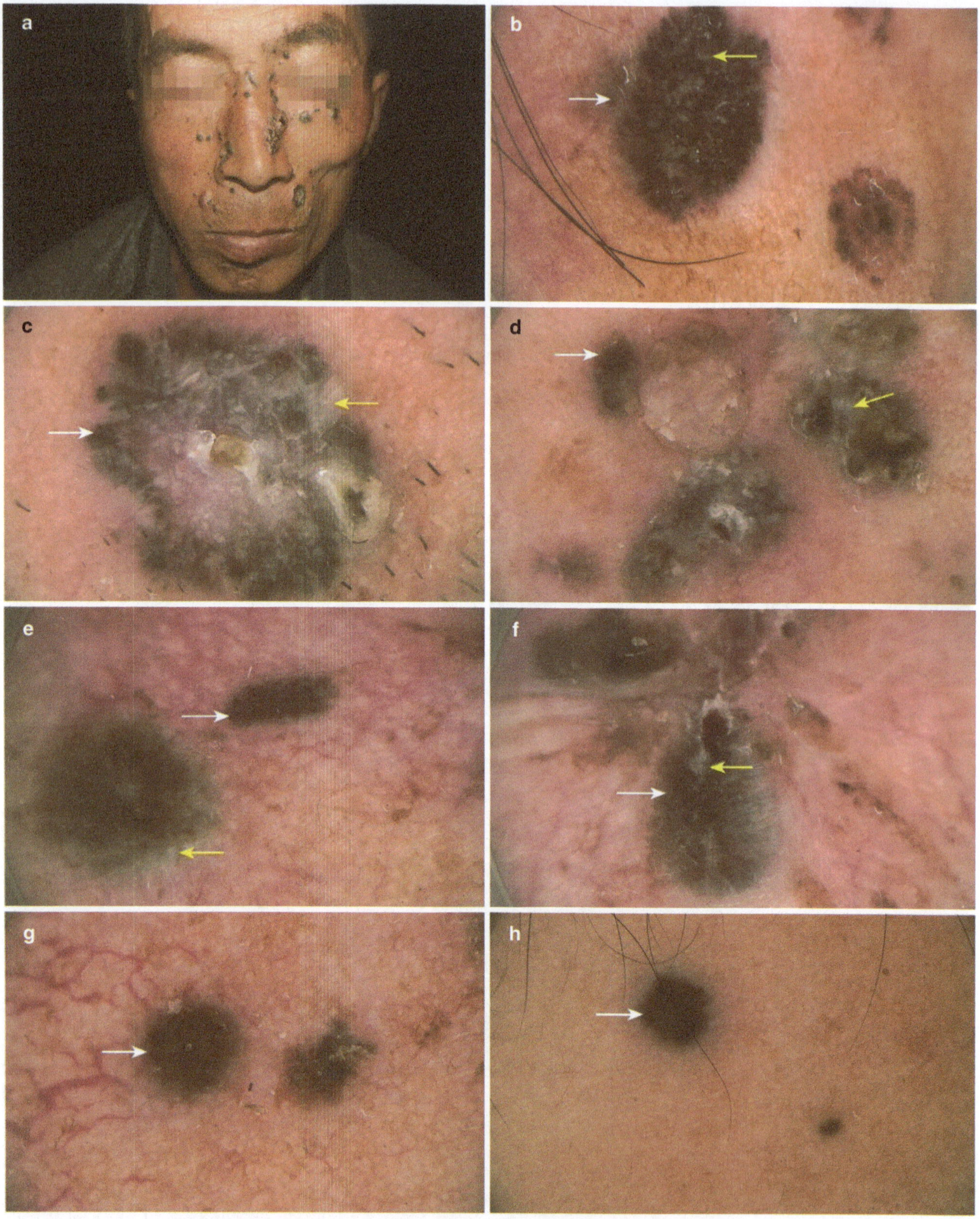

Fig. 7.25 Multiple basal cell carcinoma. (**a**) Clinical image of multiple basal cell carcinoma. (**b**) Dermoscopic image of lesion a: Large blue/gray ovoid nests (white arrow), shiny white streaks (yellow arrow) (×20). (**c**) Dermoscopic image of lesion b: Large blue/gray ovoid nests (white arrow), shiny white streaks (yellow arrow) (×20). (**d**) Dermoscopic image of lesion c: Large blue/gray ovoid nests (white arrow), shiny white streaks (yellow arrow) (×20). (**e**) Dermoscopic image of lesion d: Large blue/gray ovoid nests (white arrow), shiny white streaks (yellow arrow) (×20). (**f**) Dermoscopic image of lesion e: Large blue/gray ovoid nests (white arrow), shiny white streaks (yellow arrow), ulcerations (×20). (**g**) Dermoscopic image of lesion f: Large blue/gray ovoid nests (white arrow) (×20). (**h**) Dermoscopic image of lesion g: Large blue/gray ovoid nests (white arrow) (×20)

Further Reading

1. Devine C, Srinivasan B, Sayan A, et al. Epidemiology of basal cell carcinoma: a 10-year comparative study. Br J Oral Maxillofac Surg. 2018;56(2):101–6.
2. Lallasz A, Tellos T, Kyrgidis A, et al. Accuracy of dermoscopic criteria for discriminating superficial from other subtypes of basal cell carcinoma. J Am Acad Dermatol. 2014;70(2):303–11.
3. Urech M, Kygidisr A, Agenziano G, et al. Dermoscopic ulceration is a predictor of basal cell carcinoma response to imiquimod: a retrospective study. Acta Derm Venereol. 2017;97(1):117–9.
4. Trakatelli M, Morton C, Nagore E, et al. Update of the European guidelines for basal cell carcinoma management. Eur J Dermatol. 2014;24(3):312–29.
5. Diluvio L, Bavetta M, Di Prete M, et al. Dermoscopic monitoring of efficacy of ingenol mebutate in the treatment of pigmented and non-pigmented basal cell carcinomas. Dermatol Ther. 2017;30(1) https://doi.org/10.1111/dth.12438.
6. Menzies SW, Westerhoff K, Rabinovitz H, et al. Surface microscopy of pigmented basal cell carcinoma. Arch Dermatol. 2000;136(8):1012–6.
7. Lallas A, Argenziano G, Ioannides D. Dermoscopy for basal cell carcinoma subtype prediction. Br J Dermatol. 2016;175(4):674–5.
8. Papageorigiou V, Apalla Z, Sotiriou E, et al. The limitations of dermoscopy: false-positive and false-negative tumours. J Eur Acad Dermatol Venereol. 2018;32(6):879–88.
9. Altamura D, Menzies SW, Argenziano G, et al. Dermatoscopy of basal cell carcinoma: morphologic variability of global and local features and accuracy of diagnosis. J Am Acad Dermatol. 2010;62(1):67–75.
10. Weiwei L, Ping T, Shuxia Y, et al. Dermoscopy in the differential diagnosis of basal cell carcinoma: a preliminary study. Chin J Dermatol. 2013;46(7):480–4.
11. Arits AH, Mosterd K, Essers BA, et al. Photodynamic therapy versus topical imiquimod versus topical fluorouracil for treatment of superficial basal-cell carcinoma: a single blind, non-inferiority, randomised controlled trial. Lancet Oncol. 2013;14(7):647–54.
12. Navarrete-Dechent C, Bajaj S, Marchetti MA, et al. Association of shiny white blotches and strands with nonpigmented basal cell carcinoma: evaluation of an additional dermoscopic diagnostic criterion. JAMA Dermatol. 2016;152(5):546–52.
13. Turkmen M, Gerceker Turk B, Kilinc Karaarslan I, et al. Blue-white variant of pigmented basal cell carcinoma. Dermatologica Sinica. 2018;36(3):136–9.
14. Marghoob AA, Braun R. Atlas of dermoscopy. 2nd ed. Boca Raton, FL: CRC; 2012.
15. Trigoni A, Lazaridou E, Apalla Z, et al. Dermoscopic features in the diagnosis of different types of basal cell carcinoma: a prospective analysis. Hippokratia. 2012;16(1):29–34.
16. Pan Y, Chamberlain AJ, Bailey M, et al. Dermatoscopy aids in the diagnosis of the solitary red scaly patch or plaque-features distinguishing superficial basal cell carcinoma, intraepidermal carcinoma, and psoriasis. J Am Acad Dermatol. 2008;59(2):268–74.
17. Arpaia N, Filoni A, Bonamonte D, et al. Vascular patterns in cutaneous ulcerated basal cell carcinoma: a retrospective blinded study including dermoscopy. Acta Derm Venereol. 2017;97(5):612–6.
18. Emiroglu N, Cengiz FP, Kemeriz F. The relation between dermoscopy and histopathology of basal cell carcinoma. An Bras Dermatol. 2015;90(3):351–6.
19. Verduzco-Martinez AP, Quinones-Venegas R, Guevara-Gutierrez E, et al. Correlation of dermoscopic findings with histopathologic variants of basal cell carcinoma. Int J Dermatol. 2013;52(6):718–21.
20. Zalaudek I, Kreusch J, Giacomel J, et al. How to diagnose non-pigmented skin tumors: a review of vascular structures seen with dermoscopy: part II. Nonmelanocytic skin tumors. J Am Acad Dermatol. 2010;63(3):377–86.
21. Pyne JH, Fishburn P, Dicker A, et al. Infiltrating basal cell carcinoma: a stellate peri-tumor dermatoscopy pattern as a clue to diagnosis. Dermatol Pract Concept. 2015;5(2):21–6.
22. Zalaudek I, Moscarella E, Longo C, et al. The "signature" pattern of multiple Basal cell carcinomas. Arch Dermatol. 2012;148(9):1106.
23. Lallas A, Argenziano G, Kyrgidis A, et al. Dermoscopy uncovers clinically undetectable pigmentation in basal cell carcinoma. Br J Dermatol. 2014;170(1):192–5.
24. Tabanlioglu Onan D, Sahin S, Gokoz O, et al. Correlation between the dermatoscopic and histopathological features of pigmented basal cell carcinoma. J Eur Acad Dermatol Venereol. 2010;24(11):1317–25.

Seborrheic Keratosis and Related Disorders

8

Solar lentigo (SL), seborrheic keratosis (SK), and lichen planus-like keratosis (LPLK) are common benign epidermal proliferative diseases that mostly arise from natural epidermal aging and photoaging. Dermoscopy plays an essential role in the definitive diagnosis, differentiation from other skin tumors, the avoidance of unnecessary biopsy or surgery, and regular dynamic monitoring of lesion changes. In this chapter, the dermoscopic features of these three diseases are discussed, with a focus on SK.

8.1 Solar Lentigo

SL, also known as lentigo senilis and senile lentigo, is an early manifestation of SK whose etiology is related to ultraviolet exposure and skin aging. SL manifests as multiple light-brown patches ranging from a few millimeters to several centimeters in diameter and from light to dark brown (Fig. 8.1). SL is not a true melanocytic lesion, and its histological manifestations are increased melanin deposition in keratinocytes and a mild increase in the number of melanocytes, which are distributed linearly at the epidermal–dermal junction.

Typical dermoscopic features of SL:

1. Clear edges
2. Moth-eaten border: crenelated margins with clear edges
3. Faint pigment network: light-brown reticulated lines
4. Fingerprint-like pattern: brown parallel and curved fine lines
5. Homogenous light brown pigmentation: brown structureless areas, the "jelly sign," that appear similar to brown jelly coated on the skin
6. Pseudonetwork: brown structureless areas with interstitial hair follicles and appendage openings. Sometimes have light-brown concentric circle-like structures around hair follicles.

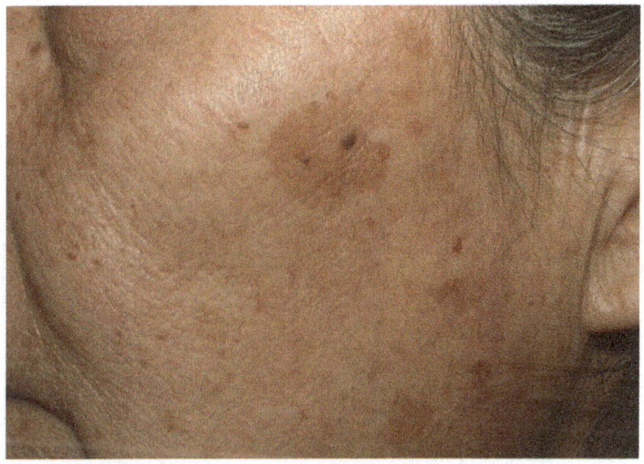

Fig. 8.1 Clinical manifestations of solar lentigo

Clear lesion edges and moth-eaten borders are the main features of SL (Fig. 8.2). The faint pigment network and fingerprint-like pattern are related to an increase in melanin in melanocytes and keratinocytes within rete ridges rather than melanocyte formation. The dermoscopic appearance of SL is related to its location: SL on the trunk may show a faint pigment network and fingerprint-like pattern in yellow to brown (Figs. 8.3 and 8.4); on the extremities, SL mostly shows a brown and homogeneous pattern (Fig. 8.5), with moth-eaten border; and on the face, SL mostly appears as a pseudonetwork, faint pigmented network and fingerprint-like pattern around the openings of the appendages (Fig. 8.6) (Table 8.1).

Sometimes SL also manifests as specific subtypes, such as lichenoid degeneration (or LPLK as described later) or ink spot lentigo. Inkspot lentigo is a kind of dark SL commonly seen in people with light skin color. The lesions are usually independent and appear as a dark-black pigment network with clear but irregular edges. Sudden interruption of the pigment network at the edge of the lesion may be mistaken for malignant melanoma, and close follow-up or biopsy is recommended if a diagnosis cannot be clearly made.

J. Liu, X. Zou, *Practical Dermoscopy*, https://doi.org/10.1007/978-981-19-1460-7_8

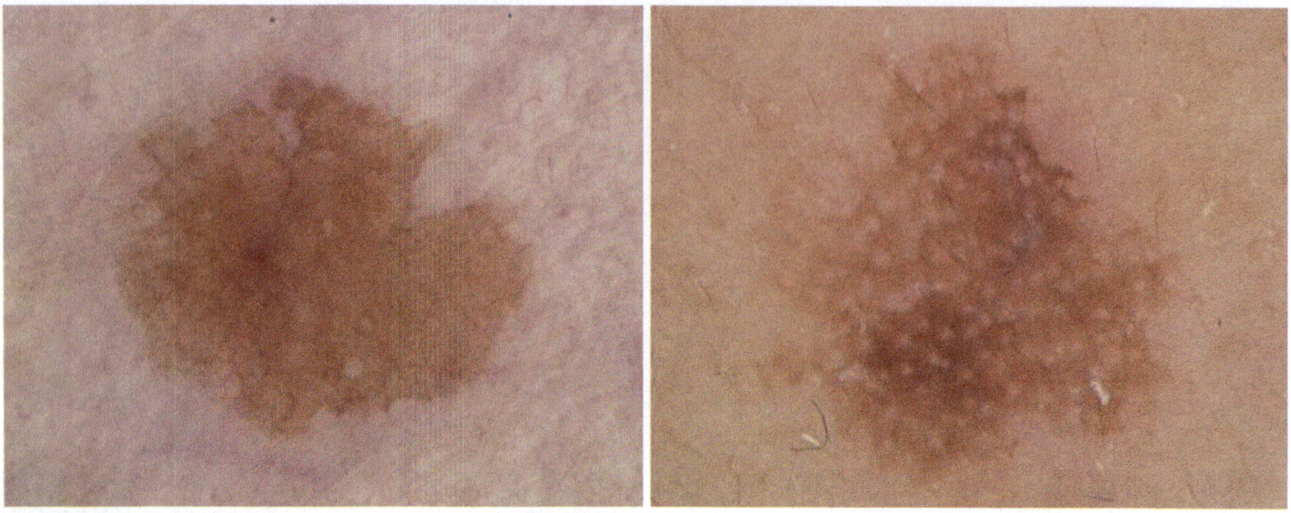

Fig. 8.2 Solar lentigo lesions have clear edges, with moth-eaten borders

Fig. 8.3 Faint pigment network

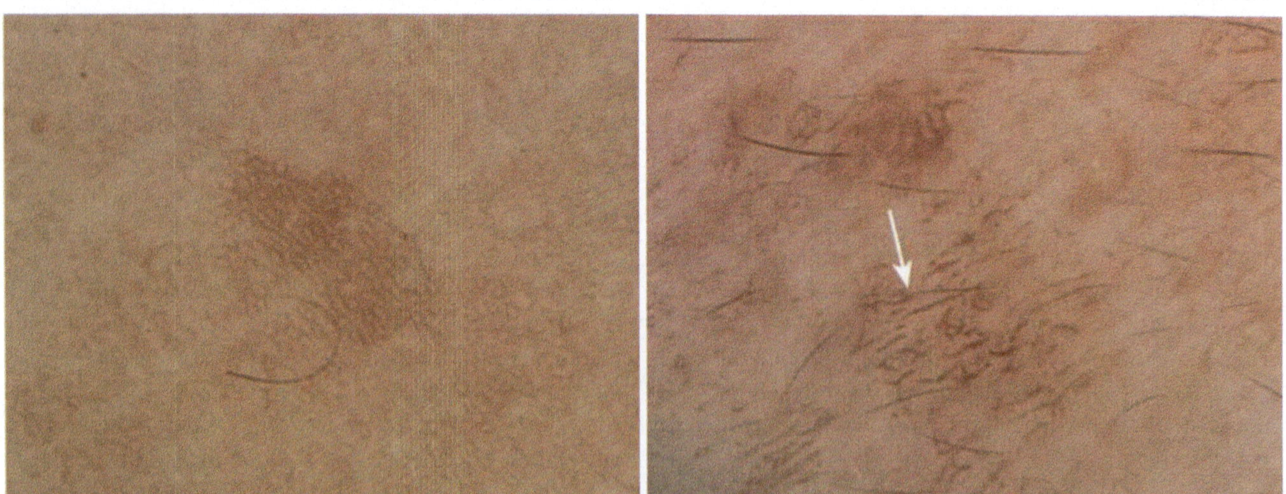

Fig. 8.4 Fingerprint-like pattern

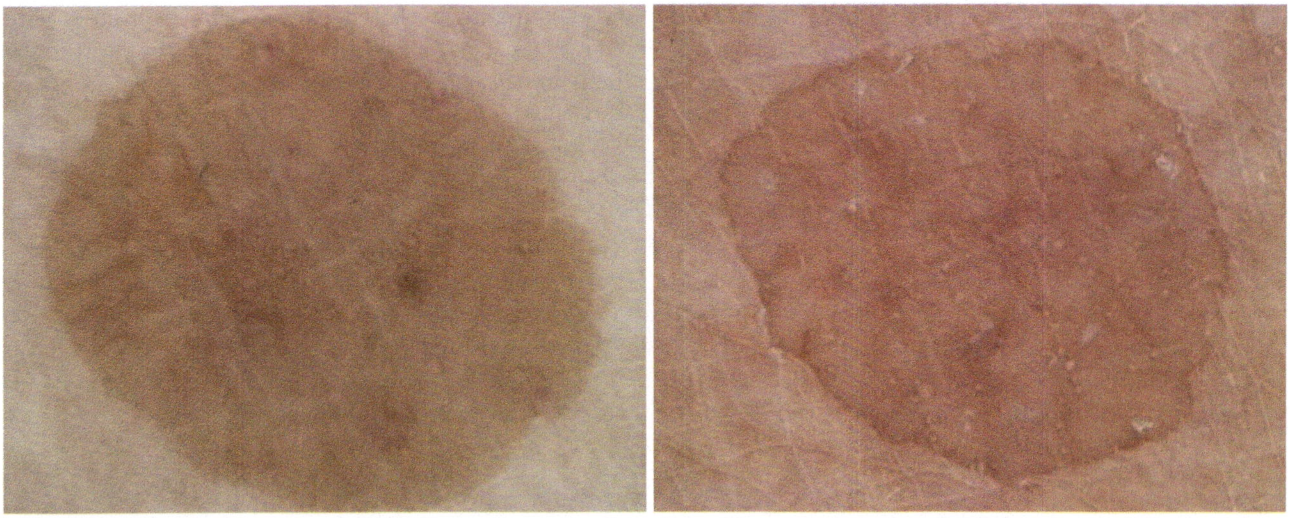

Fig. 8.5 Homogenous pattern

Fig. 8.6 Pseudonetwork

Table 8.1 Differences in the manifestations of SL in different body parts

Region	Patterns of SL
Trunk	Faint pigment network and fingerprint-like pattern
Limbs	Homogeneous brown pattern, with moth-eaten border
Face	Pseudonetwork; faint pigment network and fingerprint-like pattern can also be observed

SL solar lentigo

SL needs to be differentiated from SK, pigmented actinic keratosis (PAK), lentigo maligna (LM), and lentigo maligna melanoma. In particular, LM may similarly appear as a pseudonetwork and homogeneous structure. Attention needs to be paid to the identification of abnormal pigmented structures such as intrafollicular gray dots, asymmetrically pigmented follicular openings, rhombic patterns, and blotches under dermoscopy. LM needs to be considered if one of the following four features is present around appendage openings: ① gray dots or gray circles that differ from the surrounding light brown areas (annular-granular pattern), ② thick and variably colored reticular streaks, ③ dark brown/blue-gray bands, and ④ brown globules. In particular, the presence of blue-gray structures should be considered to possibly indicate LM (rare in SL). Clinically, SL usually manifests multiple lesions with a relatively rough surface, whereas LM is usually an isolated lesion with a smooth surface and less scales. When clinical and dermoscopic features are atypical, further biopsy is recommended to clarify the diagnosis. PAK may also present a pseudonetwork, but the lesions often have follicular openings of varying sizes with keratotic plugs; strawberry-like patterns are visible on a large scale.

8.2 Seborrheic Keratosis

SK is one of the most common benign tumors of epidermal origin, occurring in elderly individuals; therefore, SK lesions are sometimes called senile warts. SL can develop into SK (e.g., adenoid SK). Depending on the histological types, the appearance of SK is variable and may include flat black spots, uniformly thickened and raised brown plaques, verrucous black papules or verrucous tumors that clearly differ from normal skin and may have moth-eaten borders.

Under dermoscopy, SK typically exhibits one or more of the following features (some features differ in polarized and nonpolarized modes):

1. The lesions have sharp edges and moth-eaten borders.
2. Milia-like cysts (Fig. 8.7): white or yellow round structures. These structures sometimes are not easily observed in polarized mode but are clearly observed in nonpolarized (infiltrative) mode. Histopathologically, milia-like cysts appear as keratin-filled cysts within the epidermis.

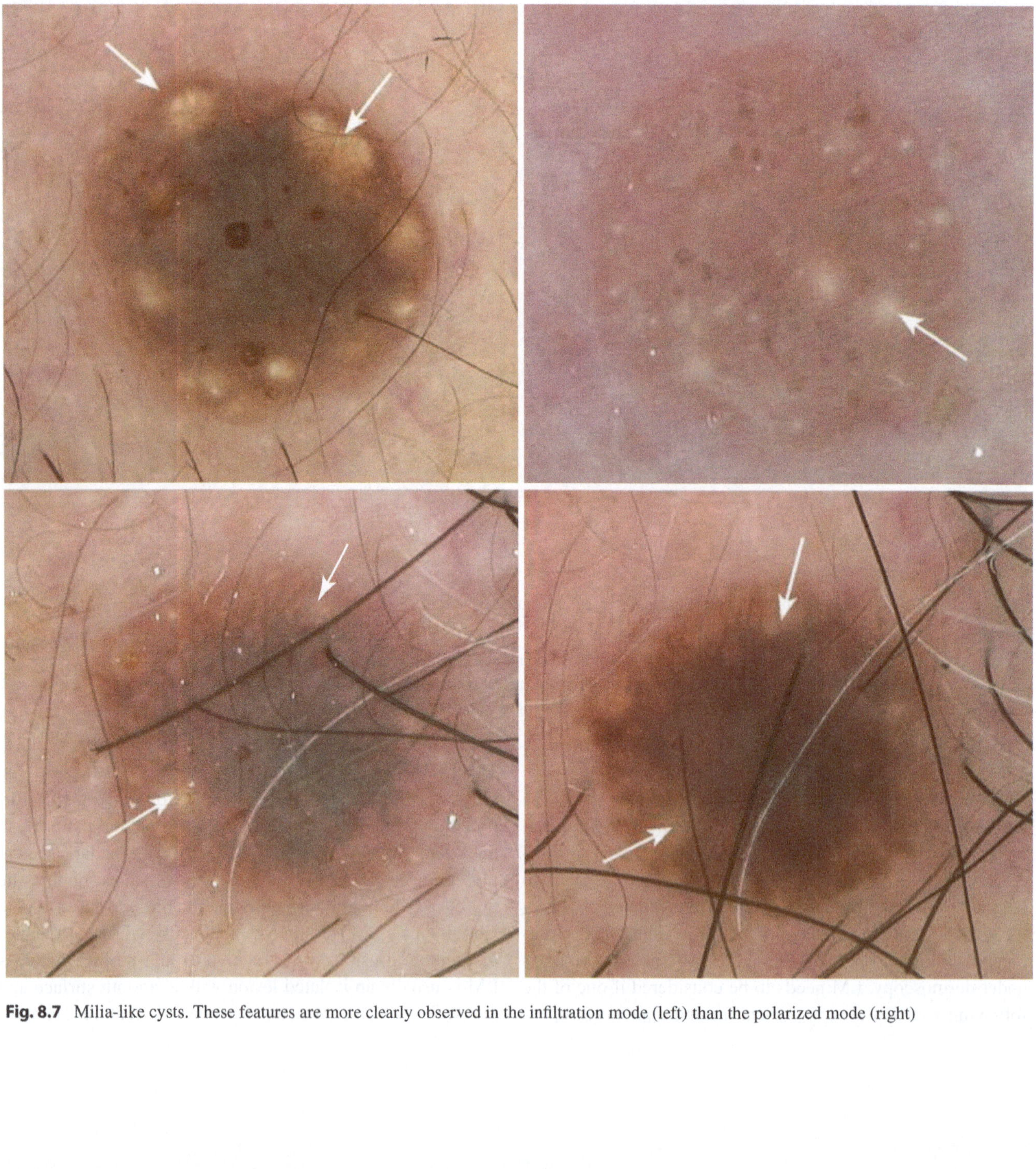

Fig. 8.7 Milia-like cysts. These features are more clearly observed in the infiltration mode (left) than the polarized mode (right)

Larger milia-like cysts are "cloudy" due to unclear edges and have a higher specificity for the diagnosis of SK; smaller and brighter cysts are "starry" and can also be observed in malignant melanoma or basal cell carcinoma.

3. Comedo-like openings (Fig. 8.8): round to ovoid keratin-filled fissures. Comedo-like openings can be brown, orange, yellow, or in rare cases black and are more visible when observed under nonpolarized dermoscopy. Histopathologically, comedo-like openings appear as keratin-filled pits on the skin surface, i.e., a pseudokeratin cyst.

4. Cerebriform pattern: a curved thick line consisting of a keratin-filled sulcus and gyrus, also known as fissures and ridges structures. The cerebriform pattern describes the morphological pattern, and the fissures and ridges describe the structural composition. In the hyperplastic stratum spinosum, elevated SK lesions may appear as thick sulci and gyri, initially as short rod-like, curved, circular, or oval thick lines (sausage-like or fat finger-like) (Fig. 8.9). With increasing hypertrophy of the stratum spinosum, the sulci and gyri may fold to form a cerebriform pattern (Figs. 8.10 and 8.11). When the hyperplasia of the stratum spinosum becomes more pronounced, the

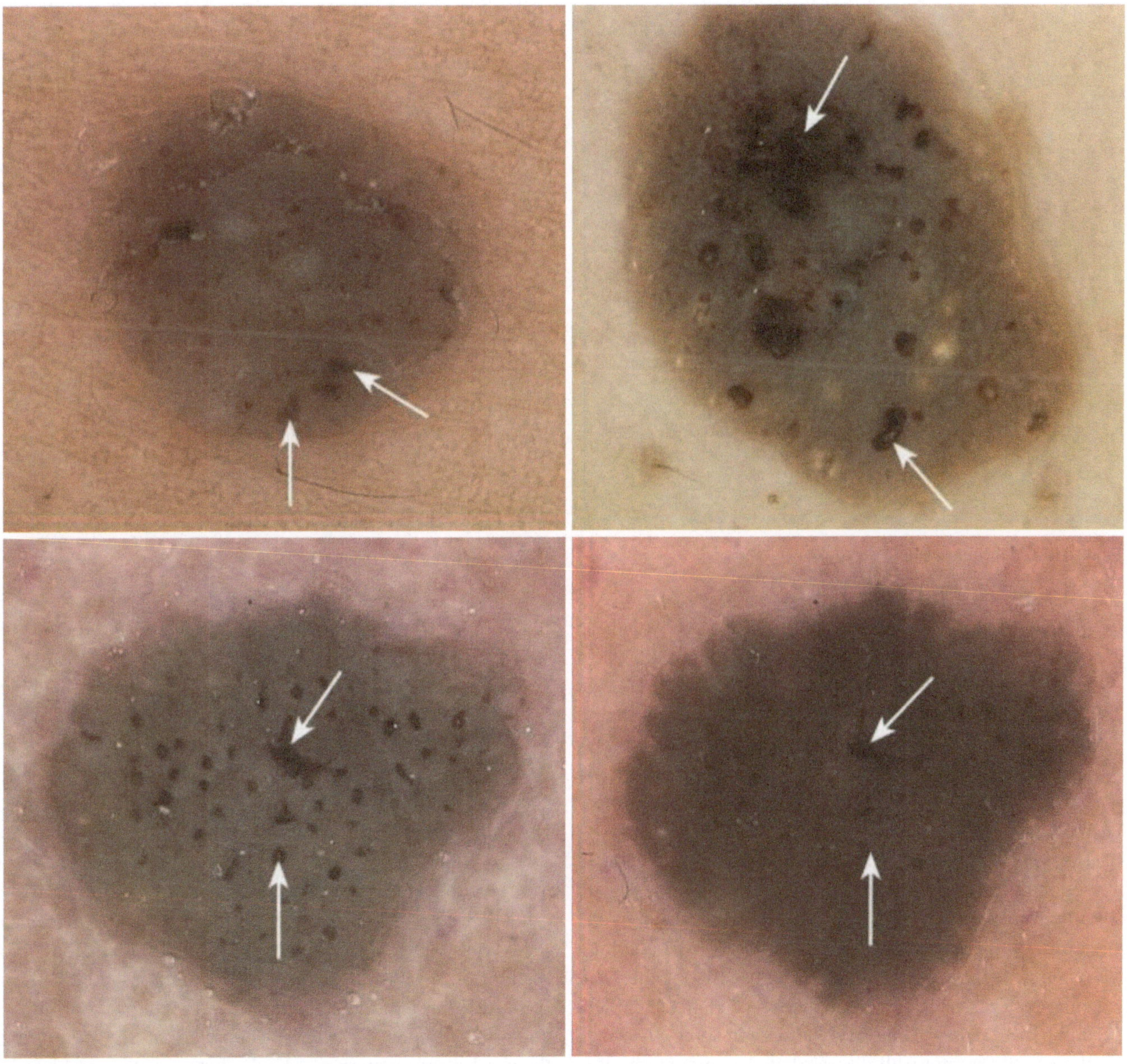

Fig. 8.8 Comedo-like openings. These features are more clearly observed in the infiltration mode (lower left) than the polarized mode (lower right), in a same lesion

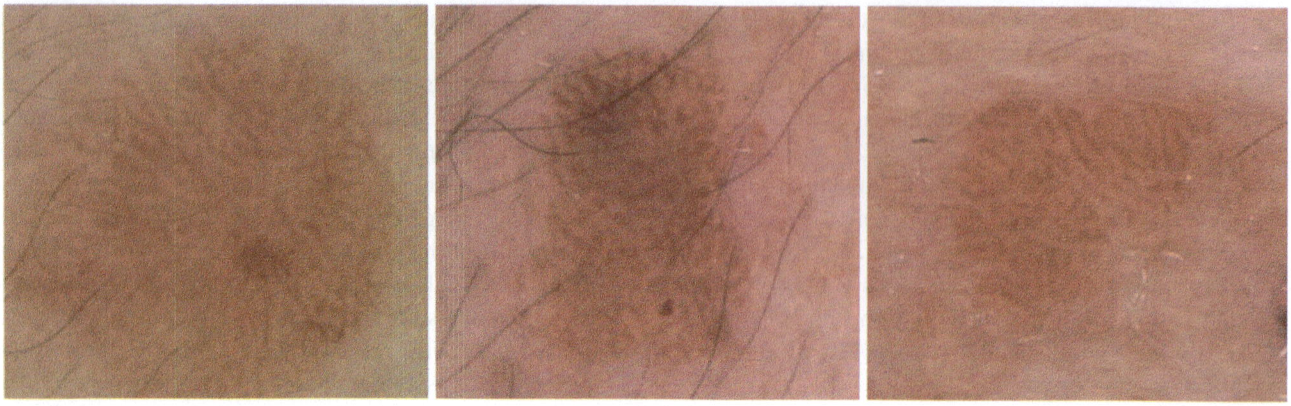

Fig. 8.9 Fat finger-like pattern

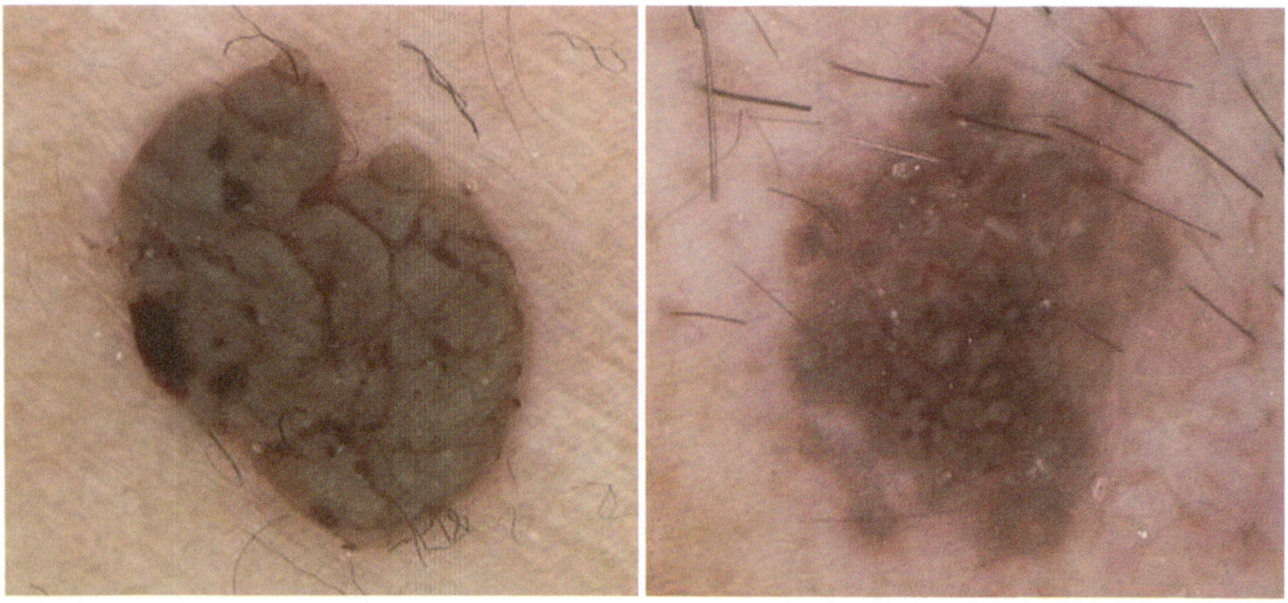

Fig. 8.10 Cerebriform pattern

pigment-rich ridges may be brown or blue-gray, and the fissures or follicular openings may be filled with dark-brown, gray, or blue-gray structureless mass-like keratin, called a crypt (a keratin-filled depression, larger than a pimple-like opening) (Fig. 8.12). The cerebriform patterns and crypts are mostly seen in acanthotic SK. Comedo-like openings and milia-like cysts are more common in these lesions.

5. Hairpin-like vessels: two parallel linear vessels forming a semicircular or looped structure. Hairpin-like vessels are often surrounded by a white halo, which is caused by the proliferation of keratinocytes and is one of the common features of thickened irritated SK (Fig. 8.13). Other vascular patterns, such as the dotted, branched, linear, coiled, and helical patterns, may also be seen in some SK. Since the vessels are not well observed after compression, it is more appropriate to use the noncontact polarized mode to observe them.
6. Overall movement of the skin lesion during the wobble test ("wobble sign"). For lesions that are examined with contact dermoscopy, the wobble test can be performed to assist in differentiating SK from intradermal nevi. SK usually slides with the contact part of the dermoscope, while an intradermal nevus does not slide as a whole.

Comedo-like openings and milia-like cysts are relatively typical structures of SK under dermoscopy and are seen in most types of SK. The more obvious acanthosis is, the more likely such structures appear. Flat SK often resembles SL in its structural pattern, showing brown, yellow, or orange curved thick lines. The fingerprint pattern of SL differs from the cerebriform pattern of SK; the former is thin and barely

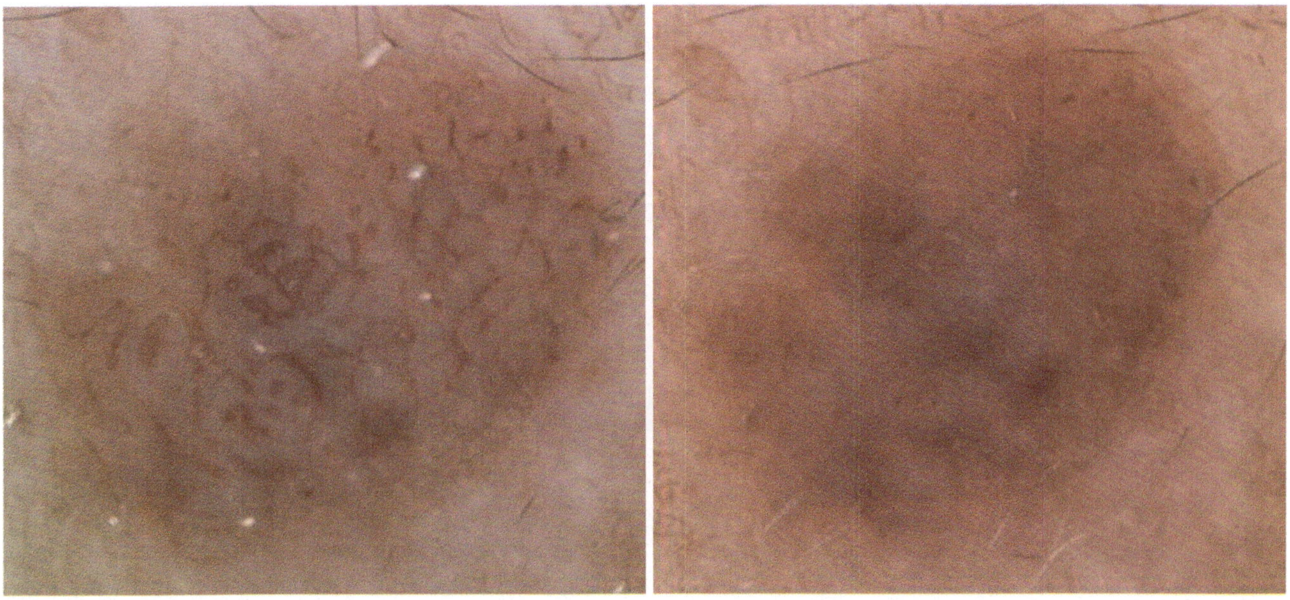

Fig. 8.11 Manifestations of the cerebriform pattern with various observation methods. The same skin lesion with various observation methods. These manifestations are more clearly observed in the infiltration mode (left) than the polarized mode (right)

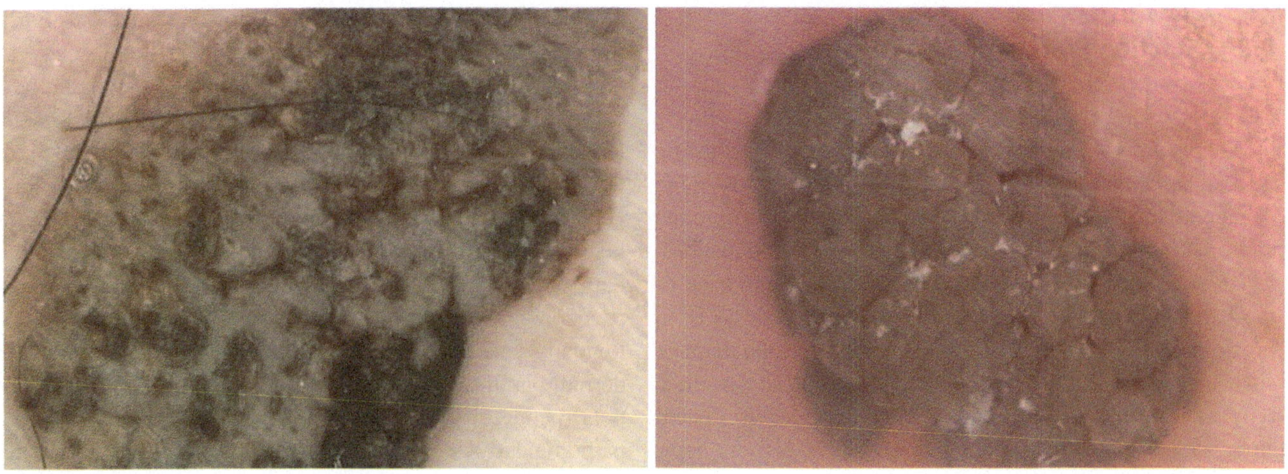

Fig. 8.12 Crypts

protrudes from the skin surface, whereas the pigment network lines of SK are much thicker than those of SL due to the thickened spinosum layer, and comedo-like openings are often seen in the lesions, mostly in reticular SK.

In addition to SL, SK should also be differentiated from verruca vulgaris, verruca plana, malignant melanoma, keratoacanthoma, and AK. Some verruca vulgaris may resemble verrucous SK, but in addition to papillomatous epidermal thickening, verruca vulgaris is characterized by multiple bleeding spots. Verruca plana is sometimes difficult to clearly distinguish from flat SK, especially if the lesions are small. Verruca plana is characterized by dots or globular vessels in a pink to light brown background with a relatively regular distribution and may have scattered bleeding spots, whereas SK is not as obvious and has a more irregular distribution. The diagnosis of malignant melanoma needs to be considered, being especially vigilant for lesions with significant pigmentation, such as the presence of an atypical pigmented network, blue-white structures, irregular dots and globules, pseudopod-like structures, and blue-black blotches. Keratoacanthomas may present with hairpin-like vessels, yet the typical lesions have a volcano-like appearance with predominantly multiple yellow-white structureless areas in the center and may present with a perifollicular white halo or white circular structures. Some AK lesions may also resemble SK lesions, but AK lesions tend to have a strawberry-like pattern and a perifollicular white or blue-gray halo and have no typical structures of SK lesions, such as comedo-like

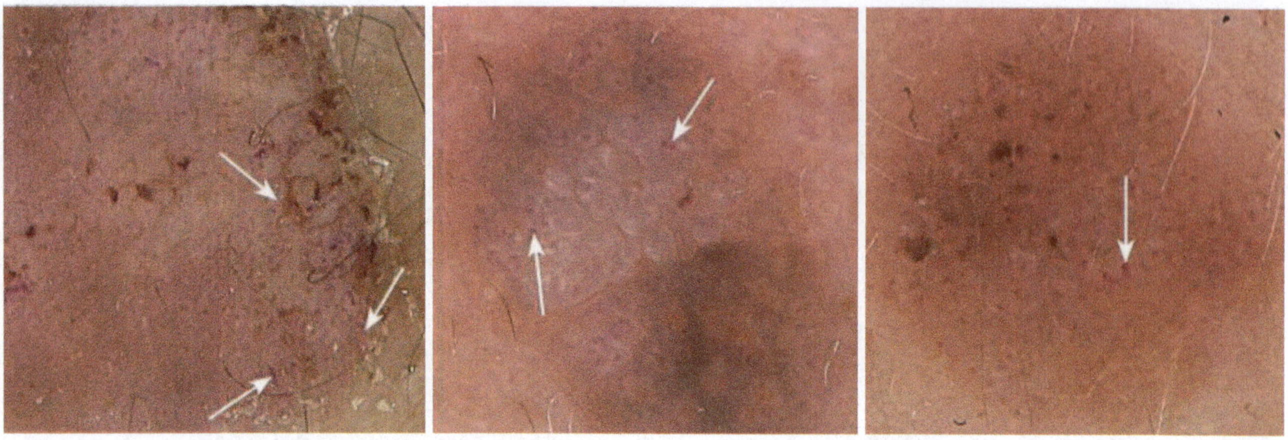

Fig. 8.13 Hairpin-like vessels

openings and milia-like cysts. Since some SKs can be confused with squamous cell carcinoma and malignant melanoma, a biopsy is still recommended for a definitive diagnosis of SK with an atypical dermoscopic presentation (Fig. 8.13).

8.3 Lichen Planus-like Keratosis

LPLK, also known as lichenoid keratosis, was first proposed by Shapiro and Ackerman in 1966. LPLK is not a specific disease but is considered a change in SL, SK, and AK in the degenerative phase, presumably associated with the immune and inflammatory response to the existing skin lesions. LPLK occurs on exposed areas such as the face and back of the hands and clinically presents as isolated pink, gray to brown papules or plaques, often surrounded by solar damage such as SL (Fig. 8.14). Clinically, LPLK can present as three types: flat erythema, flat pigmentation, and plaque. Recent studies have shown that nonpigmented LPLK is more common (61.7% of cases) than pigmented LPLK. In some cases, there is some resemblance to cutaneous malignancies; therefore, biopsy is often required to further clarify the diagnosis.

The dermoscopic features of LPLK are as follows:

1. Pepper-like or granular pattern: composed of fine blue-gray dots that are relatively typical. In completely or nearly completely degenerated LPLK, gray dots may aggregate to form small globules, streaks, or circles around hair follicles (Fig. 8.14). Histopathologically, gray dots are pigment granules or phagocytic cells in the superficial dermis, occasionally with vascular structures and shiny white streaks; the latter histopathologically reflect proliferating collagen in the superficial dermis.
2. Dermoscopic features of SL, SK, or AK are visible in the periphery (Fig. 8.15). Dermoscopic features of primary lesions such as SL, SK, or AK may be observed during degeneration from the primary lesion to LPLK.

The process of SL from onset to degeneration to LPLK has been proposed to be divided into four stages: ① Early inflammation: pink areas can be seen via dermoscopy in areas of homogeneous or pseudonetworks, histopathologically corresponding to superficial dermal and dermal papillary lymphocyte infiltration and vasodilation (Fig. 8.16). ② Early degeneration: dermoscopy can reveal a symmetric circular pigmented structure surrounding the hair follicles, with histopathologically corresponding melanophages around the hair follicles (Fig. 8.17). ③ Intermediate degeneration: a gray pseudonetwork is visible under dermoscopy with histopathologically corresponding to prominent melanophages at the dermal papillae (Fig. 8.18). ④ Late degeneration: blue-gray dots (peppering) are visible under dermoscopy with histopathologically corresponding to diffuse melanophages at the dermal papillae (Fig. 8.19).

However, recent studies have shown that these features are helpful only in distinguishing pigmented LPLK. For the majority of nonpigmented LPLK, the features are mainly scale (42.5%) and orange structureless areas (8.2%). However, these features are not very specific and therefore often need to be combined with biopsy for diagnosis.

Blue-gray fine dots may also occur in LM (annular-granular pattern), malignant melanoma (of its regression structures), and pigmented AK. Pink or near-skin colored LPLK is difficult to differentiate from basal cell carcinoma and nonpigmented melanoma due to the lack of associated dermoscopic features, especially when shiny white streaks are present in suspected LPLK lesions, in which further biopsies are needed.

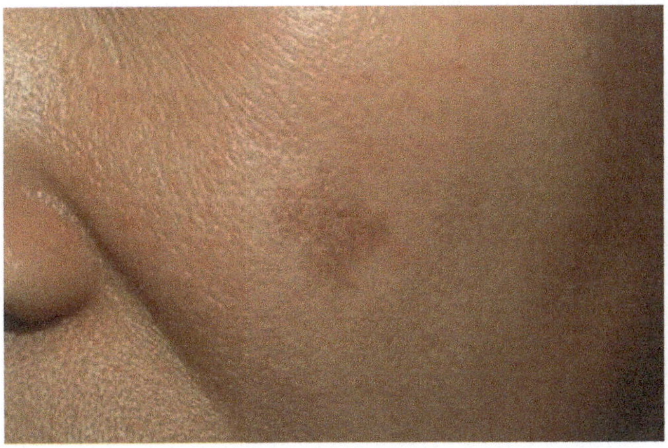

Fig. 8.14 Left: clinical appearance of LPLK. Right: pepper-like structures surrounding the hair follicles under dermoscopy

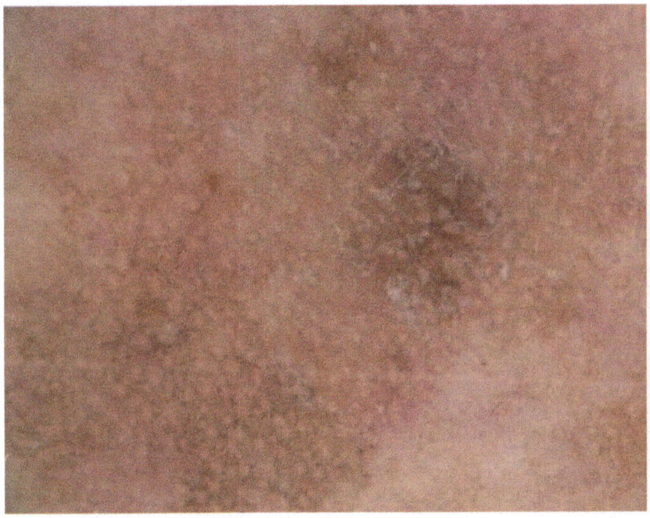
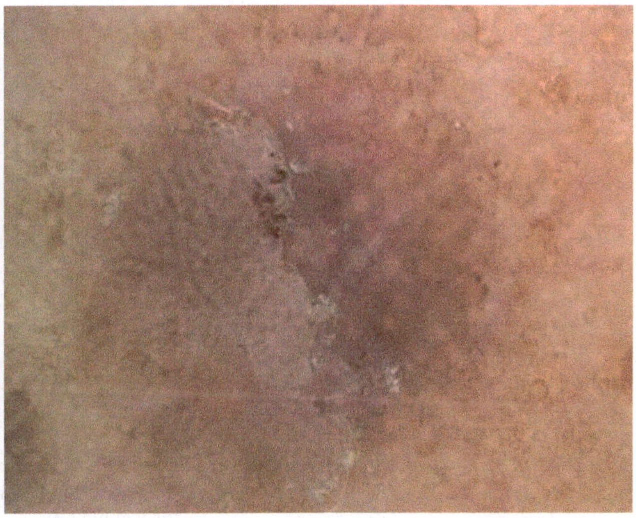

Fig. 8.15 Features of SL/SK are visible around LPLK

Fig. 8.16 LPLK early inflammation

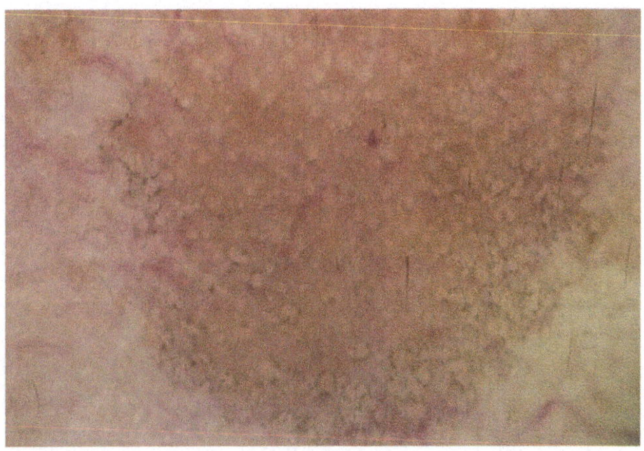

Fig. 8.17 LPLK early degeneration

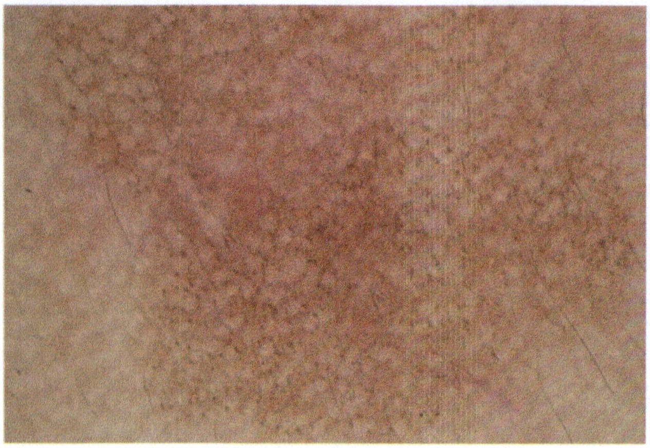

Fig. 8.18 LPLK intermediate degeneration

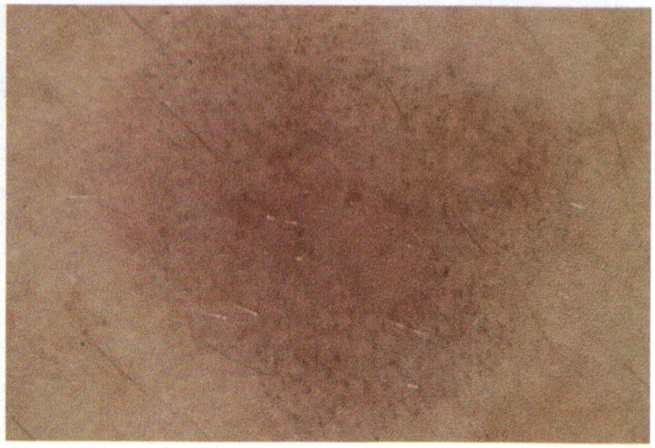

Fig. 8.19 LPLK late degeneration

Table 8.2 Differential points of keratinocyte proliferative and similar lesions

SL	LM	SK	LPLK (pigmented)	PAK
Clear lesion edges	Annular-granular pattern	Clear lesion edges ± moth-eaten border	Pepper-like or granular pattern	Strawberry pattern
Moth-eaten border	Rhomboidal structures	Milia-like cysts	Dermoscopic features of SL/SK/AK visible in the periphery	Red pseudonetwork
Faint pigmented network	Thick and variably colored pigmented network	Comedo-like openings		Variable size of follicular openings with keratotic plugs
Fingerprint pattern	Blue-gray structure	Cerebriform pattern		Perifollicular gray-brown granules
Brown homogeneous pattern	Brown globules	Hairpin-like vessels		Possible scales
Pseudonetwork	Mostly without scale	Overall movement of the skin lesion during the wobble test		
Smooth or rough	Smooth	Rough	Rough	Rough

SL solar lentigo, *LM* lentigo maligna, *SK* seborrheic keratosis, *LPLK* lichen planus-like keratosis, *PAK* pigmented actinic keratosis

A brief list of the differential diagnosis of several lesions with similar characteristics is shown in Table 8.2.

When a definite diagnosis cannot be made or malignancy is suspected based on the clinical and dermoscopic manifestations, a biopsy is recommended to verify the diagnosis.

Further Reading

1. Lallas A, Argenziano G, Moscarella E, et al. Diagnosis and management of facial pigmented macules. Clin Dermatol. 2014;32(1):94–100.
2. Menzies SW, Ingvar C, McCarthy WH. A sensitivity and specificity analysis of the surface microscopy features of invasive melanoma. Melanoma Res. 1996;6(1):55–62.
3. Schiffner R, Schiffner-Rohe J, Vogt T, et al. Improvement of early recognition of lentigo maligna using dermatoscopy. J Am Acad Dermatol. 2000;42(1 Pt 1):25–32.
4. Zaballos P, Rodero J, Pastor L, et al. Dermoscopy of lichenoid regressing solar lentigines. Arch Dermatol. 2008;144(2):284.
5. Yadav S, Vossaert KA, Kopf AW, et al. Histopathologic correlates of structures seen on dermoscopy (epiluminescence microscopy). Am J Dermatopathol. 1993;15(4):297–305.
6. Berger M, Thomas L, Dalle S. Ink spot lentigo. Ann Dermatol Venereol. 2017;144(3):225–6.
7. Bottoni U, Nistico S, Amoruso GF, et al. Ink spot lentigo: singular clinical features in a case series of patients. Int J Immunopathol Pharmacol. 2013;26(4):953–5.
8. Marulli GC, Campione E, Di Stefani A, et al. Ink spot lentigo arising on naevus spilus simulating melanoma. Acta Derm Venereol. 2004;84(2):166–7.
9. Annessi G, Bono R, Abeni D. Correlation between digital epiluminescence microscopy parameters and histopathological changes in lentigo maligna and solar lentigo: a dermoscopic index for the diagnosis of lentigo maligna. J Am Acad Dermatol. 2017;76(2):234–43.
10. Rosendahl C, Cameron A, Argenziano G, et al. Dermoscopy of squamous cell carcinoma and keratoacanthoma. Arch Dermatol. 2012;148(12):1386–92.
11. Squillace L, Cappello M, Longo C, et al. Unusual Dermoscopic patterns of seborrheic keratosis. Dermatology. 2016;232(2):198–202.

12. Braun RP, Rabinovitz HS, Krischer J, et al. Dermoscopy of pigmented seborrheic keratosis: a morphological study. Arch Dermatol. 2002;138(12):1556–60.
13. Stricklin SM, Stoecker WV, Oliviero MC, et al. Cloudy and starry milia-like cysts: how well do they distinguish seborrheic keratoses from malignant melanomas? J Eur Acad Dermatol Venereol. 2011;25(10):1222–4.
14. Kopf AW, Rabinovitz H, Marghoob A, et al. "Fat fingers:" a clue in the dermoscopic diagnosis of seborrheic keratoses. J Am Acad Dermatol. 2006;55(6):1089–91.
15. Argenziano G, Soyer HP, Chimenti S, et al. Dermoscopy of pigmented skin lesions: results of a consensus meeting via the internet. J Am Acad Dermatol. 2003;48(5):679–93.
16. Lin J, Han S, Cui L, et al. Evaluation of dermoscopic algorithm for seborrhoeic keratosis: a prospective study in 412 patients. J Eur Acad Dermatol Venereol. 2014;28(7):957–62.
17. Goncharova Y, Attia EA, Souid K, et al. Dermoscopic features of facial pigmented skin lesions. ISRN Dermatol. 2013;2013:1–7. Article ID: 546813
18. Wang S, Jie L, Liu Z, et al. High-frequency skin ultrasonographic and dermoscopic features of seborrheic keratosis. Chin J Dermatol. 2018;51(11):815–9.
19. Braun RP, Krischer J, Saurat JH. The "wobble sign" in epiluminescence microscopy as a novel clue to the differential diagnosis of pigmented skin lesions. Arch Dermatol. 2000;136(7):940–2.
20. Shapiro L, Ackerman AB. Solitary lichen planus-like keratosis. Dermatologica. 1966;132(5):386–92.
21. Zaballos P, Blazquez S, Puig S, et al. Dermoscopic pattern of intermediate stage in seborrhoeic keratosis regressing to lichenoid keratosis: report of 24 cases. Br J Dermatol. 2007;157(2):266–72.
22. Bugatti L, Filosa G. Dermoscopy of lichen planus-like keratosis: a model of inflammatory regression. J Eur Acad Dermatol Venereol. 2007;21(10):1392–7.
23. Liopyris K, Navarrete-Dechent C, Dusza SW, et al. Clinical and dermoscopic features associated with lichen planus-like keratoses that undergo skin biopsy: a single-center, observational study. Australas J Dermatol. 2018;60(2):e119–26.
24. Watanabe S, Sawada M, Dekio I, et al. Chronology of lichen planus-like keratosis features by dermoscopy: a summary of 17 cases. Dermatol Pract Concept. 2016;6(2):29–35.
25. Lallas A, Apalla Z, Moscarella E, et al. Extensive regression in pigmented skin lesions: a dangerous confounding feature. Dermatol Pract Concept. 2012;2(2):202–8.
26. Elgart GW. Seborrheic keratoses, solar lentigines, and lichenoid keratoses. Dermatoscopic features and correlation to histology and clinical signs. Dermatol Clin. 2001;19(2):347–57.
27. Chan AH, Shulman KJ, Lee BA. Differentiating regressed melanoma from regressed lichenoid keratosis. J Cutan Pathol. 2017;44(4):338–41.

9 Vascular Diseases

Vascular diseases mainly involve vascular disorders and lymphatic disorders. While vascular diseases are heterogeneous and have complex classifications, they can be divided into vascular tumors and vascular malformations according to clinical manifestations and skin imaging, hemodynamic, and histopathology findings. Vascular tumors are also called hemangiomas, which are caused by abnormal proliferation of vascular endothelial cells and neoangiogenesis. Vascular tumors can be divided into benign and malignant tumors. Common hemangiomas include infantile hemangiomas (IHs), congenital hemangiomas, cherry angiomas, pyogenic granulomas (PGs), angiokeratomas, Kaposi's sarcoma (KS), etc. Vascular malformations are due to morphological and structural abnormalities in the process of vascular development and differentiation. Port-wine stains are common vascular malformations. Lymphatic diseases can be divided into lymphangiomas and lymphatic malformations. Localized lymphangiomas are a common type of lymphatic disease.

Most vascular diseases can be diagnosed by clinical manifestation and physical examination. However, when the clinical manifestations of vascular diseases are not typical or are easily misdiagnosed as other diseases, dermoscopy and other skin imaging tools can be used as auxiliary examination methods, which also play an important role in the curative effect observation and follow-up of hemangioma before and after treatment. This chapter focuses on the dermoscopic features of several common vascular and lymphatic diseases.

9.1 Cherry Angioma

Cherry angioma is the most common acquired skin vascular proliferative disease. Cherry angioma occurs in middle-aged and elderly people. The lesions, also known as Campbell De Morgan spots, are characterized by clear boundaries and round, oval, or polygonal red papules (Fig. 9.1). Cherry angiomas most often appear on the trunk and can fade when pressed, but some lesions have more fibrous components, which will not fade completely under pressure.

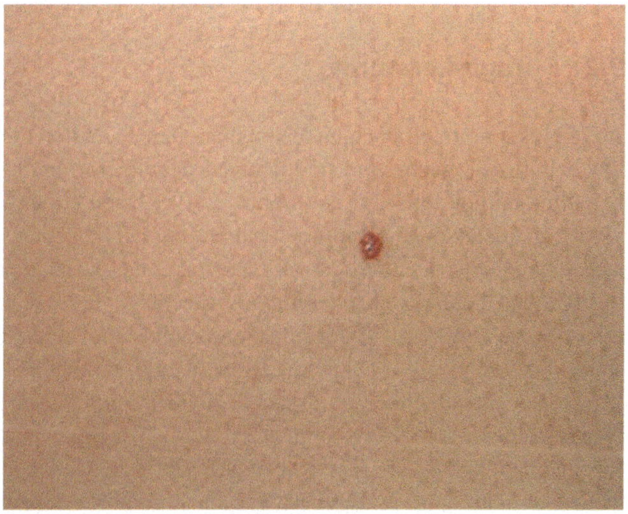

Fig. 9.1 Clinical manifestations of cherry hemangioma: red papules on the chest with clear boundaries

The dermoscopic characteristics of cherry hemangiomas are as follows (Fig. 9.2):

1. Red, purple and reddish-brown lacunae
2. Isolated dilated blood vessels
3. White fibrous septation
4. Blue-black coloring when thrombosed

Recent studies have found that the white halo around cherry hemangioma lesions is associated with an onset age later than 60 years, more than 4 lesions, and a lesion diameter greater than 3 mm.

J. Liu, X. Zou, *Practical Dermoscopy*, https://doi.org/10.1007/978-981-19-1460-7_9

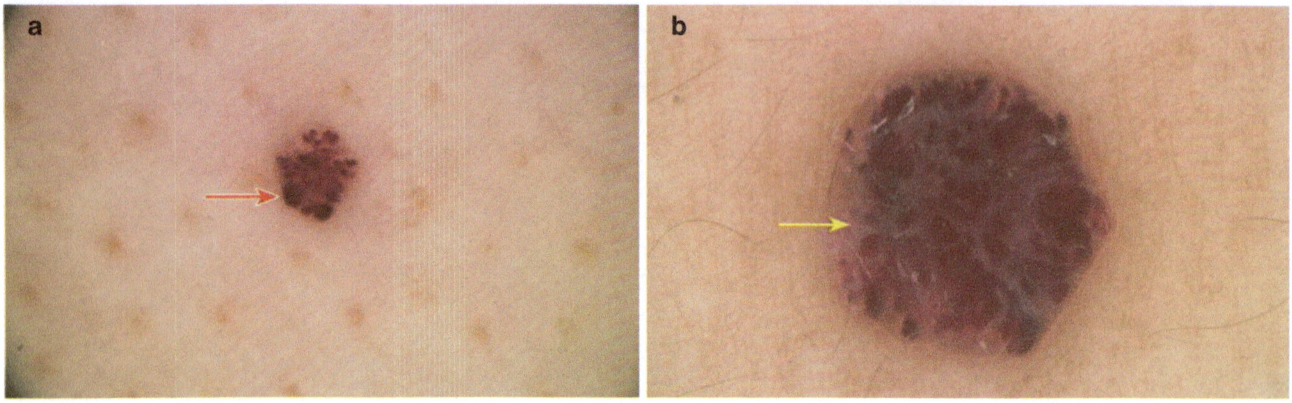

Fig. 9.2 Dermoscopic characteristics of cherry hemangioma: (**a**) Red and reddish-brown lacunae can be seen (red arrow, × 20). (**b**) White fibrous septation (yellow arrow, × 30)

9.2 Angiokeratoma

An angiokeratoma is a benign lesion that often occurs on the lower limbs of young and middle-aged people. An angiokeratoma initially presents as smooth, soft, crimson papules with a diameter of 2–10 mm and then gradually becomes larger and harder, presenting as dark-red, blue-purple, or black round hard papules. Secondary bleeding may occur after trauma (Fig. 9.3). The lesions are composed of dilated superficial blood vessels and covered with epidermal hyperkeratosis. Clinically, the lesions can be divided into five subtypes: solitary, extremity angiokeratomas (Mibelli type), scrotal angiokeratomas (Fordyce type), and localized and diffuse somatic angiokeratomas. The most common lesion subtype is a solitary angiokeratoma.

The dermoscopic characteristics of angiokeratoma are as follows (Fig. 9.4):

1. Dark lacunae: round or oval, dark-blue, dark-purple, or black areas of different sizes
2. Red lacunae
3. Blue-white veil in the center of the lesion
4. Erythema around the lesion
5. Blood crusts
6. Rainbow pattern

The corresponding relationships between the dermoscopic findings and histopathology of angiokeratoma are as follows:

1. The "dark lacunae" under dermoscopy corresponds to dilated blood vessels in the middle and upper dermis, which can be partially or completely blocked.
2. The "blue-white veil" under dermoscopy corresponds to the hyperkeratosis and thickening of the spinous layer.
3. The "blood scab" under dermoscopy corresponds to the bleeding area.

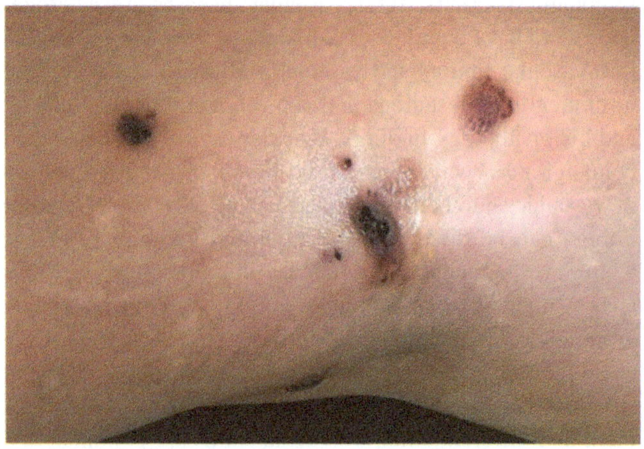

Fig. 9.3 Clinical manifestations of angiokeratoma: multiple dark-red papules, plaques, crusts, and surgical scars were found on the right thigh

9.3 Pyogenic Granuloma

A PG is a kind of benign vascular tumor of the skin or mucosa that can occur at any age, especially in children and young adults. The commonly involved sites are the hands, face, and lips. The clinical manifestations of PG are rapidly growing red papules or polyps with glossy surfaces (Fig. 9.5) and a tendency for recurrence and bleeding, which is usually an indication for surgical treatment.

The dermoscopic findings of PG are as follows (Fig. 9.6):

1. Red homogeneous area
2. White-collar-like structure
3. White streaks
4. Various vascular patterns
5. Ulcers

The corresponding relationships between the dermoscopic findings and histopathology of PG are as follows:

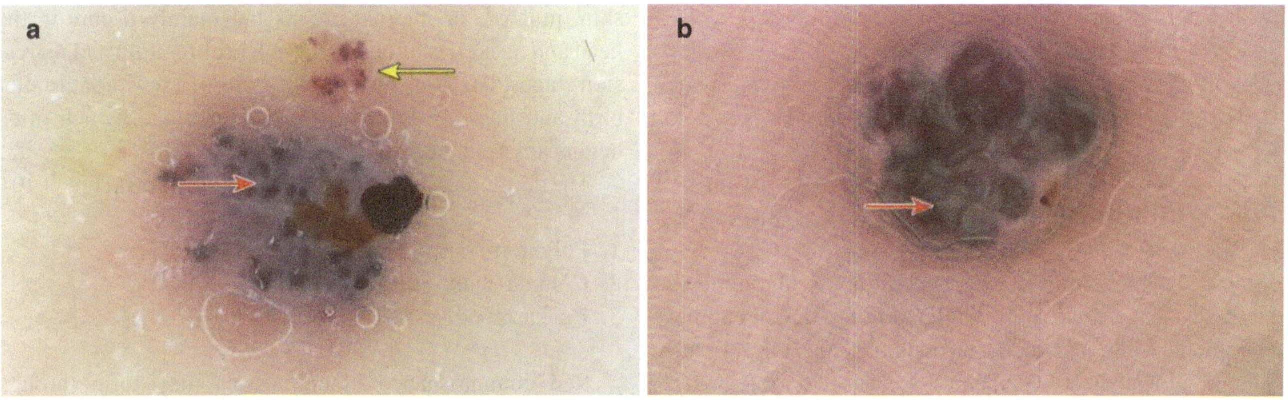

Fig. 9.4 Dermoscopic characteristics of angiokeratoma: (**a**) Dark lacunae, blue-white veil (red arrow), red lacunae (yellow arrow), blood scab, and erythema around the lesion (× 30). (**b**) Dark lacunae and the rainbow pattern (red arrow) can be seen (× 30)

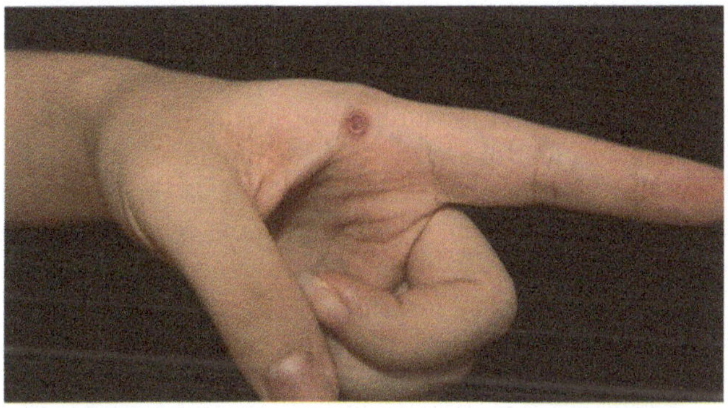

Fig. 9.5 Clinical manifestation of pyogenic granuloma: a red papule on the left hand surrounded by white scales

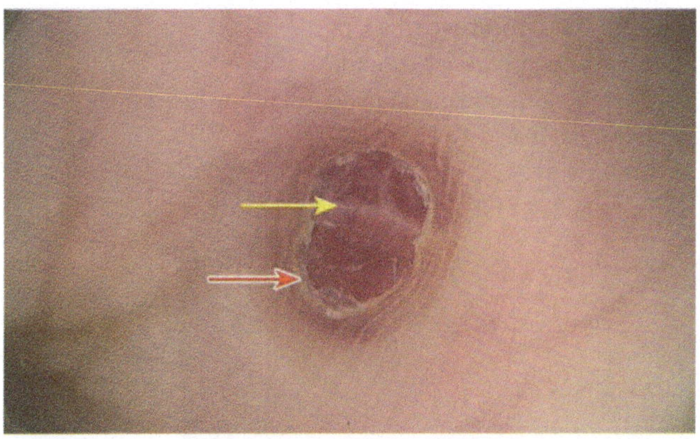

Fig. 9.6 Dermoscopic findings of pyogenic granuloma: a red homogeneous area, a white-collar-like structure (red arrow) and white streaks (yellow arrow) (× 20)

1. The "red homogeneous area" under dermoscopy correlates with the proliferating capillaries and veins.
2. The "white-collar-like structure" under dermoscopy corresponds to the surrounding epithelium.
3. The "white streaks" under dermoscopy correspond to fibrous septation around the capillary plexus.

9.4 Port-Wine Stain

A port-wine stain is a congenital capillary malformation characterized by pink, red or purple patches (Fig. 9.7). Port-wine stain can be treated by pulsed dye laser and photodynamic therapy.

The dermoscopic findings of port-wine stain are as follows (Fig. 9.8):

1. Superficial lesions: diffuse distribution of dotted or globular blood vessels.
2. Deep lesions: linear or curved blood vessels, a gray-white veil, a central brown punctate area with a peripheral white halo.

The corresponding relationships between the dermoscopic findings and histopathology of port-wine stain are as follows:

1. The globular blood vessels under dermoscopy correspond to the vertical dilated capillaries in the dermal papilla. The globular blood vessels indicate that the lesion is shallow, further indicating that the lesion is suitable for laser therapy.
2. The linear blood vessels under dermoscopy correspond to the horizontal dilated capillaries in the reticular layer of the dermis.

9.5 Angioma Serpiginosum

Angioma serpiginosum (AS) is a kind of abnormal telangiectasia involving the superficial dermis, especially the papillary layer. AS is rare and often occurs in young women. AS skin lesions are more commonly found on the limbs, presenting as red or dark red macules in a serpentine arrangement, on which there are clusters of red papules of needle size, which do not fade when pressed.

The dermoscopic findings of AS are as follows:

1. Multiple small, well-defined, round, or oval red lacunae.
2. Comma-shaped and hairpin-like blood vessels.

9.6 Infantile Hemangiomas

Infantile hemangiomas (IHs) are common vascular tumors in newborns that are caused by benign proliferation of capillary endothelial cells and their surrounding connective tissues. The initial lesions are congestive, scratch-like, or telangiectatic patches.

The early proliferative stage of IHs is during the first three months after birth, when the lesion proliferates rapidly, forming a strawberry-like plaque or tumor (Fig. 9.9), after which proliferation slows down. IH can occur in any area of skin, mucosa, or internal organs but mainly occurs in the head and neck. IHs often go through proliferation and regression stages. IHs grow most rapidly within a few months after birth and then go through a regression stage, which often begins after one year of age.

The dermoscopic findings of IHs are as follows (Fig. 9.10):

1. Polymorphous globular vessels
2. Comma-shaped blood vessels
3. Linear blood vessels

Red comma-shaped blood vessels may form through dilated superficial vertical capillaries in the papillary layer of the dermis transforming into the deep papillary layer of the dermis.

9.7 Verrucous Vascular Malformations

A verrucous vascular malformation is a kind of vascular malformation with typical clinical manifestations of blue-red well-defined papules or nodules, most of which are located on the lower extremities, but they can also appear on the chest and forearm. Verrucous hyperkeratosis occurs in the late stage (Fig. 9.11). Histological changes include epidermal hyperkeratosis, papillomatous hyperplasia, spinous layer hypertrophy, and capillary and venous malformations in the dermis and subcutaneous tissue.

The dermoscopic findings of a verrucous vascular malformation are as follows:

1. Alveolar appearance
2. Oval and polygonal structure
3. Peripheral pigmentation and a shallow groove
4. Dark lacunae
5. Blue-white veil

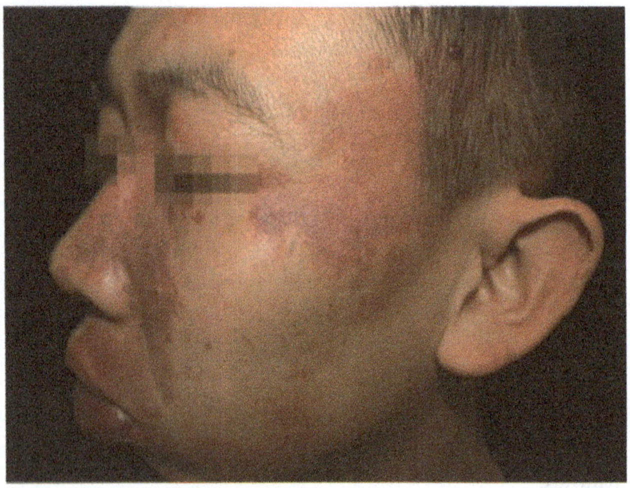

Fig. 9.7 Clinical manifestations of port-wine stain: purplish-red patches on the face

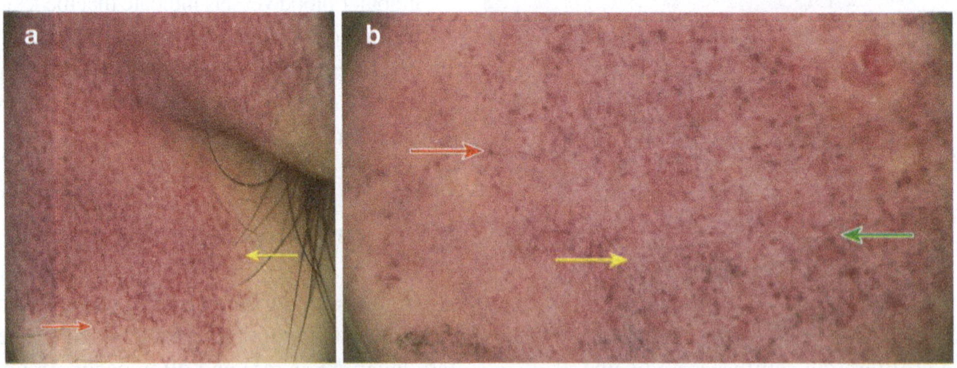

Fig. 9.8 Dermoscopic findings of port-wine stain. (**a**). (superficial lesions) There are dotted and globular blood vessels (red arrow) and linear blood vessels (yellow arrow) (× 20). (**b**). (deep lesions) There are globular blood vessels (red arrow), curved linear blood vessels, a gray-white veil (yellow arrow), and a central brown punctate area with peripheral white halo (green arrow) (× 20)

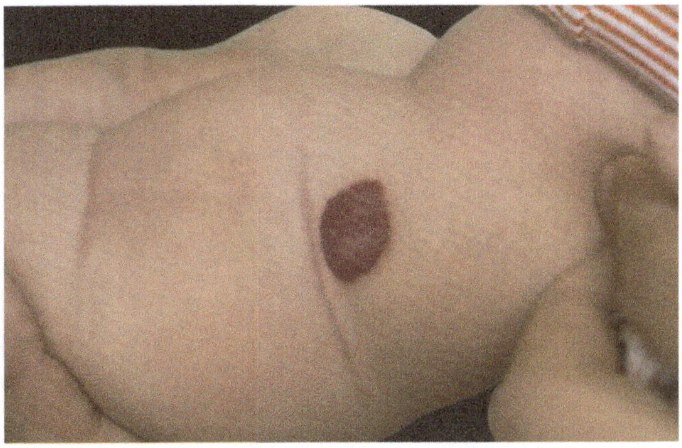

Fig. 9.9 Clinical manifestations of infantile hemangioma: a red plaque in the right cubital fossa

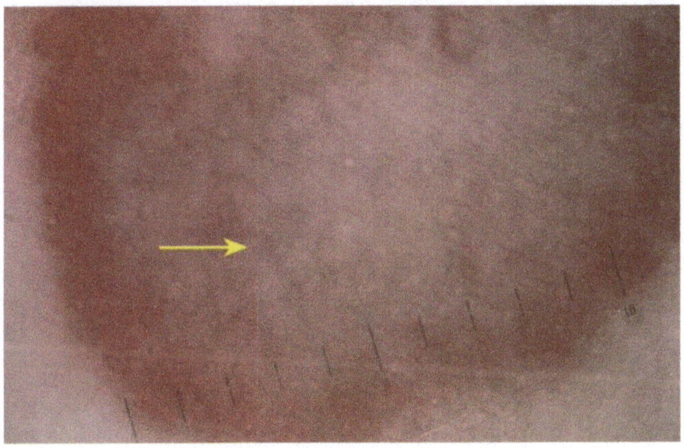

Fig. 9.10 Dermoscopic findings of infantile hemangioma: dilated linear blood vessels (yellow arrow, ×20)

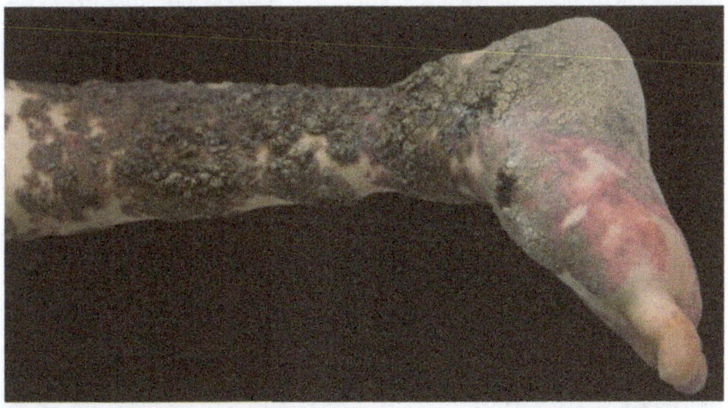

Fig. 9.11 Clinical manifestations of a verrucous vascular malformation: dark, purplish-red patches diffusely distributed on the right lower limb and verrucous proliferative papules and plaques densely distributed on the surface

9.8 Hobnail Hemangioma

Hobnail hemangioma, also known as targetoid hemosiderotic hemangioma, mainly involves the trunk and extremities. Hobnail hemangioma often appears as a solitary lesion and presents with a target-like appearance, which has a central brown-purple area, a peripheral brown or pale area, and an outside congestion circle.

The dermoscopic findings of hobnail hemangioma are as follows:

1. Homogeneous area, mostly red, purplish-red, or brown
2. Central red and dark lacunae
3. Peripheral homogeneous area or pigment network
4. White structureless area, including shiny white streaks

9.9 Venous Lakes

Venous lakes are significant varicose veins caused by chronic sunlight damage. The lesions are dark-blue, purple, or black papules with a diameter of 2–10 mm, which are soft and easy to compress. Severe bleeding may occur after injury (Fig. 9.12).

The dermoscopic findings of a venous lake are as follows (Fig. 9.13):

1. Purple, red, and blue structureless areas
2. Globules and clods
3. White structure

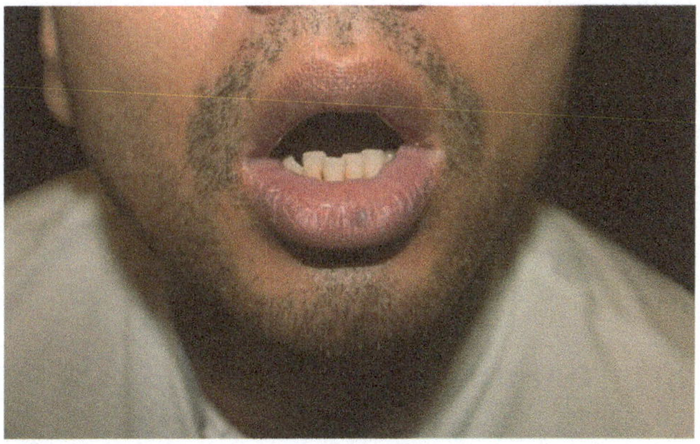

Fig. 9.12 Clinical manifestations of a venous lake: blue-purple papules on lips

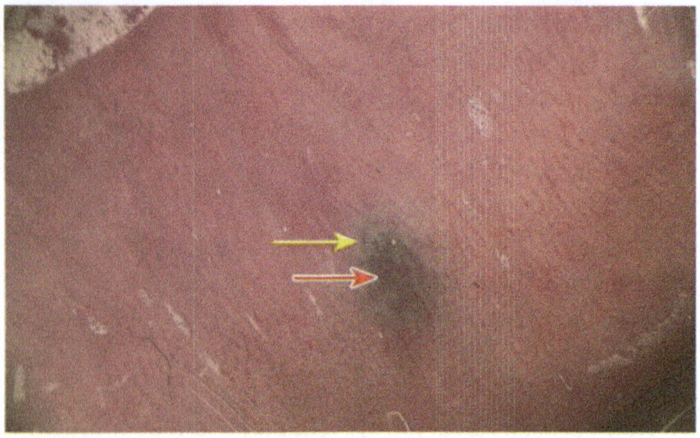

Fig. 9.13 Dermoscopic findings of a venous lake: purple and blue structureless area (red arrow) and white structure (yellow arrow) (× 20)

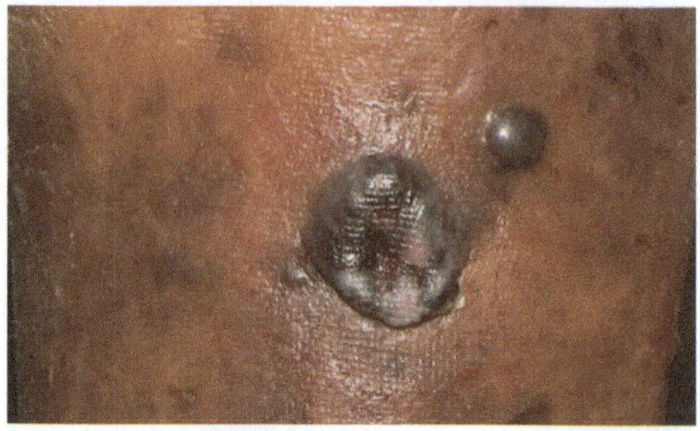

Fig. 9.14 Clinical manifestations of Kaposi's sarcoma: multiple red and blue-purple nodules on the leg

9.10 Kaposi's Sarcoma

KS lesions are spindle cell tumors derived from malignant endothelial cells. KS can be divided into four subtypes: classic, endemic, iatrogenic and acquired immune deficiency syndrome related. The clinical manifestations of KS vary in different subtypes and clinical stages and can manifest as isolated or multiple pink, blue-purple or black nodules, plaques, and polyps (Fig. 9.14).

The dermoscopic findings of KS are as follows (Fig. 9.15):

1. Rainbow pattern
2. Blue-red, multi-colored area
3. Scales
4. Brown globules
5. White collarette
6. Structureless area
7. Vascular structure

It should be noted that the rainbow pattern is not a unique manifestation of KS under dermoscopy. The rainbow pattern can also be seen in some other skin conditions and diseases, such as hypertrophic scarring, angiokeratoma, and pseudo-KS.

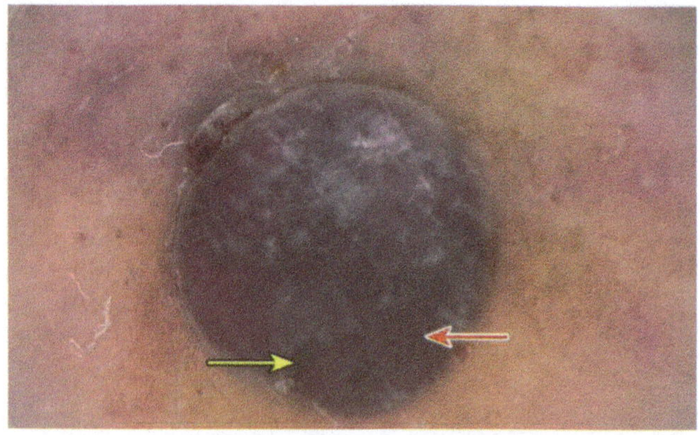

Fig. 9.15 Dermoscopic features of Kaposi's sarcoma: a blue-red area (red arrow) and brown globules (yellow arrow) (×20)

9.11 Cutaneous Angiosarcoma

A cutaneous angiosarcoma (AS) is a rare soft-tissue malignant tumor that mainly occurs on the head and face of elderly individuals. Cutaneous AS presents as dark-red plaques or nodules with infiltrative growth (Fig. 9.16), which may rupture and bleed or metastasize to lymph nodes and viscera.

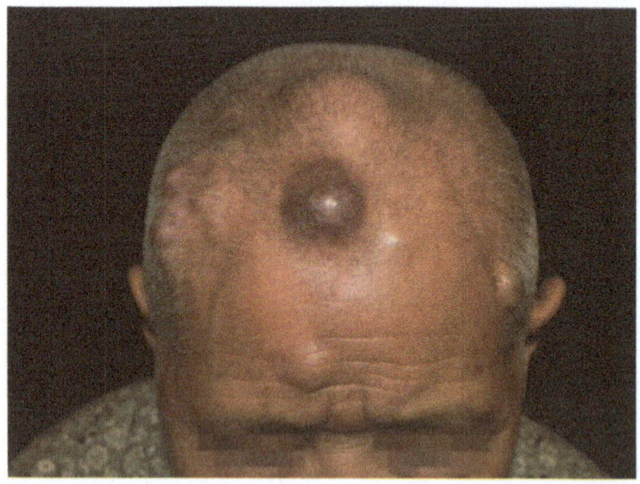

Fig. 9.16 Clinical manifestations of classic angiosarcoma: multiple purplish-red nodules on the scalp

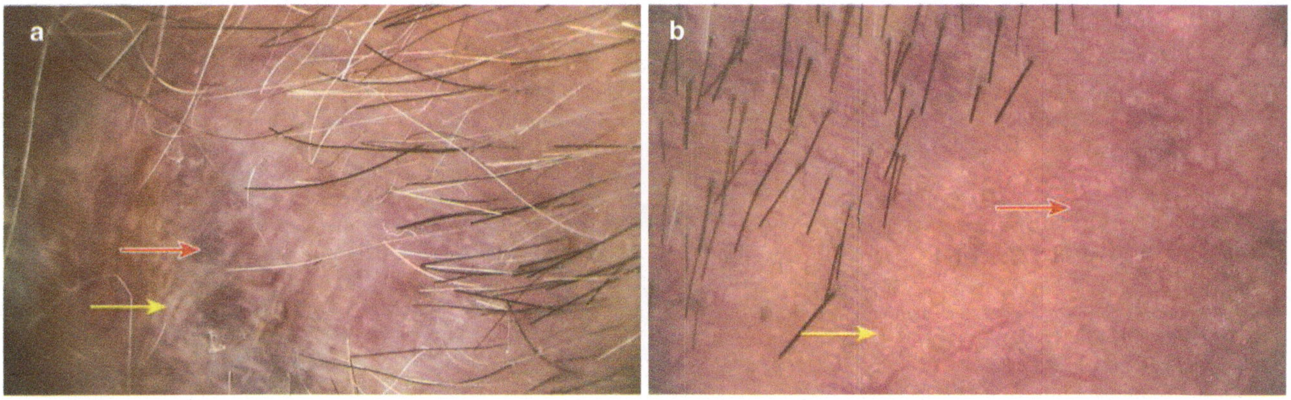

Fig. 9.17 Dermoscopic findings of classic angiosarcoma: (**a**). Purplish-red structureless area (red arrow) and shiny white streaks (yellow arrow) (× 20). (**b**). Pink homogeneous area (red arrow) and hair follicular plugs (yellow arrow) (× 20)

Clinically, there are three AS subtypes: classic AS (head and neck type), lymphedema-associated AS (Stewart–Treves syndrome), and radiation-induced AS.

The dermoscopic findings of AS are as follows (Fig. 9.17):

Classic type (head and neck type)

1. Pink, red to purple areas
2. White area around hair follicles and follicular plugs
3. Shiny white streaks

Radiation-induced type:

1. Pink and white homogeneous areas
2. Purplish-red or pink smoky areas
3. The surrounding color deepens

9.12 Cutaneous Lymphangioma Circumscriptum

Cutaneous lymphangioma circumscriptum (CLC) is the most common type of cutaneous lymphangioma. CLC lesions, also known as superficial lymphatic malformations (SLMs), can occur on any area of the body, presenting as needle- to pea-sized blister-like lesions on skin and mucosa, with clear boundaries, and in scattered or linear arrangements or clustered in frog-egg-like structures (Fig. 9.18). The blisters are translucent milky white or light yellow, are often found to be light red, red, blue, or black due to the blood, and sometimes can be misdiagnosed as warts.

The dermoscopic findings of CLC are as follows (Fig. 9.19):

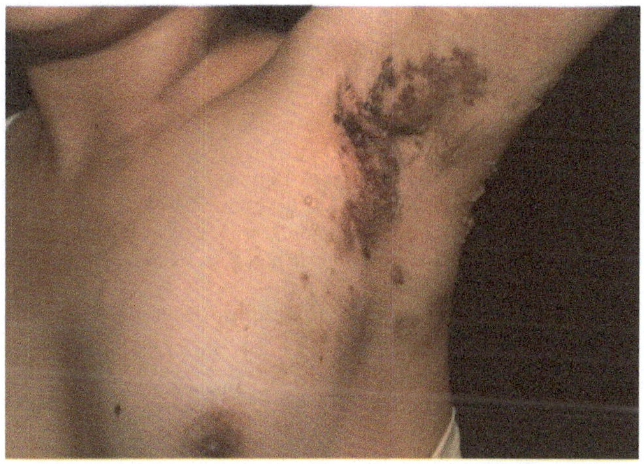

Fig. 9.18 Clinical manifestations of cutaneous lymphangioma circumscriptum: multiple transparent blisters and blood blisters in the left armpit, which clustered in a frog-egg-like pattern

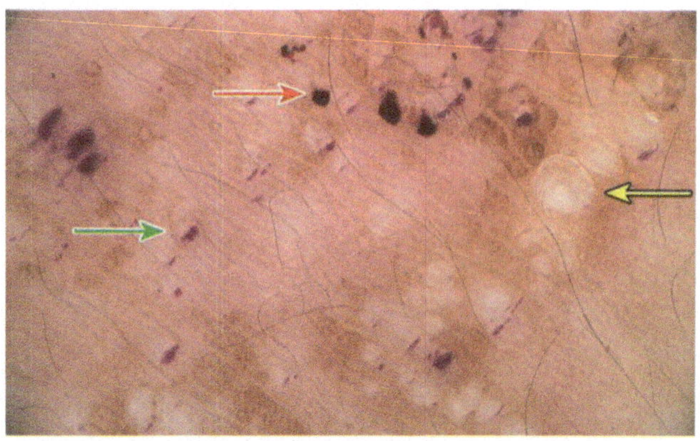

Fig. 9.19 Dermoscopic findings of cutaneous lymphangioma circumscriptum: dark lacuna (red arrow), white lacuna (yellow arrow), and "empyema of anterior chamber" sign (green arrow), (× 20)

1. Lacunae: red, dark, yellow, white, or a variety of colors
2. Vascular structure
3. White line
4. “Empyema of anterior chamber” sign
5. Light background

Further Reading

1. Taghinia AH, Upton J. Vascular anomalies. J Hand Surg Am. 2018;43(12):1113–21.
2. Piccolo V, Russo T, Moscarella E, et al. Dermatoscopy of vascular lesions. Dermatol Clin. 2018;36(4):389–95.
3. Grazzini M, Stanganelli I, Rossari S, et al. Dermoscopy, confocal laser microscopy, and hi-tech evaluation of vascular skin lesions: diagnostic and therapeutic perspectives. Dermatol Ther. 2012;25(4):297–303.
4. Fettahlioglu KB. Halo formation around cherry angiomas: a rare but substantial finding. Med Sci Monit. 2018;24:5050–3.
5. Jha AK, Sonthalia S, Jakhar D. Dermoscopy of angiokeratoma. Indian Dermatol Online J. 2018;9(2):141–2.
6. Pinos Leon VH, Granizo Rubio JD. Acral pseudolymphomatous angiokeratoma of children with rainbow pattern: a mimicker of Kaposi sarcoma. J Am Acad Dermatol. 2017;76(2S1):S25–7.
7. Jha AK, Sonthalia S, Khopkar U. Dermoscopy of pyogenic granuloma. Indian Dermatol Online J. 2017;8(6):523–4.
8. Shirakawa M, Ozawa T, Wakami S, et al. Utility of Dermoscopy before and after laser irradiation in port wine stains. Ann Dermatol. 2012;24(1):7–10.
9. Ghanadan A, Kamyab-Hesari K, Moslehi H, et al. Dermoscopy of angioma serpiginosum: a case report. Int J Dermatol. 2014;53(12):1505–7.
10. Munden A, Butschek R, Tom WL, et al. Prospective study of infantile haemangiomas: incidence, clinical characteristics and association with placental anomalies. Br J Dermatol. 2014;170(4):907–13.
11. Prabhakar V, Kaliyadan F. A case of verrucous hemangioma and its dermoscopic features. Indian Dermatol Online J. 2015;6(Suppl 1):S56–8.
12. Popadic M. Dermoscopic diagnosis of a rare, congenital vascular tumor: verrucous hemangioma. J Dermatol. 2012;39(12):1049–50.
13. Zaballos P, Llambrich A, Delpozo LJ, et al. Dermoscopy of targetoid Hemosiderotic Hemangioma: a morphological study of 35 cases. Dermatology. 2015;231(4):339–44.
14. Lee JS, Mun JH. Dermoscopy of venous lake on the lips: a comparative study with labial melanotic macule. PLoS One. 2018;13(10):e0206768.
15. Gulec AT. Videodermoscopy enhances the ability to diagnose Kaposi's sarcoma by revealing its vascular structures. J Am Acad Dermatol. 2016;74(6):e117–8.
16. Kelati A, Mernissi FZ. The rainbow pattern in dermoscopy: a zoom on nonkaposi sarcoma skin diseases. Biom J. 2018;41(3):209–10.
17. Minagawa A, Koga H, Okuyama R. Vascular structure absence under dermoscopy in two cases of angiosarcoma on the scalp. Int J Dermatol. 2014;53(7):e350–2.
18. Cozzani E, Chinazzo C, Ghigliotti G, et al. Cutaneous angiosarcoma: the role of dermoscopy to reduce the risk of a delayed diagnosis. Int J Dermatol. 2018;57(8):996–7.
19. Zaballos P, Del P, Argenziano G, et al. Dermoscopy of lymphangioma circumscriptum: a morphological study of 45 cases. Australas J Dermatol. 2018;59:e189–93.
20. Jha Abhijeet K, Lallas A, Sonthalia S. Dermoscopy of cutaneous lymphangioma circumscriptum. Dermatol Pract Concept. 2017;7:37–8.

10 Squamous Cell Neoplasms

Squamous cell neoplasms are an important type of nonmelanocyte-derived skin tumors. The dermoscopic characteristics of nonmelanocyte tumors are more difficult to evaluate than those of melanocyte-derived tumors. The squamous cell neoplasms introduced here include actinic keratosis (AK), Bowen's disease (BD), keratoacanthoma (KA), and squamous cell carcinoma (SCC). The characteristic dermoscopic patterns of squamous cell tumors are related to disease progression and staging and can be used as a supplement to clinical observations, assist in biopsy positioning and help in making preliminary judgments. However, it should be noted that squamous cell tumors may be viewed in a spectrum of keratinocyte dysplasia. Therefore, the clinical and dermoscopic features of these squamous cell tumors do show some overlaps. A comprehensive judgment should be made based on the patient's age, medical history, and clinical manifestations. Histopathological examination is needed to confirm the diagnosis when considering this group of diseases.

10.1 Actinic Keratosis

AK, also known as solar keratosis, is a kind of premalignant lesion caused by long-term sun damage. AK is more common in exposed areas such as the face, ears, forearms, and back of hands, presenting as scattered skin-colored or pink-to-red papules, plaques, or small nodules, with adhesive scales on the surface.

10.1.1 According to the Degree of the Lesion, AK Can Be Divided into Three Grades, Each with Different Dermoscopic Characteristics

Grade I AK lesions are slightly palpable, and the dermoscopic features are as follows:

(i) Red pseudo-network pattern: uninvolved openings of hair follicles on a red background.
(ii) Dotted and linear vessels around the hair follicles, distributed in a network (Fig. 10.1).

Grade II AK lesions are moderately thick, and the manifestations under dermoscopy are as follows:

(i) Strawberry pattern
(ii) Yellow-white, keratinized, and enlarged follicular openings on a red background
(iii) White halo around the openings of hair follicles
(iv) Dotted and irregular linear vessels (Fig. 10.2)

Grade III AK lesions show obvious hyperkeratosis, and the manifestations under dermoscopy are as follows:

(i) Yellow-white structureless area
(ii) Enlarged follicular openings filled with keratotic plugs
(iii) Surface is covered with yellow-white scales (Fig. 10.3).

The red pseudo-network pattern combined with the enlargement of the hair follicle openings has a high sensitivity (95.6%) and specificity (95.0%) for the diagnosis of AK.

The rosette sign (Fig. 10.4) is characterized by four white spots in a follicle opening, arranged in a square, which is similar to a four-leaf clover and can be seen only with polarized dermoscopy. The rosette sign was previously thought to be common in AK, superficial SCC, and sun-damaged skin. Recent studies have shown that this structure can be seen in a variety of tumors and inflammatory diseases. The rosette sign probably represents an optical effect of polarized light interacting with keratinization and fibrosis around hair follicles arranged in concentric circles, and this sign is not disease-specific.

J. Liu, X. Zou, *Practical Dermoscopy*, https://doi.org/10.1007/978-981-19-1460-7_10

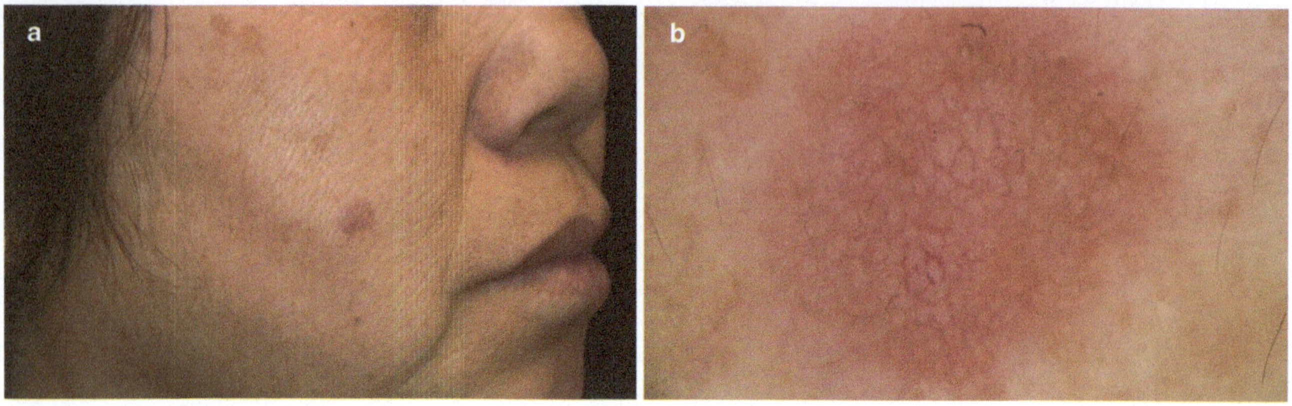

Fig. 10.1 Clinical and dermoscopic images of grade I actinic keratosis. (**a**) A dark red patch on the right cheek. (**b**) Under dermoscopy, a red pseudonetwork pattern can be seen, as well as the openings of the nonpigmented hair follicles on a red background and the dotted, globular and short linear blood vessels around the hair follicles distributed in a network (×30)

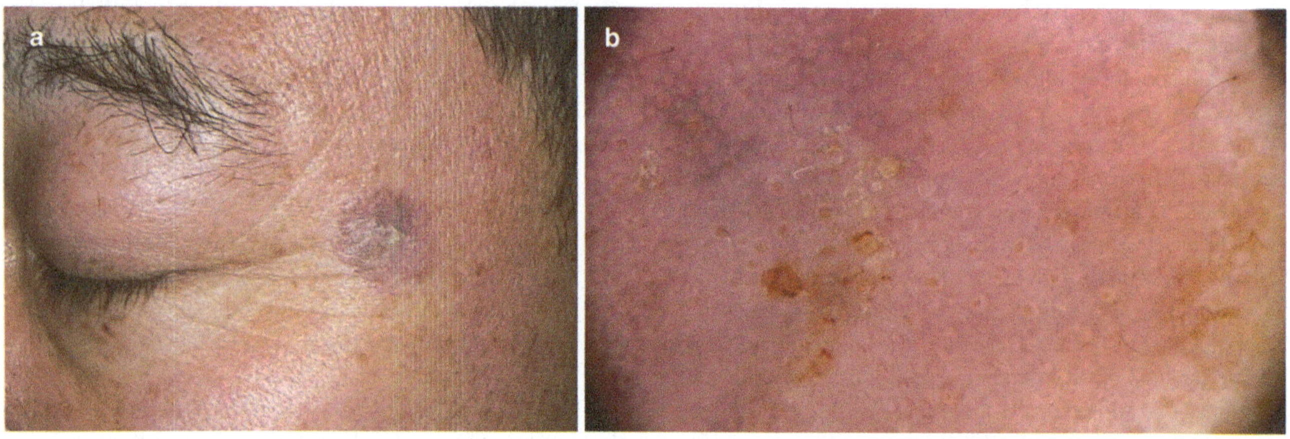

Fig. 10.2 Clinical and dermoscopic images of grade II actinic keratosis. (**a**) A dark red plaque on the left temporal area with adhesive scales on the surface. (**b**) Strawberry patterns can be seen under dermoscopy, with a red background, yellow follicular keratotic plugs, a white halo around the hair follicle, and dotted and irregular linear vessels (×20)

10.1.2 Differential Diagnosis Between AK and Discoid Lupus Erythematosus (DLE) Under Dermoscopy

(i) Both AK and DLE have hair follicle keratotic plugs.

(ii) AK manifests white keratinized target-like hair follicle openings on a red background, also known as the "red strawberry sign."

(iii) DLE presents with a white to pink background mixed with large red hair follicle openings of various shapes and white halos around them, also known as the "white strawberry sign."

10.1.3 Dermoscopic Manifestations of Pigmented AK (pAK)

In addition to the dermoscopic features of AK above, gray-brown dots around the hair follicles distributed in a pseudonetwork structure can be seen in pAK (Fig. 10.5).

10.1.4 Differentiation Between pAK and Lentigo Maligna under Dermoscopy (Fig. 10.6)

The structures in pAK may overlap with those in early lentigo maligna, which include rhomboidal structures, an annular–granular pattern, and gray-brown dots. pAK and lentigo maligna can be distinguished by the features listed in Table 10.1.

> **Tip**
> PAK and lentigo maligna can be distinguished by palpation. The former is rough on palpation, and the latter has a smooth surface. Although dermoscopy sometimes cannot completely differentiate pAK from lentigo maligna, it may help guide biopsy positioning.

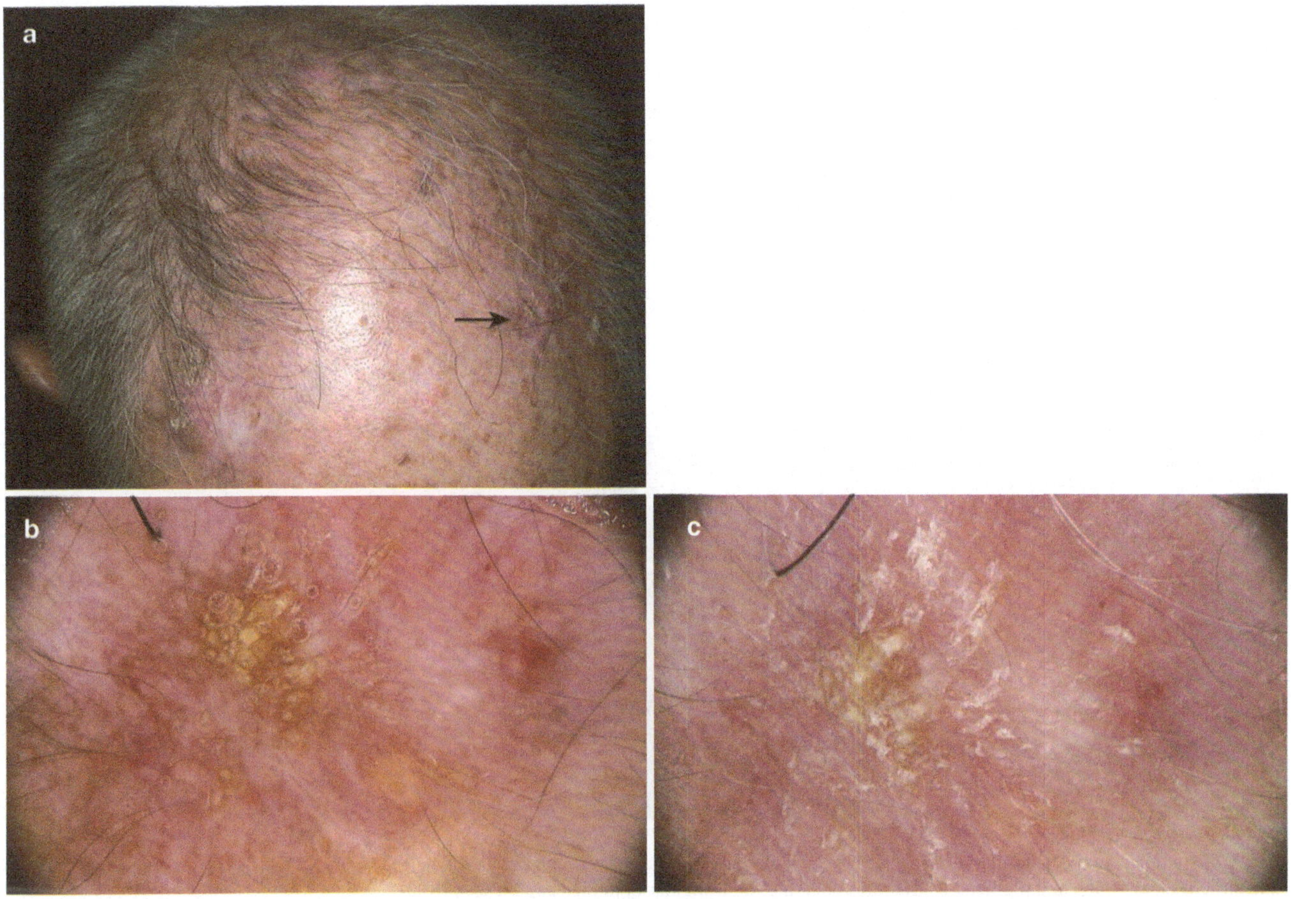

Fig. 10.3 Clinical and dermoscopic images of grade III actinic keratosis. (**a**) Multiple red plaques on the forehead with significant keratinization on the surface. (**b**) Under dermoscopy, dense yellow keratotic plugs in the hair follicle openings and yellow-white structureless areas can be seen (×20). (**c**) Yellow-white scales can also be seen under polarized mode (×20)

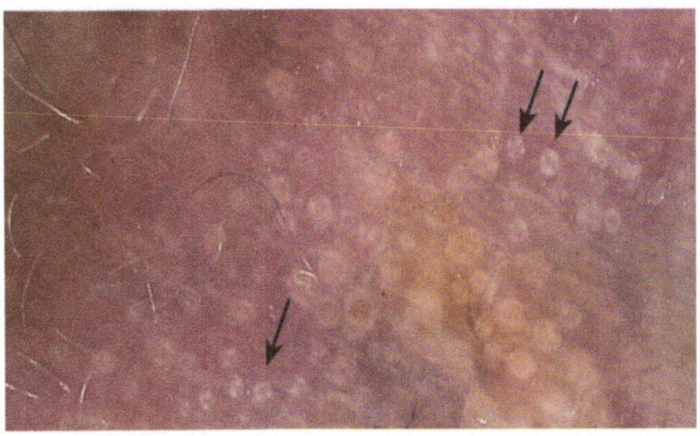

Fig. 10.4 Typical rosette sign under dermoscopy (black arrow, ×20)

10.1.5 The Relationships Between the Dermoscopic Findings and Histopathology of AK (Fig. 10.7)

(i) Grade I AK shows atypical keratinocytes in the lower one-third of the epidermis, and follicular plugs are not yet formed, which corresponds to the red pseudo-network pattern under dermoscopy.

(ii) Grade II AK presents atypical keratinocytes in the lower two-thirds of the epidermis, with focal hyperkeratosis and parakeratosis, significant acanthosis, and epidermal buds extending into the dermal papillary layer. At this stage, follicular plugs can be seen obviously, which corresponds to the strawberry pattern under dermoscopy.

(iii) Grade III AK is characterized by atypical keratinocytes in the full thickness of the epidermis, with increased mitotic activity, hyperkeratosis and parakeratosis, papilloma-like hyperplasia, and adnexa also involved. Follicular openings disappear due to diffuse keratinization, corresponding to yellow-white structureless areas under dermoscopy.

10.2 Bowen's Disease

BD is considered SCC in situ that grows slowly and typically manifests as a brownish-red scaly patch or plaque with a sharp boundary.

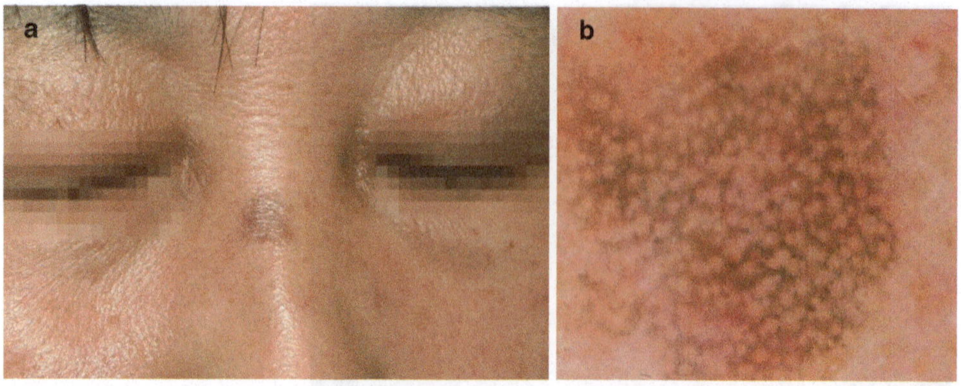

Fig. 10.5 Clinical and dermoscopic images of pigmented actinic keratosis. (**a**) Scaly brown patches on the radix nasi. (**b**) Under dermoscopy, gray-brown dots distributed regularly around the hair follicles can be seen, showing a pseudo-network structure (×20)

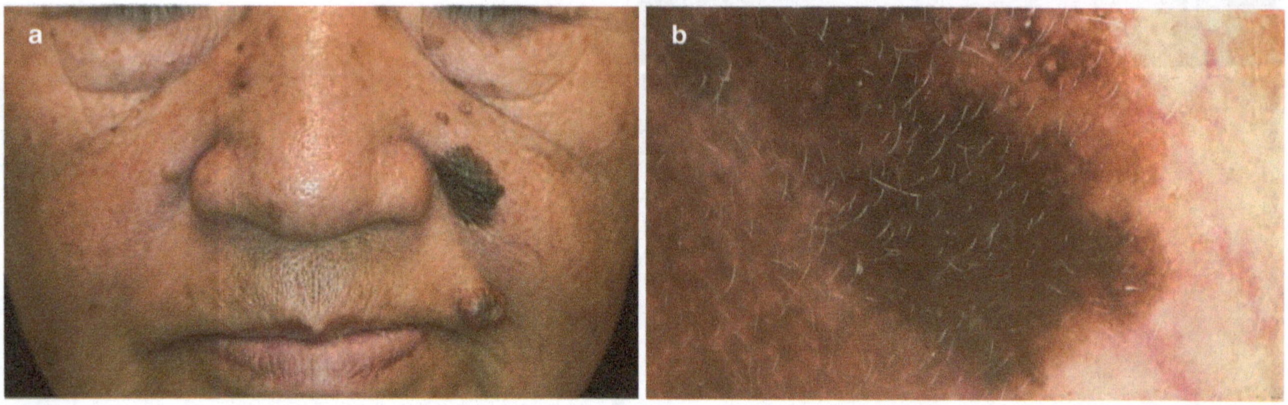

Fig. 10.6 Clinical and dermoscopic images of lentigo maligna. (**a**) A dark brown plaque on the left face. (**b**) Under dermoscopy, a homogeneous and structureless blotch and pigmented structures covering the follicular openings can be seen (×30)

Table 10.1 Differentiation signs of pAK and lentigo maligna under dermoscopy

Dermoscopic features	pAK	Lentigo maligna
Distribution of gray-brown dots	Around the hair follicles	Diffuse
Broken-up pseudo-network structure	Common	Rare
Strawberry pattern combined with a pseudo-network structure	Common	Pigmented structures may cover the hair follicular openings, and a homogeneous, structureless blotch can be seen
Surface scales	Common	Absent
Vascular pattern	Often monotonous	Polymorphous
Small black dot in the center of the follicular opening at early stage	Absent	Common

pAK pigmented actinic keratosis

10.2.1 Dermoscopic Manifestations of BD (Fig. 10.8)

(i) Coiled vessels, also known as glomerular vessels, are tightly coiled like a glomerulus.
(ii) Blood vessels distributed in clusters.
(iii) Yellow-white scales on the surface.
(iv) Red background.

The simultaneous presence of the first three items indicates a 98% probability of BD.

Tip
Coiled vessels need to be observed under high-magnification dermoscopy. Only dotted vessels are displayed under dermoscopy at lower magnification.

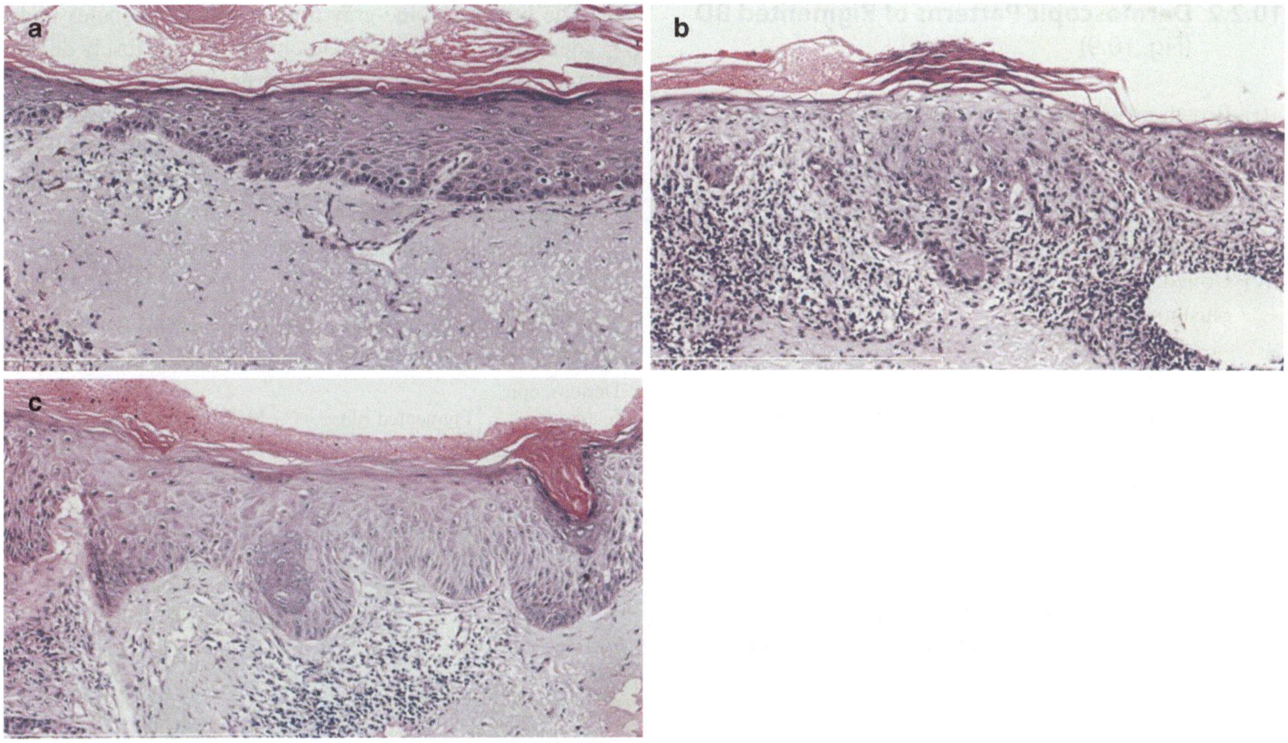

Fig. 10.7 Pathological grading of actinic keratosis. (**a**) Grade I, atypical keratinocytes in the lower one-third of the epidermis, without follicular plugs (hematoxylin and eosin, ×200). (**b**) Grade II, atypical keratinocytes in the lower two-thirds of the epidermis, with focal hyperkeratosis and parakeratosis, marked acanthosis, and epidermal buds extending into the dermal papillary layer (hematoxylin and eosin, ×200). (**c**) Grade III hyperkeratosis and parakeratosis can be seen, with follicular plugs, and atypical keratinocytes in the full thickness of the epidermis, which show active mitosis (hematoxylin and eosin, ×200)

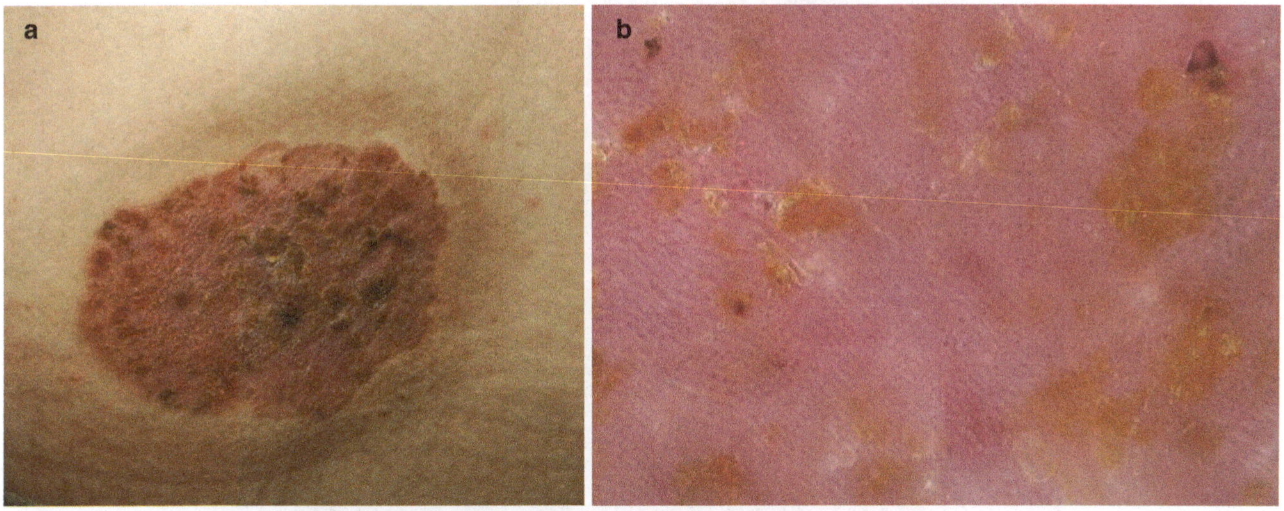

Fig. 10.8 Clinical and dermoscopic images of Bowen's disease. (**a**) A well-circumscribed brownish-red plaque on the back with scales and crusts on the surface. (**b**) A red background, yellow-white scales, and dotted and coiled (glomerular) vessels distributed in clusters under polarized dermoscopy (×20)

10.2.2 Dermoscopic Patterns of Pigmented BD (Fig. 10.9)

(i) Brown or gray dots or globules are a strong indication of BD when radially arranged at the periphery of the lesion.
(ii) Gray-brown structureless pigmented areas.
(iii) Pink or skin-colored eccentric structureless areas.
(iv) Coiled vessels, arranged randomly, radially or in clusters.

10.2.3 Dermoscopic Differential Diagnosis of Pigmented BD and Malignant Melanoma (Table 10.2)

10.2.4 The Relationship between the Dermoscopic Findings and Histopathology of Pigmented BD

(i) The brown or blue-gray dots and small globules under dermoscopy correspond to clustered or diffusely distributed melanophages in the superficial dermis.
(ii) Homogeneous, structureless, pigmentation areas under dermoscopy correspond to the increased pigmentation of the basal layer and the disappearance of the rete ridges due to remarkable acanthosis, leading to the absence of the normal network structures formed by epidermal melanin.

Table 10.2 Differentiation points between pigmented BD and malignant melanoma under dermoscopy

Dermoscopic features	Pigmented BD	Malignant melanoma
Brown or gray dots	Radially arranged at the periphery of the lesion	Irregularly arranged
Vessels	Coiled vessels distributed in clusters	Dotted, hairpin polymorphic vascular pattern, irregularly distributed

BD Bowen's disease

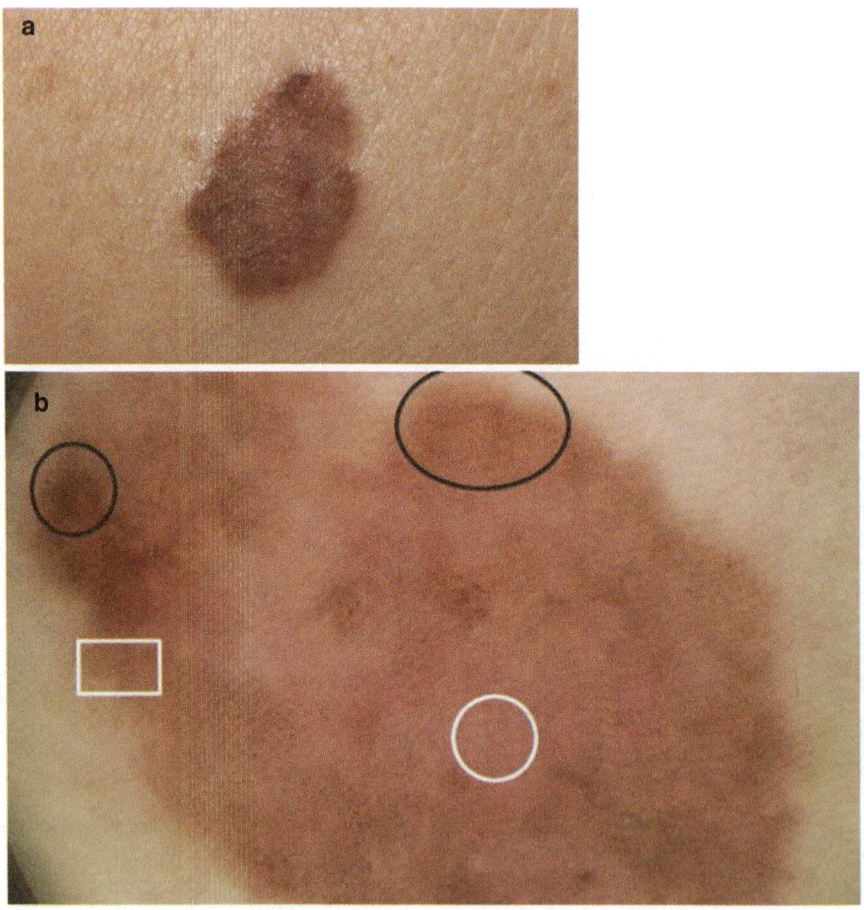

Fig. 10.9 Clinical, dermoscopic, and histopathological manifestations of pigmented Bowen's disease. (**a**) A scaly brown plaque with a sharp boundary on the back. (**b**) Under dermoscopy, brown dots or small globules at the periphery of the lesion, distributed radially (black circles and ovals); light-brown pigmentation structureless areas (white rectangles); and pink or skin-colored eccentric structureless areas (white circle) (×20). (**c**) Under dermoscopy, clusters of coiled vessels can also be seen (white arrow, ×30). (**d**). Histopathology shows epidermal parakeratosis, acanthosis, and obviously atypical cells varying in size throughout the epidermis, with a disordered arrangement. Melanophages and lymphocyte infiltration can be seen in the superficial dermis (hematoxylin and eosin, ×100)

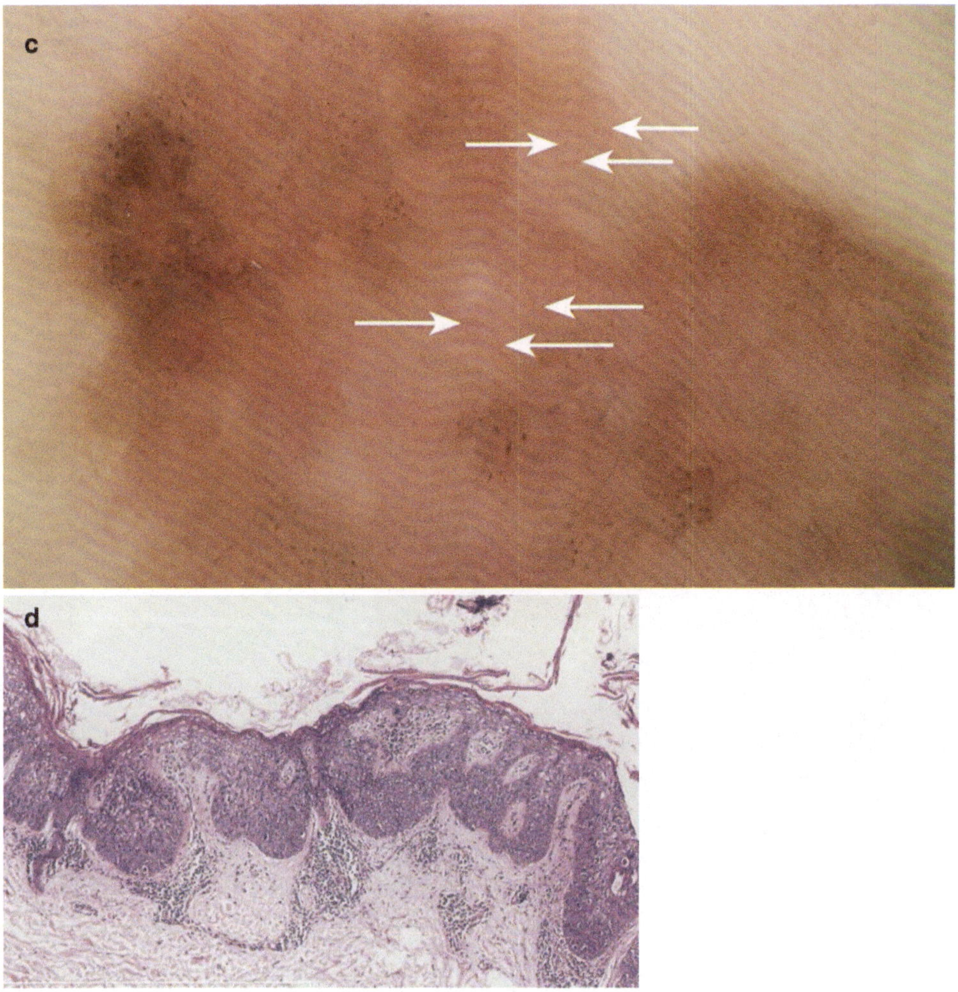

Fig. 10.9 (Continued)

10.3 Keratoacanthoma

KA is similar to well-differentiated SCC clinically and pathologically. KA is characterized by initial rapid growth followed by spontaneous involution over a period of a few months.

10.3.1 Dermoscopic Features of KA (Fig. 10.10)

(i) Central yellow-white structureless keratin
(ii) Keratinized scales
(iii) Vessels may be hairpin, linear-irregular or coiled. These vessels are large, rarely branched and usually distributed peripherally, with white halos surrounding them.
(iv) Yellow opaque center, also known as a pearl-like structure, is surrounded by white halos.
(v) Blood crusts

10.3.2 Differential Diagnosis

Dermoscopy cannot distinguish KA from well-differentiated nodular SCC, but it may help distinguish KA from other non-pigmented nodular tumors, such as nodular basal cell carcinomas, which show arborizing vessels and no keratin.

10.3.3 The Relationship Between the Dermoscopic Findings and Histopathology of KA

The pearl-like structures correspond to the histopathological endoepidermal keratin pearls, which are characteristics of KA and nodular SCC.

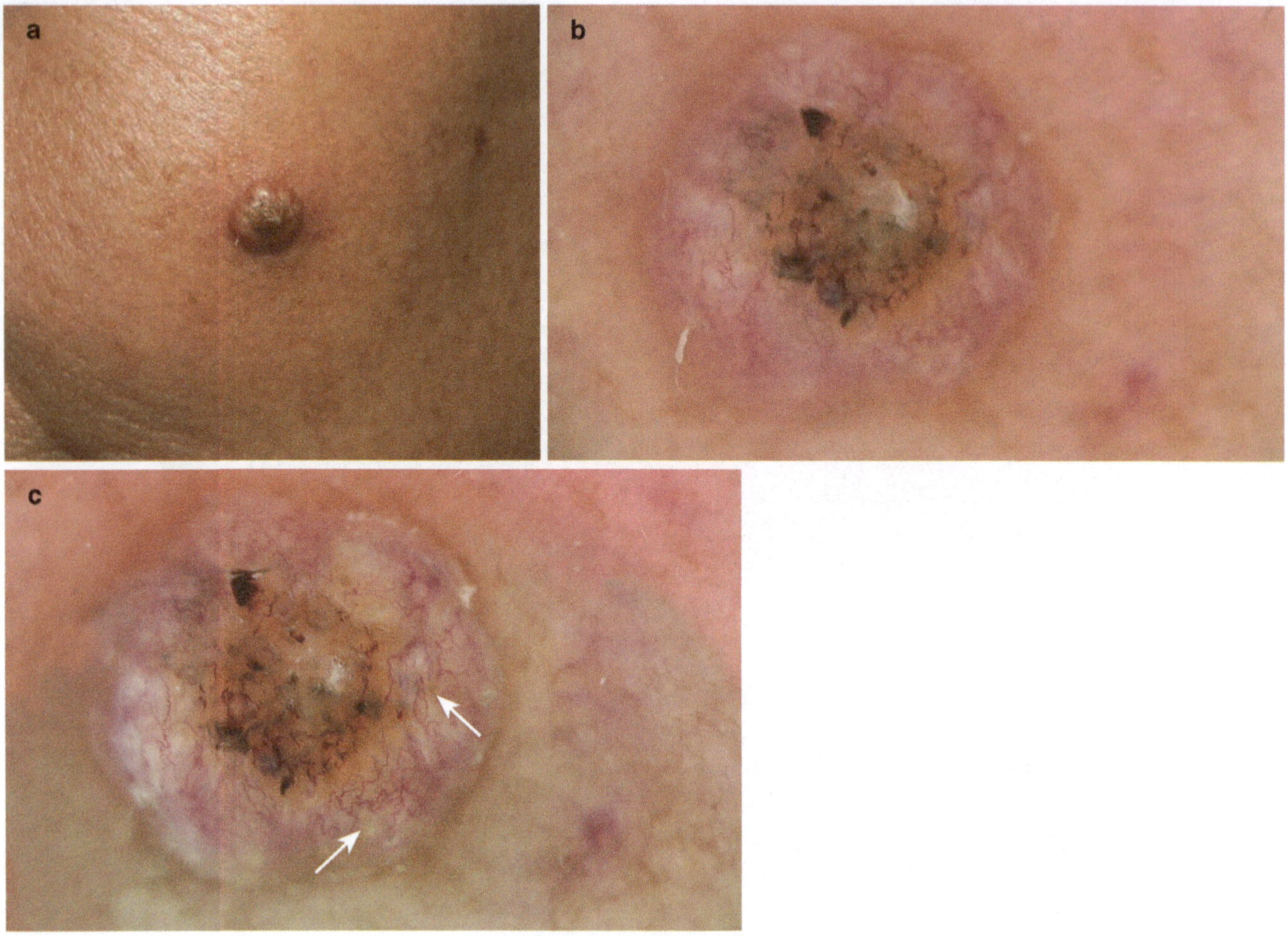

Fig. 10.10 Clinical and dermoscopic manifestations of keratoacanthoma. (**a**) An isolated red hemispherical mass on the left cheek, with a "crater-like" structure in the center; keratin and crusts can be seen. (**b**) Under dermoscopy, the central yellowish structureless mass of keratin, blood crusts, white scales, and enlarged and irregular linear vessels with white halos located peripherally can be seen (×30). (**c**) Pearl-like structures (white arrows, ×30)

10.4 Squamous Cell Carcinoma

An SCC is usually a nodular plaque or mass with exophytic growth on an original skin lesion, and a diagnosis of SCC needs to be confirmed by histopathology.

10.4.1 Dermoscopic Manifestations of Highly Differentiated SCC (Fig. 10.11)

(i) Similar to KA under dermoscopy
(ii) Yellow-white keratin in the center
(iii) Hairpin, linear-irregular, coiled vessels distributed peripherally and irregularly
(iv) Pearl-like structures
(v) The dermoscopic features of AK can be seen if SCC develops from AK

10.4.2 Dermoscopic Manifestations of Moderately Differentiated SCC (Fig. 10.12)

(i) Peripheral hairpin vessels and diffuse yellow to light-brown structureless areas
(ii) Often accompanied by large ulcers
(iii) Pearl-like structures can still be seen.

10.4.3 Dermoscopic Manifestations of Poorly Differentiated SCC (Fig. 10.13)

(i) Often lack keratinized structures
(ii) A polymorphic vascular pattern (>50% lesion area) with numerous small linear, hairpin, and coiled vessels on a red background
(iii) Peripheral white structureless areas are occasionally seen as important diagnostic clues.

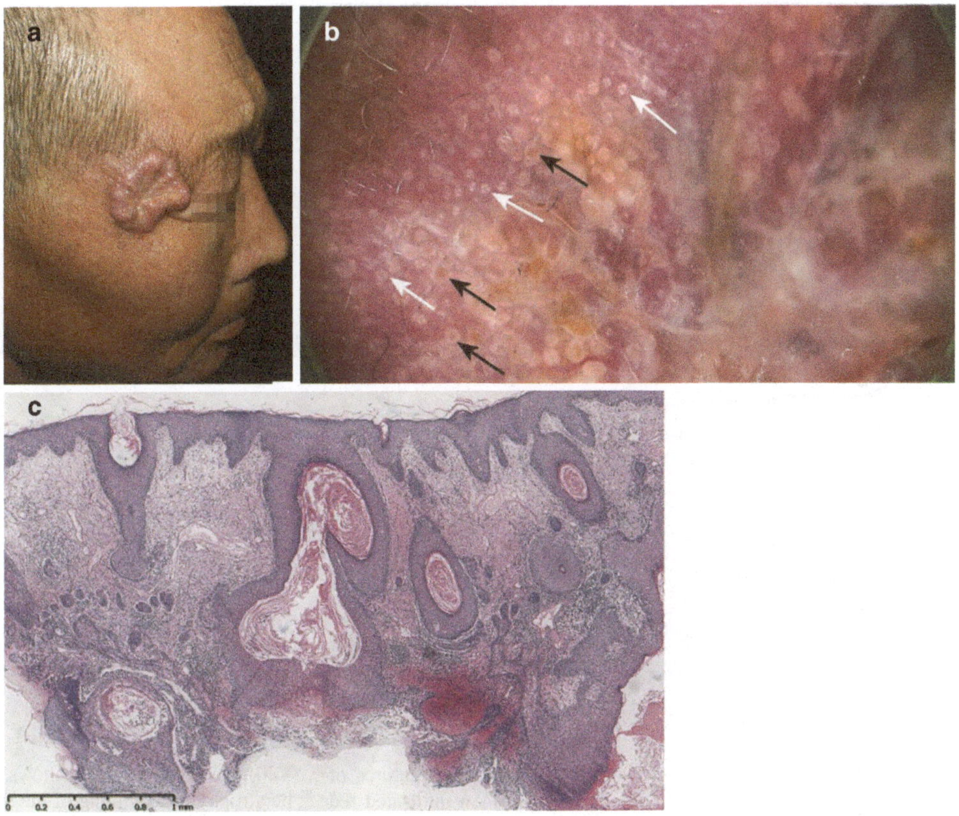

Fig. 10.11 Clinical, dermoscopic, and histopathological features of highly differentiated squamous cell carcinoma. (**a**) A red mass on the right temporal area, with a raised border and erosion on the surface. (**b**) Dermoscopy shows pearl-like structures (black arrows), rosette signs (white arrows), and irregular linear vessels (× 20). (**c**) Histopathology shows that the layer of spinous cells is thickened, the epidermis suddenly extends downward, and squamous cell masses are seen in the dermis; cellular atypia can be seen, and multiple obvious keratin pearls are formed (hematoxylin and eosin, ×50)

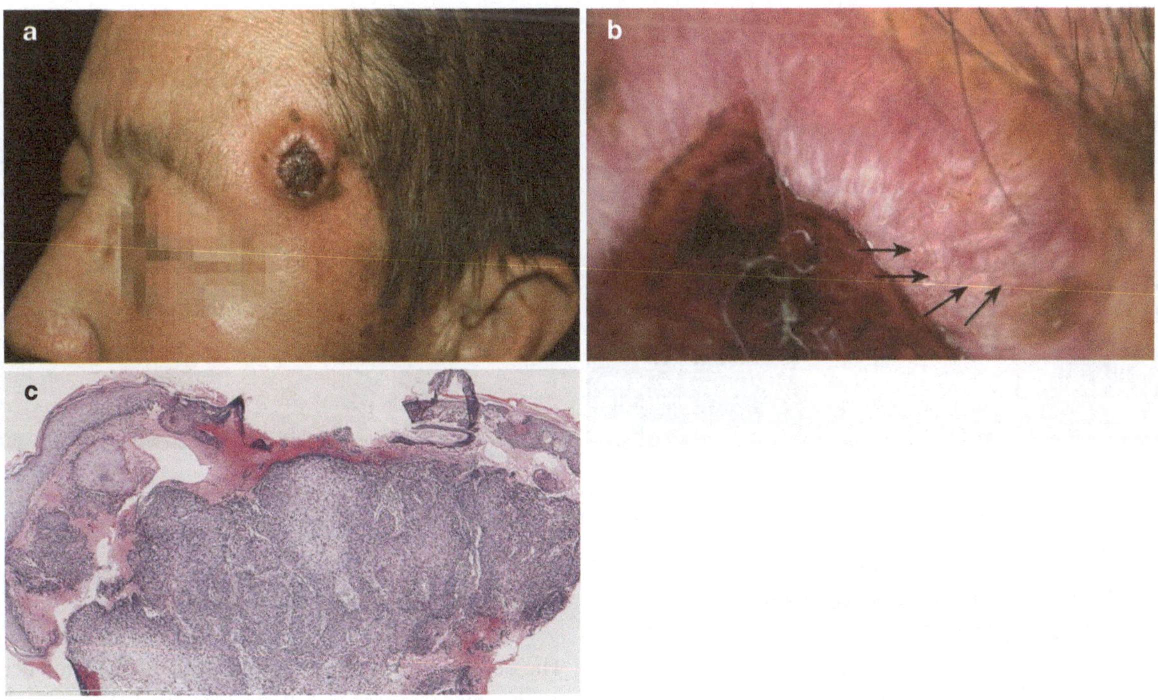

Fig. 10.12 Clinical, dermoscopic and histopathological features of moderately differentiated squamous cell carcinoma. (**a**). An isolated red mass, 4 cm in diameter with central ulceration and crusts on the left temporal region. (**b**) Under dermoscopy, ulceration and blood crusts are seen in the center of the tumor, with polymorphic vascular patterns, pearl-like structures (black arrows) and shiny white streaks (×20). (**c**) Histopathology shows necrosis, squamous cell masses in the epidermis and dermis, cellular atypia, with deep-dyed and enlarged nuclei. Keratosis is still visible (hematoxylin and eosin, ×40)

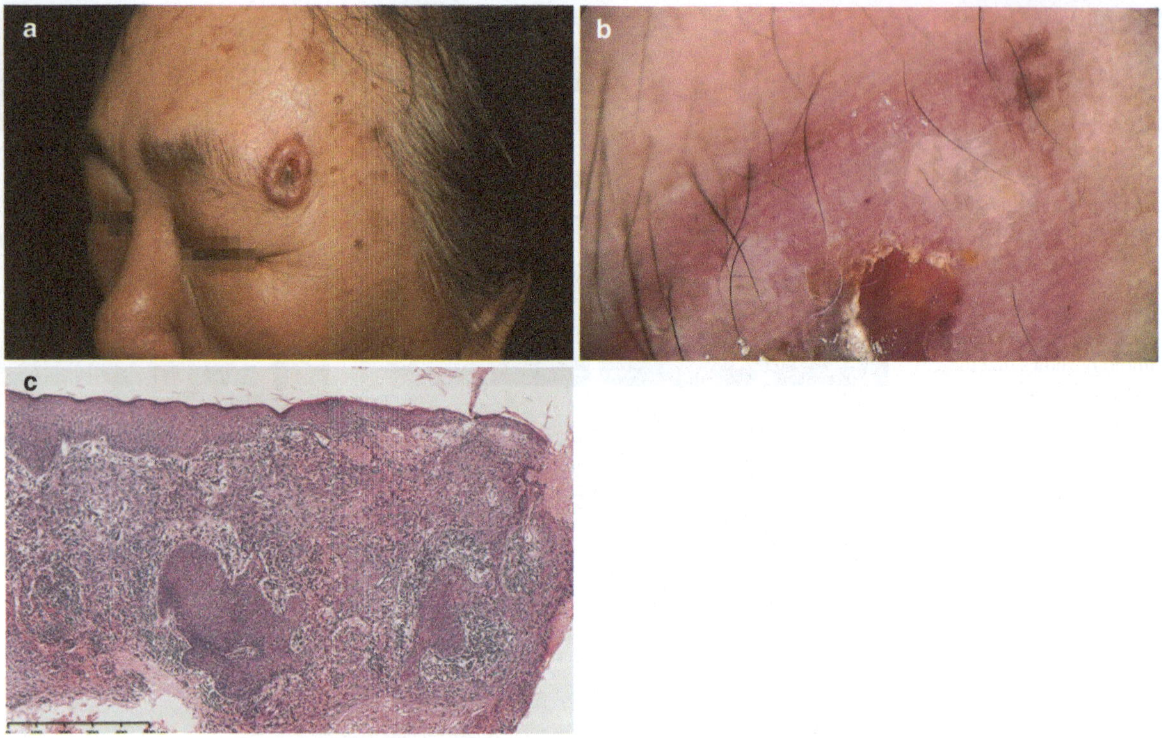

Fig. 10.13 Clinical, dermoscopic, and histopathological features of poorly differentiated squamous cell carcinoma. (**a**) An infiltrated red mass on the left superciliary arch, with ulceration in the center and a raised border. (**b**) Dermoscopy presents a central ulcer with a lack of keratosis and numerous polymorphic vessels on a red background (×20). (**c**) Histopathology shows mild hyperkeratosis in the epidermis, the atrophy and thinning of the spinous layer, a mass of tumor cells in the dermis, and chronic inflammatory cell infiltration, without keratin pearls (hematoxylin and eosin, ×100)

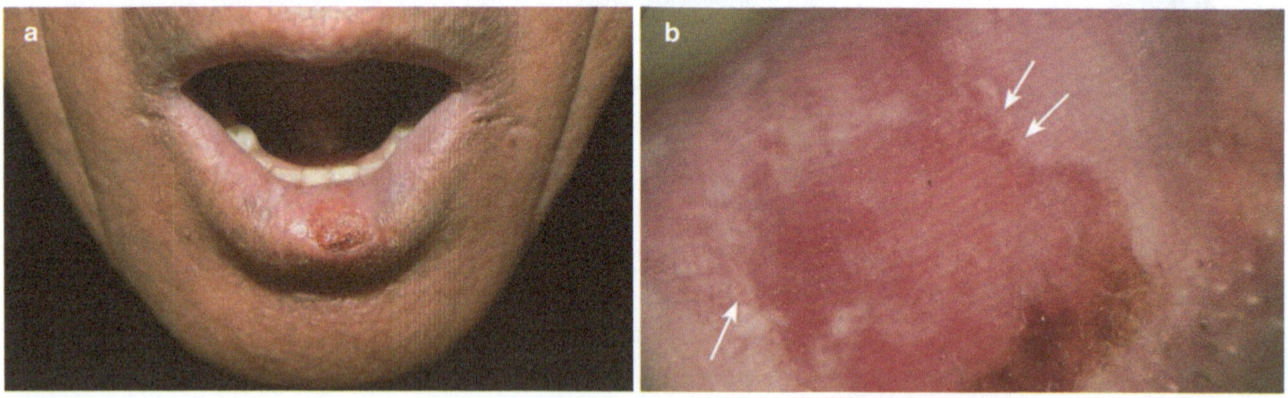

Fig. 10.14 Clinical and dermoscopic features of squamous cell carcinoma of the lip. (**a**). Erythema and ulcer on the lower lip. (**b**). Dermoscopy shows scales, ulcerations, scattered small polymorphous vessels, and yellow-white structures (white arrows) (×20)

10.4.4 Dermoscopic Manifestations of Pigmented SCC

(i) Diffuse homogeneous blue pigmentation
(ii) Irregularly distributed blue-gray granular structures
(iii) If ulcerated, dark brown to black crusts are visible.
(iv) Due to pigmentation, vascular structures are usually not seen.

10.4.5 SCC on Special Locations

The dermoscopic manifestations of lip SCC (often occurring on the lower lip) are as follows (Fig. 10.14):

(i) Scales and ulcers
(ii) Scattered small polymorphous vessels
(iii) Red or yellow to white structures

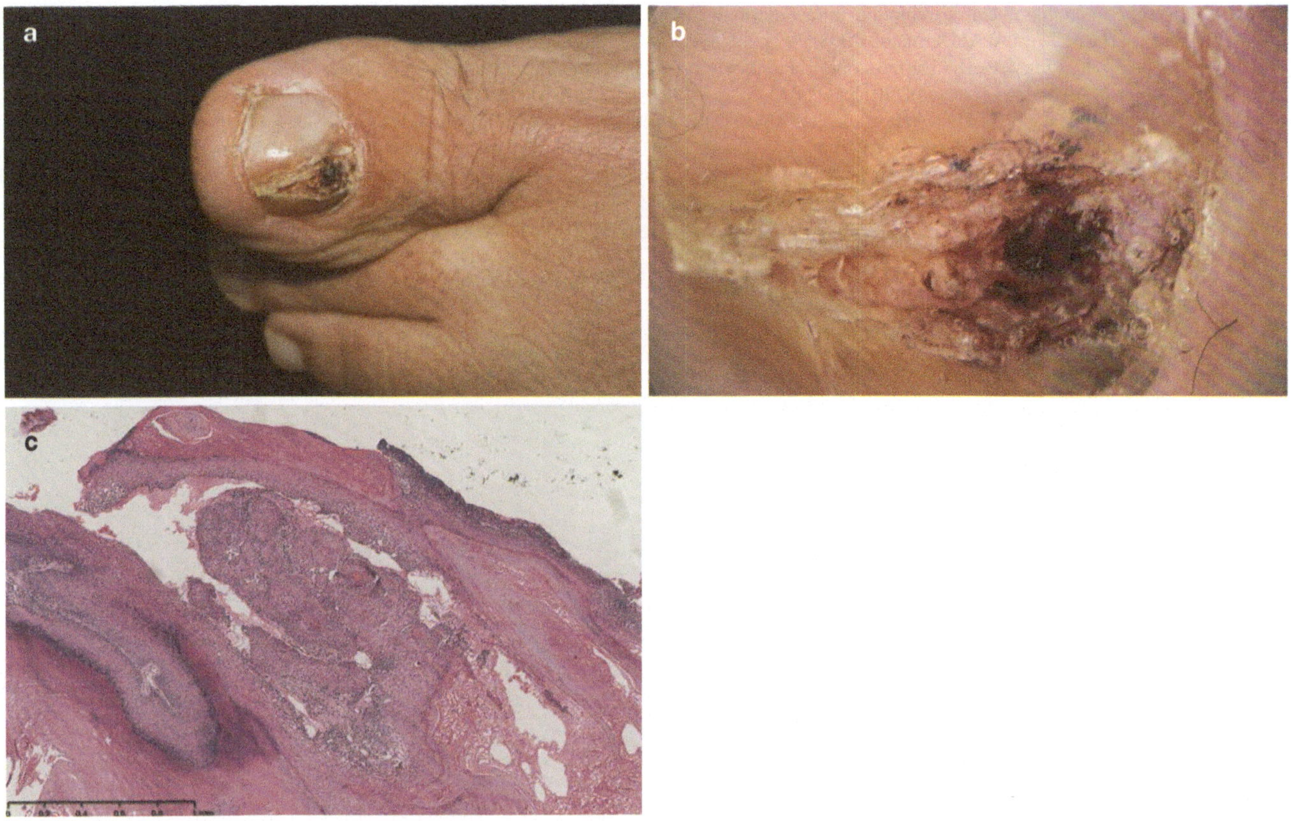

Fig. 10.15 Clinical, dermoscopic, and histopathological features of nail squamous cell carcinoma. (**a**). Erythematous ulcer of the left toenail with partial loss of the nail plate. (**b**). Dermoscopy shows partial onychomadesis, longitudinal nail red bands, irregular vessels, and patchy hemorrhage (× 20). (**c**). Histopathology shows verrucous hyperplasia of the epidermis, hyperkeratosis, parakeratosis, acanthosis, squamous cell masses extending into the dermis, and keratin pearls; and some present cellular atypia (hematoxylin and eosin, ×50)

10.4.6 Dermoscopic Manifestations of Nail Squamous Cell Carcinoma (Fig. 10.15)

(i) Manifests as longitudinal black or red bands
(ii) Irregular vessels
(iii) Patchy hemorrhage

Some scholars have proposed a pattern of evolution from AK to SCC. In this process, the initial dotted vessels gradually expand, coil (such as form globular vessels), and gather. During this time, the hair follicles in this region shrink and even disappear. These represent that the lesion evolves to SCC in situ, namely BD; and then may progress to aggressive SCC, with clinically thickened lesions, dermoscopic hairpin and/or irregular linear vessels, and sometimes central keratotic plugging or ulceration.

Further Reading

1. Skin Imaging Group. Dermatology branch of China international exchange and promotion association for medical and healthcare. Expert consensus on dermoscopic features of squamous cell tumors (2017). Chin J Dermatol. 2018;2:87–91.
2. Zalaudek I, Giacomel J, Schmid K, et al. Dermatoscopy of facial actinic keratosis, intraepidermal carcinoma, and invasive squamous cell carcinoma: a progression model. J Am Acad Dermatol. 2012;66(4):589–97.
3. Zalaudek I, Piana S, Moscarella E, et al. Morphologic grading and treatment of facial actinic keratosis. Clin Dermatol. 2014;32(1):80–7.
4. Huerta-Brogeras M, Olmos O, Borbujo J, et al. Validation of dermoscopy as a real-time noninvasive diagnostic imaging technique for actinic keratosis. Arch Dermatol. 2012;148(10):1159–64.
5. Cuellar F, Vilalta A, Puig S, et al. New dermoscopic pattern in actinic keratosis and related conditions. Arch Dermatol. 2009;145(6):732.
6. Haspeslagh M, Noe M, De Wispelaere I, et al. Rosettes and other white shiny structures in polarized dermoscopy: histological correlate and optical explanation. J Eur Acad Dermatol Venereol. 2016;30(2):311–3.
7. Lallas A, Apalla Z, Argenziano G, et al. Clues for differentiating discoid lupus erythematosus from actinic keratosis. J Am Acad Dermatol. 2013;69(1):e5–6.
8. Ciudad C, Aviles JA, Suarez R, et al. Diagnostic utility of dermoscopy in pigmented actinic keratosis. Actas Dermosifiliogr. 2011;102(8):623–6.
9. Giacomel J, Lallas A, Argenziano G, et al. Dermoscopic "signature" pattern of pigmented and nonpigmented facial actinic keratoses. J Am Acad Dermatol. 2015;72(2):e57–9.
10. Lallas A, Tschadl P, Kyrgidis A, et al. Dermoscopic clues to differentiate facial lentigo maligna from pigmented actinic keratosis. Br J Dermatol. 2015;174(5):1079–85.
11. Pan Y, Chamberlain AJ, Bailey M, et al. Dermatoscopy aids in the diagnosis of the solitary red scaly patch or plaque-features distin-

guishing superficial basal cell carcinoma, intraepidermal carcinoma, and psoriasis. J Am Acad Dermatol. 2008;59(2):268–74.
12. Payapvipapong K, Tanaka M. Dermoscopic classification of Bowen's disease. Australas J Dermatol. 2015;56(1):32–5.
13. Mota AN, Pineiro-Maceira J, Alves MF, et al. Pigmented Bowen's disease. An Bras Dermatol. 2014;89(5):825–7.
14. Zalaudek I, Argenziano G. Dermoscopy of actinic keratosis, intraepidermal carcinoma and squamous cell carcinoma. Curr Probl Dermatol. 2015;46(46):70–6.
15. Kuonen F, Durack A, Gaide O. Clues in DeRmoscopy: Dermoscopy of keratoacanthoma. Eur J Dermatol. 2016;26(4):419–20.
16. Lin MJ, Pan Y, Jalilian C, et al. Dermoscopic characteristics of nodular squamous cell carcinoma and keratoacanthoma. Dermatol Pract Concept. 2014;4(2):9–15.
17. Lallas A, Pyne J, Kyrgidis A, et al. The clinical and dermoscopic features of invasive cutaneous squamous cell carcinoma depend on the histopathologic grade of differentiation. Br J Dermatol. 2014;172(5):1308–15.
18. Benatie E, Rsechino F, Piana S, et al. Dermoscopic features of squamous cell carcinoma on the lips. Br J Dermatol. 2017;177(3):e41–3.
19. Dika E, Fantia PA, Patrizi A, et al. Mohs surgery for squamous cell carcinoma of the nail unit: 10 years of experience. Dermatol Surg. 2015;41(9):1015–9.
20. Kupsae R, Deinlein T, Woltsche N, et al. Dermoscopy of keratinocyte skin cancer. G Ital Dermatol Venereol. 2016;151(6):649–62.

Other Neoplasms

11

This chapter focuses on pathological changes of adnexal neoplasms and other skin tumors that are not discussed in the preceding chapters. These neoplastic diseases can be a major diagnostic challenge due to their rarity and nonspecific clinical manifestations. However, as a noninvasive supplementary tool, dermoscopy can lead to improved description and identification of these diseases, as well as improved differentiation of these diseases from other diseases.

11.1 Sebaceous Adenoma/Sebaceoma

Sebaceous adenomas and sebaceomas are benign neoplasms with sebaceous differentiation, which usually present as yellowish, reddish, or skin-colored nodules on the head and neck region but also can display a lobular pattern (Fig. 11.1a). Histopathological changes are mainly characterized by a well-circumscribed tumor that consists of basaloid seboblastic cells and mature sebocytic cells in certain proportions. The term sebaceous adenoma is used when mature sebocytes predominate, while the term sebaceoma is used when basaloid seboblasts predominate (Fig. 11.1b).

The dermoscopic features of sebaceous adenoma/sebaceomas are as follows (Fig. 11.1c):

1. Clinically pink to white papules/nodules with a central crater, dermoscopically characterized by elongated crown vessels surrounding opaque structureless yellow areas, at times covered by blood crusts.
2. Clinically pink to yellow papules/nodules without a central crater, dermoscopically exhibiting a few, loosely arranged yellow comedo-like globules and arborizing vessels.

J. Liu, X. Zou, *Practical Dermoscopy*, https://doi.org/10.1007/978-981-19-1460-7_11

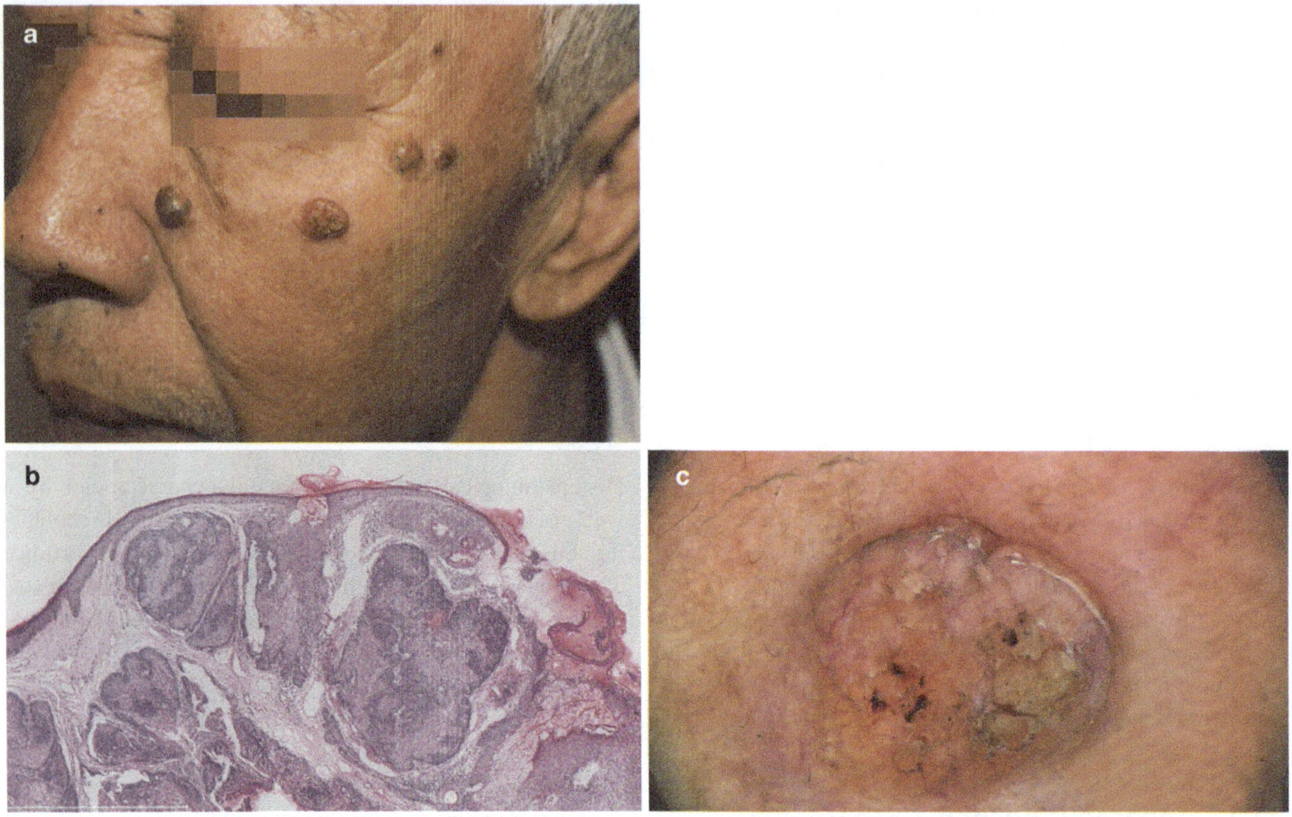

Fig. 11.1 Clinical, pathological and dermoscopic features of sebaceous adenoma. (**a**). A red nodule with a crater in the left zygomatic area. (**b**). Skin biopsy shows epidermal atrophy and increased sebaceous lobules of various sizes and shapes in the dermis that are constituted by mature sebocytes in the central area and basaloid seboblasts in the outer layer, a few of which show mitosis (hematoxylin and eosin, ×40). (**c**). Under dermoscopy, the lesion presents an opaque structureless yellow area with yellow comedo-like globules in the center, surrounded by radially arranged arborizing vessels (×20)

11.2 Desmoplastic Trichilemmoma

Desmoplastic trichilemmoma is a variant of trichilemmoma that is usually distributed on the face or on genital skin, presenting as a skin-colored to reddish, elevated papule or nodule, sometimes with hyperkeratosis or a verrucous surface (Fig. 11.2a). Histopathological changes include verrucous hyperplasia and hypergranulosis, lobular tumor clusters arrayed in an infiltrative pattern with enveloping sclerotic stroma, and commonly seen squamous eddies (Fig. 11.2b).

The dermoscopic features of desmoplastic trichilemmomas are as follows (Fig. 11.2c):

1. Crown vessels
2. Unspecific amorphous white areas
3. Central hyperkeratotic area of regression
4. Shiny white streaks
5. Blue-gray globules

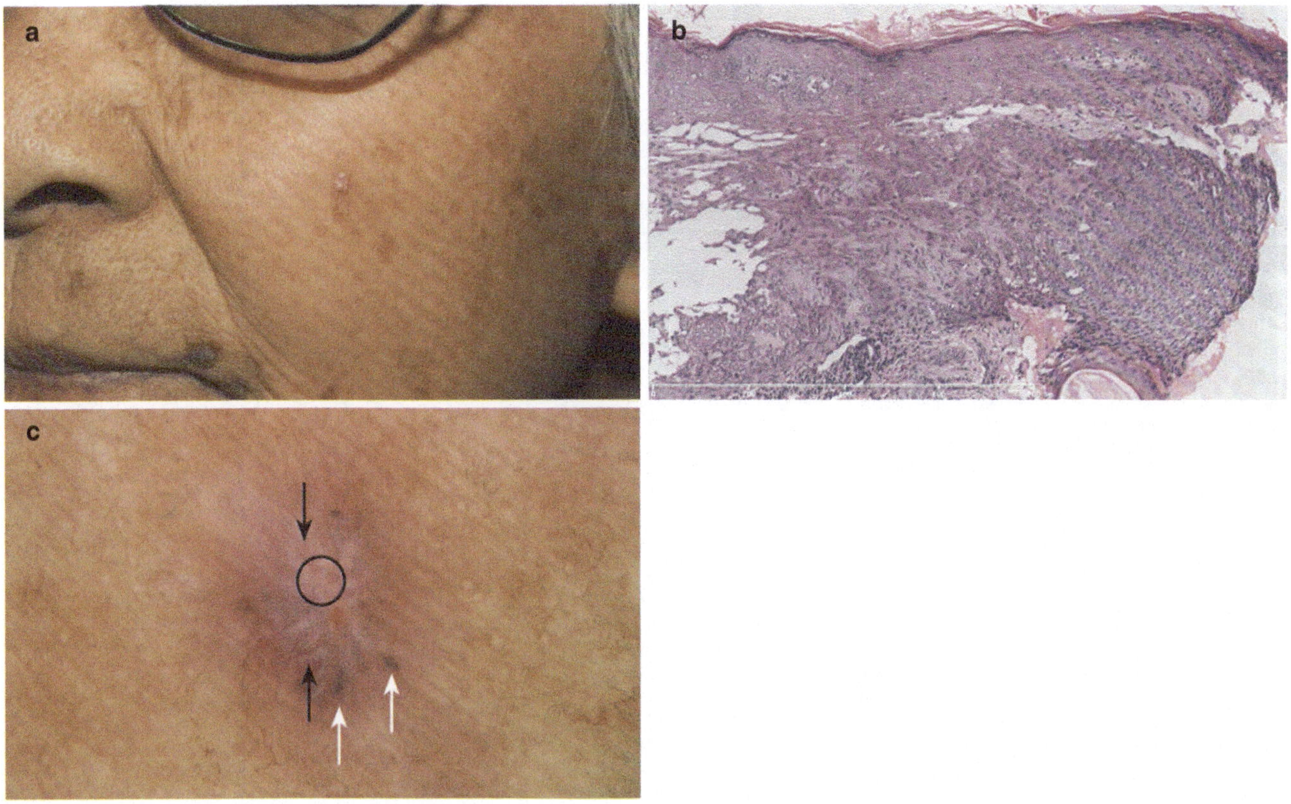

Fig. 11.2 Clinical, pathological, and dermoscopic features of desmoplastic trichilemmoma. (**a**) A small pink papule in the left zygomatic area. (**b**). Histopathological examination shows typical lobular structures of trichilemmoma on the periphery, and in the central region, an area of pseudoepitheliomatous hyperplasic epidermis is inserted into the stroma (hematoxylin and eosin, ×100). (**c**). Dermoscopic findings are characterized by a central amorphous white area with shiny white streaks (circle); radially arranged linear and hairpin-like vessels (black arrow); and peripheral, multiple, blue-gray globules (white arrow) (×40)

11.3 Trichoepithelioma

A trichoepithelioma is a benign neoplasm with follicular germinative differentiation, and trichoepithelioma is currently considered to be a variant of trichoblastoma. Classic trichoepithelioma conventionally manifests as a papule or small nodule with skin coloration on the face, especially the nose or upper trunk (Fig. 11.3a), which histopathologically consists of clusters of follicular germinative cells and conspicuous fibrous stroma (Fig. 11.3b).

The dermoscopic features of trichoepitheliomas are as follows (Fig. 11.3c):

1. Fine arborizing vessels
2. Shiny white streaks or areas
3. Milia-like cysts
4. Blue-gray dots/globules

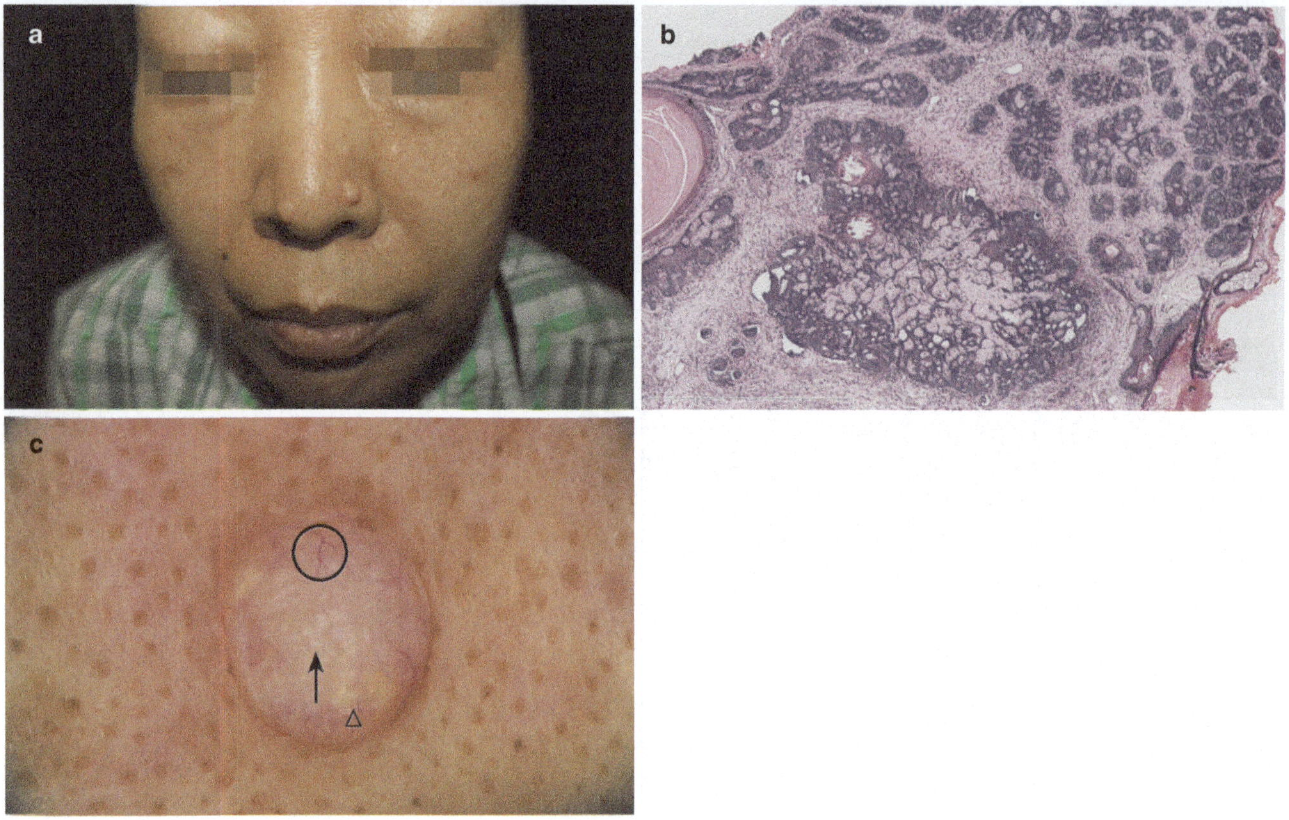

Fig. 11.3 Clinical, pathological, and dermoscopic features of trichoepithelioma. (**a**). Two dome-shaped, skin-colored papules on the nose. (**b**). Histopathological examination shows the presence of basaloid follicular germinative cells that are arrayed in a cribriform pattern and connected with surrounding fibrous stroma (hematoxylin and eosin, ×40). (**c**). Dermoscopy shows peripheral fine arborizing vessels (circle), shiny white streaks (arrow), and milia-like cysts (triangle) (×20)

11.4 Poroma

Poromas are a group of benign adnexal neoplasms with poroid (terminal ductal) differentiation that can be a proliferation of either apocrine or eccrine lineage. Poromas clinically present as solitary papules, plaques, or nodules (Fig. 11.4a). Sessile vascular plaques surrounded by indented moats on the palms and soles are highly suggestive of poroma. Histopathologically, a poroma is composed of a circumscribed proliferation of compact cuboidal keratinocytes with various degrees of ductal differentiation (Fig. 11.4b).

The dermoscopic features of poromas are as follows (Fig. 11.4c, d):

1. White interlacing areas around vessels
2. Yellow structureless areas
3. Milky-red globules
4. Poorly visualized vessels
5. Branched vessels with rounded endings and atypical hairpin vessels

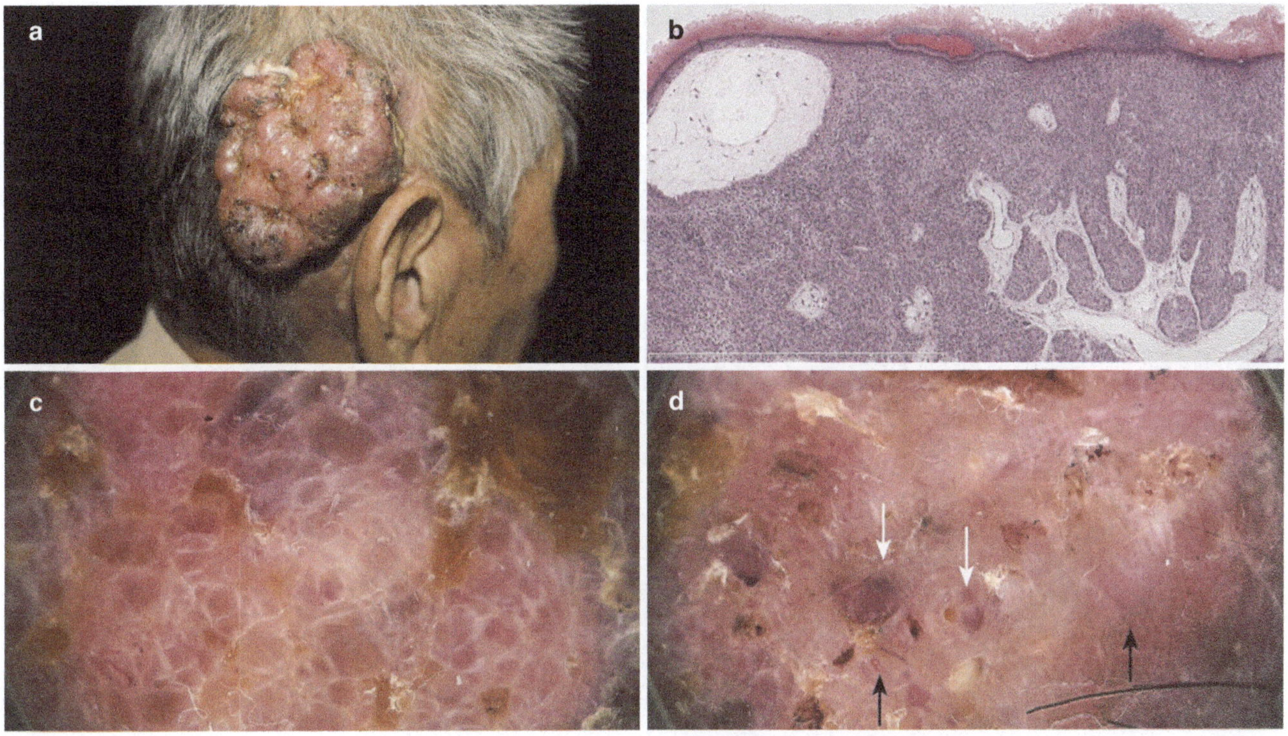

Fig. 11.4 Clinical, pathological, and dermoscopic features of poroma. (**a**). A 9 × 6 cm, red, exophytic mass with ulceration and suppuration on the surface in the right postauricular area. (**b**). Histopathological examination shows hyperplastic interanastomosing cords composed of basaloid cells with the formation of a lumen (hematoxylin and eosin, ×100). (**c** and **d**). Dermoscopy shows the presence of white interlacing areas around vessels, milky-red globules (white arrow), and atypical hairpin vessels (black arrow) (×20)

11.5 Porocarcinoma

A porocarcinoma is the most common type of sweat gland carcinoma that may develop de novo or in association with an existing poroma. The clinical manifestation of a porocarcinoma is a pink nodule with or without ulceration (Fig. 11.5). In histopathology, a porocarcinoma consists of eosinophilic or pallid cuboidal cell nests with conspicuous ductal differentiation infiltrating the dermis.

The dermoscopic features of porocarcinomas are as follows:

1. Polymorphous vessels including hairpin, linear-irregular and dotted vessels
2. Round to oval, pink or white structureless areas
3. White to pink halos around vessels or structureless areas

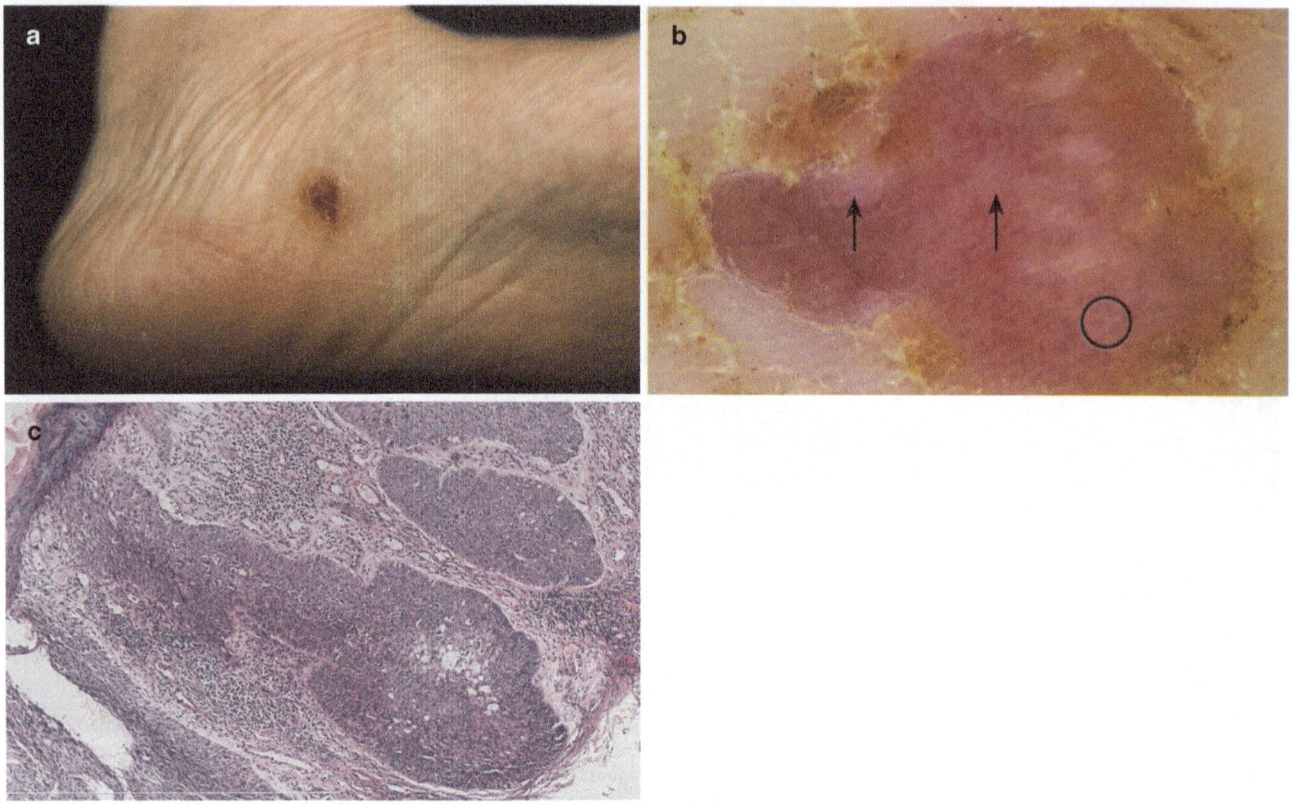

Fig. 11.5 Clinical, pathological and dermoscopic features of porocarcinoma. (**a**). Red plaque in the interior area of the left sole. (**b**). Dermoscopy shows irregular-linear vessels with surrounding white halos (circle) and pink structureless areas (arrow) (×30). (**c**). Skin biopsy shows intradermal cords and clusters of poroid eosinophilic tumor cells with remarkable atypia, accompanied by the infiltration of surrounding chronic inflammatory cells. The tendency toward ductal differentiation is also observable (hematoxylin and eosin, ×100)

11.6 Apocrine Hidrocystoma

Apocrine hidrocystomas are less common, benign, cystic tumors of the apocrine gland that often occur solitarily and usually on the head and neck, with a propensity to involve the cheek and eyelid. Skin lesions present as millet- to bean-sized, dome-shaped, semitranslucent nodules with cystic rigidity and brown, blue, or skin coloration. The surface of apocrine hidrocystomas is tense and smooth (Fig. 11.6a). Histopathologically, these lesions are characterized by single or occasionally multiple dilated cystic ducts and cyst lumens with light-red amorphous contents. Decapitation secretion is usually present (Fig. 11.6b).

The dermoscopic features of apocrine hidrocystomas are as follows (Fig. 11.6c):

1. Blue-gray, semitranslucent, homogeneous area that occupies the whole lesion
2. Arborizing vessels
3. Rosette sign

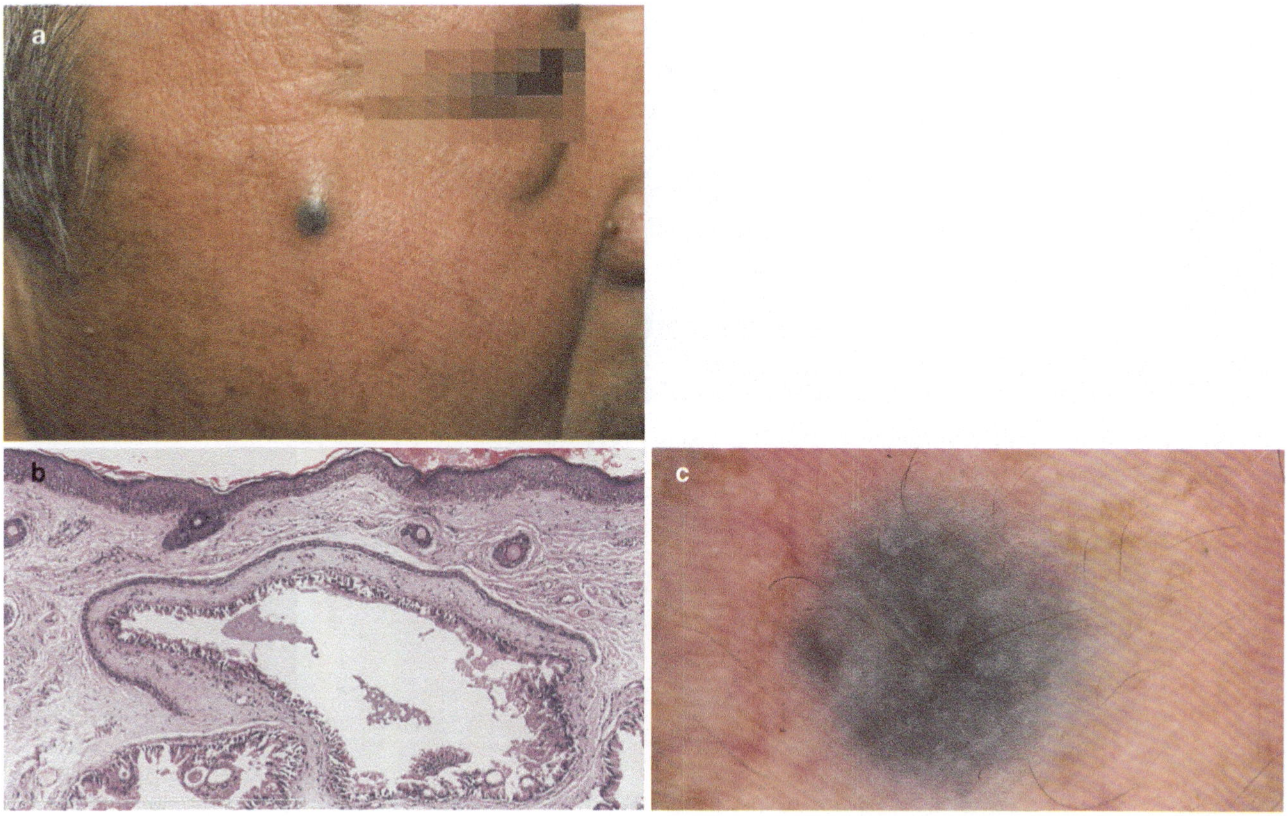

Fig. 11.6 Clinical, pathological, and dermoscopic features of apocrine hidrocystoma. (**a**). A pea-sized, blue-black, semitranslucent nodule with a smooth surface on the right zygomatic area. (**b**). Skin biopsy displays multiple intradermal cysts, the wall of which consists of a double layer of epithelial cells with the outer layer being myoepithelial cells and the inner layer being tall columnar cells. Decapitation secretion is also shown (hematoxylin and eosin, ×100). (**c**). Under dermoscopy, the whole lesion is covered by a blue-gray, semitranslucent, homogeneous area. Arborizing vessels and the rosette sign are also featured (×30)

11.7 Eccrine Hidrocystoma

Eccrine hidrocystomas are uncommon benign skin neoplasms that are caused by cystic dilation of eccrine ducts due to sweat retention. Eccrine hidrocystomas commonly present on the face, especially in the periorbital area. The cheek and nose are also frequently involved. Eccrine hidrocystomas manifest as dome-shaped, translucent, cystic papules with a diameter of 1 to 6 mm, showing yellowish, bluish, or brownish color (Fig. 11.7a). These lesions often occur or are exacerbated in hot and humid environments. Histopathologically, eccrine hidrocystomas are characterized by unilocular cysts containing clear fluids that are lined by two layers of cuboidal to flattened epithelial cells (Fig. 11.7b).

The dermoscopic features of eccrine hidrocystomas are as follows (Fig. 11.7c):

1. Well-demarcated, blue-purple, homogeneous, structureless area with an enveloping white halo.
2. No or only a few vascular structures can be found.

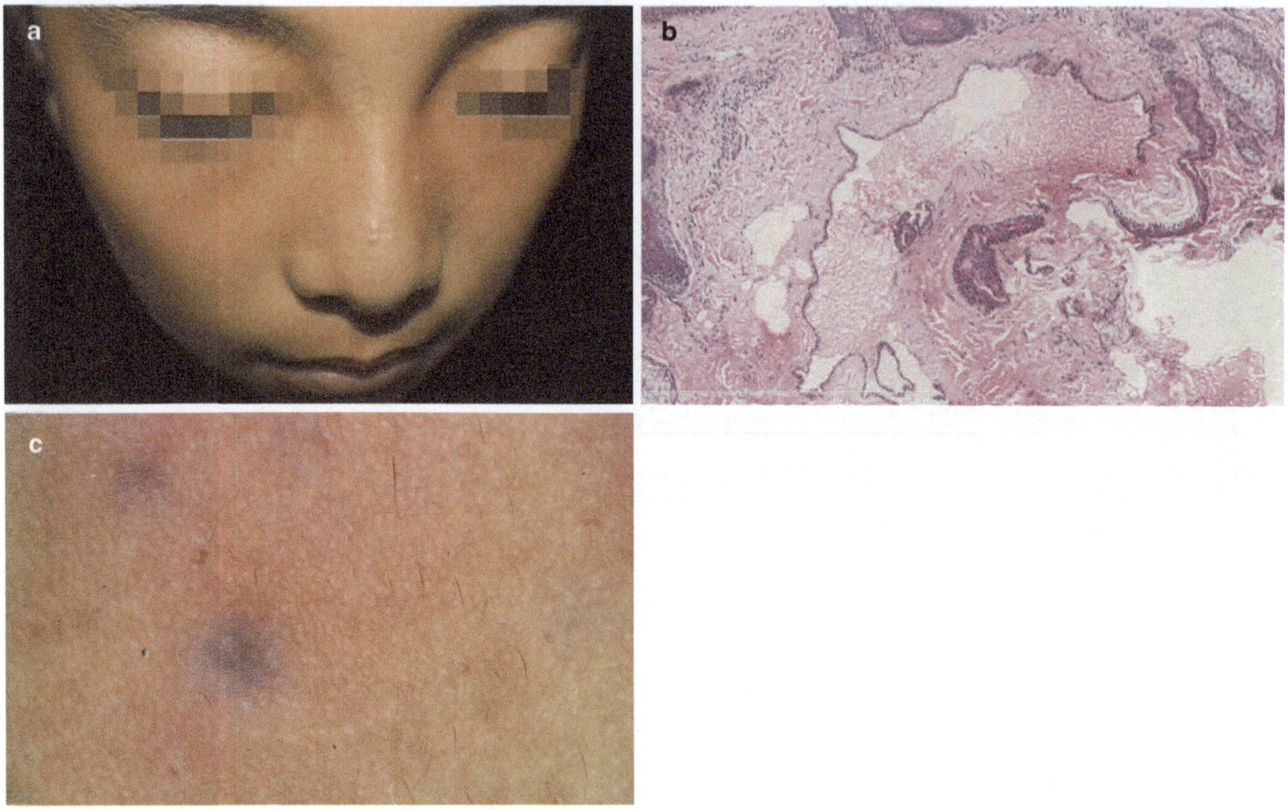

Fig. 11.7 Clinical, pathological, and dermoscopic features of eccrine hidrocystoma. (**a**). Multiple, small, cystic, skin-colored to taupe papules with smooth surfaces are scattered on the nose. (**b**). Histopathological examination shows an intradermal unilocular cyst with reddish contents lined by two layers of cuboidal to flattened epithelial cells (hematoxylin and eosin, ×100). (**c**). Dermoscopy shows well-defined, blue-purple, homogeneous, structureless areas surrounded by a white halo, but no obvious vascular structure is seen (×40)

11.8 Syringocystadenoma Papilliferum

Syringocystadenoma papilliferum is a type of apocrine adenoma presenting as a papule or nodule with a crusted surface almost exclusively on the head or neck (Fig. 11.8a). Histopathologically, syringocystadenoma papilliferum is composed of papillary fronds lined by double layers of columnar cells with prominent apocrine differentiation, and the cores of fronds contain a dense infiltration of lymphocytes and plasma cells (Fig. 11.8b).

The dermoscopic features of syringocystadenoma papilliferum are as follows (Fig. 11.8c):

1. Exophytic papillary structure
2. Yellow, white, or pink structureless areas
3. Vascular structures can be hairpin-like, linear, comma-like, or polymorphous
4. Erosion, crust, and ulceration

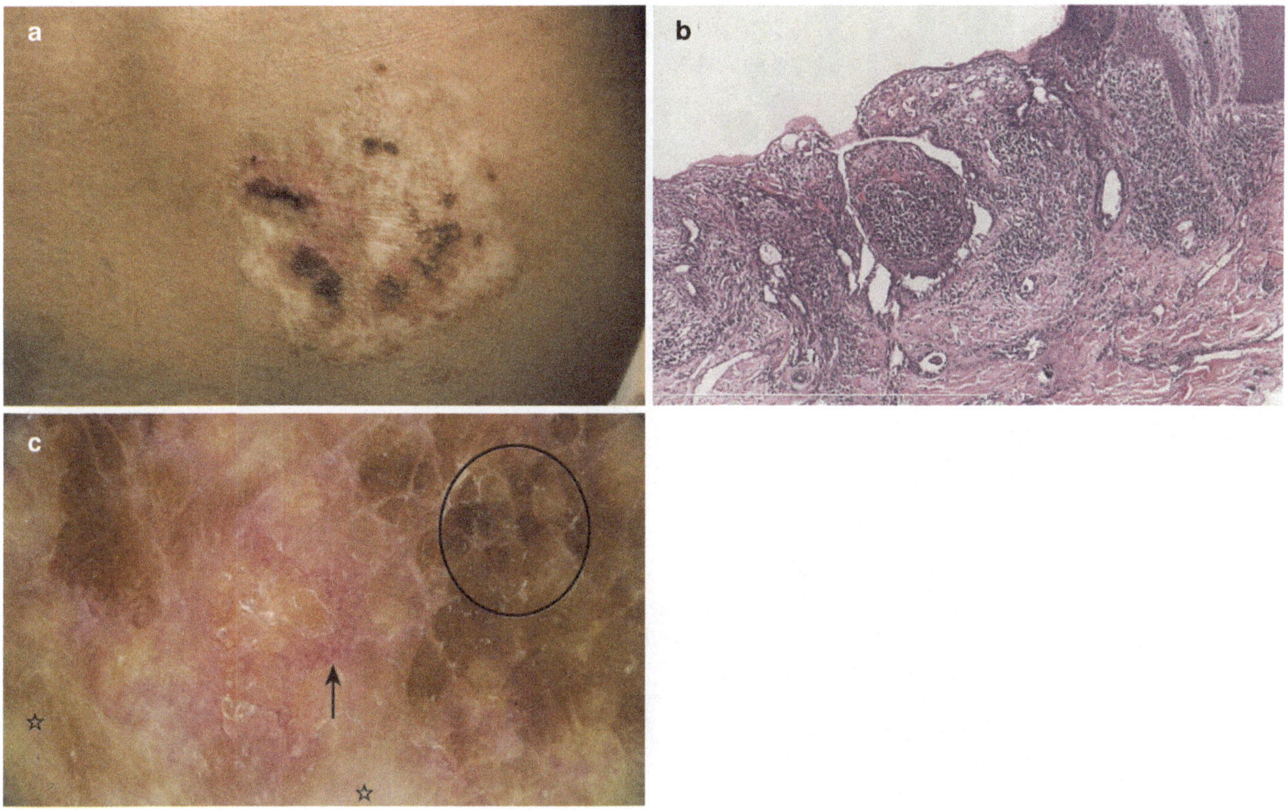

Fig. 11.8 Clinical, pathological and dermoscopic features of syringocystadenoma papilliferum. (**a**). A crusted plaque with a diameter of 10 cm on the right lumbar region. (**b**). Skin biopsy shows adenoid tumor clusters in the dermis, the luminal layer of which consists of columnar cells with decapitation secretion. The infiltration of plasma cells in the stoma is dense (hematoxylin and eosin, ×100). (**c**). Dermoscopy shows umber, papillary lobules (circle), comma-like or irregular-linear vessels (arrow), and yellowish-white structureless areas (asterisk) (×20)

11.9 Epidermoid Cysts

Epidermoid cysts are the most common cutaneous cysts and can occur anywhere on the skin. Epidermoid cysts present as well-demarcated, dermal nodules, sometimes with a clinically visible punctum (Fig. 11.9a). Histologically, epidermoid cysts are characterized by cystic cavities filled with laminated keratin lined by a stratified squamous epithelium, including a granular layer (Fig. 11.9b).

The dermoscopic features of epidermoid cysts are as follows (Fig. 11.9c):

1. Ivory-white background
2. Pore sign
3. Blue-white veil, more frequent in unruptured cysts
4. Red lacunae, more frequent in ruptured cysts
5. Unruptured cysts show arborizing vessels or no vascular structure, while in ruptured cysts, peripheral linear branched vessels are common.

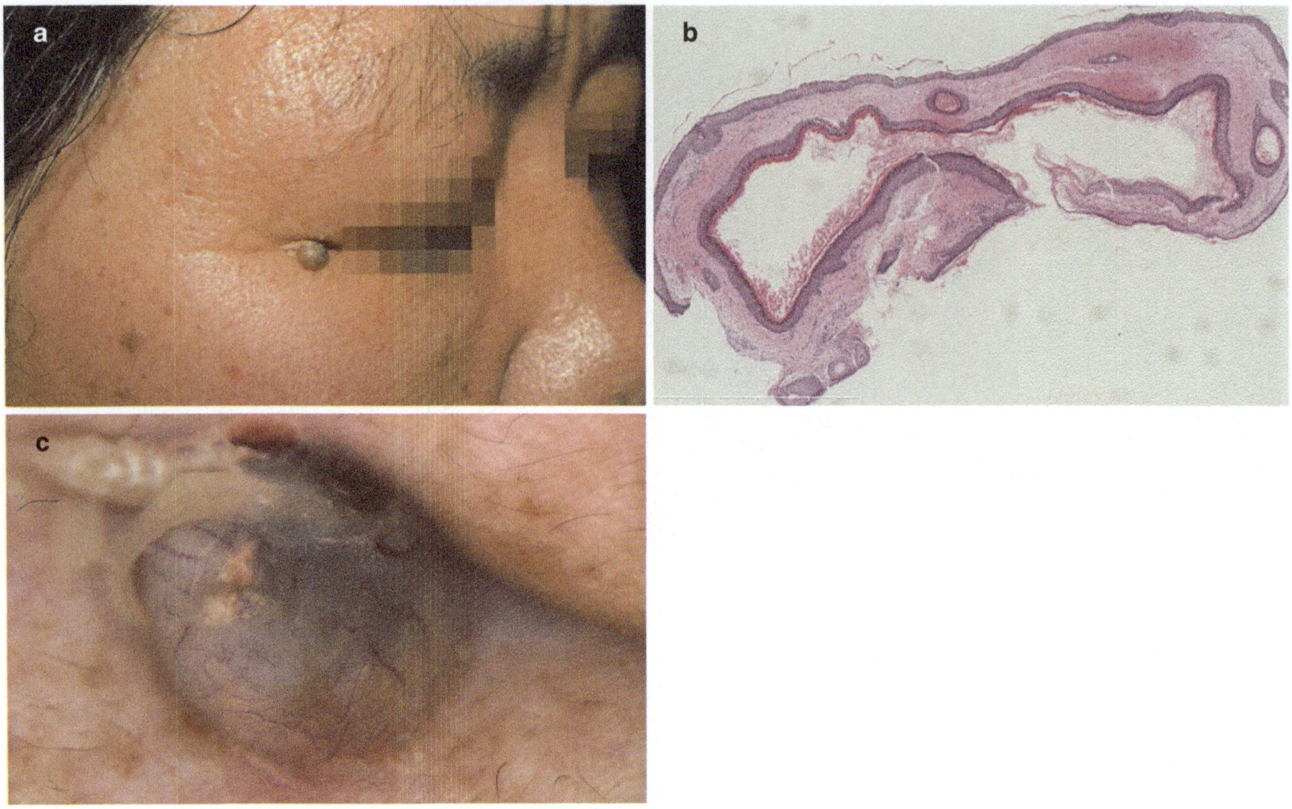

Fig. 11.9 Clinical, pathological, and dermoscopic features of epidermoid cysts. (**a**). An elevated grayish-blue nodule on the right lateral canthus. (**b**). Histopathological examination shows a dermal cyst lined by a stratified squamous epithelium that contains keratin in the cavity (hematoxylin and eosin, ×40). (**c**). Dermoscopically, a blue-white veil, and linear branched vessels are present on an ivory-white background (×30)

11.10 Nipple Adenoma

A nipple adenoma is a rare benign tumor of the nipple derived from the nipple ducts or lactiferous sinus. Nipple adenoma is also known as erosive adenomatosis of the nipple. In the early stage, a nipple adenoma is clinically characterized by an erosive nipple with serous discharge, and nodular hyperplasia of the nipple may occur as the lesion progresses (Fig. 11.10a). Histopathologically, a nipple adenoma includes a proliferation of glandular structures lined by dual layers of epithelial and myoepithelial cells within the nipple stroma, with varying degrees of ductal hyperplasia (Fig. 11.10b).

The dermoscopic features of nipple adenomas are as follows (Fig. 11.10c):

1. Light-red background
2. Yellow-white hyperkeratosis
3. Dotted, irregular-linear vessels

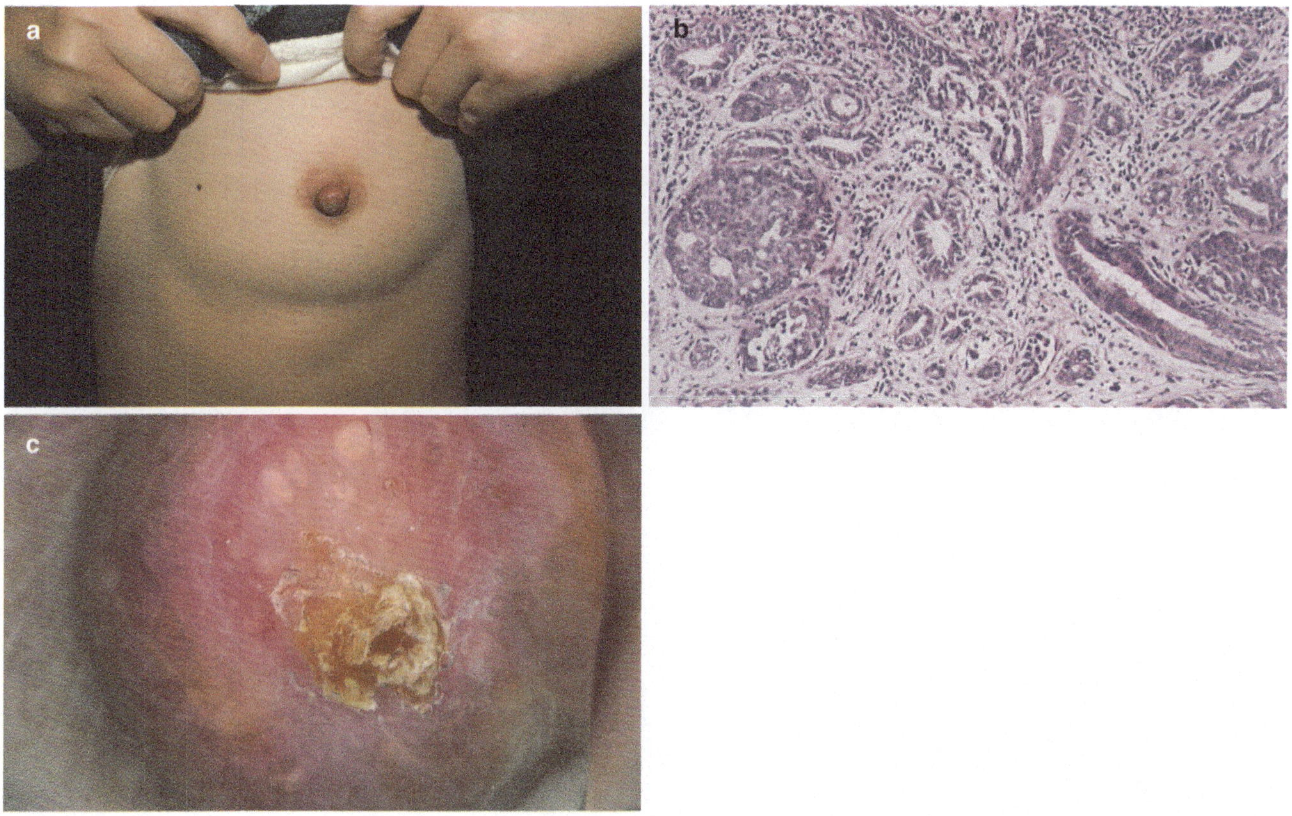

Fig. 11.10 Clinical, pathological, and dermoscopic features of nipple adenoma. (**a**). Erythema with crust on the left nipple. (**b**). Histopathological examination shows numerous glandular lacunae with papillary neoplastic cells protruding into the lumen, where decapitation secretion is also present. Lymphocytes and plasma cells infiltrate the periphery (hematoxylin and eosin, ×200). (**c**). Dermoscopy shows dotted and irregular-linear vessels and central yellow keratinization on a red background (×20)

11.11 Mammary Paget's Disease

Mammary Paget's disease is an intraepidermal adenocarcinoma of the nipple and areola, an uncommon form of breast cancer that results from the invasion of underlying intraductal in situ carcinoma into the epidermis. Clinical manifestations resemble eczema, including scales, erosion, effusion, etc. (Fig. 11.11); therefore, mammary Paget's disease is also called "mammary eczematoid carcinoma." The most characteristic histopathological feature is the presence of Paget cells in the epidermis.

The dermoscopic features of mammary Paget's disease are as follows:

1. Irregular-linear vessels
2. Pepper-like, blue-gray dots
3. Shiny white streaks

The clinical and dermoscopic features of the rarer pigmented form of mammary Paget's disease are similar to those of melanoma, which under dermoscopy shows diffuse irregular brown pigmentation or an atypical pigment network, irregular dots/globules, blue-white structures, etc. Therefore, biopsy and immunohistochemistry are required to distinguish pigmented mammary Paget's disease and melanoma.

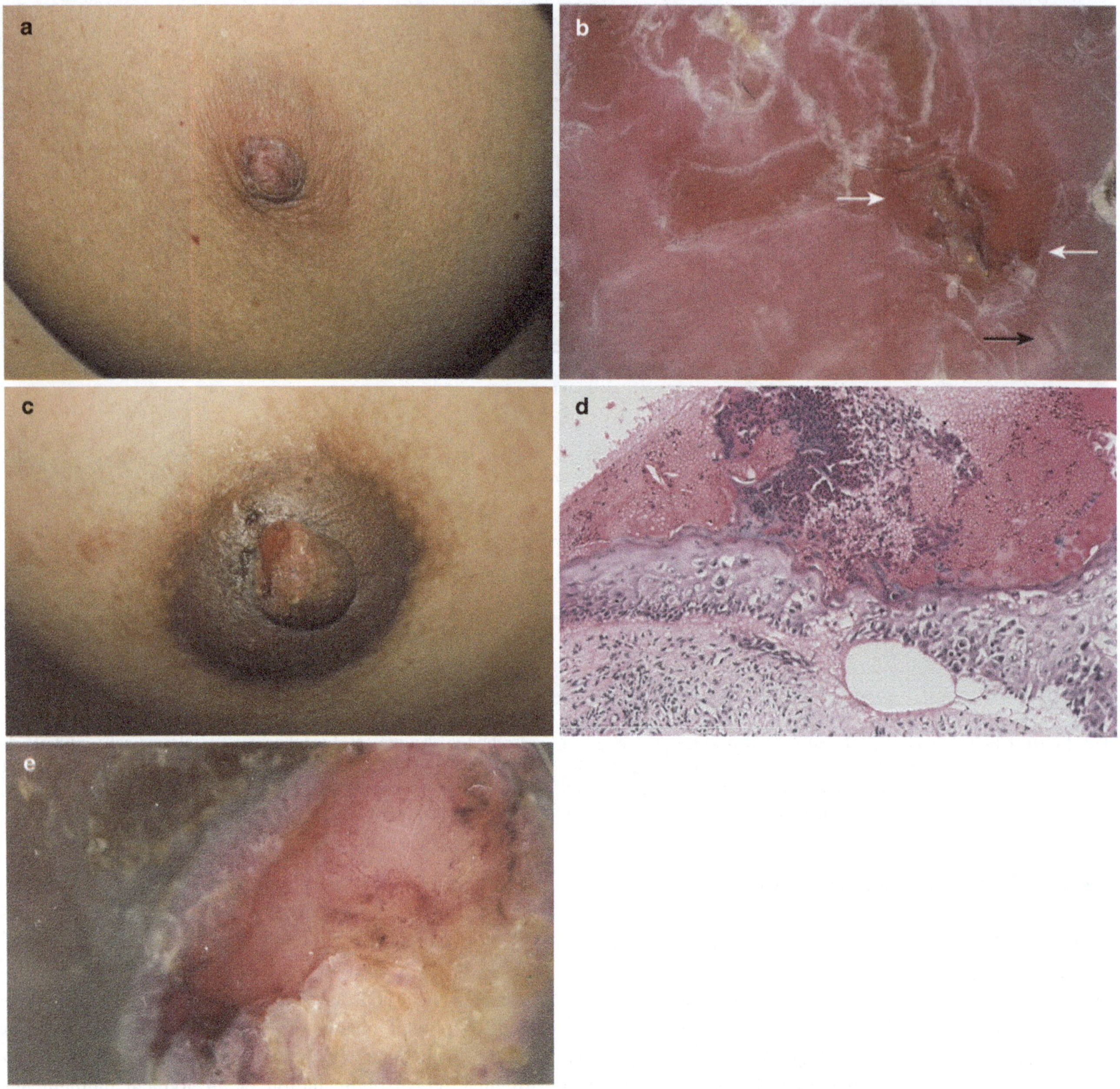

Fig. 11.11 Clinical, pathological, and dermoscopic features of mammary Paget's disease. (**a**). Erythema with erosion and crust on the left nipple. (**b**). Dermoscopy shows irregular-linear vessels; shiny white streaks (black arrow); and pepper-like, blue-gray dots (white arrow) (×30). (**c**). An ulcerated red plaque with effusion and crust on the right nipple. (**d**). Histopathological examination shows irregular acanthosis and many nested or scattered Paget cells in the epidermis; the cytoplasm of these Paget cells is lightly stained. Lymphocytes and histiocytes infiltrate the upper dermis (hematoxylin and eosin, ×200). (**e**). Irregular-linear and spiral vessels are detected via dermoscopy (×20)

11.12 Extramammary Paget's Disease

Extramammary Paget's disease is an intraepithelial adenocarcinoma of the apocrine gland that is associated with other internal malignancies. Primary extramammary Paget's disease originates from pluripotent stem cells in the genital skin, while secondary extramammary Paget's disease usually results from direct extension of or metastasis from an underlying adnexal adenoma of the skin or other internal carcinomas. The lesion often presents on vulval or perianal skin as a well-demarcated, red plaque, giving a "strawberries and cream" appearance, with white scales and erosion (Fig. 11.12a). Histopathological features include the occurrence of varying numbers of specific Paget cells in the epidermis (Fig. 11.12b).

The dermoscopic features of extramammary Paget's disease are as follows (Fig. 11.12c, d):

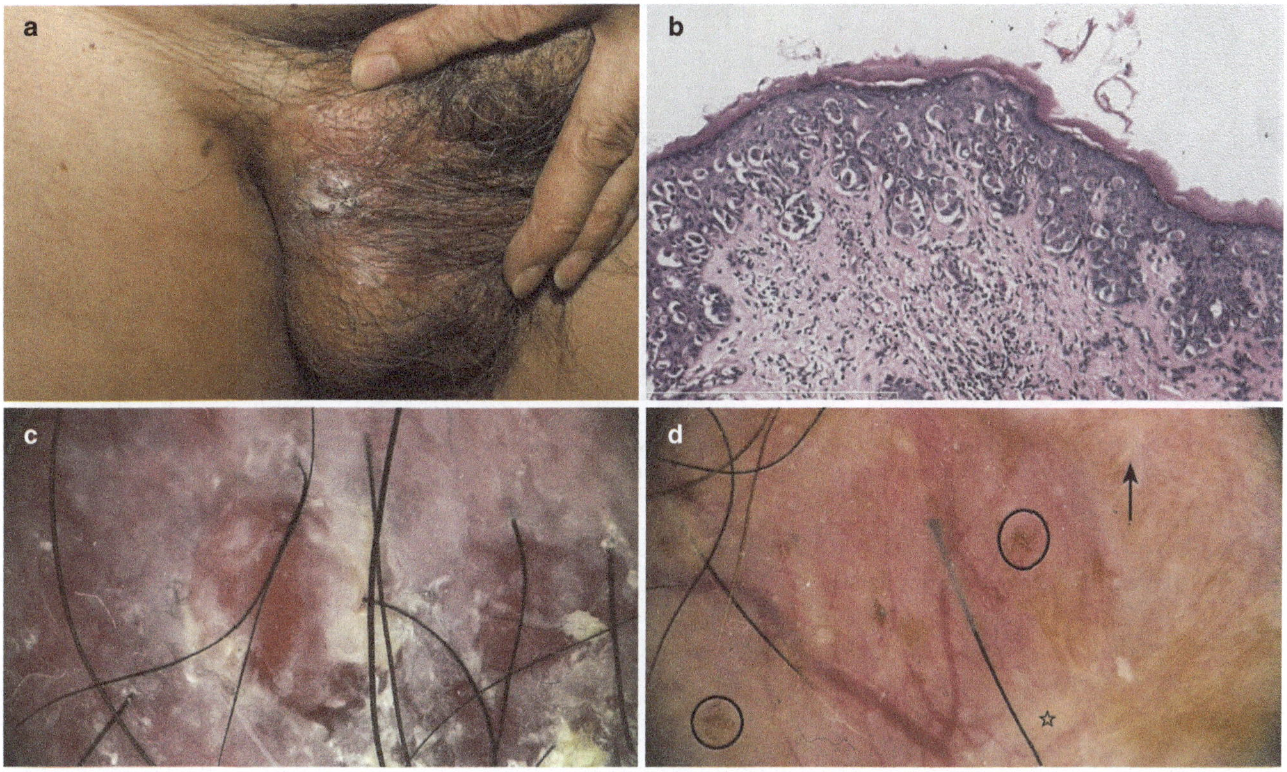

Fig. 11.12 Clinical, pathological, and dermoscopic features of extramammary Paget's disease. (**a**). Red plaques and papules with white crusts on the right aspect of scrotum. (**b**). Histopathologically, single scattered or clustered Paget cells with lightly stained cytoplasm are distributed in stratum spinosum, and the upper and middle dermis is infiltrated by lymphocytes (hematoxylin and eosin, ×200). (**c** and **d**). Dermoscopy shows a milky-red area; erosion; superficial crusts (**c**); dotted, linear, and arborizing vessels; brown dots (circle); shiny white streaks (arrow); and a white structureless area (asterisk) (**d**) (×20)

1. Milky-red area
2. Surface scales
3. Dotted, glomerular, irregular-linear, and polymorphous vessels
4. Gray/brown dots or structures area
5. Shiny white streaks
6. White structureless area
7. Ulcers or erosions

11.13 Rosai–Dorfman Disease

The characteristic clinical manifestation of Rosai–Dorfman disease, also known as sinus histiocytosis with massive lymphadenopathy, is massive, painless bilateral cervical lymphadenopathy. Concomitant symptoms include fever, an increased erythrocyte sedimentation rate (ESR), anemia, neutrophilia, and polyclonal hypergammaglobulinemia. A protracted course marked by alternating remission and exacerbation occurs in many patients. Virtually any organ can be involved, but the skin can also be the only site of involvement, which is designated as cutaneous Rosai–Dorfman disease. Approximately 10% of patients with the systemic form of Rosai–Dorfman disease have cutaneous lesions that present as multiple, red to red-brown or xanthomatous macules, papules, nodules, or plaques, with a predilection for the eyelids and zygomatic area (Fig. 11.13a). Histopathologically, cutaneous lesions demonstrate a dense dermal infiltrate of histiocytes that express S100 and CD68 but not CD1a, with scattered lymphocytes, plasma cells, and neutrophils. Due to the unspecific clinical features, the diagnosis of Rosai–Dorfman disease relies on histopathological and immunohistochemical examination, while dermoscopy can provide some clues.

The dermoscopic features of Rosai–Dorfman disease are as follows:

1. Red or orange background
2. Arborizing vessels
3. Yellow homogeneous area

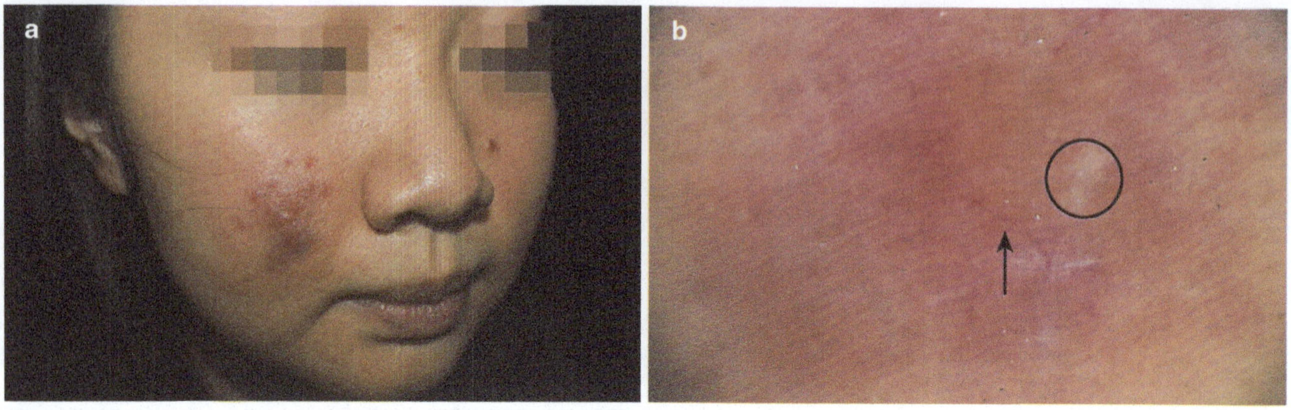

Fig. 11.13 Clinical and dermoscopic features of Rosai–Dorfman disease. (**a**). Yellow-red plaques and nodules surrounded by satellite papules on the right cheek. (**b**). Dermoscopy shows an orange background, arborizing vessels (arrow), and a yellow homogeneous area (circle) (×20)

11.14 Juvenile Xanthogranuloma

Juvenile xanthogranuloma is the most common non-Langerhans histiocytosis that usually affects infants and young children. Cutaneous lesions present as single or multiple red-brown or yellow papules or nodules that are most commonly located on the head and neck, followed by the upper torso and the distal limbs, and can regress spontaneously (Fig. 11.14a). Other organs, such as the eyes and lungs, can also be involved. The infiltration of foamy histiocytes and Touton giant cells is a characteristic histopathological finding in juvenile xanthogranuloma lesions (Fig. 11.14b).

The dermoscopic features of juvenile xanthogranuloma are as follows (Fig. 11.14c):

1. Setting sun sign: a central yellow-orange background with a subtle erythematous border, the specific feature of juvenile xanthogranuloma.
2. Pale to yellowish cloudy area
3. Linear and arborizing vessels
4. Shiny white streaks
5. Subtle pigment networks

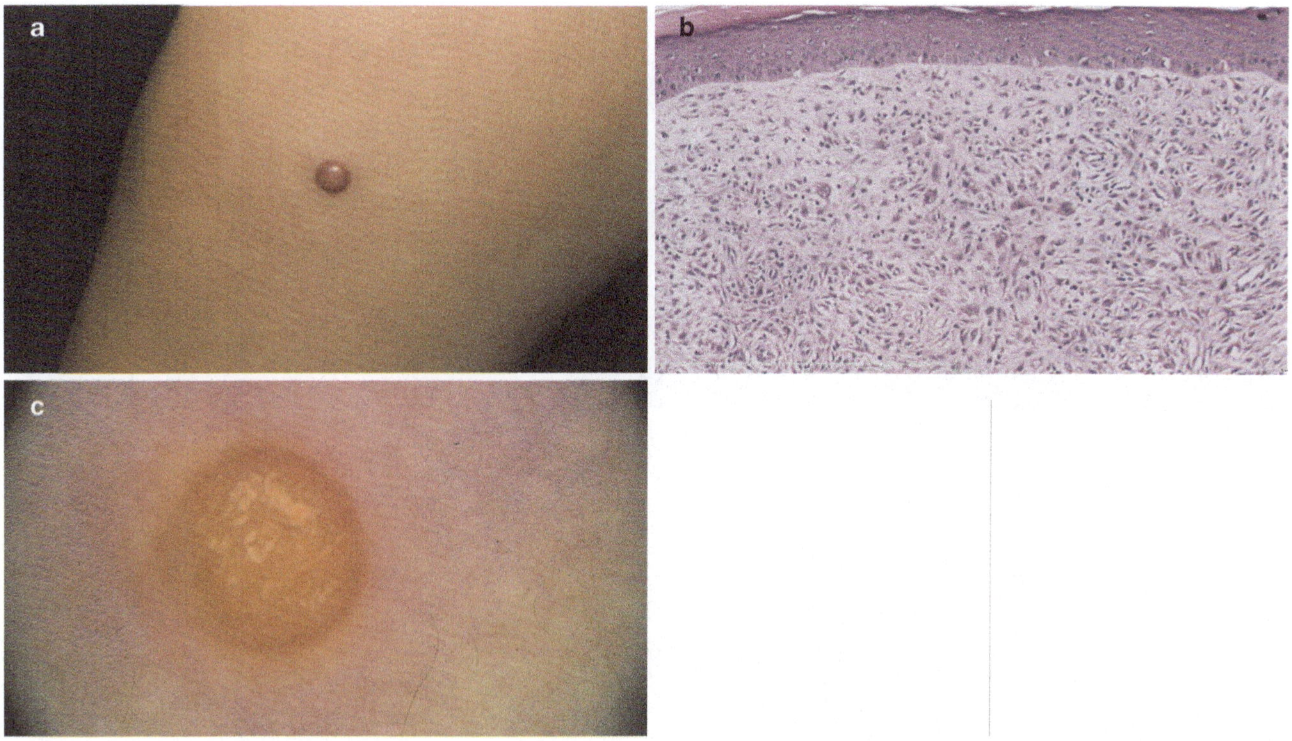

Fig. 11.14 Clinical, pathological and dermoscopic features of juvenile xanthogranuloma. (**a**). A red-brown, dome-shaped papule on the anteromedial aspect of the right knee. (**b**). Histopathological examination shows an abundant, nodular, histiocytic infiltrate in the dermis, including spindled histiocytes, foamy histiocytes, and Touton giant cells, as well as fibrohistiocytic hyperplasia (hematoxylin and eosin, ×100). (**c**). Dermoscopic findings are the setting sun sign, a yellowish cloudy area, shiny white streaks, and dotted and linear vessels (×20)

11.15 Foreign Body Granuloma

Foreign body granulomas are chronic granulomatous reactions induced by foreign bodies in the skin. Foreign body granulomas have diverse clinical features, with the most common manifestation being red to red-brown papules, nodules, or plaques (Fig. 11.15a). Histopathologically, there are two types of granulomas: the allergic type, which is characterized by the presence of collections of epithelioid histiocytes, and the nonallergic type, which is characterized by conspicuous infiltration of foreign body giant cells (Fig. 11.15b).

The dermoscopic features of foreign body granulomas are as follows (Fig. 11.15c):

1. Orange-yellow background
2. Shiny white streaks
3. Arborizing and irregular-linear vessels

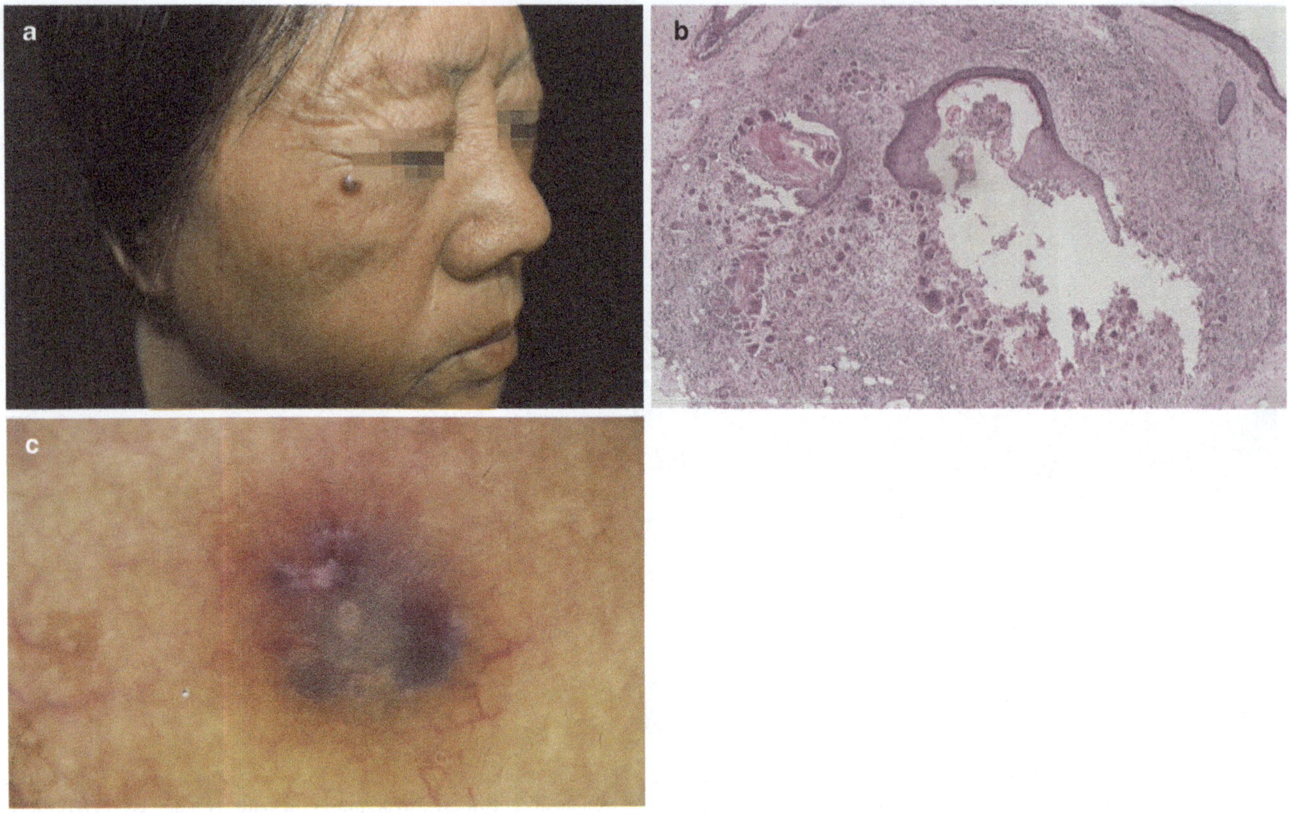

Fig. 11.15 Clinical, pathological, and dermoscopic features of foreign body granuloma. (a). A small, dark-red papule in the right zygomatic area. (b). Histopathological examination shows epidermal atrophy, an intradermal ruptured follicle surrounded by numerous foreign body giant cells, histiocytes and lymphocytes, and fibroblast hyperplasia (hematoxylin and eosin, ×40). (c). Dermoscopy shows the presence of arborizing and irregular-linear vessels and shiny white streaks, in addition to a central keratotic plug and hemorrhage (×30)

11.16 Kimura's Disease

Kimura's disease is a chronic inflammatory disorder that often involves the salivary glands. Kimura's disease is characterized by painless subcutaneous nodules or masses on the face or neck (Fig. 11.16a), with benign, reactive, regional lymphadenopathy, peripheral eosinophilia, and elevated IgE levels. Histopathological features are dense lymphocytic infiltration, lymphoid follicle hyperplasia, and peripheral eosinophil aggregation. The vessels are also proliferated (Fig. 11.16b).

The dermoscopic features of Kimura's disease are as follows (Fig. 11.16c):

1. Dotted, glomerular, and linear vessels
2. Shiny white streaks
3. Brown pigmentation and pigment networks
4. Milia-like cysts

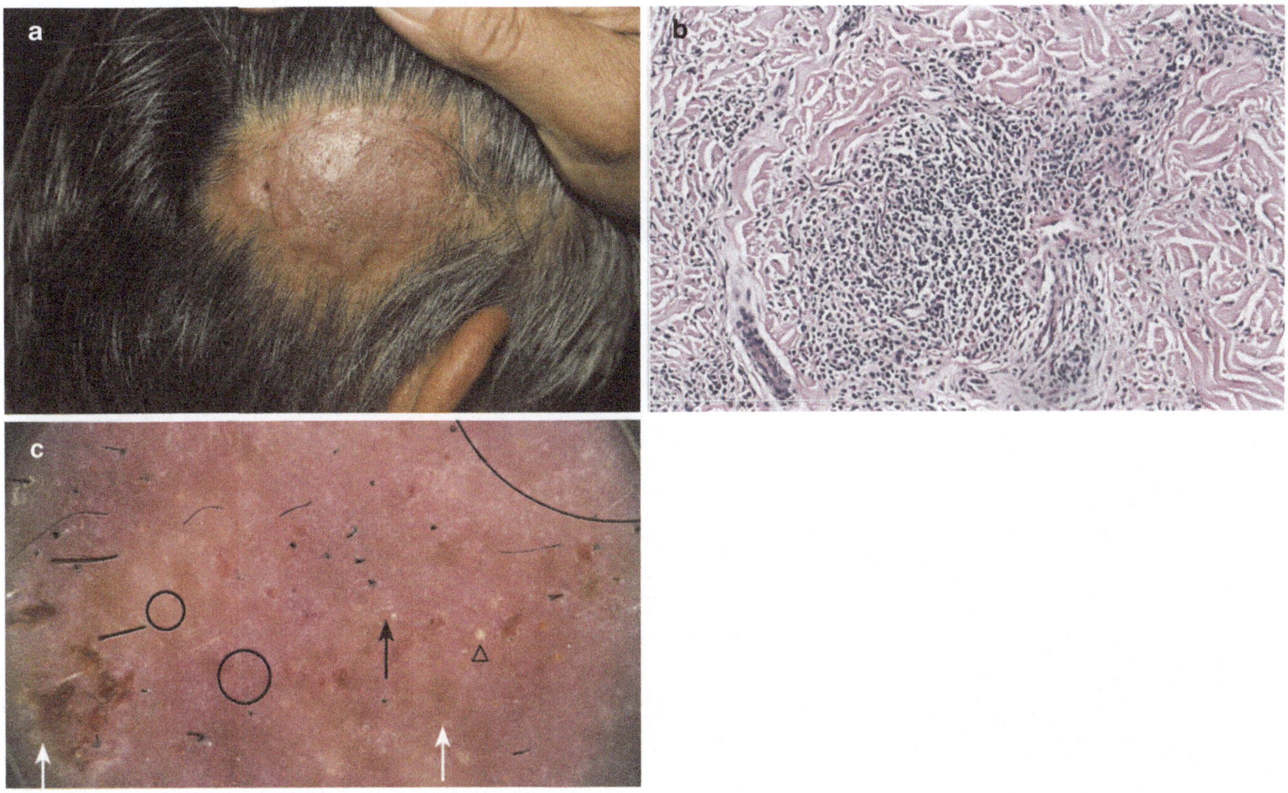

Fig. 11.16 Clinical, pathological, and dermoscopic features of Kimura's disease. (**a**). An elevated dark-red mass with scales and crusts on the right aspect of the head. (**b**). Skin lesion biopsy shows clumps of dense lymphocytes infiltrating the dermis surrounded by many eosinophils (hematoxylin and eosin, ×100). (**c**). Dermoscopy shows brown pigmentation and pigment networks (white arrow); dotted, glomerular, and linear vessels (circle); shiny white streaks (black arrow); and milia-like cysts (triangle) (×20)

11.17 Angiolymphoid Hyperplasia with Eosinophilia

Angiolymphoid hyperplasia with eosinophilia (AHE) may be related to trauma and arteriovenous shunting. Typical skin lesions of AHE present as pink to dull-red, angiomatoid papules or nodules that often occur in clusters and predominantly on the head and neck region, especially around the ears and on the scalp (Fig. 11.17a). Some patients have regional lymph node enlargement and peripheral eosinophilia. Histopathologically, AHE is characterized by lobular proliferation of capillary-sized vessels composed of epithelioid (hobnail-like or cobblestone-like) endothelial cells surrounding larger vessels with thick walls, accompanied by an infiltration of lymphocytes and eosinophils (Fig. 11.17b).

The dermoscopic features of AHE are as follows (Fig. 11.17c):

1. Red background
2. Reddish purple lacunae
3. Polymorphous vessels: dotted, spiral, and irregular-linear vessels
4. Shiny white streaks or white structureless areas

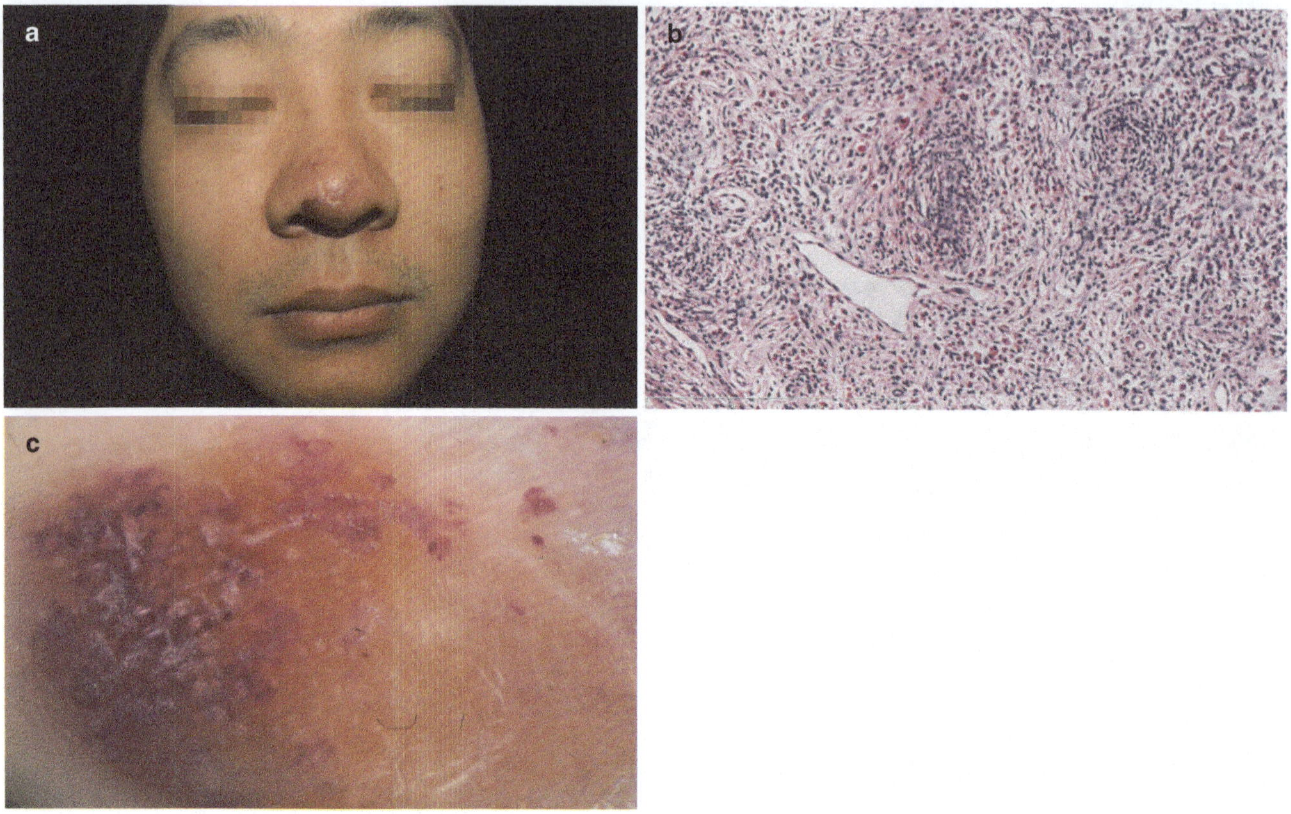

Fig. 11.17 Clinical, pathological and dermoscopic features of angiolymphoid hyperplasia with eosinophilia. (**a**). Multiple dull-red papules and nodules on the nose. (**b**). Histopathological examination demonstrates intradermal hyperplasic vessels lined by swollen endothelial cells with dilated lumens and infiltrated by dense eosinophils and plasma cells, as well as lymphocytes and histiocytes (hematoxylin and eosin, ×100). (**c**). Dermoscopy shows reddish-purple lacunae, polymorphous vessels, and shiny white streaks (×20)

11.18 Urticaria Pigmentosa

Mastocytosis represents a rare spectrum of disorders characterized by mast cell hyperplasia and aggregation in multiple tissues and organs (such as the skin, bone marrow, skeletal system, gastrointestinal tract, spleen, lymph nodes, and liver). Urticaria pigmentosa is the most common cutaneous lesion in mastocytosis, and it presents as a positive Darier sign, round to oval macule, plaque, or nodule with a red to brown-red coloration that might be darkened due to hyperpigmentation (Fig. 11.18a).

The dermoscopic features of urticaria pigmentosa are as follows (Fig. 11.17b):

1. Brown pigment network
2. Brown or orange-yellow, homogenous dots
3. Occasionally, a vascular network ("reticular vessel" pattern) interlaced by linear vessels

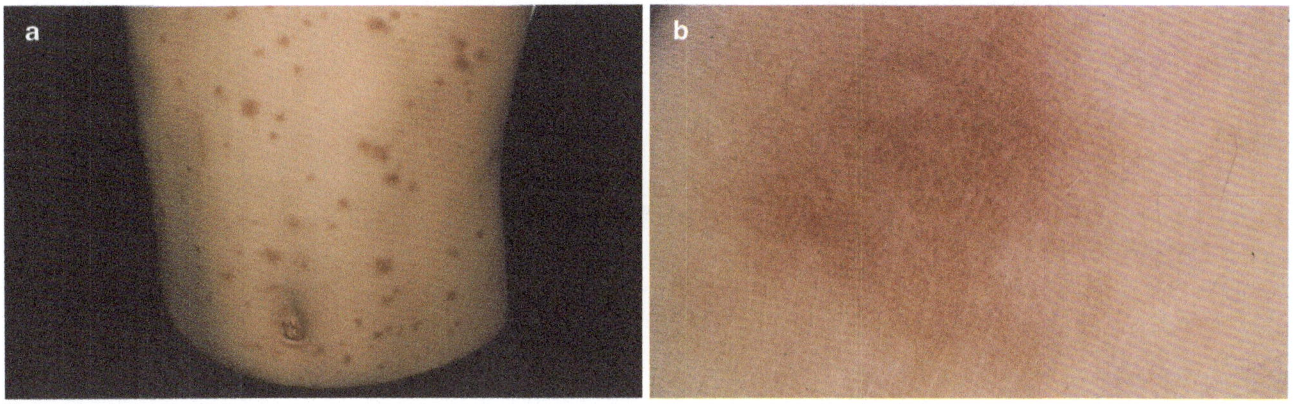

Fig. 11.18 Urticaria pigmentosa. (**a**). Brown macules of varying sizes with a positive Darier sign on the trunk and extremities. (**b**). Brown pigment network (×20)

Further Reading

1. Moscarella E, Argenziano G, Longo C, et al. Clinical, dermoscopic and reflectance confocal microscopy features of sebaceous neoplasms in Muir-Torre syndrome. J Eur Acad Dermatol Venereol. 2013;27(6):699–705.
2. Navarrete-Dechent C, Uribe P, Gonzalez S. Desmoplastic trichilemmoma dermoscopically mimicking molluscum contagiosum. J Am Acad Dermatol. 2017;76(2s1):S22–s24.
3. Ardigo M, Zieff J, Scope A, et al. Dermoscopic and reflectance confocal microscope findings of trichoepithelioma. Dermatology. 2007;215(4):354–8.
4. Pitarch G, Botella-Estrada R. Dermoscopic findings in Trichoblastoma. Actas Dermosifiliogr. 2015;106(9):e45–8.
5. Lazaridou E, Fotiadou C, Patsatsi A, et al. Solitary trichoepithelioma in an 8-year-old child: clinical, dermoscopic and histopathologic findings. Dermatol Pract Concept. 2014;4(2):55–8.
6. Marchetti MA, Marino ML, Virmani P, et al. Dermoscopic features and patterns of poromas: a multicentre observational case-control study conducted by the International Dermoscopy Society. J Eur Acad Dermatol Venereol. 2018;32(8):1263–71.
7. Edamitsu T, Minagawa A, Koga H, et al. Eccrine porocarcinoma shares dermoscopic characteristics with eccrine poroma: a report of three cases and review of the published work. J Dermatol. 2016;43(3):332–5.
8. Pinheiro R, Oliveira A, Mendes-Bastos P. Dermoscopic and reflectance confocal microscopic presentation of relapsing eccrine porocarcinoma. J Am Acad Dermatol. 2017;76(2S1):S73–5.
9. Zaballos P, Banuls J, Medina C, et al. Dermoscopy of apocrine hidrocystomas: a morphological study. J Eur Acad Dermatol Venereol. 2014;28(3):378–81.
10. Duman N, Duman D, Sahin S. Pale halo surrounding a homogeneous bluish-purplish central area: dermoscopic clue for eccrine hidrocystoma. Dermatol Pract Concept. 2015;5(4):43–5.
11. Zaballos P, Serrano P, Flores G, et al. Dermoscopy of tumours arising in naevus sebaceous: a morphological study of 58 cases. J Eur Acad Dermatol Venereol. 2015;29(11):2231–7.
12. Lombardi M, Piana S, Longo C, et al. Dermoscopy of syringocystadenoma papilliferum. Australas J Dermatol. 2018;59(1):e59–61.
13. Suh KS, Kang DY, Park JB, et al. Usefulness of dermoscopy in the differential diagnosis of ruptured and unruptured epidermal cysts. Ann Dermatol. 2017;29(1):33–8.
14. Takashima S, Fujita Y, Miyauchi T, et al. Dermoscopic observation in adenoma of the nipple. J Dermatol. 2015;42(3):341–2.
15. Errichetti E, Avellini C, Pegolo E, et al. Dermoscopy as a supportive instrument in the early recognition of erosive adenomatosis of the nipple and mammary Paget's disease. Ann Dermatol. 2017;29(3):365–7.
16. Crignis GS, Abreu L, Bucard AM, et al. Polarized dermoscopy of mammary Paget disease. An Bras Dermatol. 2013;88(2):290–2.
17. Brugues A, Iranzo P, Diaz A, et al. Pigmented mammary Paget disease mimicking cutaneous malignant melanoma. J Am Acad Dermatol. 2015;72(4):e97–8.
18. Yanagishita T, Tamada Y, Tanaka M, et al. Pigmented mammary Paget disease mimicking melanoma on dermatoscopy. J Am Acad Dermatol. 2011;64(6):e114–6.
19. Mun JH, Park SM, Kim GW, et al. Clinical and dermoscopic characteristics of extramammary Paget disease: a study of 35 cases. Br J Dermatol. 2016;174(5):1104–7.
20. Wang F, Zhou H, Luo DQ, et al. Dermatoscopic findings in cutaneous Rosai-Dorfman disease and response to low-dose thalidomide. J Dtsch Dermatol Ges. 2014;12(4):350–2.
21. Aviles-Izquierdo JA, Parra Blanco V, Alfageme F, Roldan. Dermoscopic features of cutaneous Rosai-Dorfman disease. Actas dermosifiliograficas. 2012;103(5):446–8.
22. Palmer A, Bowling J. Dermoscopic appearance of juvenile xanthogranuloma. Dermatology. 2007;215(3):256–9.
23. Rubegni P, Mandato F, Fimiani M. Juvenile xanthogranuloma: dermoscopic pattern. Dermatology. 2009;218(4):380. author reply 381
24. Hussain SH, Kozic H, Lee JB. The utility of dermatoscopy in the evaluation of xanthogranulomas. Pediatr Dermatol. 2008;25(4):505–6.
25. Bombonato C, Argenziano G, Lallas A, et al. Orange color: a dermoscopic clue for the diagnosis of granulomatous skin diseases. J Am Acad Dermatol. 2015;72(1 Suppl):S60–3.
26. Rodriguez-Lomba E, Aviles-Izquierdo JA, Molina-Lopez I, et al. Dermoscopic features in 2 cases of angiolymphoid hyperplasia with eosinophilia. J Am Acad Dermatol. 2016;75(1):e19–21.
27. Bastug NB, Duman N, Tokyol C, et al. Angiolymphoid hyperplasia with eosinophilia: two case reports. Australas J Dermatol. 2019;60(3):e236–7.
28. Miller MD, Nery NS, Gripp AC, et al. Dermatoscopic findings of urticaria pigmentosa. An Bras Dermatol. 2013;88(6):986–8.
29. Vano-Galvan S, Alvarez-Twose I, De Las Heras E, et al. Dermoscopic features of skin lesions in patients with mastocytosis. Arch Dermatol. 2011;147(8):932–40.
30. Akay BN, Kittler H, Sanli H, et al. Dermatoscopic findings of cutaneous mastocytosis. Dermatology. 2009;218(3):226–30.

12 Inflammatory Diseases

Over the last few years, dermoscopy has been increasingly used in the field of inflammatory diseases, such as papulosquamous disorders, vasculitis, autoimmune diseases, and inherited diseases. According to the most recent consensus of the International Dermoscopy Society, the main dermoscopic finding categories are as follows: vessels (morphology, distribution), scales (color, distribution), follicular findings, other structures (color, distribution), and specific clues. Vessel morphologic types can be dotted, linear, linear with branches, or linear curved. Vessel distribution can be uniform, clustered, peripheral, reticular, or nonspecific. Scale color can be white, yellow, or brown. Scale distribution can be diffuse, central, peripheral, or patchy. Follicular findings include follicular plugs, follicular red dots, perifollicular white color, and perifollicular pigmentation. Other structure categories include color (white, brown, gray, blue, orange, yellow, or purple) and morphology (structureless areas, dots/globules, lines, or circles). Specific clues include Wickham striae (lichen planus (LP)), peripheral keratotic structures with two free edges (porokeratosis), and spongiotic vesicles (eczema). Of note, the diagnosis of inflammatory diseases should not be based on only dermoscopic examination findings. A combination of clinical history and macroscopic, dermoscopic, and even histopathological examination findings is needed to reach the final diagnosis.

12.1 Erythematous and Papulosquamous Disorders

12.1.1 Introduction

These entities represent a group of inflammatory disorders that present with erythematous papules with/without scales, including psoriasis, dermatitis/eczema, lichen planus, pityriasis rubra, and pityriasis rosea. Untypical cases are often difficult to distinguish because of their similar clinical manifestations. Dermoscopy can be a useful tool in the diagnosis and differential diagnosis of the above diseases. In addition, early-stage mycosis fungoides (MF) also manifests squamous patches and plaques, which are often misdiagnosed as inflammatory diseases. Dermoscopy can help identify erythematous and papulosquamous disorders and promote further targeted laboratory and histopathological examinations. Consequently, MF is also listed in this section.

12.1.2 Psoriasis

Psoriasis is a common, recurrent papulosquamous disorder that can be classified into four main types according to its clinical features: psoriasis vulgaris, erythrodermic psoriasis, psoriatic arthritis, and pustular psoriasis. Dermoscopy can be adopted in the differential diagnosis of psoriasis and other erythematous and papulosquamous disorders, such as eczema, seborrheic dermatitis, and early-stage MF. Additionally, dermoscopy can be useful for monitoring the therapeutic effects and side effects of drugs.

12.1.2.1 Dermoscopic Features of Psoriasis Vulgaris

1. **The dermoscopic features of plaque psoriasis are as follows** (Figs. 12.1, 12.2 and 12.3):
   (a) Dotted vessels (including dots and globules)
   (b) Linear curved vessels (including looped and hairpin-like vessels)
   (c) Looped and hairpin-like vessels, highly predictive of a diagnosis of plaque psoriasis (more observable under higher magnifications)
   (d) Uniform distribution of vessels
   (e) Diffuse/patchy distribution of white scales
   (f) Other features, including a light-red background and punctate hemorrhages (dermoscopic "Auspitz sign")

J. Liu, X. Zou, *Practical Dermoscopy*, https://doi.org/10.1007/978-981-19-1460-7_12

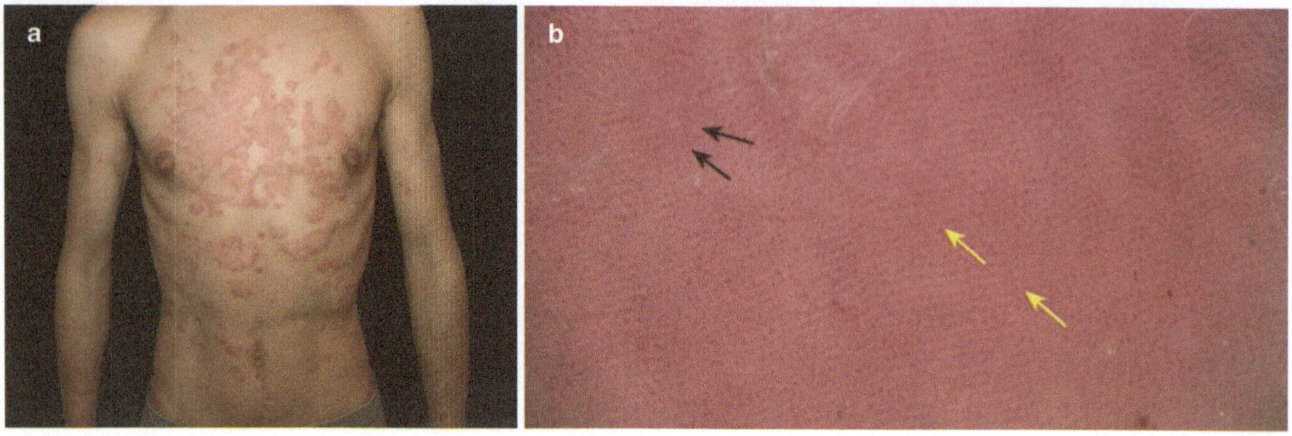

Fig. 12.1 Plaque psoriasis. (**a**). Generalized scaly plaques on trunk and limbs. (**b**) Regularly distributed dotted, looped (yellow arrows), and hairpin-like vessels (black arrows) on a light-red background (×30)

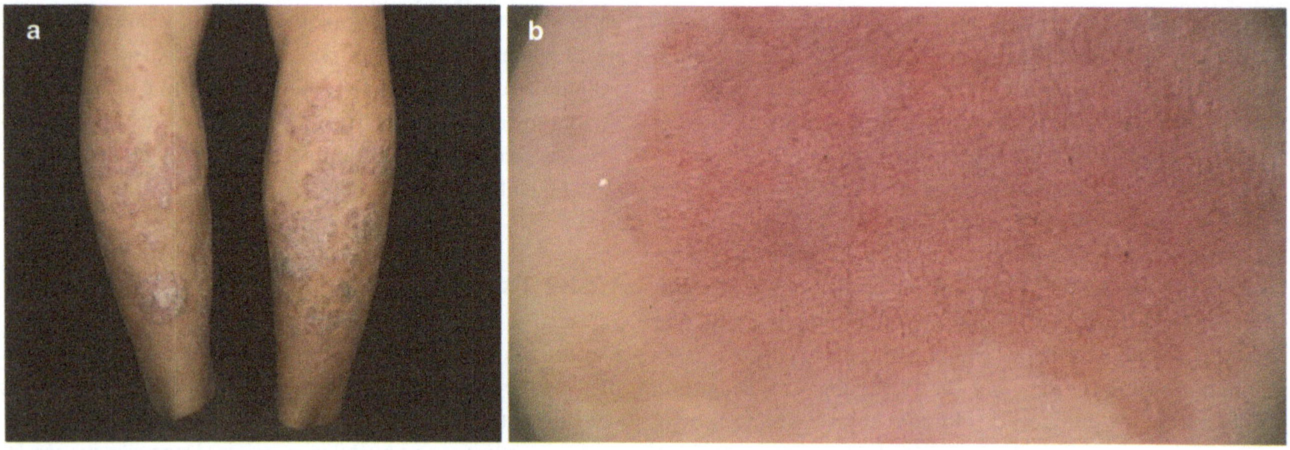

Fig. 12.2 Plaque psoriasis. (**a**). Multiple red plaques with white scales on the lower limbs. (**b**). Dotted and looped vessels arranged uniformly or in a "string of pearls" distribution; patchily distributed white scales on a light-red background (×20)

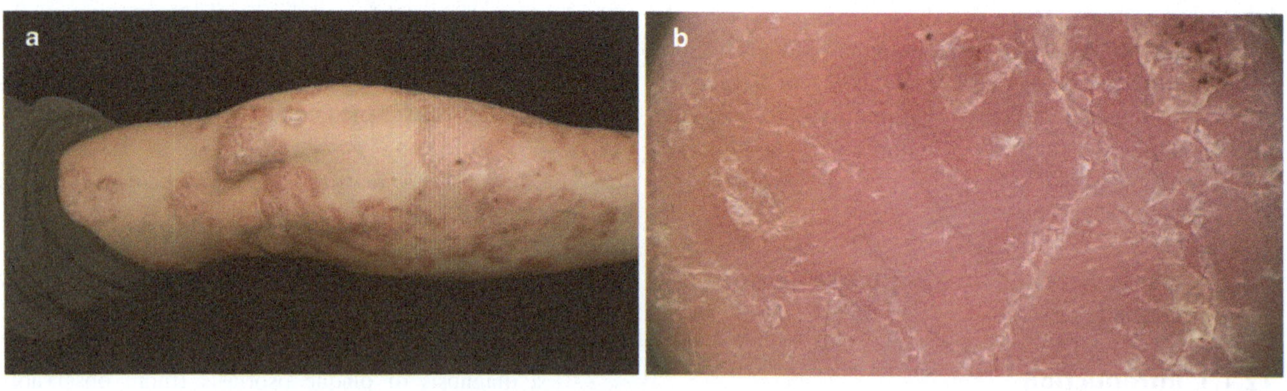

Fig. 12.3 Plaque psoriasis. (**a**). Multiple red patches and plaques with white scales on the upper limbs. (**b**). Uniformly distributed dotted vessels and patchily distributed white scales on a light-red background. Punctate hemorrhages can also be seen (×30)

2. **The dermoscopic features of guttate psoriasis are as follows** (Fig. 12.4):
   (a) Few reports thus far. Similar to those of plaque psoriasis according to our experiences.
   (b) Dermoscopy can be used in the differentiation of guttate psoriasis and pityriasis lichenoides chronica.

12.1.2.2 Dermoscopic Features of Erythrodermic Psoriasis (Fig. 12.5)

1. Few reports thus far. Similar to those of plaque psoriasis according to our experiences.
2. Dermoscopy can be used for differentiation from other causes of erythroderma, such as dermatitis, pityriasis rubra, and MF.

12.1.2.3 Psoriasis on Special Body Sites

1. **The dermoscopic features of scalp psoriasis are as follows** (Figs. 12.6 and 12.7):
   (a) Similar to those of plaque psoriasis. Perifollicular regions can be involved.
   (b) Uniformly distributed dotted, looped, and hairpin-like vessels.
   (c) Looped and hairpin-like vessels are highly predictive of a diagnosis of psoriasis.
   (d) Diffusely/patchy distribution of white scales.
   (e) Light-red background.
   (f) Punctate hemorrhages (dermoscopic Auspitz sign).

In a previous study, the videodermoscopy scalp psoriasis severity index (VSCAPSI) was created. The VSCAPSI can provide important evidence for the differential diagnosis, screening, and follow-up of scalp psoriasis. The VSCAPSI takes into account the scalp affected by psoriasis and the presence and morphology of vascular patterns, erythema, and desquamation. The scalp is divided into four areas: the left side (L), the right side (R), the front (F), and the back (B). Each area is assigned a different percentage value. In each area, the presence and morphology of vascular patterns (dotted, looped, and hairpin-like vessels) (PV) and the severity of erythema (E) and desquamation (D) are graded separately. The final score is calculated using the following formula:

$$\mathrm{VSCAPSI} = \mathrm{L}(\mathrm{EL}+\mathrm{DL}+\mathrm{PVL})+\mathrm{R}(\mathrm{ER}+\mathrm{DR}+\mathrm{PVR})+\mathrm{F}(\mathrm{EF}+\mathrm{DF}+\mathrm{PVF})+\mathrm{B}(\mathrm{EB}+\mathrm{DB}+\mathrm{PVB})$$

2. **The dermoscopic features of psoriatic nails are as follows** (see Chap. 14) (Fig. 12.8):
   (a) Dilated, tortuous, and elongated capillaries on the nail bed and proximal nail fold.
   (b) Nail plate pitting.
   (c) Nail fragmentation, onycholysis, and pustules under the nail plate.
   (d) Nail plate crumbling is a sign of severe psoriasis. Scales on the proximal part of the nail plate indicate nail matrix involvement.

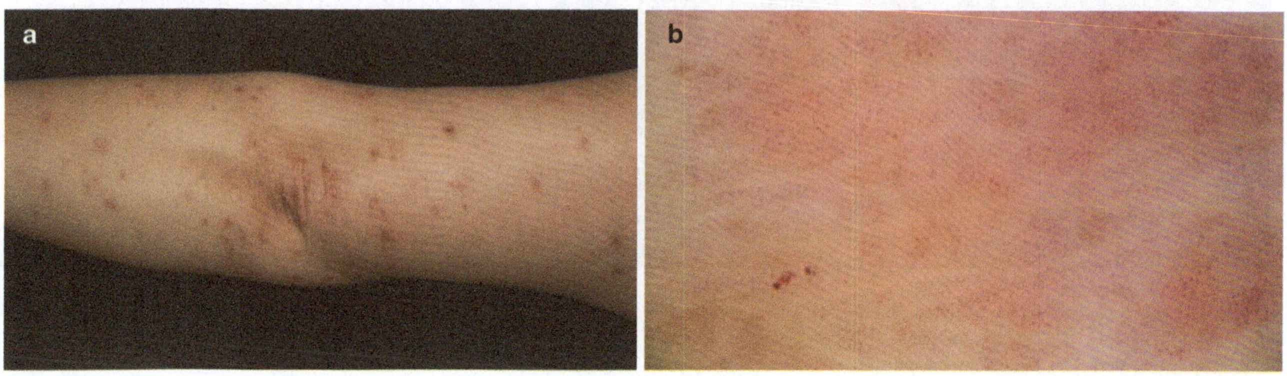

Fig. 12.4 Guttate psoriasis. (**a**). Multiple red papules with white scales on the upper limbs. (**b**). Dotted and looped vessels under dermoscopy (×30)

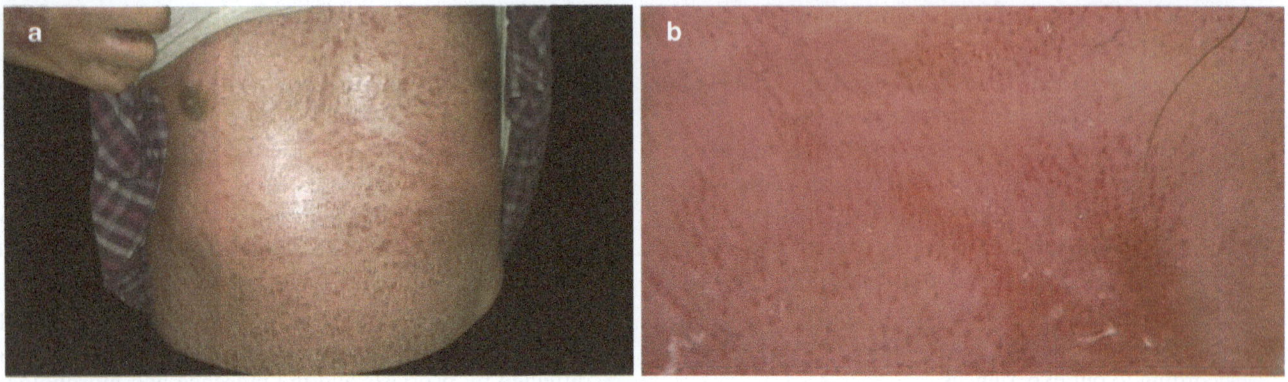

Fig. 12.5 Erythrodermic psoriasis. (**a**). Generalized edematous erythema with white scales on the trunk. (**b**). Uniformly distributed dotted, looped, and hairpin-like vessels (×40)

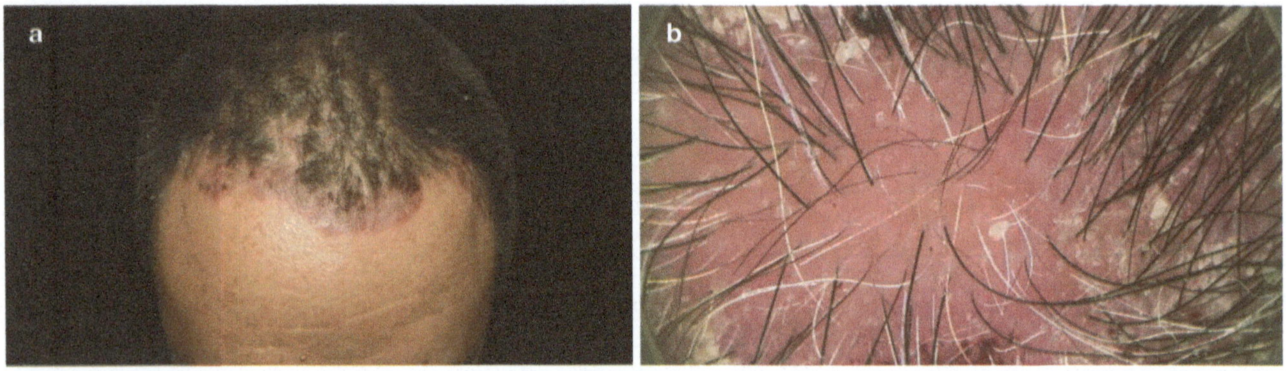

Fig. 12.6 Scalp psoriasis (**a**). Dull-red plaques with adhesive scales on the scalp. (**b**). Perifollicular uniformly distributed dotted vessels and patchily distributed white scales on a light-red background. Punctate hemorrhages can also be seen (×20)

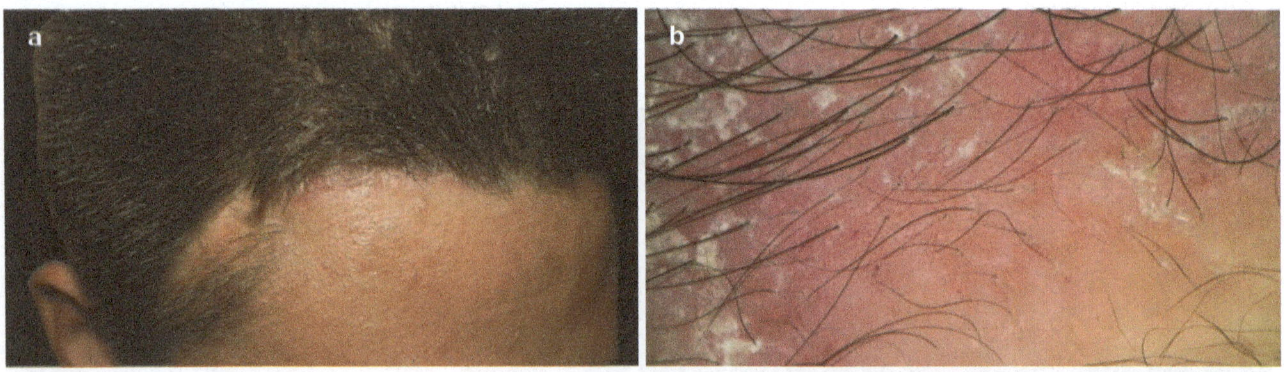

Fig. 12.7 Scalp psoriasis. (**a**). Dull-red plaques with adhesive scales on the scalp. (**b**). Perifollicular uniformly distributed dotted, looped, and hairpin-like vessels. Looped and hairpin-like vessels are highly predictive of a diagnosis of plaque psoriasis. Patchily distributed white scales can also be seen (×40)

3. **The dermoscopic features of palmar psoriasis are as follows** (Fig. 12.9):
   (a) Uniformly distributed dotted vessels.
   (b) Diffusely distributed white scales. Yellow scales are rare and are significant in chronic hand eczema.

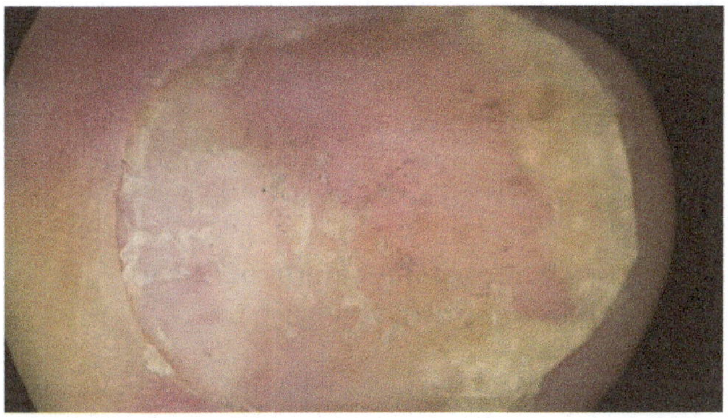

Fig. 12.8 A psoriatic nail. Dermoscopy shows onycholysis, scales, and pits on the nail plate and dilated, tortuous, and elongated capillaries on the nail bed. Scales on the proximal part of the nail plate indicate nail matrix involvement (×20)

12.1.2.4 Correlations Between the Dermoscopic and Histopathological Findings (Fig. 12.10)

1. Uniformly distributed vessel patterns represent dilated capillaries within regularly elongated dermal papillae.
2. Dotted or globular vessels can be seen when the dermoscope is perpendicular to the dilated capillaries in the dermal papillae.
3. Looped or hairpin-like vessels indicate a slope angle.
4. Diffusely distributed white scales represent coalescing parakeratosis.

Investigations have indicated that dermoscopy can be useful in monitoring the effects and side effects of topical corticosteroids in patients with psoriasis. The reduced number of vessels (dotted, hairpin-like vessels, etc.) in lesions represents an effective response. Linear vessels outside of the lesion represent early steroid-induced skin atrophy (Fig. 12.11). Another investigation revealed that the dermoscopic appearance of hemorrhagic dots represented a robust predictor of subsequent response to treatment with biologi-

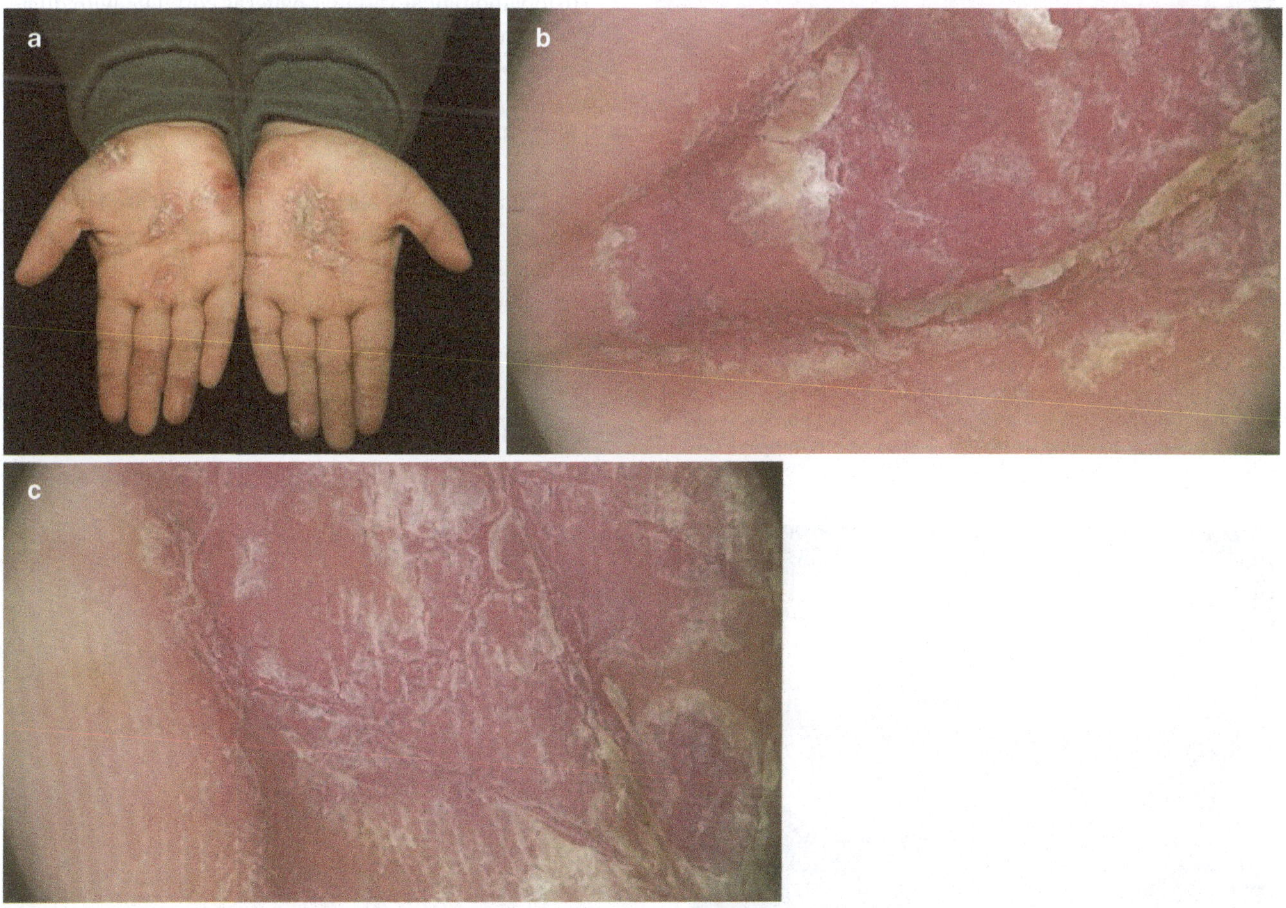

Fig. 12.9 Palmar psoriasis. (**a**). Multiple well-demarcated red plaques with white scales. (**b**). Uniformly distributed dotted vessels and white scales on a light-red background (×20). (**c**). Diffusely distributed white scales on a light-red background (×20)

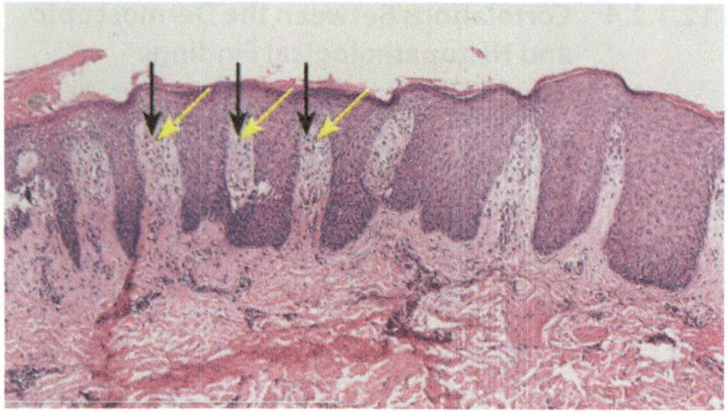

Fig. 12.10 Histopathological findings of plaque psoriasis. Histopathology shows psoriasiform epidermal hyperplasia and dilated capillaries in the papillary dermis (hematoxylin and eosin, ×100). Uniformly distributed vessel patterns represent dilated capillaries within regularly elongated dermal papillae. Vessel patterns differ when the dermoscope is placed at a different angle to dilated capillaries within dermal papillae. Dotted or globular vessels are present when the dermoscope is placed in the direction indicated by the black arrow. Looped or hairpin-like vessels are present when the dermoscope is placed in the direction indicated by the yellow arrow. Diffusely distributed white scales represent coalescing parakeratosis

Fig. 12.11 Psoriatic lesion under treatment with topical steroids. The reduced number of dotted vessels in the lesion indicates a positive treatment response; however, the large number of dilated linear vessels outside of the lesion indicates early steroid-induced skin atrophy (×20)

cal agents. On the other hand, the persistent existence of dotted vessels predicts prolonged disease or a recurrence of the disease.

12.1.3 Dermatitis and Eczema

Dermatitis and eczema are allergic diseases caused by various internal and external factors. Skin lesions are polymorphic depending on the clinical stages. In the acute phase, lesions present erythema, vesicles, oozing, and crusts, while lesions in the chronic phase are typified by the presence of thickening, lichenification, and scales.

12.1.3.1 Dermoscopic Features of Acute Dermatitis/Eczema (Fig. 12.12)

1. Red patches
2. Yellow scales/crusts (yellow clod sign)

12.1.3.2 Dermoscopic Features of Chronic Dermatitis/Eczema (Figs. 12.13, 12.14, and 12.15)

1. Irregular or patchy arrangement of dotted vessels.
2. Histopathological vascular patterns correlate with dilated capillaries in rete ridges with irregular acanthosis.
3. Spongiotic vesicles.
4. Patchily/diffusely distributed yellow scales.
5. Dull-red background.

At special sites, such as the palms, vascular patterns are hard to see because of the thick corneum. In addition to the abovementioned vascular structures, brownish-salmon-colored dots/globules, yellow scales, and orange-yellow crusts can also be detected under close observation (Fig. 12.16). These features can help differentiate between hand eczema and palmar psoriasis, which typically does not have these findings.

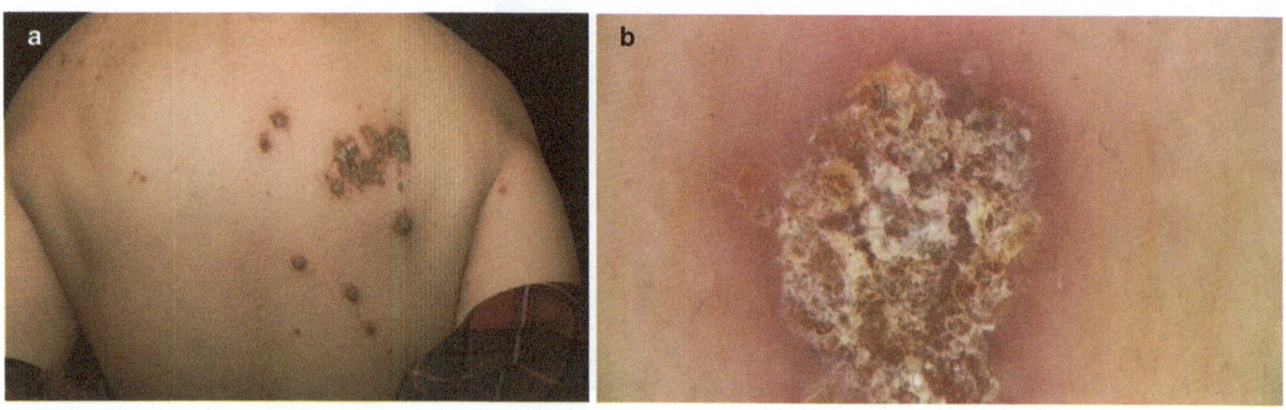

Fig. 12.12 Acute dermatitis. (**a**). Multiple erythematous patches with oozing and crusts on the back. (**b**). Red patches and diffusely distributed yellow-white scales/crusts (×30)

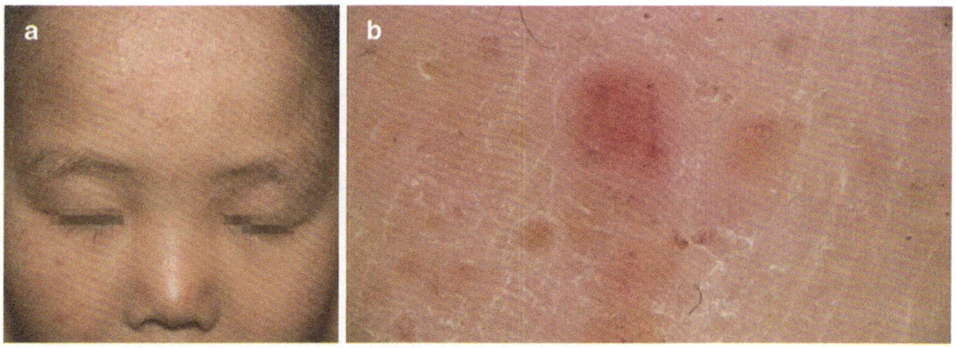

Fig. 12.13 Facial chronic dermatitis. (**a**). Chronic dermatitis in a patient with atopic dermatitis. (**b**). Patchily distributed dotted vessels, spongiotic vesicles, and diffusely distributed yellow-white scales on a dull-red background (×30)

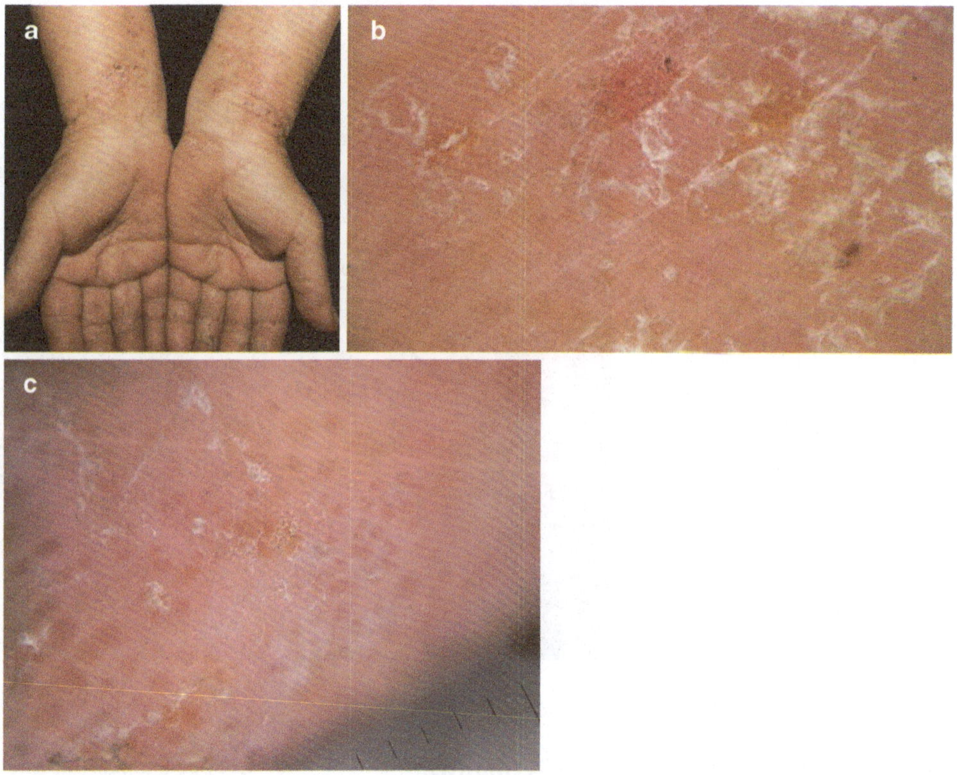

Fig. 12.14 Chronic dermatitis on wrists and palms. (**a**). Lichenoid papules on wrists and plaques with crusts on fingers and palms. (**b**). Irregularly distributed dotted vessels, yellow scales, and blood crusts on a dull-red background. (**c**). Spongiotic vesicles (×30)

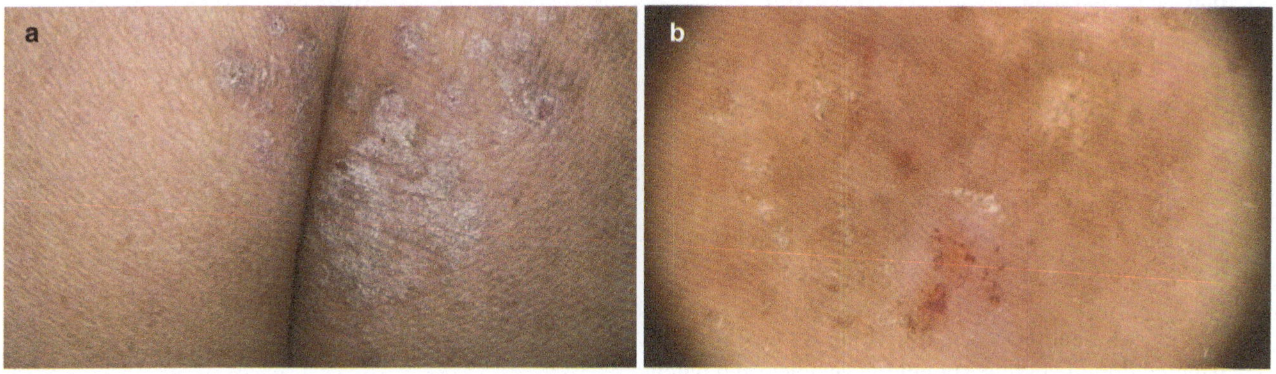

Fig. 12.15 Chronic dermatitis on the buttocks. (**a**) Lichenoid dark-red plaques on the buttocks. (**b**). Irregularly distributed dotted vessels, patchy arrangement of yellow scales, and blood crusts on a dull-red background (×20)

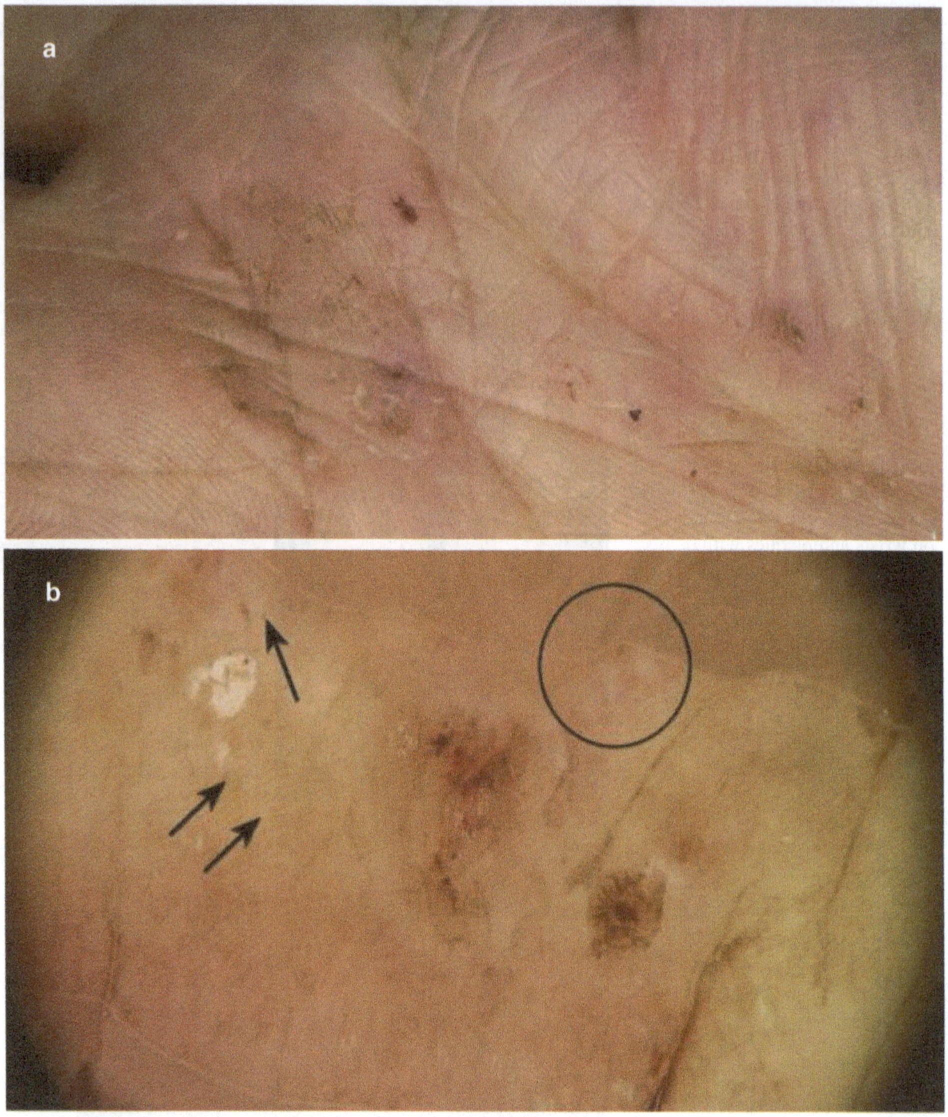

Fig. 12.16 Hand chronic dermatitis/eczema. (**a**). Erythematous patches, scales, and scratches on the palm. (**b**). Irregularly distributed vascular patterns (circle), yellow scales/crusts, and brownish-salmon-colored dots/globules (arrow). Blood crusts could also be observed (×20)

12.1.3.3 Erythroderma Due to Dermatitis/Eczema

1. Patchily distributed dotted vessels.
2. Pinkish background.
3. Yellowish scales/serocrusts, and sparse whitish scales.

12.1.3.4 Dermoscopy as an Auxiliary Tool in the Differential Diagnosis of Plaque Psoriasis and Chronic Dermatitis/Eczema (Fig. 12.17) (Table 12.1)

1. Plaque psoriasis presents as uniformly distributed dotted vessels and diffusely distributed white scales on a light-red background.
2. Chronic dermatitis/eczema presents as patchily distributed dotted vessels, spongiotic vesicles, and patchily distributed yellow scales on a dull-red background.
3. Looped and hairpin-like vessels are highly predictive of a diagnosis of plaque psoriasis (sensitivity and specificity of 91.9% and 94.6%, respectively).

12.1.4 Seborrheic Dermatitis

Seborrheic dermatitis is characterized by yellowish erythema with greasy scales/crusts with a predilection for seborrheic areas, such as the scalp, face, and upper chest (for facial seborrheic dermatitis, please refer to 12.2.1).

12.1.4.1 Dermoscopic Features of Scalp Seborrheic Dermatitis (Figs. 12.18, 12.19, and 12.20)

1. Irregularly distributed linear vessels with branches and linear curved vessels.

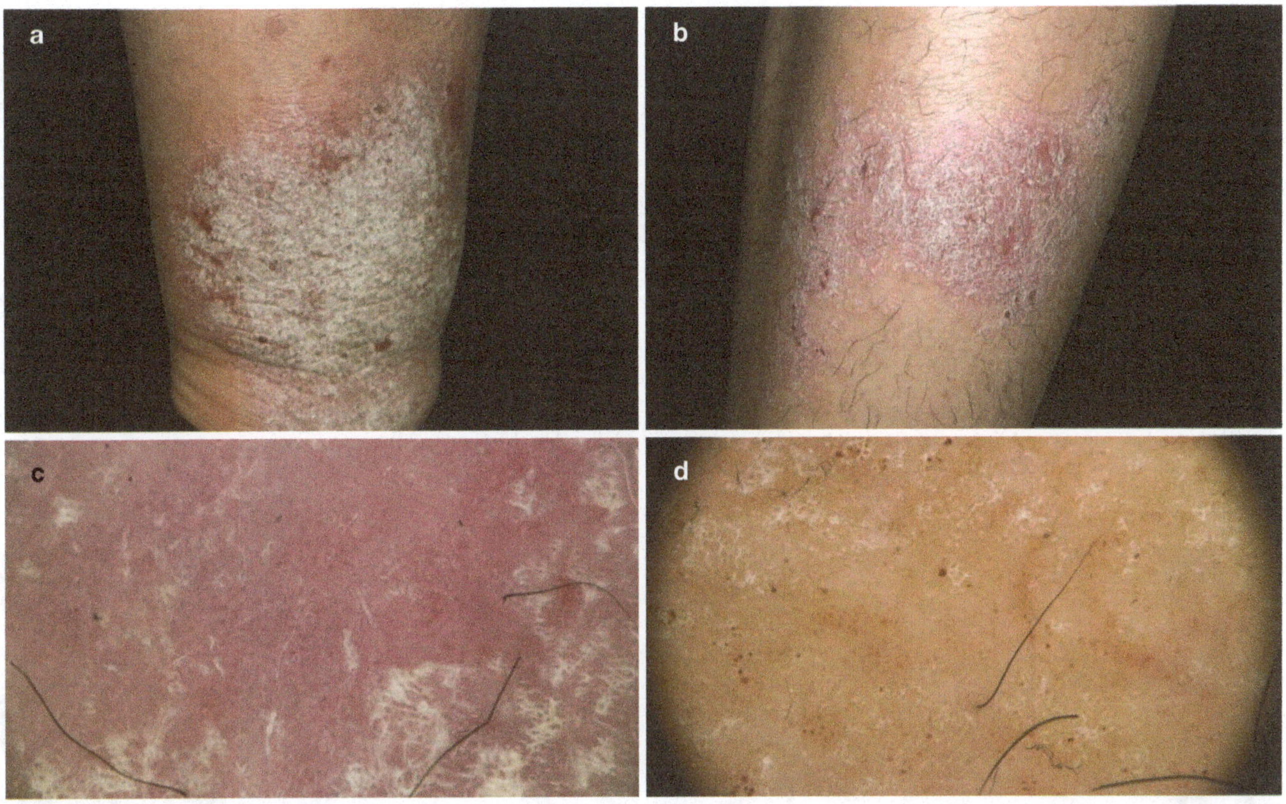

Fig. 12.17 Clinical and dermoscopic pictures of plaque psoriasis and chronic dermatitis/eczema, which have similar clinical manifestations. (**a, b**). Both cases present red patches and plaques with white scales. However, their dermoscopic manifestations differ. (**c**). Uniformly distributed dotted vessels and diffusely distributed white scales on a light-red background indicate plaque psoriasis (×30). (**d**). Irregularly distributed dotted vessels and yellow scales on a dull-red background indicate chronic dermatitis/eczema (×20)

Table 12.1 Dermoscopic feature comparison between plaque psoriasis and chronic dermatitis/eczema

Dermoscopic features	Plaque psoriasis	Chronic dermatitis/eczema
Background color		
Light red	+++	+
Dull red	+	++
Vascular pattern		
Dotted	+++	+++
Looped/hairpin-like	++	+
Distribution of vessels		
Regular	+++	+
Irregular	+	+++
Nonvascular structures		
White scales	+++	+
Yellow scales	+	++

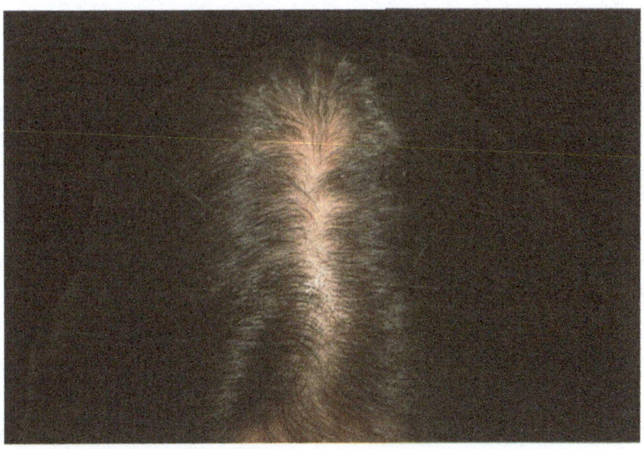

Fig. 12.18 Clinical manifestations of scalp seborrheic dermatitis. Light-red patches with tiny greasy scales and prominent androgenetic alopecia on the scalp

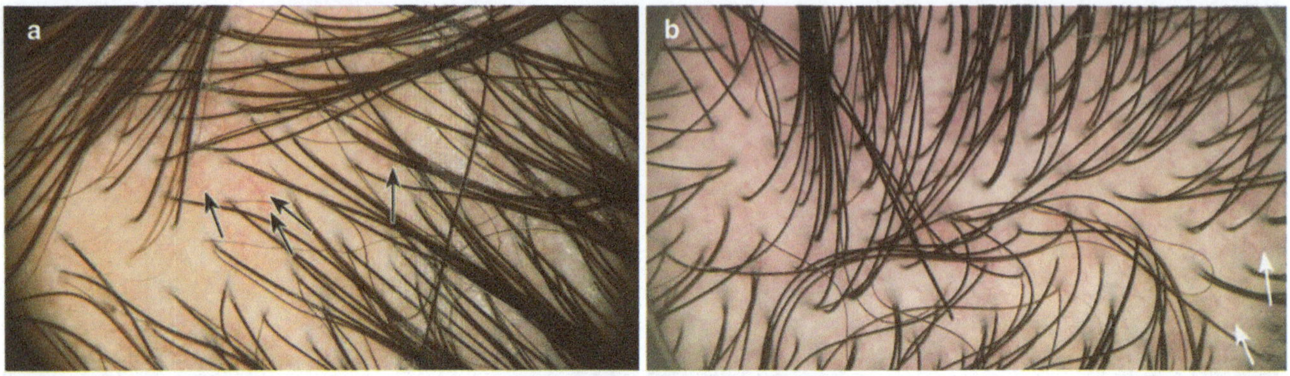

Fig. 12.19 Dermoscopic manifestations of scalp seborrheic dermatitis. (**a**). Irregularly distributed linear vessels with branches and linear curved vessels (black arrows) (×20). (**b**) Irregularly distributed linear vessels with branches and linear curved vessels (white arrows) on a dull-red background (×20)

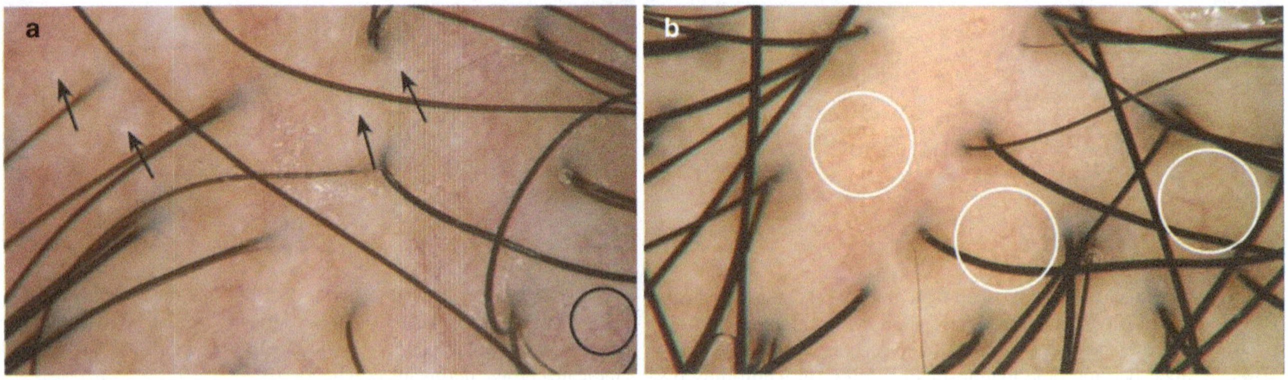

Fig. 12.20 Dermoscopic manifestations of scalp seborrheic dermatitis. (**a**). Irregularly distributed linear vessels with branches and linear curved vessels (black circle) and prominent white structureless areas (black arrows). (**b**). Honeycomb pigment network (white circle) (×50)

2. Perifollicular white or yellowish structureless regions.
3. Honeycomb pigment network, composed of hypopigmented holes and dark reticulate lines, which may be related to the concurrence of androgenetic alopecia.
4. Vascular patterns correspond to the ectatic subpapillary vascular plexus.

12.1.4.2 Dermoscopy as an Auxiliary Tool in the Differential Diagnosis of Scalp Psoriasis and Seborrheic Dermatitis (Fig. 12.21) (Table 12.2)

1. Linear vessels with branches, linear curved vessels, white or yellowish structureless regions, and honeycomb pigment networks indicate seborrheic dermatitis.
2. Dotted vessels; globular vessels; looped, hairpin-like vessels; white scales; and the Auspitz sign indicate scalp psoriasis.

12.1.5 Pityriasis Rosea

Pityriasis rosea is a common acute inflammatory skin disorder. Most cases initially manifest as a single mother patch. Typical lesions present as oval erythematous patches with peripheral scales that present a "Christmas tree-like" distribution. The histopathological changes of pityriasis rosea are nonspecific. Furthermore, pityriasis rosea can be easily confused with psoriasis, seborrheic dermatitis, and pityriasis lichenoides chronica. Dermoscopy can be useful in the noninvasive differential diagnosis of pityriasis rosea and other inflammatory diseases.

The dermoscopic features of pityriasis rosea are as follows (Figs. 12.22, 12.23, and 12.24):

1. Peripheral white scales ("collarette" sign).
2. Yellowish background.
3. Irregular/patchy arrangement of dotted vessels and linear vessels.

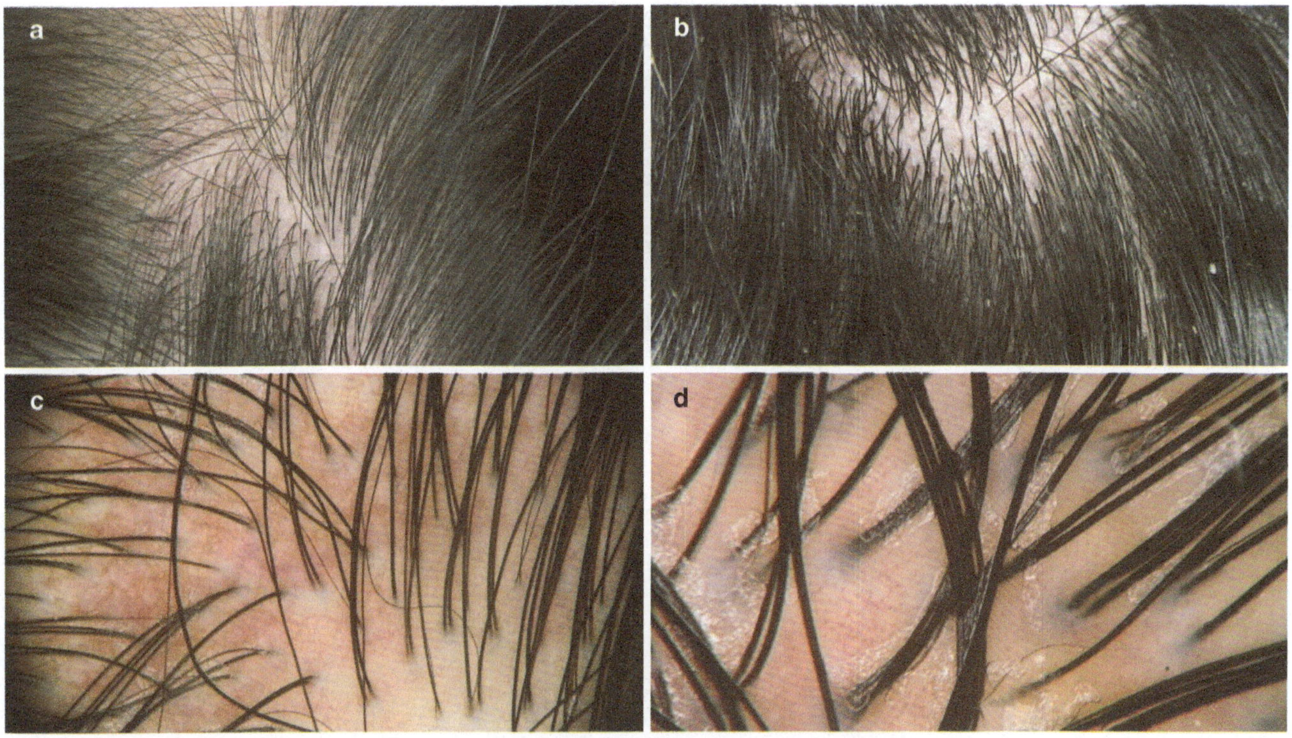

Fig. 12.21 Clinical and dermoscopic images of seborrheic dermatitis and scalp psoriasis, which have similar clinical manifestations. (**a, b**). Scalp seborrheic dermatitis and scalp psoriasis, which are indistinguishable on the basis of clinical manifestations. (**c, d**). Dermoscopic images of **a** and **b**. (**c**). Linear vessels with branches and honeycomb pigment networks indicate seborrheic dermatitis (×20). (**d**). Dotted, looped, and hairpin-like vessels indicate scalp psoriasis (×50)

Table 12.2 Dermoscopic feature comparison between scalp seborrheic dermatitis and scalp psoriasis

Dermoscopic features	Scalp seborrheic dermatitis	Scalp psoriasis
Vascular structures		
Dotted vessels	+	++
Hairpin-like vessels	+	+++
Linear curved vessels	++	+
Linear vessels with branches	+++	–
Nonvascular structures		
White scales	+	++
Yellow scales	++	+
White or yellowish structureless regions	++	–
Auspitz sign	–	++
Honeycomb pigment networks	++	–

12.1.6 Mycosis Fungoides and Parapsoriasis

MF is the most common type of cutaneous T-cell lymphoma (CTCL). Because early-stage MF (patch stage and early plaque stage) typically manifests as scaly infiltrated erythematous patches or plaques, it is difficult to differentiate MF from other inflammatory skin diseases. Additionally, some subtypes of parapsoriasis, such as pityriasis lichenoides chronica, can also be confused with psoriasis. Consequently, we discuss the two entities in together in this section. Dermoscopy can help differentiate MF and parapsoriasis from other inflammatory skin diseases and promote further targeted histopathological examinations.

12.1.6.1 Dermoscopic Features of Early-Stage Mycosis Fungoides (Figs. 12.25 and 12.26)

1. Dull-red background.
2. Regularly distributed dotted vessels.
3. Linear curved vessels: formerly called spermatozoa-like vessels, which are characterized by short, thin, and slightly curved linear vessels, which might be combined with dotted vessels to form peculiar structures reminiscent of a spermatozoon. Spermatozoa-like vessels are highly predictive of a diagnosis of early-stage MF.
4. Orange-yellowish patchy areas.
5. Patchy distributed white scales.
6. Petechiae-like dots.

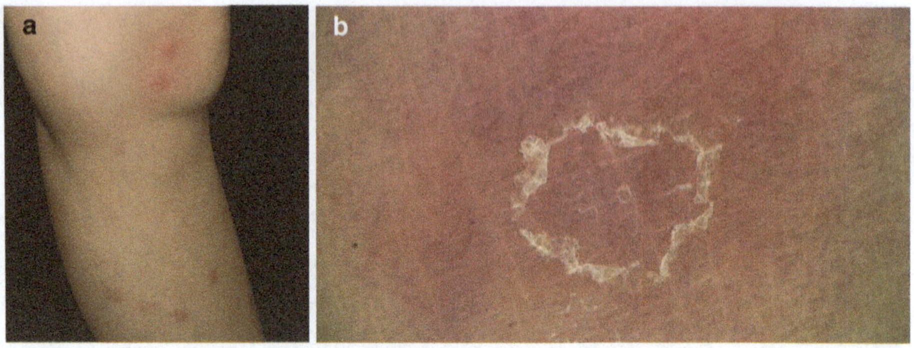

Fig. 12.22 Pityriasis rosea. (**a**). Multiple oval erythematous patches with peripheral scales on legs. (**b**). Patchy arrangement of dotted vessels, linear vessels, and peripheral white scales (collarette sign) (×30)

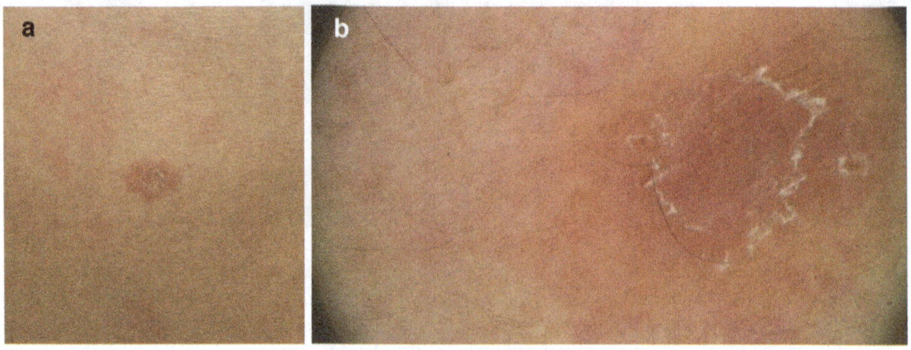

Fig. 12.23 Pityriasis rosea. (**a**). Edematous erythema with peripheral scales. (**b**). Peripheral white scales (collarette sign) on a yellowish background (×20)

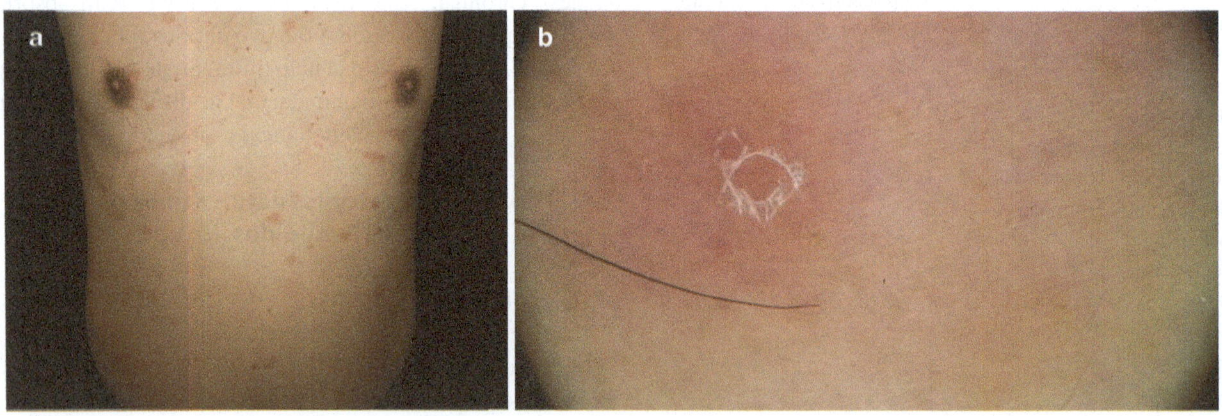

Fig. 12.24 Pityriasis rosea. (**a**). Multiple oval erythematous patches with peripheral scales on the trunk. (**b**). Prominent peripheral white scales (collarette sign) (×20)

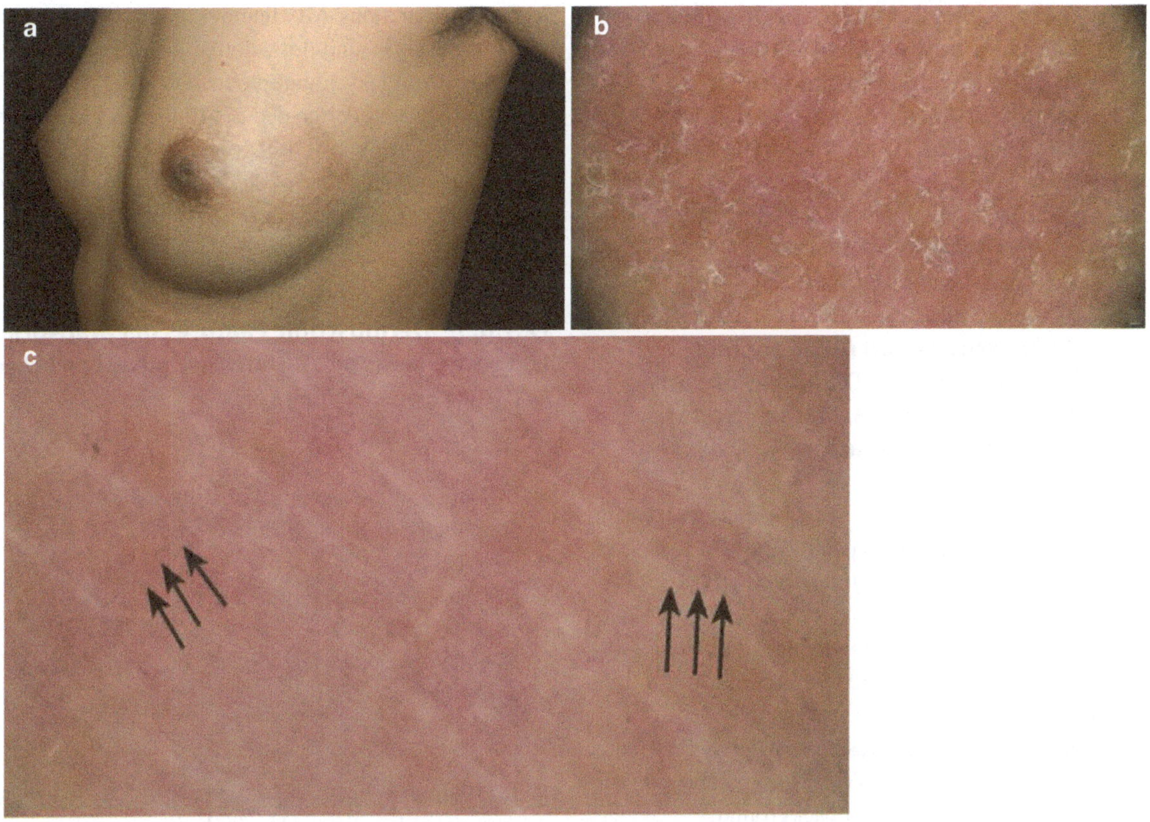

Fig. 12.25 Patch stage mycosis fungoides. (**a**). Infiltrative light-red patches with white scales on the left breast. (**b**). Uniformly distributed dotted vessels, orange-yellowish patchy areas, and white scales on a dull-red background (×20). (**c**). Prominent dotted vessels, linear curved vessels, and spermatozoa-like vessels (arrows) are shown at a higher magnification (×40)

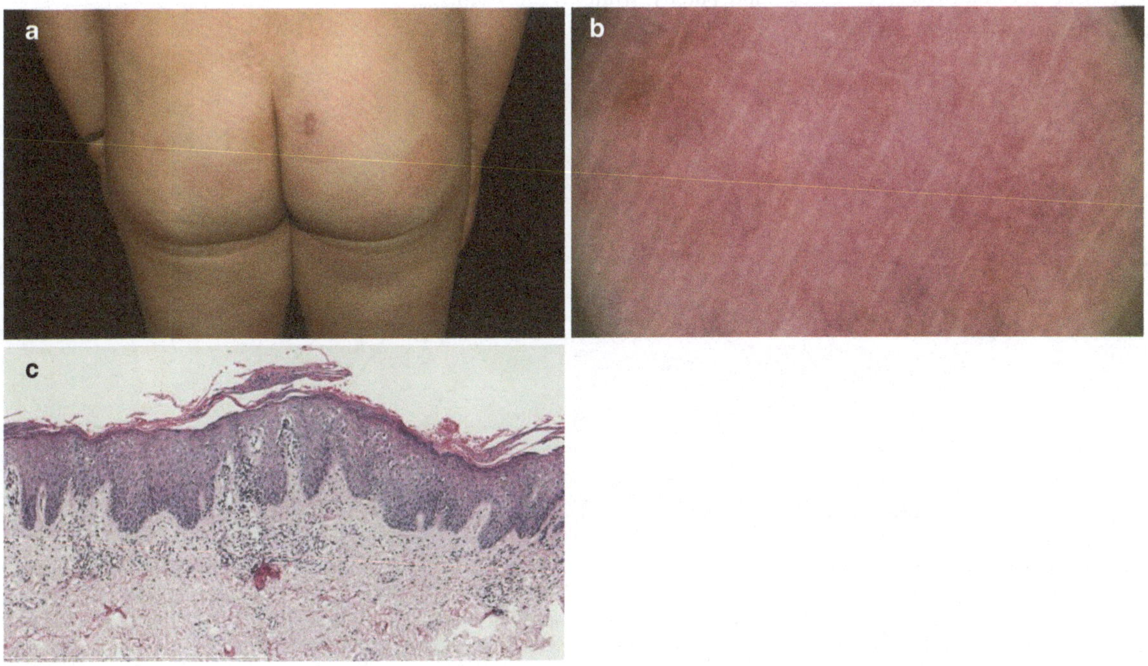

Fig. 12.26 Early-stage mycosis fungoides. (**a**). Infiltrative dark-red to brown patches with white scales on the buttocks and legs. (**b**). Regularly distributed dotted vessels, linear curved vessels, spermatozoa-like vessels, and orange-yellowish patchy areas on a dull-red background (×20). (**c**). Histopathological examination shows hyperkeratosis; parakeratosis; acanthosis; atypical lymphoid cells within the epidermis, some forming "Pautrier's microabscess"; liquefaction degeneration of basal cells; and bandlike lymphohistiocytic infiltration. Combined with further immunohistochemical examination findings (CD4+++, CD8+), the diagnosis of mycosis fungoides was made (HE ×100)

12.1.6.2 Correlations Between the Dermoscopic and Histopathological Findings of Early Mycosis Fungoides (Fig. 12.27)

1. Short linear vessels might correlate with a dilated subpapillary vascular plexus.
2. Spermatozoa-like vessels correspond to capillaries that proliferate vertically along the dermal papillae and extend horizontally into the subpapillary dermis.
3. White scales correspond to parakeratosis.

12.1.6.3 Dermoscopy as an Auxiliary Tool in the Differential Diagnosis of Early Mycosis Fungoides, Plaque Psoriasis, and Chronic Dermatitis (Fig. 12.28) (Table 12.3)

1. Early MF presents short linear vessels, spermatozoa-like vessels, and orange-yellowish patchy areas.
2. Spermatozoa-like vessels are highly predictive of a diagnosis of early-stage MF.
3. Plaque psoriasis presents as uniformly distributed dotted vessels and diffusely distributed white scales on a light-red background.
4. Chronic dermatitis/eczema present as patchily distributed dotted vessels, spongiotic vesicles, and patchily distributed yellow scales on a dull-red background.

12.1.6.4 Dermoscopic Features of Other Subtypes of Mycosis Fungoides

1. Erythrodermic MF presents as regularly distributed dotted vessels, spermatozoa-like vessels, and patchy white scales on a white-pink background.
2. Poikilodermatous MF features areas of polygonal pigment networks and dots, dotted and hairpin-like vessels, and structureless orange-yellowish areas.
3. Acquired keratoderma due to MF presents as amber scales on a white-to-pinkish background, which could distinguish it from other causes of keratoderma, such as psoriasis, chronic dermatitis/eczema, and pityriasis rubra pilaris (PRP).

12.1.6.5 Dermoscopic Features of Parapsoriasis

1. **The dermoscopic features of pityriasis lichenoides chronica are as follows** (Fig. 12.29):
   (a) Orange-yellowish structureless areas (diffused/focal)
   (b) Diffusely/peripherally distributed white scales
   (c) Patchy distributed dotted vessels and linear curved vessels
   (d) Milky-red areas/globules

2. The dermoscopic features of pityriasis lichenoides et varioliformis acuta (PLEVA) are as follows (Fig. 12.30):

   (a) Purpuric aspect in early-stage lesions (correlate with somewhat diffuse hemorrhagic areas due to erythrocyte extravasation).
   (b) Central amorphous brownish crusts in mature lesions (correlate with epidermal necrosis).
   (c) Central white area in healing lesions (correlate with fibrosis).

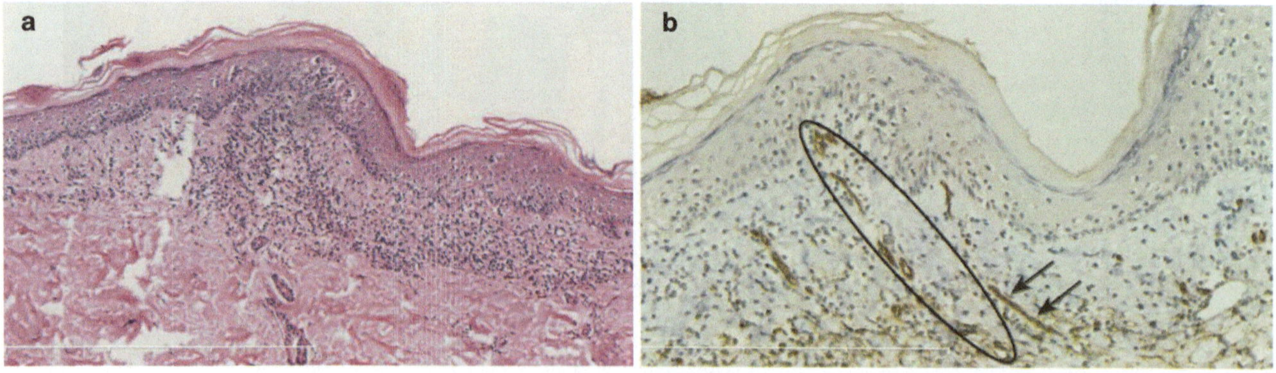

Fig. 12.27 Histological findings of early-stage mycosis fungoides. (**a**). Histopathological examination shows hyperkeratosis, parakeratosis, acanthosis, and liquefaction degeneration of basal cells. Atypical lymphoid cells infiltrated within the epidermis, and some formed Pautrier's microabscess. Bandlike lymphohistiocytic infiltration of the upper dermis. Histological changes were coincident with the diagnosis of mycosis fungoides (HE ×100). (**b**). CD34 immunohistochemistry indicated that the short linear vessels might correlate with a dilated subpapillary vascular plexus (circle), while spermatozoa-like vessels might correlate with capillaries that proliferated along the dermal papillae and extended horizontally into the subpapillary dermis (arrow) (CD34 × 100)

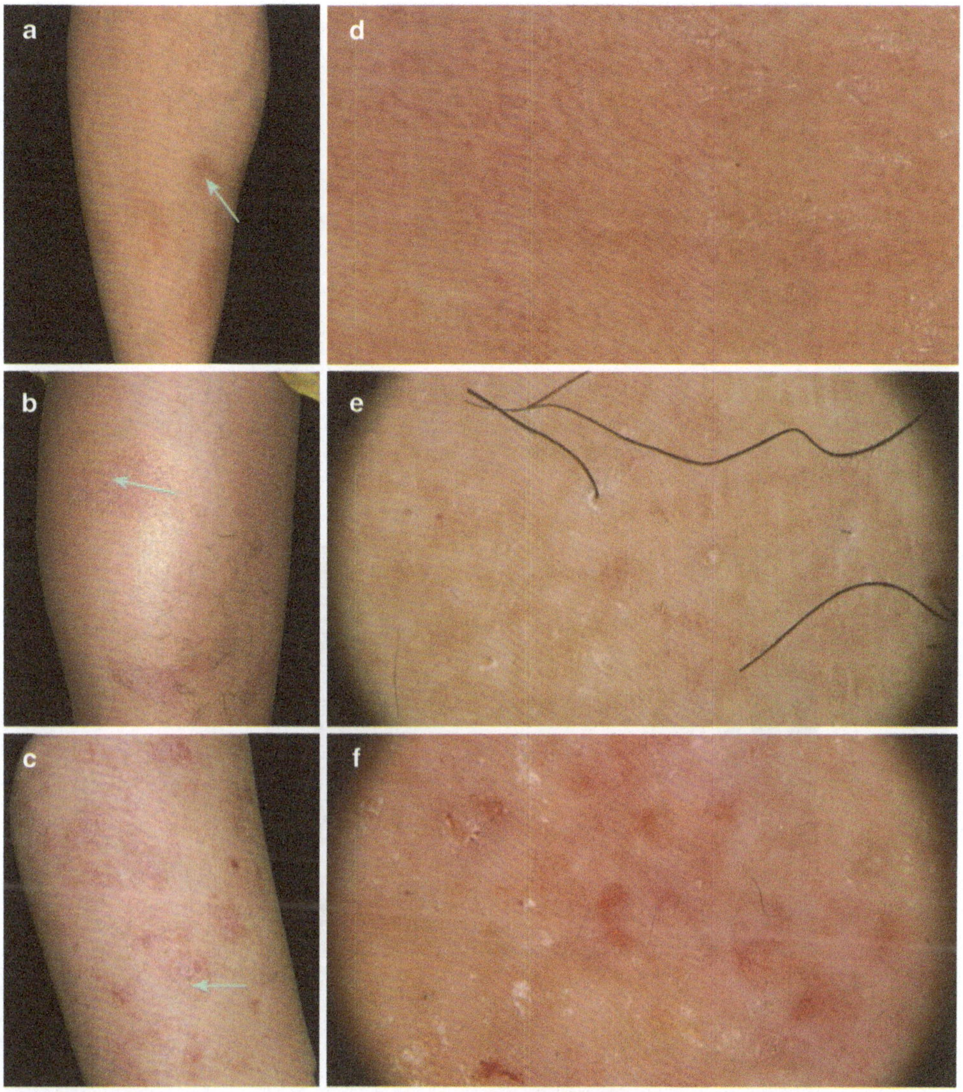

Fig. 12.28 Clinical and dermoscopic images of early mycosis fungoides, plaque psoriasis, and chronic dermatitis, which have similar clinical manifestations. (**a, b, c**). Three entities that are similar clinically. (**d, e, f**). Dermoscopic images of the three entities. (**d**). Uniformly distributed short linear vessels and spermatozoa-like vessels indicate early mycosis fungoides (×20). (**e**). Irregularly distributed dotted vessels and yellow scales indicate chronic dermatitis/eczema (×20). (**f**). Regularly distributed dotted vessels, white scales, and the Auspitz sign on a light-red background indicate plaque psoriasis (×20)

Table 12.3 Dermoscopic feature comparison between early mycosis fungoides and other clinically similar inflammatory skin diseases (plaque psoriasis and chronic dermatitis/eczema)

Dermoscopic features	Early mycosis fungoides	Plaque psoriasis and chronic dermatitis
Background color		
Light red	+	++
Dull red	+	+
Vessel structures		
Dotted	+	++
Looped/hairpin-like	+	++
Linear curved	+++	+
Spermatozoa-like	+++	–
Distribution of vascular structures		
Uniform	+	++
Clustered	+	+
Irregular	+	+
Nonvascular dermoscopic structures		
White scales	+	+
Yellow scales	–	+
Orange-yellowish patchy areas	+++	+

(d) A rim of pinpoint and/or linear vessels to form a targetoid manifestation at the periphery of the lesions.
(e) Peripheral collarette scaling with an inner free edge can be seen in all the stages.

12.1.7 Lichen Planus

LP is an idiopathic mucocutaneous inflammatory disorder. Typical lesions of classic LP present with violaceous papules with shiny tiny white crossing lines (Wickham striae) on the flexure surfaces of extremities. Wickham striae are of high sensitivity and specificity in the diagnosis of LP. Clinically invisible delicate Wickham striae and other specific features in most active lesions can be seen with dermoscopy to enhance diagnostic accuracy. Dermoscopic features differ depending on the subtypes and stages of the disease.

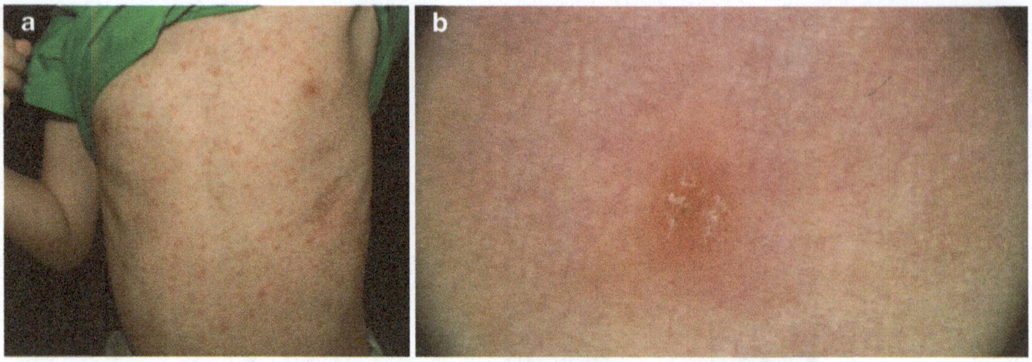

Fig. 12.29 Pityriasis lichenoides chronica. (**a**). Generalized yellowish-red plaques with tiny scales on the trunk and extremities. (**b**). Orange-yellowish structureless area, peripherally distributed white scales, and patchy distributed dotted vessels (×20). (**c**). Orange-yellowish structureless area, patchy distributed dotted vessels, and linear curved vessels (×20)

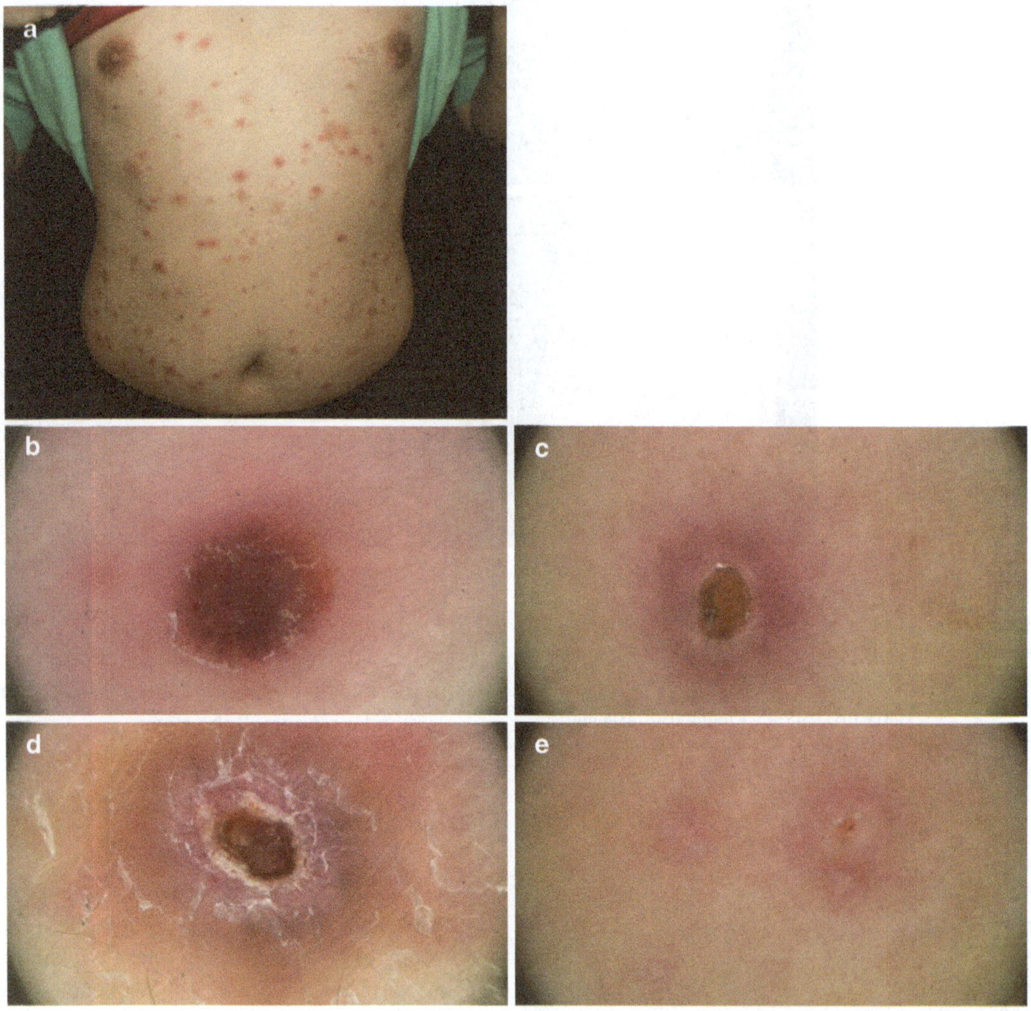

Fig. 12.30 Pityriasis lichenoides et varioliformis acuta. (**a**). Red-brownish papules with central necrosis and crusts on the trunk and extremities. (**b**). Early-stage lesion presents with purpuric aspect, peripheral dotted vessels, and peripheral collarette scaling with an inner free edge (×20). (**c**). Mature-stage lesion presents with central amorphous brownish crusts and rims of pinpoint/linear vessels to form a targetoid aspect (×20). (**d**). Mature-stage lesion presents with central amorphous brownish crusts, rims of pinpoint/linear vessels, and peripheral collarette scaling with an inner free edge (×20). (**e**). Healing-stage lesion presents with central white area and rim of pinpoint/linear vessels to form a targetoid aspect (×20)

12.1.7.1 Dermoscopic Features of Lichen Planus and Their Correlations with Dermoscopic Histological Findings

1. Wickham striae: correspond to compact hyperkeratosis, hypergranulosis, and acanthosis.
2. Dotted/linear vessels: correspond to an ectatic subpapillary vascular plexus.
3. Pigmented structures: correspond to the hyperpigmentation of the basal layer, pigmentary incontinence, and melanophages in the superficial dermis.

12.1.7.2 Dermoscopic Features of Lichen Planus in Different Stages

1. Active lesions
   ① Wickham striae, ② Peripheral dotted/linear vessels.
2. Revolving lesions
   Different pigmented structures

12.1.7.3 Dermoscopic Features of Classic Lichen Planus (Figs. 12.31 and 12.32)

1. Common features
   (a) Wickham striae (reticular, annular, round, radial streaming, and linear)
   (b) Several morphological types of vessels (dotted, linear, linear with branches, and linear curved vessels)
   (c) Radial distribution (common) or diffuse distribution of vessels surrounding Wickham striae
   (d) Blue-gray and yellow-brown pigmented structures (dots/globules, reticular, and cloud-like)
2. Uncommon features
   (a) Blue-white structures
   (b) Follicular plugs

12.1.7.4 Dermoscopic Features of Lichen Planus Pigmentosus (Fig. 12.33, Table 12.4)

1. Common features

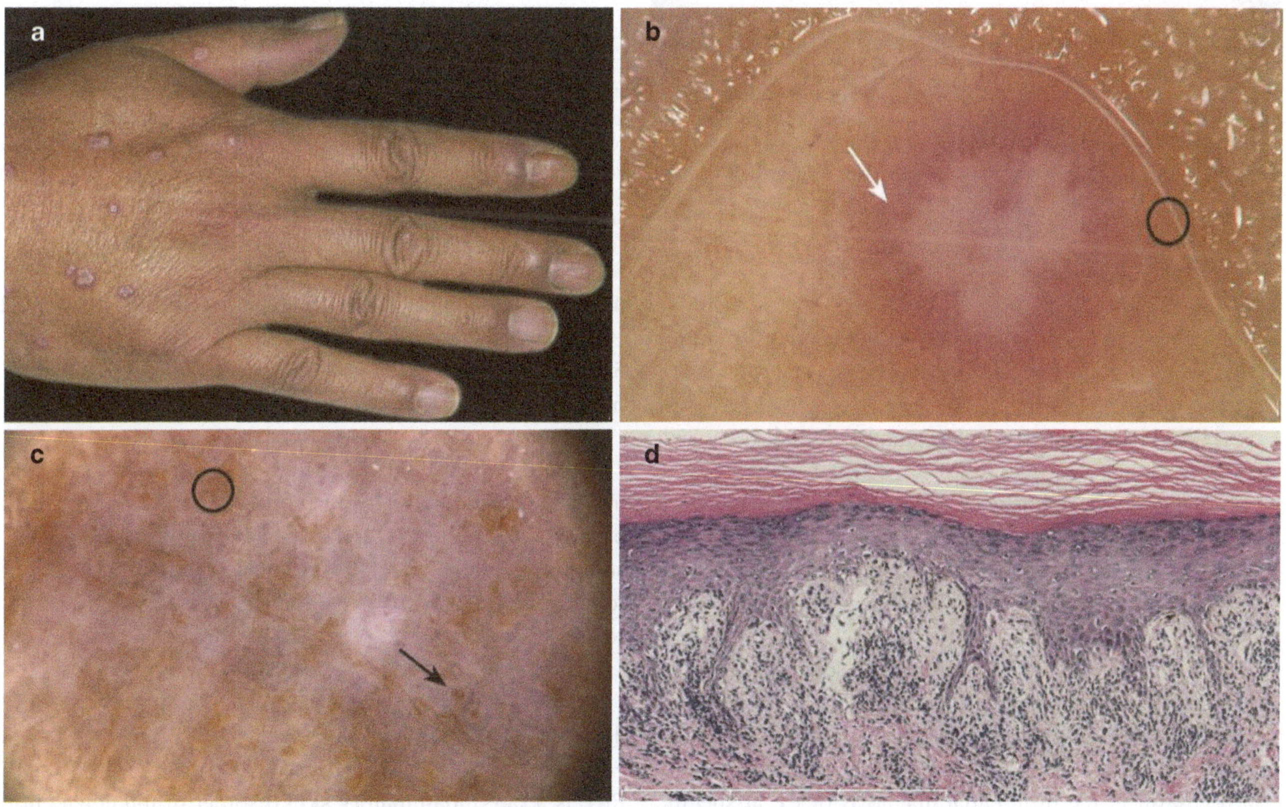

Fig. 12.31 Classic lichen planus. (**a**). Polygonal papules on the right dorsal hand. (**b**). Round Wickham striae, radial distribution surrounding Wickham striae of dotted and linear vessels (white arrow), and patchy yellow-brownish homogeneous pigmented structures (black arrow) (×40). (**c**). Patchy yellow-brownish homogeneous pigmented structures (black circle), blue-white structures, and follicular plugs (black arrow) (×20). (**d**). Histopathological examination shows hyperkeratosis, hypergranulosis, liquefaction degeneration of the basal layer, and bandlike infiltration of lymphocytes and histocytes in the superficial dermis (HE, ×100)

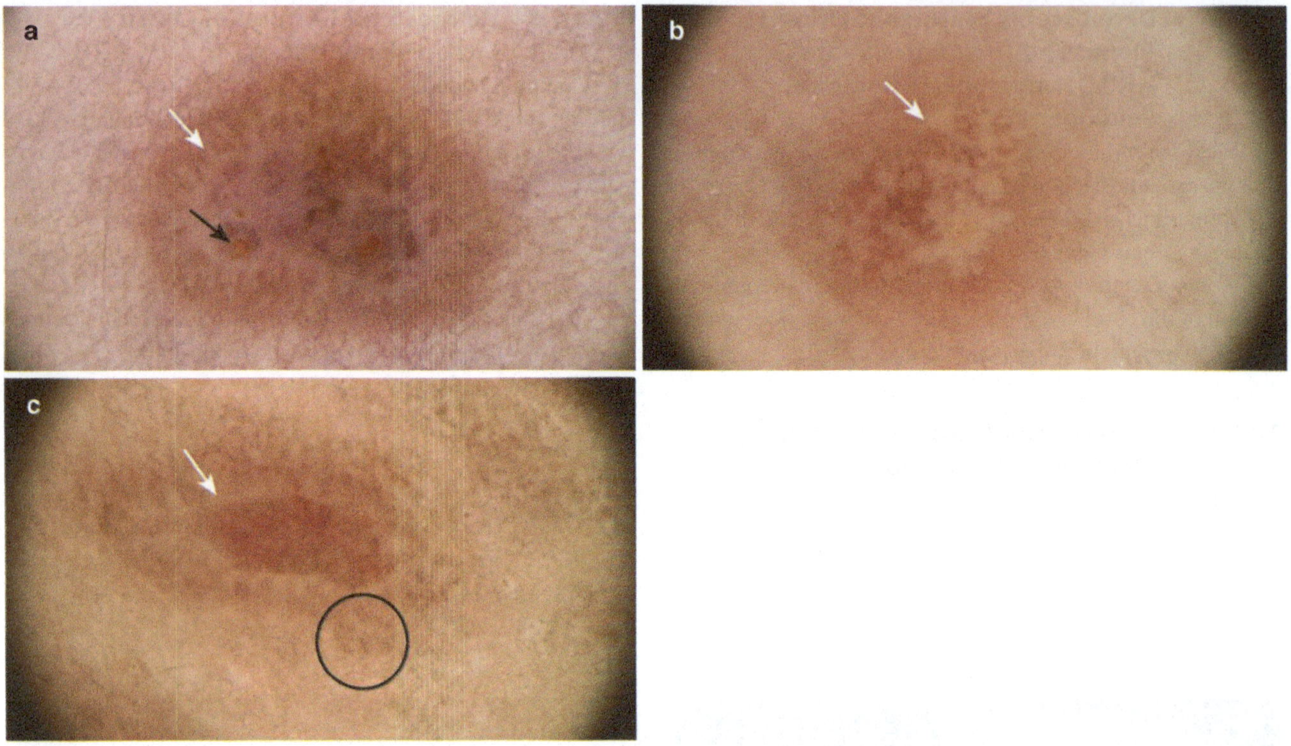

Fig. 12.32 Dermoscopic patterns of Wickham striae in classic lichen planus. (a). Reticular Wickham striae. Peripheral radial distribution surrounding Wickham striae of dotted and linear vessels (white arrow) and follicular plugs (black arrow) (×40). (b). Round, branched Wickham striae. Peripheral radial distribution surrounding Wickham striae of dotted and linear vessels (white arrow) (×40). (c). Annular Wickham striae (white arrow). Dotted/globule blue-gray pigmented structures and yellow-brownish homogeneous pigmented structures (black circle) (×20)

   (a) Blue-white structures
   (b) Follicular plugs
   (c) Blue-gray and yellow-brown pigmented structures (dots/globules, patchy homogeneous, and reticular)
2. Uncommon features
   (a) Wickham striae (reticular, annular, round, branched, and linear)
   (b) Dotted, linear, linear with branches, and linear curved vessels
   (c) Peripheral radial distribution (common) or diffuse distribution surrounding Wickham striae of vessels

Notably, at specific sites, such as the scalp and mucous membranes, lesions can also present with Wickham striae, linear vessels, and other dermoscopic features of classic LP (Figs. 12.34, 12.35, and 12.36). Consequently, dermoscopy can be useful in the differential diagnosis of LP at specific sites.

12.1.7.5 Dermoscopic Features of Hypertrophic Lichen Planus (Fig. 12.37)

1. Wickham striae
2. Comedo-like openings
3. Follicular plugs
4. Dotted/globular blue-gray to brown-black pigmented structures
5. Dotted vessels
6. Occasional yellow structures

Dermoscopy can be useful in the differentiation of hypertrophic LP from nodular prurigo, which presents with non-pigmented structures, comedo-like openings, and white starburst patterns (radially arranged whitish lines) surrounded by reddish/brown-yellowish crusts, erosions, and/or scales.

12.1.8 Pityriasis Rubra Pilaris

PRP is a rare inflammatory skin disorder of unknown etiology. The typical manifestations of PRP are papulosquamous erythema with unaffected skin islands and palmoplantar keratoderma. Untypical cases might be misdiagnosed as plaque psoriasis. Dermoscopy can be useful in the differentiation of PRP and plaque psoriasis.

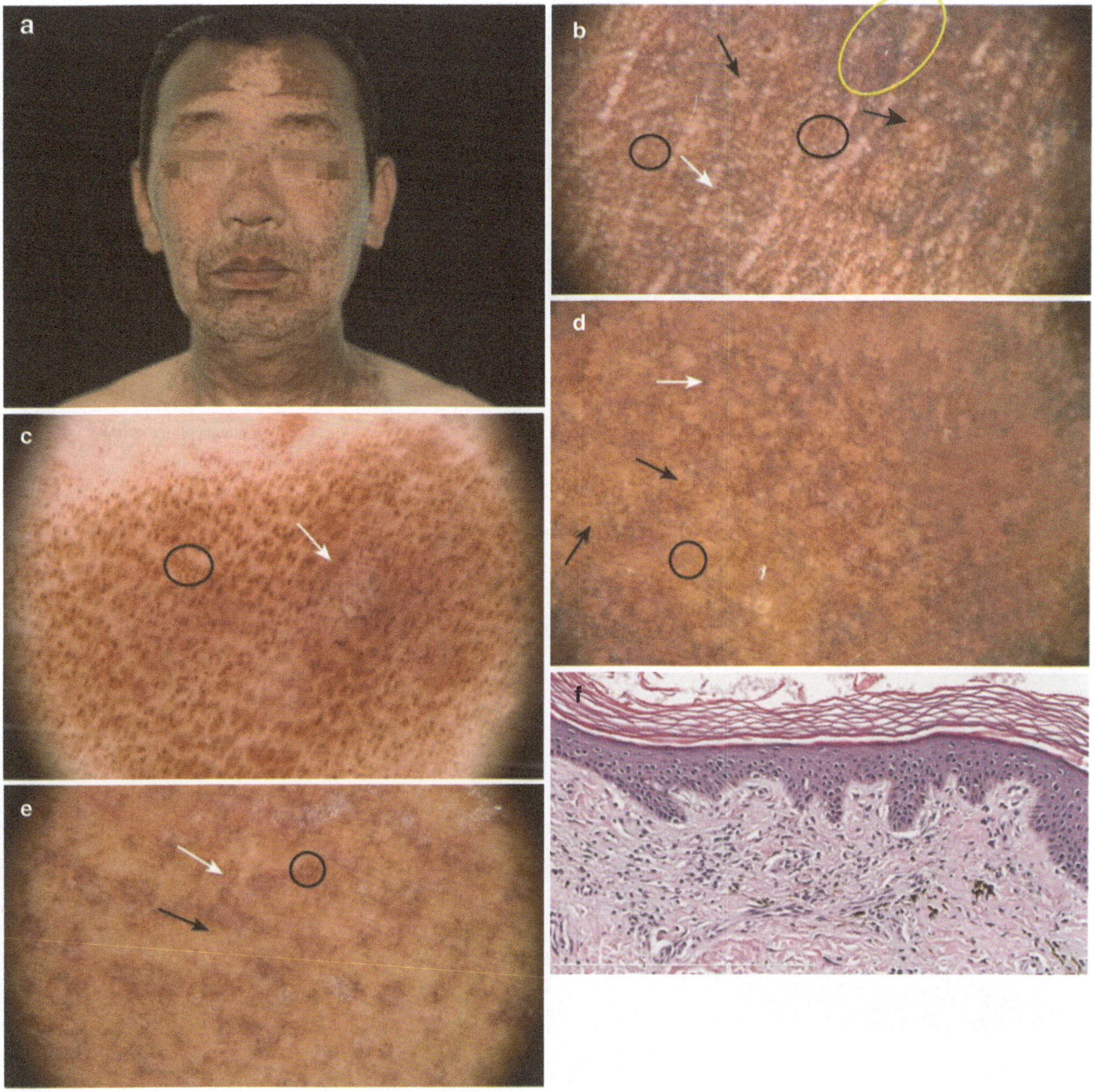

Fig. 12.33 Lichen planus pigmentosus. (**a**). Bilateral multiple brown patches on the face and neck. (**b**). Blue-white structures (yellow circle), follicular plugs (black arrow), dotted/globular blue-gray pigment granules (white arrow), and patchy yellow-brownish homogeneous pigmented structures (black circle) (×20). (**c**). Reticular Wickham striae. Dotted blue-gray pigment granules (white arrow) and dotted/globular/patchy yellow-brownish homogeneous pigmented structures (black circle) (×20). (**d**). Globular blue-gray pigment granules (white arrow) and dotted/globular/patchy yellow-brownish homogeneous pigmented structures (black circle) and follicular plugs (black arrow) (×40). (**e**). Dotted/globular blue-gray pigment granules (white arrow) and patchy yellow-brownish homogeneous pigmented structures (black circle) and follicular plugs (black arrow) (×20). (**f**). Histopathological examination shows hyperkeratosis; stratum spinosum atrophy; liquefaction degeneration of the basal layer; and a bandlike infiltration of lymphocytes, histocytes, and many melanophages in the superficial dermis (hematoxylin and eosin, ×100)

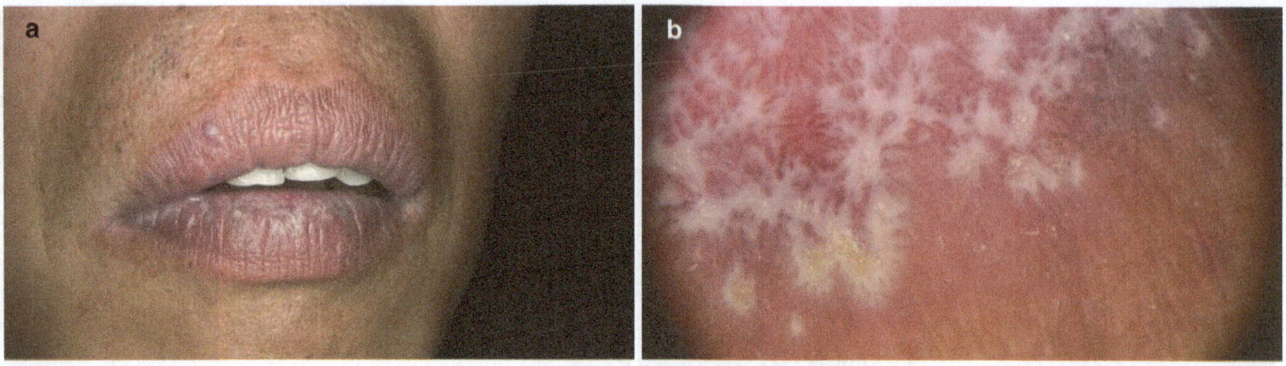

Fig. 12.34 Lichen planus of the lip. (**a**). Violaceous patches on the lower lip. (**b**). Striking radial streaming Wickham striae (×20)

Table 12.4 Comparison of dermoscopic features of classic lichen planus and lichen planus pigmentosus

Dermoscopy	Classic lichen planus	Lichen planus pigmentosus
Wickham striae	+++	+
Blue-white structures	+	++
Blue-gray and yellow-brown pigmented structures	+++ Mainly yellow-brown patchy homogeneous pattern	+++ Mainly blue-gray dotted/globule pattern
Follicular plugs	+	+++
Vascular structures	+++ Peripheral radial distribution surrounding Wickham striae	+

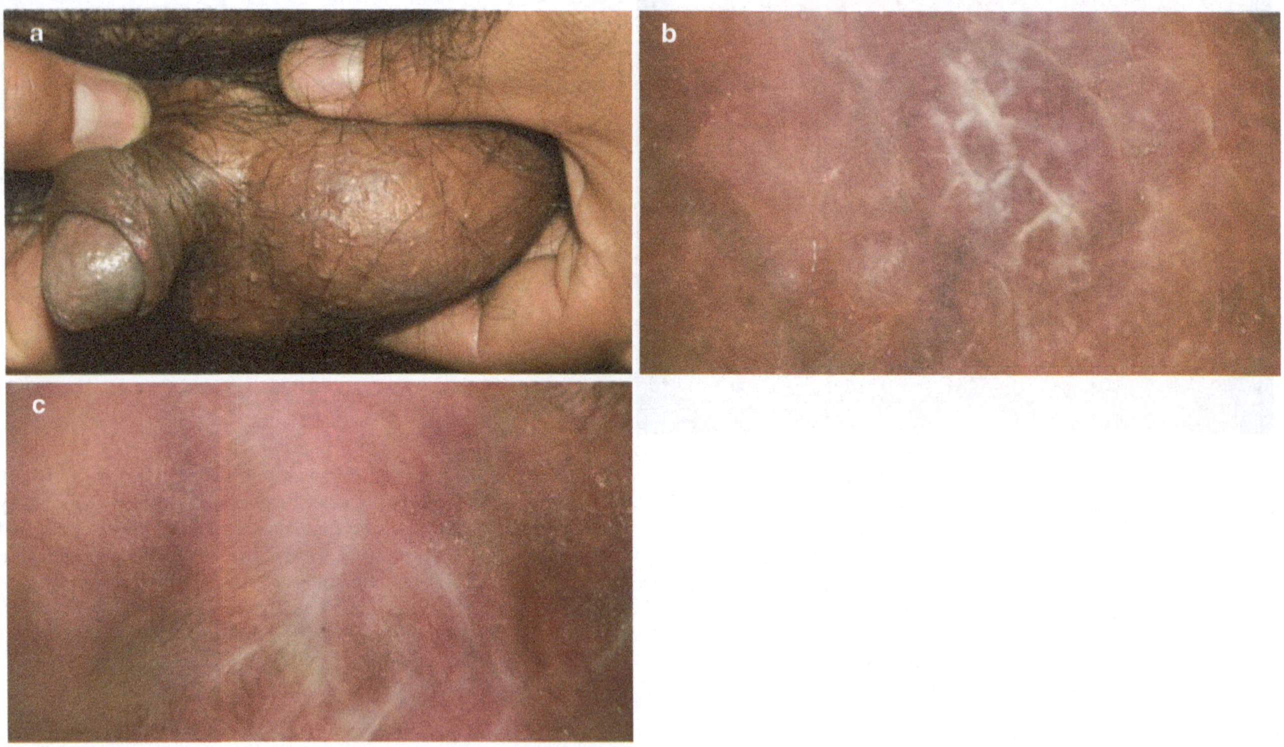

Fig. 12.35 Lichen planus of the scrotum. (**a**). Violaceous patches on the scrotum; (**b, c**). Branched Wickham striae and linear vessels (×50)

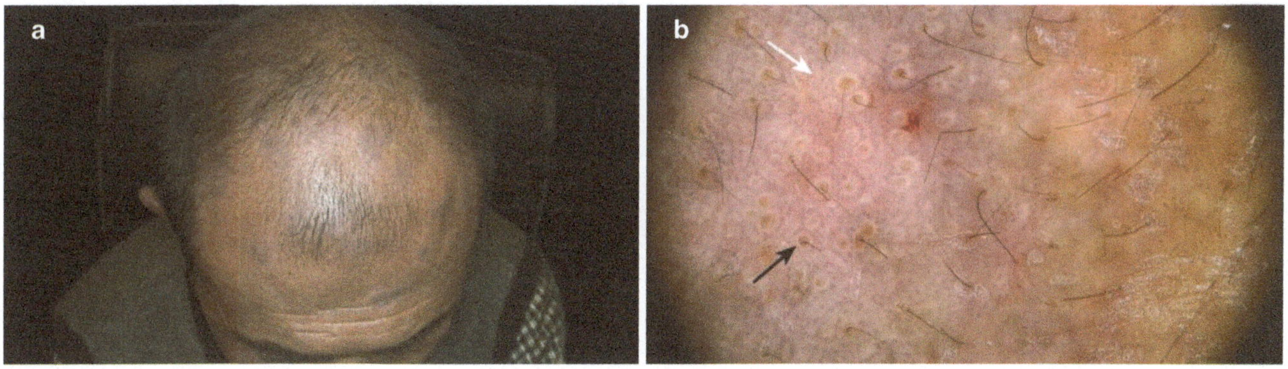

Fig. 12.36 Lichen pilaris. (**a**). Lesions of lichen pilaris. (**b**). Reticular Wickham striae, follicular plugs (black arrow), and diffusely distributed dotted/linear vessels (white arrow) (×20)

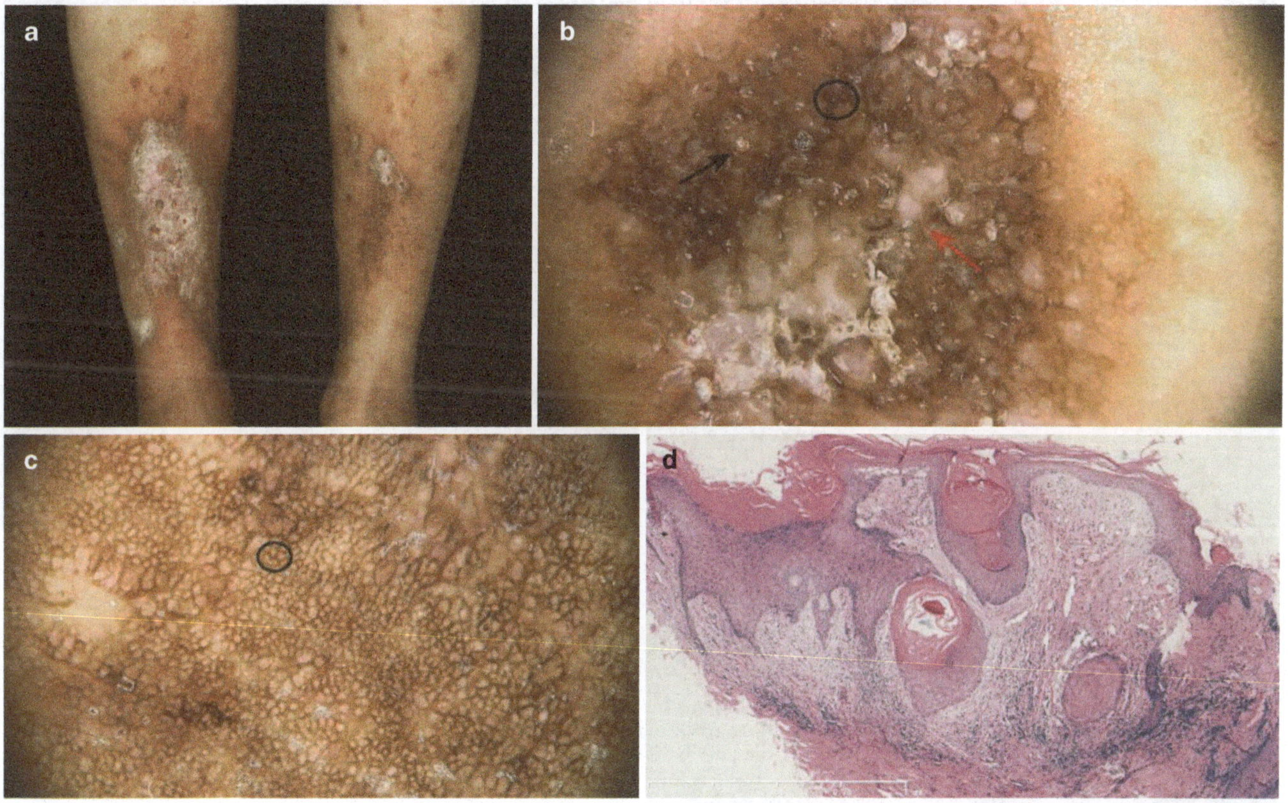

Fig. 12.37 Hypertrophic lichen planus. (**a**). Verrucous violaceous plaques on the lower extremities. (**b**). Follicular plugs (black arrows), brown-black patchy homogeneous patterns (black circle), and yellow structures (red arrow) (×20). (**c**). Reticular brown-black pigmentation (black circle) (×20) . (**d**). Histopathological examination shows hyperkeratosis, follicular plugs, irregular acanthosis, focal liquefaction degeneration of basal cells, and bandlike infiltration of lymphocytes in the superficial dermis (hematoxylin and eosin, ×40)

12.1.8.1 Dermoscopic Features of the Classic Form Pityriasis Rubra Pilaris (Figs. 12.38 and 12.39)

1. Central round/oval yellowish areas surrounded by dotted/linear vessels
2. Keratin plugs in the center of some round/oval yellowish areas
3. Patchy whitish scales

12.1.8.2 Dermoscopic Features of Erythroderma Due to Pityriasis Rubra Pilaris (Fig. 12.40)

1. Reddish background
2. Scattered dotted vessels
3. Orange blotches
4. Diffuse whitish scales
5. Reticular vessels in islands of non-erythematous (spared) skin

12.1.8.3 Dermoscopic Features of Palmoplantar Keratoderma Due to Pityriasis Rubra Pilaris (Fig. 12.41)

1. Patchily distributed homogeneous orange structureless areas of different sizes
2. Patchy white scales

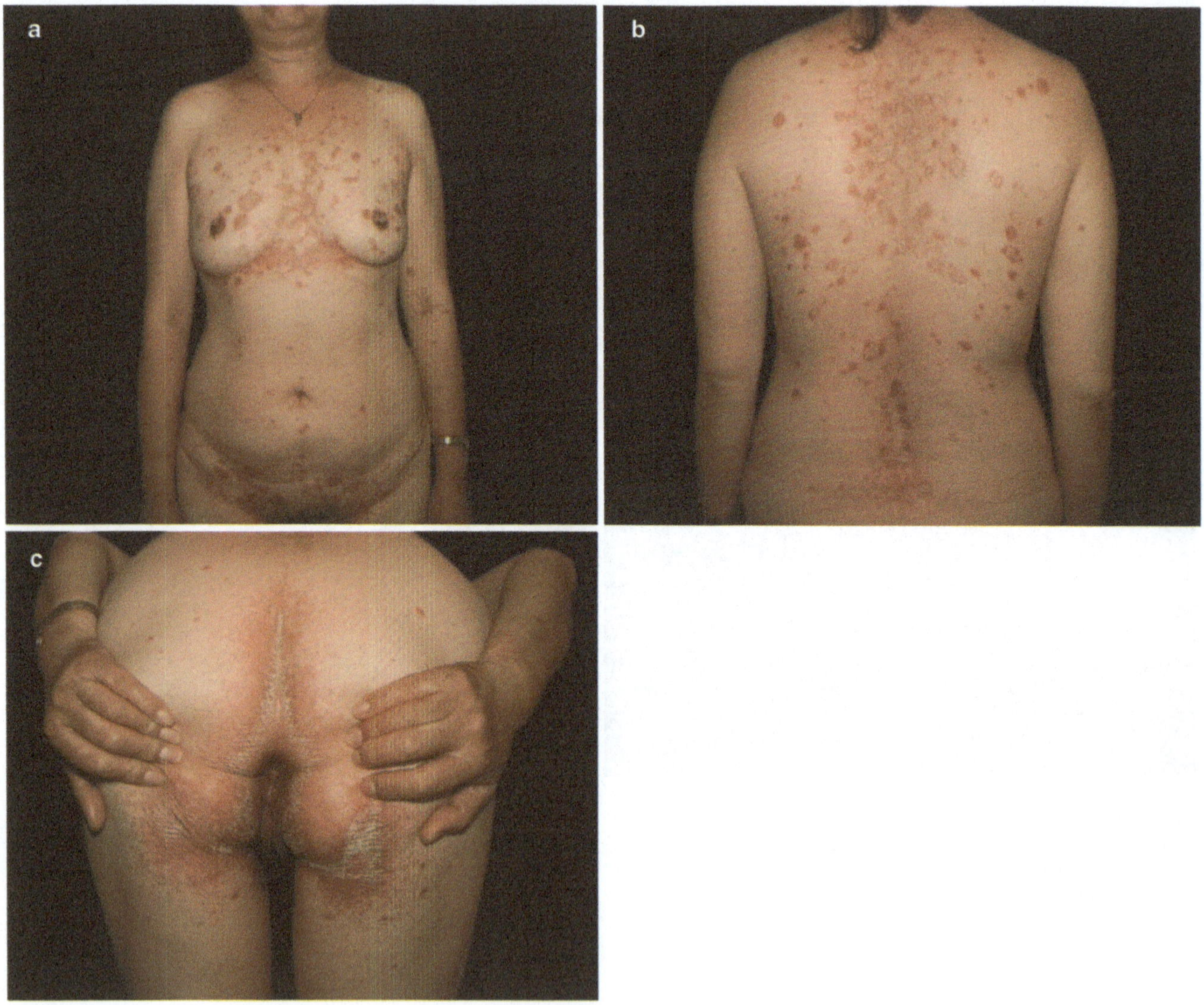

Fig. 12.38 Clinical manifestations of classic pityriasis rubra pilaris. (**a-c**). Salmon-colored scaly patches on the trunk, extremities, dorsal hands, and perianal area with peripheral follicular hyperkeratotic papules

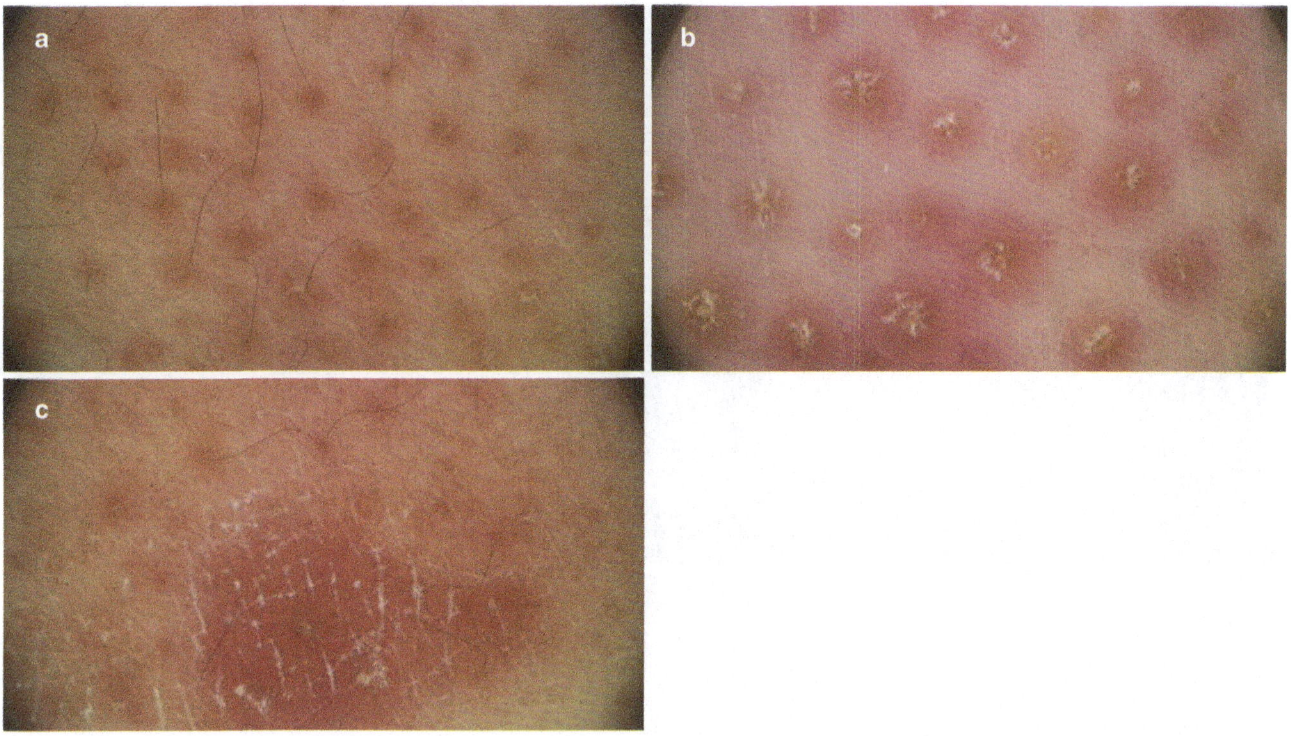

Fig. 12.39 Dermoscopic manifestations of the classic form of pityriasis rubra pilaris. (**a**). Central round/oval yellowish areas surrounded by dotted/linear vessels. Some yellowish areas are associated with central keratotic plugs (×20). (**b**). Round/oval yellowish areas associated with pinpoint-like central keratotic plugs are surrounded by dotted/linear vessels (×20). (**c**). Yellowish area with a central keratotic plug with peripheral dotted vessels and white scales distributed patchily along the furrow (×20)

12.1.8.4 Dermoscopy as an Auxiliary Tool in the Differential Diagnosis of Pityriasis Rubra Pilaris and Plaque Psoriasis (Fig. 12.42) (Table 12.5)

1. Linear vessels and follicular plugs on a yellowish-red background indicate PRP.
2. Dotted vessels and diffusely distributed white scales on a light-red background indicate plaque psoriasis.

12.1.9 Erythema Multiforme

Erythema multiforme is a self-limited disease caused by infections, drugs, and autoimmune disorders. Typical "target" or "iris" lesions consist of three zones: an inner dark-red zone surrounded by a pale edematous zone and an outer erythematous ring. Reports about the dermoscopic features of erythema multiforme are few.

The dermoscopic features of erythema multiforme are as follows (Fig. 12.43):

1. Central dusky zone
2. Peripheral plain edematous structureless zone
3. Outer red rim
4. Some linear vessels

12.1.10 Graft-Versus-Host Disease

Graft-versus-host disease (GVHD) is an immunological disorder caused by a graft-versus-host response, which is a common complication of allogenic hematopoietic stem cell transplantation. Acute GVHD occurs within 100 days of transplantation and presents as itching or painful red papules and bulla or epidermolysis in severe cases. Chronic GVHD typically occurs 100 days after transplantation, presenting as LP-like, scleroderma-like, or poikiloderma-like lesions, ultimately resulting in skin sclerosis and pigmentation. Until recently, reports of GVHD have been few. Dermoscopy can help in the noninvasive and differential diagnosis of GVHD.

12.1.10.1 Dermoscopic Features of Acute Graft-Versus-Host Disease

1. Pink to red background
2. Dilated capillaries

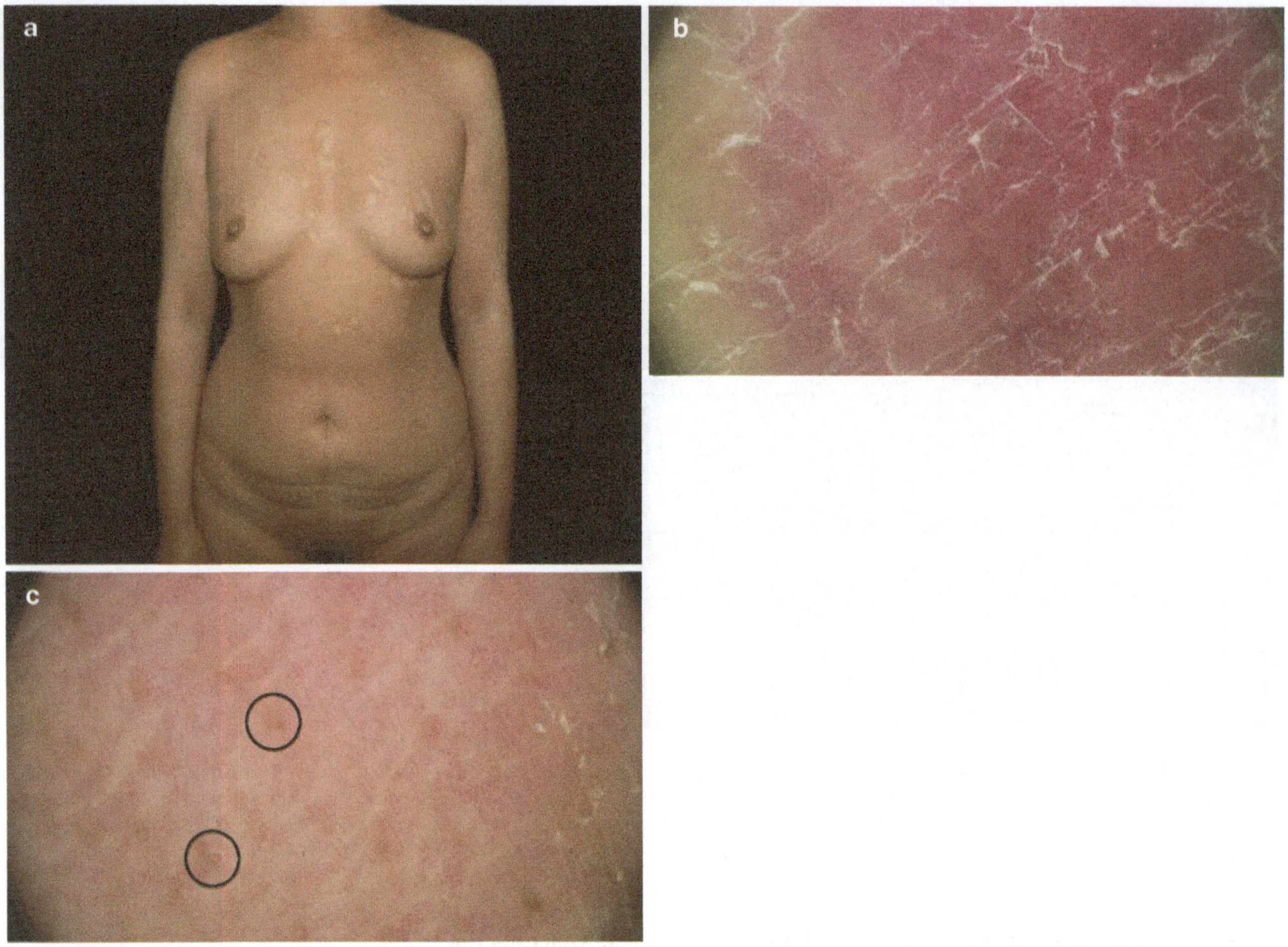

Fig. 12.40 Erythroderma due to pityriasis rubra pilaris. (**a**). Generalized yellowish-red patches with scales on trunk and extremities. Islands of spared skin are evident in some regions. (**b**). Scattered dotted vessels with diffuse whitish scales on a reddish background (×20). (**c**). Orange blotches (circle) can also be seen apart from dotted vessels and a few linear vessels (×20)

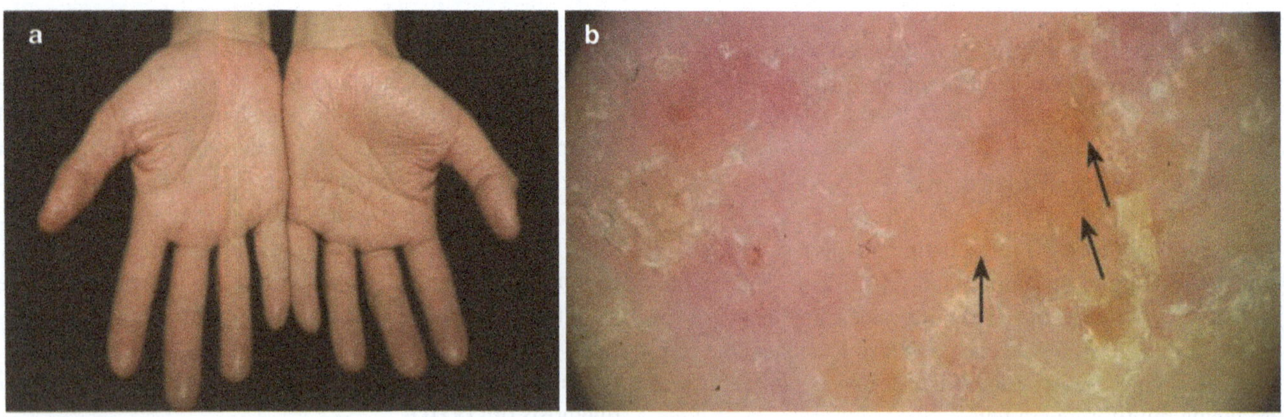

Fig. 12.41 Pityriasis rubra pilaris on palms. (**a**). Diffuse erythematous keratoderma on palms. (**b**). Patchily distributed homogeneous orange structureless areas in different sizes (arrow) and white to white-yellowish scales and milky-red patches (×20)

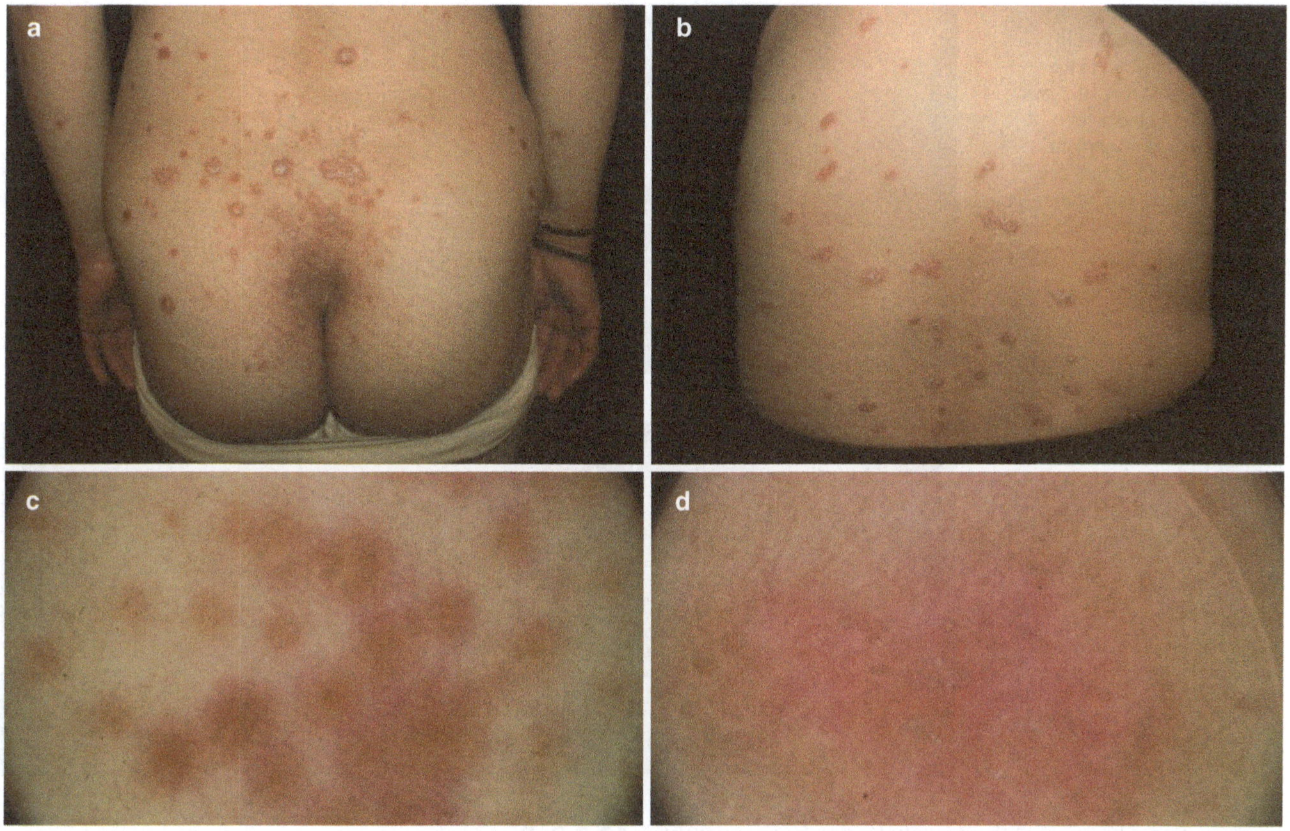

Fig. 12.42 Clinical and dermoscopic images of pityriasis rubra pilaris and plaque psoriasis, which have similar clinical manifestations. (**a, b**). Pityriasis rubra pilaris and plaque psoriasis lesions, which are similar clinically. (**c**). Central round/oval yellow area, follicular plugs, and peripheral dotted/linear vessels indicate pityriasis rubra pilaris (×20). (**d**). Dotted vessels with a light-red background indicate plaque psoriasis (×20)

Table 12.5 Comparison of dermoscopic features between pityriasis rubra pilaris and plaque psoriasis

Dermoscopic features	Pityriasis rubra pilaris	Plaque psoriasis
Background color		
Light red	–	+++
Yellowish red	+++	+
Vascular patterns		
Dotted	+	+++
Linear	++	–
Dotted+linear	++	+
Vascular arrangement		
Uniform	+	+++
Peripheral	++	–
Additional features		
White scales	++	+++
Yellow scales	+	+
Clustered distribution of scales	++	+
Diffused distribution of scales	+	++
Keratotic plugs	+++	–

Dermoscopy can detect telangiectasia that is not detectable by the naked eye, which is of great importance in the early detection of acute GVHD.

12.1.10.2 Dermoscopic Features of Chronic Graft-Versus-Host Disease (Squamopapular Lesions)

1. Mixed vascular structures, mainly dotted and linear vessels
2. White scales

12.2 Facial Skin Disorders

Seborrheic dermatitis, rosacea, acne vulgaris, and lupus miliaris disseminatus faciei (LMDF) are a group of common facial skin disorders that present as facial erythematous patches, papules, and plaques. The diagnosis of this group of diseases often relies on clinical manifestations. Invasive histopathological examinations are often refused

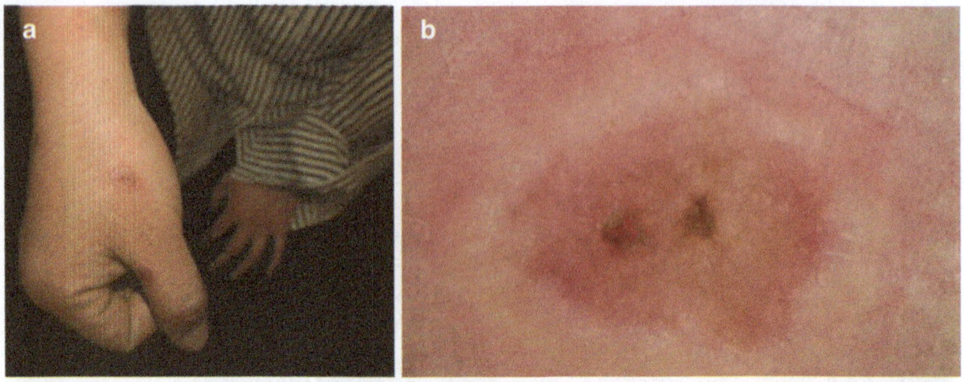

Fig. 12.43 Erythema multiforme. (**a**). Targetoid erythematous lesion on the hand. (**b**). Three typical zones under dermoscopy, namely, a central dusky zone, a plain edematous structureless zone, and an outer red rim. Some linear vessels can also be seen (×20)

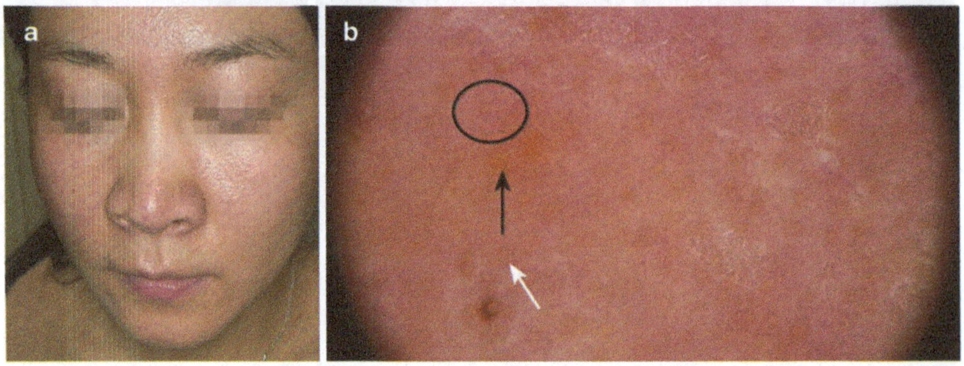

Fig. 12.44 Facial seborrheic dermatitis. (**a**). Light-red patches with small scales on the cheeks and intercilium. (**b**). Patchy white-yellowish scales, perifollicular faint yellow halos (black arrow), follicular plugs (white arrow), and blurred branched vessels (circle) on a light-red background (×20)

by the patients because of the potential risks. Consequently, dermoscopy has great value as a noninvasive tool in the diagnosis and differential diagnosis of facial skin disorders.

12.2.1 Seborrheic Dermatitis

Seborrheic dermatitis is a common inflammatory skin disorder that presents as light-red patches with greasy scales with a predilection for seborrheic areas, such as the scalp (see scalp seborrheic dermatitis in Sect. 12.1), face, chest, and back. Seborrheic dermatitis can occur in both adults and neonates. Dermoscopy can be used in the differential diagnosis of facial seborrheic dermatitis and other facial disorders.

The dermoscopic features of facial seborrheic dermatitis are as follows (Fig. 12.44):

1. Patchy arrangement of yellowish, tiny scales with/without white scales.
2. Unspecific distribution of vascular patterns (dotted, linear with branches, linear curved).
3. Red/light-red background.
4. Perifollicular faint yellow halo-like oil drops.
5. White structureless areas and follicular plugs are rare.

12.2.2 Rosacea

The pathogenesis of rosacea remains unknown and may be associated with abnormal vasomotor response and recurrent *Demodex folliculorum* infection. The three clinical stages of rosacea are the erythematotelangiectatic, papulopustular, and glandular rosacea stages. No distinct developmental boundaries exist between the different stages of rosacea. This section mainly discusses the dermoscopic features of the erythematotelangiectatic and papulopustular rosacea stages.

12.2.2.1 Dermoscopic Features of Rosacea (Fig. 12.45)

1. Linear vessels arranged in polygons (reticular vessels).
2. Purple-red background.
3. Gray-white follicular plugs and white linear structures.
4. Additional features include rosettes, orange-yellowish areas, dilated follicles, and follicular pustules.

12.2.2.2 Dermoscopy as an Auxiliary Tool in the Differential Diagnosis of Facial Seborrheic Dermatitis and Rosacea (Table 12.6)

1. Facial seborrheic dermatitis presents as an unspecific arrangement of dotted/branched vessels and perifollicular faint yellow oil droplet halos with yellowish-whitish scales on a red/light-red background.

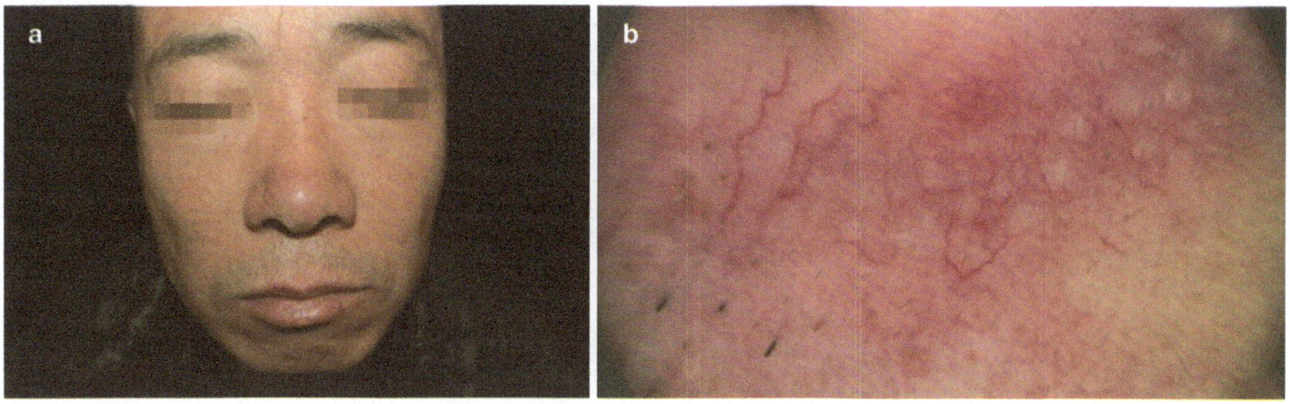

Fig. 12.45 Rosacea. (**a**). Telangiectasia on the nose. (**b**). Reticular vessels, dilated follicles, and follicular plugs on a purple-red background (×20)

Table 12.6 Comparison of dermoscopic features between facial seborrheic dermatitis and rosacea

Dermoscopic features	Seborrheic dermatitis	Rosacea
Background color		
Light red/yellowish red	+++	+
Purple red	+	++
Vascular structures		
Linear curved	+++	+++
Linear with branches	++	+++
Reticular (polygonal)	+	+++
Dotted	+	+
Nonvascular structures		
Perifollicular yellow halos	+++	+
Follicular plugs	++	++
Pustules	–	++

2. Rosacea presents as linear vessels arranged in polygons on a purple-red background and follicular pustules in some patients.

Some reports indicated that gray-white follicular plugs and white linear structures (white masses projecting out of each hair follicle) correspond to demodecidosis. Furthermore, dermoscopy can be utilized in the evaluation of treatment effectiveness and follow-up.

12.2.3 Acne Vulgaris

Acne vulgaris is a common chronic pilosebaceous inflammatory disease with a predilection in adolescents. The clinical manifestations of acne include comedones, inflammatory papules, pustules, nodules, and cysts. The diagnosis of acne vulgaris mainly relies on clinical features. Dermoscopy can be used for the differentiation of acne vulgaris from other diseases, such as eruptive vellus hair cysts.

The dermoscopic features of acne vulgaris are as follows:

1. Inflammatory acne presents as a well-demarcated yellow-whitish round structure in the center with a fine brown linear boundary surrounded by an erythematous halo (Fig. 12.46).
2. Comedonal acne presents as central brown-yellowish follicular plugs and scattered inflammatory erythema (Fig. 12.47).

Dermoscopy can be used in the differential diagnosis of acne vulgaris from several conditions, such as eruptive vellus hair cysts (Fig. 12.48) and molluscum contagiosum. The dermoscopic features of eruptive vellus hair cysts include a roundish, light-brown to gray-blue structure centered by blue-gray lines or multiple yellowish globular structureless areas. Patchy brown-yellowish pigmented structures with clear hair are also seen in some lesions. Molluscum contagiosum appears as a white-yellow amorphous area and crown-like vessels under dermoscopy (see related chapters).

12.2.4 Lupus Miliaris Disseminatus Faciei

LMDF is an uncommon chronic inflammatory disease of unknown etiology that has been considered to be a form of a tuberculid in the past. However, a purified protein derivative (PPD) test is negative in LMDF. Therefore, the disease is considered to be irrelevant to tuberculosis. LMDF typically manifests as roundish red to brown papules or nodules on the face, particularly around the eyelids and nose, which leave atrophic scars after healing.

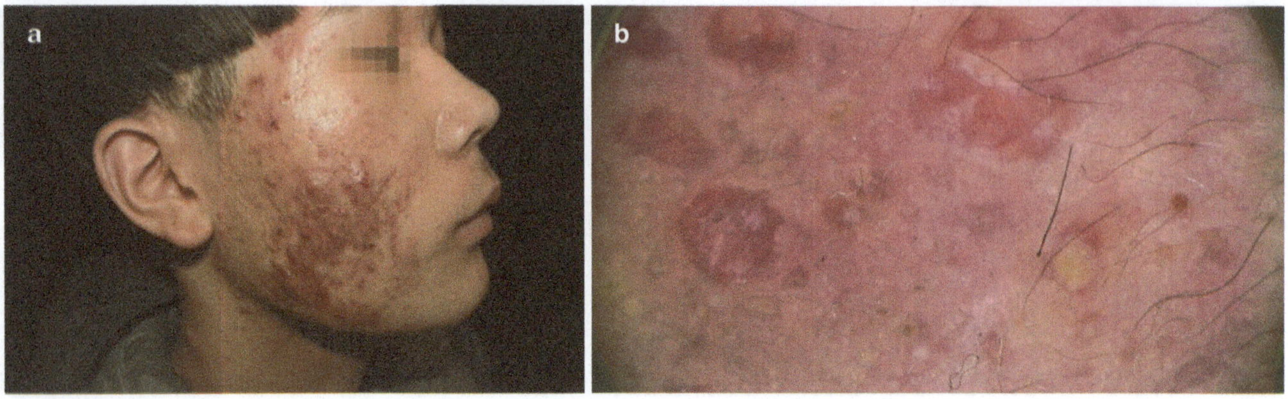

Fig. 12.46 Inflammatory acne. (**a**). Facial inflammatory papules, pustules, nodules, cysts, and focal scar formation. (**b**). Dermoscopy shows a well-demarcated yellow-whitish round structure in the center with a fine brown linear boundary surrounded by an erythematous halo. Follicular plugs and branched vessels can also be seen (×20)

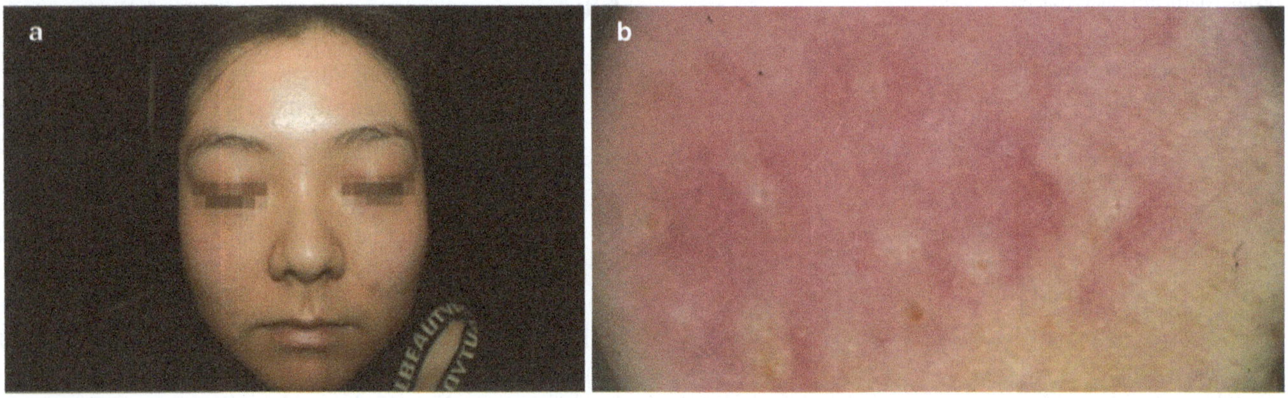

Fig. 12.47 Comedonal acne. (**a**). Multiple comedones on the face. (**b**). Multiple brownish-yellowish follicular plugs and scattered inflammatory erythema (×20)

The dermoscopic features of LMDF are as follows (Fig. 12.49):

1. Orange-yellow/erythematous background
2. Targetoid follicular plugs
3. Radial arrangement of hairpin-like and linear vessels

12.2.5 Granuloma Faciale

Granuloma faciale is a facial chronic inflammatory disorder of unknown etiology that often presents as facial infiltrative nodules or plaques with no ruptures or crusts. Histological examination of granuloma faciale shows the infiltration of a large number of neutrophils and eosinophils as well as leukocytoclastic vasculitis in the early stage.

The dermoscopic features of granuloma faciale are as follows (Fig. 12.50):

1. Dilated follicular openings.
2. Linear/linear with branched vessels.
3. Pinkish background.
4. Less common findings include whitish perifollicular halos, shiny white streaks, follicular plugs, and pigmented structures.

12.3 Noninfectious Granulomatous Skin Disorders

Sarcoidosis, granuloma annulare, and necrobiosis lipoidica are common granulomatous skin diseases that dermoscopically appear as yellowish or orange-yellowish structureless areas. Dermoscopy can assist clinicians in the diagnosis of the aforementioned granulomatous diseases, but differentiation among them is difficult. Histopathological examination is needed to reach an accurate clinical diagnosis.

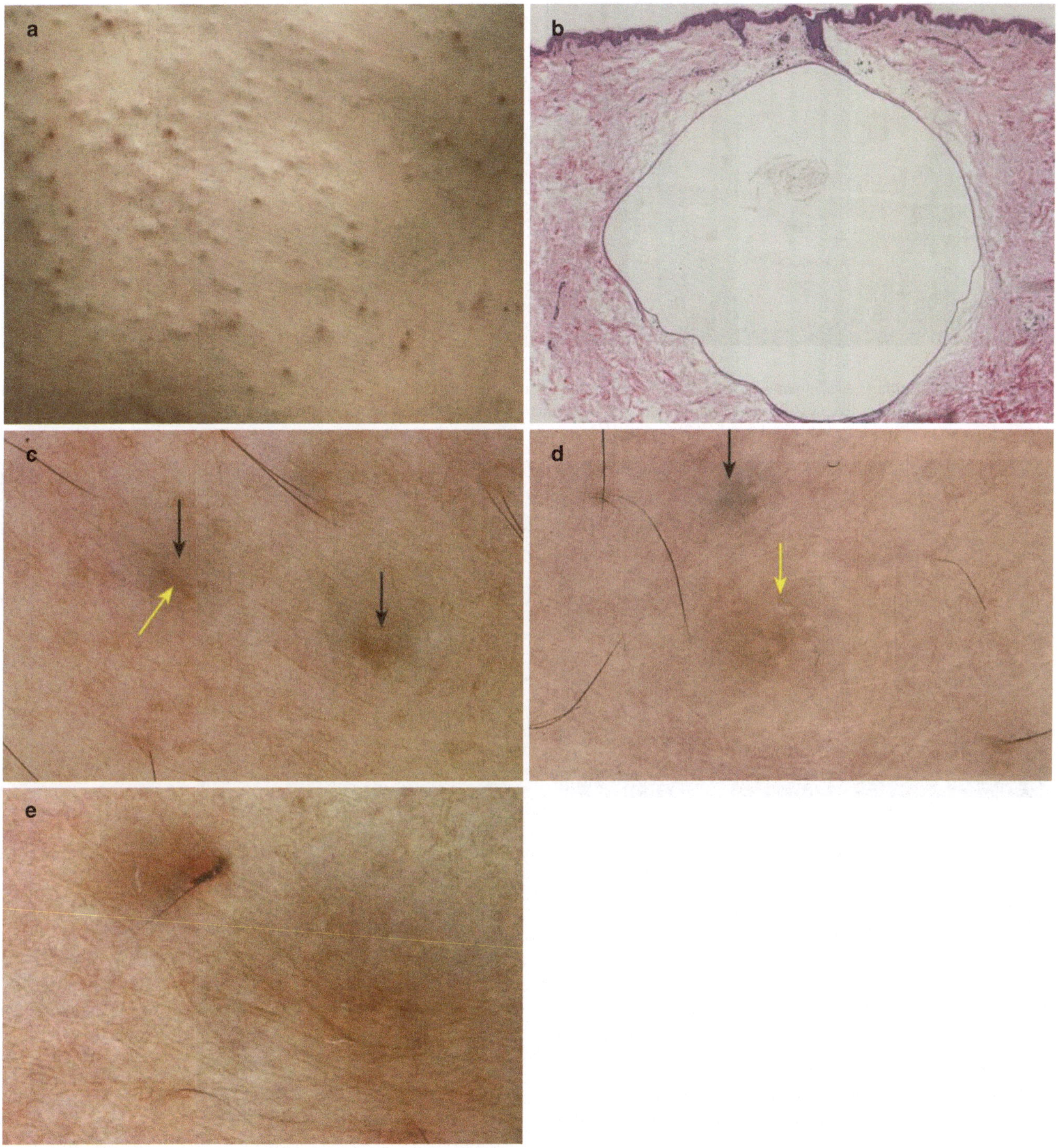

Fig. 12.48 Eruptive vellus hair cysts. (**a**). Multiple skin-colored to yellowish papules and subcutaneous nodules. (**b**). Histopathological examination shows a cyst with stratified squamous epithelial cyst wall and vellus hairs inside in the dermis, corresponding to the diagnosis of eruptive vellus hair cysts (hematoxylin and eosin, ×40). (**c**). Light-brown round structures (black arrow) centered by blue-gray linear pigmentation (yellow arrow) (×50). (**d**). Roundish, light-brown to gray-blue structures (black arrow) centered by multiple yellowish globular structureless areas (yellow arrow) (×50). (**e**). Brown-yellowish pigmented structures with clear hair (×70). The aforementioned dermoscopic features are helpful in the differential diagnosis

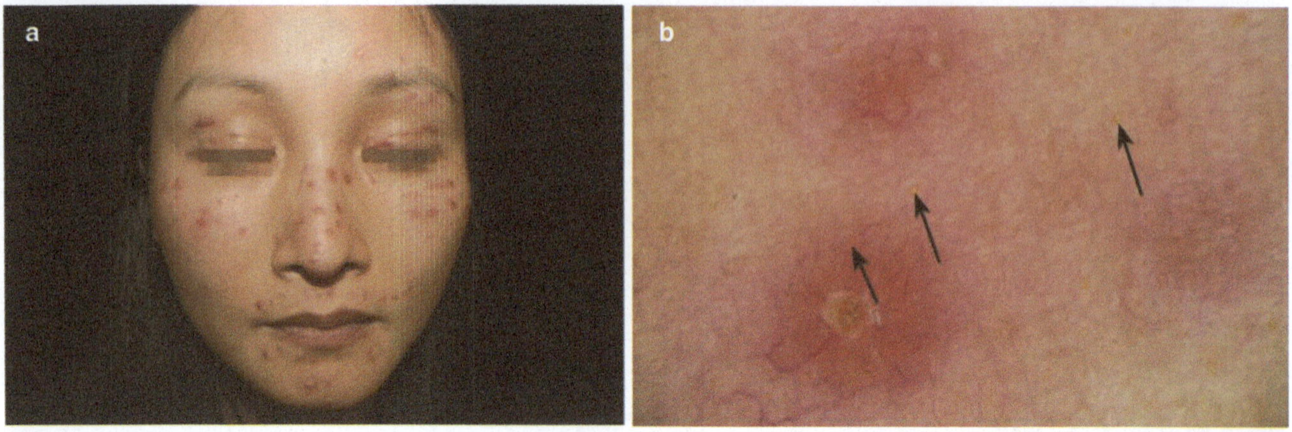

Fig. 12.49 Lupus miliaris disseminatus faciei. (**a**). Red papules and nodules on the face. (**b**). Yellow homogeneous structureless areas surrounded by linear/branched/hairpin-like vessels and targetoid follicular plugs (arrow) on an erythematous background (×50)

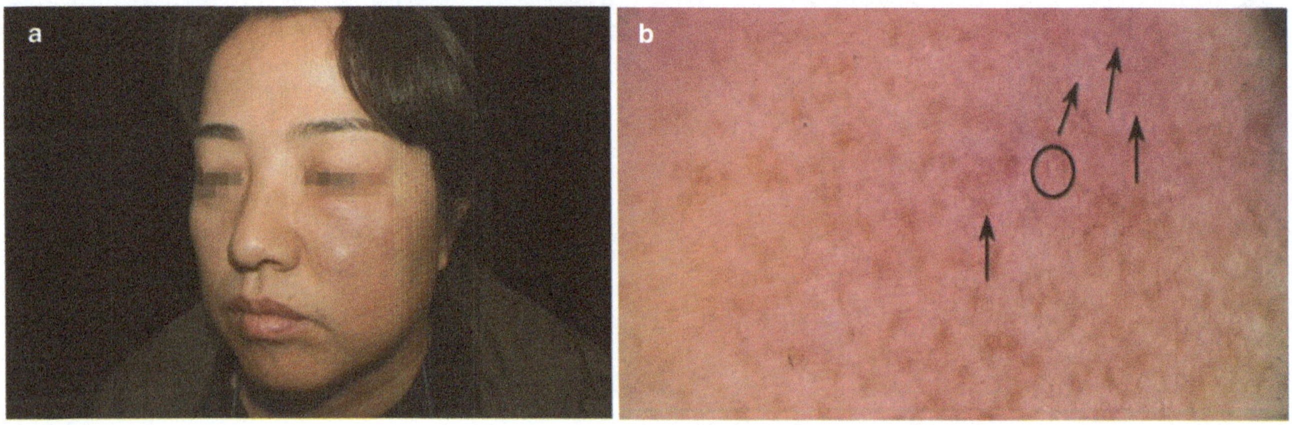

Fig. 12.50 Granuloma faciale. (**a**). Infiltrative edematous plaque on the face. (**b**). Dermoscopy shows dilated follicular openings (arrow) and branched vessels (circle) on a pinkish background. A perifollicular whitish halo and brownish pigmented structures can also be seen (×20)

12.3.1 Sarcoidosis

Sarcoidosis is a systemic granulomatous disease of unknown etiology that involves the skin, lungs, lymph nodes, liver, and kidneys. Severe cases of sarcoidosis can be life-threatening. Since skin lesions may be the initial signs of sarcoidosis, early diagnosis is the predominant factor in prognosis.

The dermoscopic features of sarcoidosis are as follows (Fig. 12.51):

1. Focal orange lobular structureless areas
2. Linear/linear with branches vessels
3. White scaring-like centers in some lesions

Orange structureless areas often indicate granulomatous diseases, such as sarcoidosis, granuloma annulare, lupus vulgaris, and cutaneous leishmaniasis.

Furthermore, dermoscopy can be utilized in the differential diagnosis of sarcoidosis and necrobiosis lipoidica. A pinkish background, orange lobular structures, and white scarring-like centers are more prominent in sarcoidosis than in necrobiosis lipoidica.

12.3.2 Granuloma Annulare

Granuloma annulare is a self-limited dermatosis of uncertain etiology that may be related to diabetes, thyroid diseases, and hematological diseases. The characteristic lesions of granuloma annulare are generalized papules, which may coalesce to form annular plaques.

The dermoscopic features of granuloma annulare (presenting as palisading granuloma histologically) are as follows (Figs. 12.52 and 12.53):

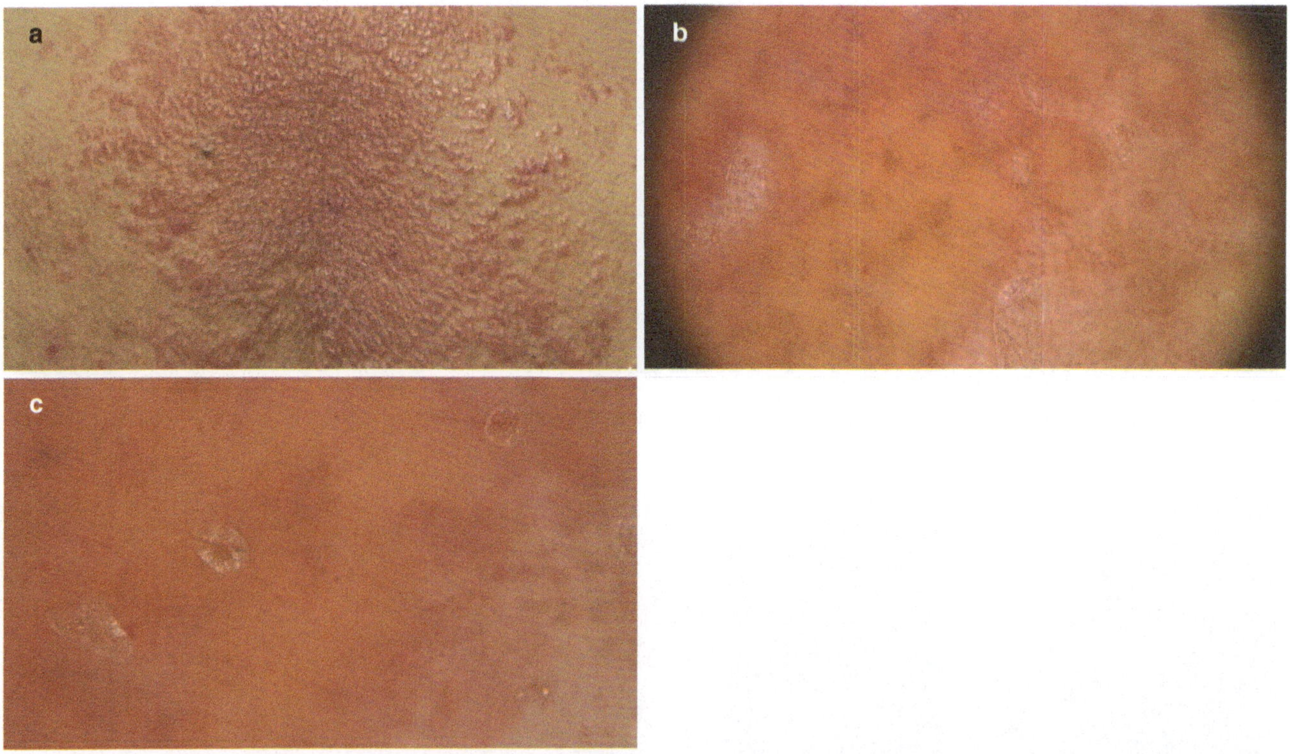

Fig. 12.51 Sarcoidosis. (**a**). Dense yellow-reddish papules on the back, with some coalescing into plaques. (**b**). Focal orange lobular structureless area and peripheral linear vessels (×20). (**c**). Orange structureless area, with linear and branched vessels distributed on/around the area (×50)

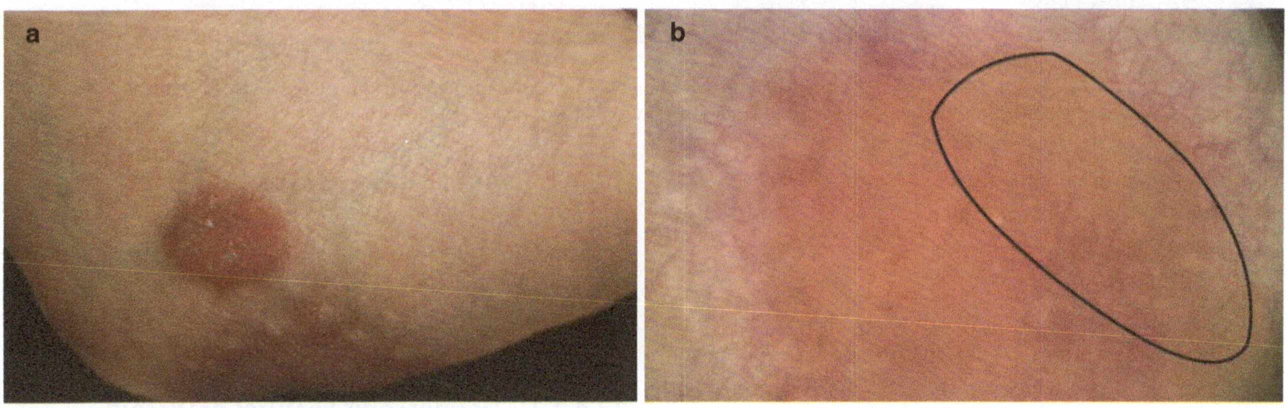

Fig. 12.52 Granuloma annulare. (**a**). Annular dull-red plaques on the trunk. (**b**). Orange structureless area (circle) and peripheral arrangement of linear/branched vessels on a pinkish-red background (×20)

1. Orange structureless areas
2. Red-whitish/pinkish/reddish/whitish/yellow-whitish background
3. Dotted/linear/branched vessels
4. Pigmented structures

12.3.3 Necrobiosis Lipoidica

Necrobiosis lipoidica often presents as pretibial sclerotic yellow-reddish plaques with ulceration or scarring sometimes. Necrobiosis lipoidica most commonly occurs in diabetic patients, and chronic lesions may result in secondary squamous cell carcinoma.

The dermoscopic features of necrobiosis lipoidica are as follows (Fig. 12.54):

1. Multimorphological vascular structures according to disease stages. Dotted and comma-shaped vessels are more common in early stages, while reticular and hairpin-like vessels are more frequent in more developed (mature) lesions and branched or serpentine vessels are more common in advanced lesions.
2. Orange-yellowish/pink-whitish background.

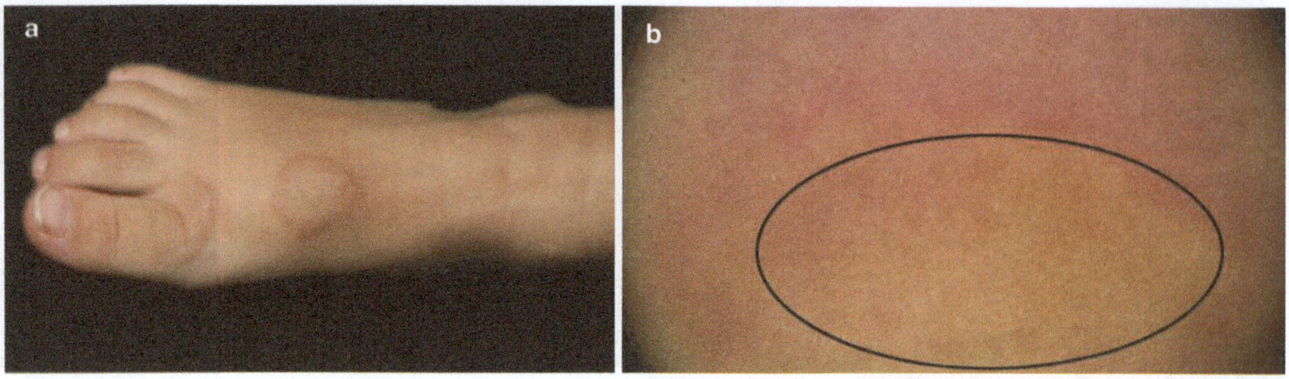

Fig. 12.53 Granuloma annulare. (**a**). A coin-sized plaque with peripheral annular rim on the dorsal foot. (**b**). Orange structureless area (circle) on a pinkish-red background (×20)

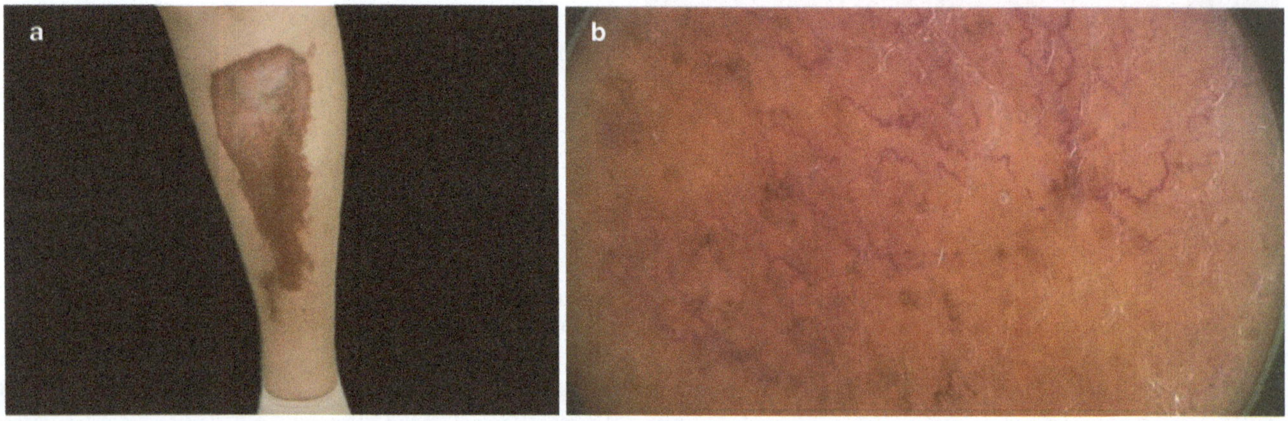

Fig. 12.54 Necrobiosis lipoidica (advanced lesion). (**a**). Pretibial yellow-brownish atrophic telangiectatic plaques. (**b**). Prominent branched vessels and scattered honeycomb pigmentation network on an orange-yellowish background (×20)

3. Orange-yellowish structureless areas.
4. Additional findings include ulceration and yellow crusts.

The key point of differentiation between necrobiosis lipoidica and sarcoidosis is that the former has more prominent telangiectasia, which often forms linear vessels with branches, while the latter presents as scattered linear vessels or branched vessels. Granuloma annulare presents fewer branched vessels than necrobiosis lipoidica.

12.4 Connective Tissue Diseases

Connective tissue diseases are a group of heterogenetic and overlapping diseases caused by multiple factors, including lupus erythematous, dermatomyositis, rheumatoid arthritis, and scleroderma. Among these, the dermoscopic features of lupus erythematous and morphea have been reported.

12.4.1 Lupus Erythematosus

Lupus erythematosus (LE) is a spectrum of autoimmune diseases, including discoid LE (DLE), subacute cutaneous LE, systemic LE, and LE profundus, among which the dermoscopic features of DLE have been most reported.

12.4.1.1 Dermoscopic Features of Discoid Lupus Erythematosus and Their Correlations with Histopathological Findings

1. **The dermoscopic features of early lesions are as follows** (Figs. 12.55, 12.56, and 12.57):
   (a) Follicular red dots (corresponding to perifollicular telangiectasis, evacuation of erythrocytes, and infiltration of inflammatory cells histopathologically)
   (b) Perifollicular whitish halos (Corresponding to perifollicular fibrosis)
   (c) Follicular keratotic plugs
   (d) Dotted/branched/linear curved vessels
   (e) White scales

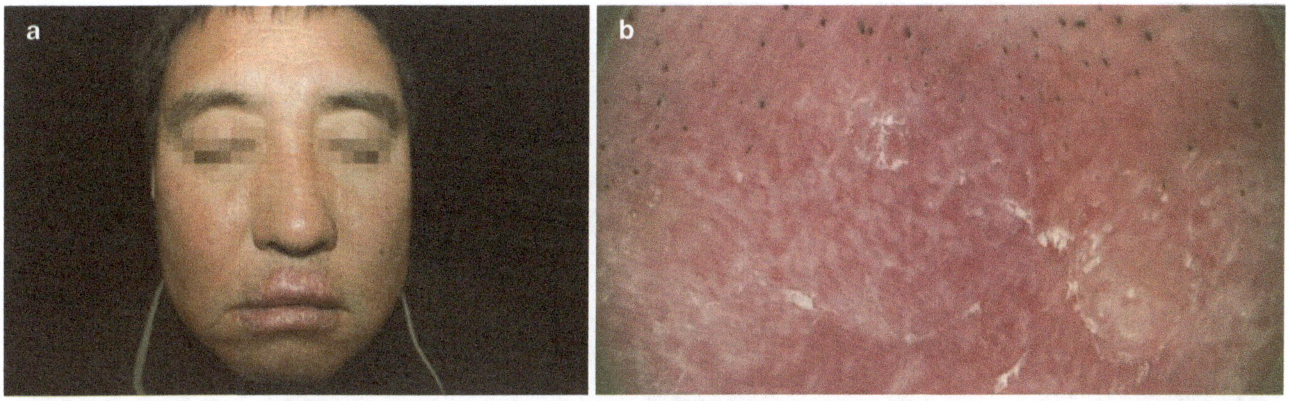

Fig. 12.55 Discoid lupus erythematosus. (**a**). A discoid plaque with scales on the lip. (**b**). Dotted/linear curved vessels with follicular keratotic plugs, perifollicular halos, and white scales (×20)

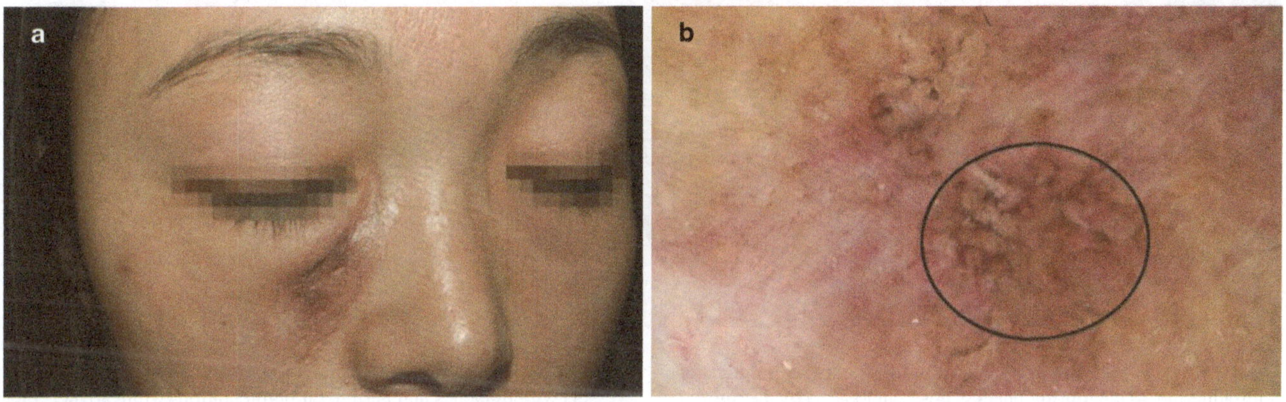

Fig. 12.56 Discoid lupus erythematosus. (**a**). Dull-red atrophic patches on the right cheek. (**b**). Linear branched vessels with follicular keratotic plugs, whitish perifollicular halos, honeycomb networks (circle), and whitish structureless areas (×30)

2. **The dermoscopic features of long-lasting lesions are as follows:**

   (a) Linear vessels with branches
   (b) Whitish structureless areas (corresponding to diffuse fibrosis in the dermis histologically)
   (c) Hyperpigmentation (honeycomb network/blue-gray pigment dots, corresponding to pigmentary incontinence)
   (d) Blue-white structures on the scalp lesions (related to pigmentary incontinence)

Dermoscopy can be utilized in the differential diagnosis of DLE and actinic keratosis. DLE presents as follicular red dots, follicular keratotic plugs, and perifollicular whitish halos on a whitish background ("inverse strawberry pattern"), whereas actinic keratosis presents the "strawberry pattern."

12.4.1.2 Dermoscopic Features of Subacute Cutaneous Lupus Erythematosus

1. Pink-whitish background.
2. Diffusely or peripherally distributed white scales.
3. At least two among dotted, linear, branched, and linear curved vessels exist.
4. Focally distributed orange-yellowish structureless areas can occasionally be seen.

12.4.2 Morphea and Lichen Sclerosus

Morphea, also called localized scleroderma, classically presents as an erythematous, edematous plaque in the inflammatory phase that develops into wax-colored sclerosis in the sclerotic phase. These lesions often appear on the head, neck, and extremities without systemic involvement. Lichen sclerosus is a chronic inflammatory disorder of unknown etiology that can affect any part of the body, especially the anogenital region. Lichen sclerosus can be divided into anogenital and extragenital types according to the areas involved. Since differentiation between morphea and lichen sclerosus is sometimes clinically difficult, histological and dermoscopic examinations should be combined to confirm the

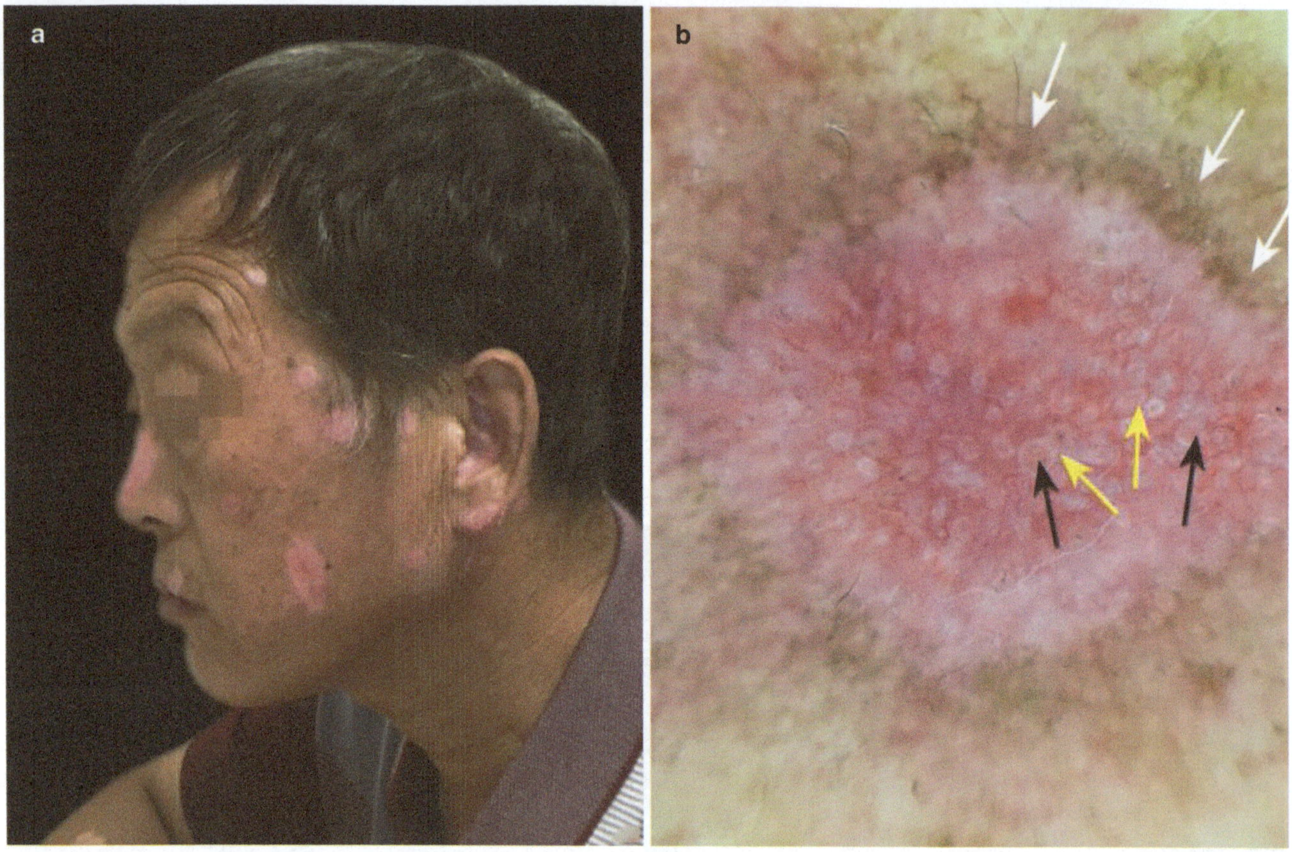

Fig. 12.57 Discoid lupus erythematosus. (**a**). Pinkish atrophic patches with adhering scales on the cheeks, nose, and ears. (**b**). Dermoscopy shows follicular red dots and follicular keratotic plugs (black arrow) surrounded by perifollicular whitish halos (yellow arrow) on a whitish background, forming the so-called inverse strawberry pattern. Linear vessels with branches and peripheral pigmentation (white arrow) could also be seen (×30)

Table 12.7 Comparison of dermoscopic features between extragenital lichen sclerosus and morphea

Dermoscopic features	Lichen sclerosus	Morphea
White-yellow structureless areas	+++	–
White clouds	–	+++
Purpuric spots	+	–
Vascular patterns	++	++
Pigmented structures	++	++
Follicular plugs	++	+
Comedo-like openings	++	+

diagnosis. Consequently, the two entities are listed together in this section (Table 12.7).

12.4.2.1 Dermoscopic Features of Localized Scleroderma (Morphea) (Fig. 12.58)

1. White clouds, previously known as white fiber bundles, histologically corresponding to fibrosis in the dermis
2. Linear/linear with branches vessels
3. Comedo-like openings and follicular keratotic plugs
4. Pigmented structures.

12.4.2.2 Dermoscopic Features of Lichen Sclerosus

1. The dermoscopic features of anogenital lichen sclerosus (Fig. 12.59) are as follows:
   (a) Common features
   - White-yellow structureless areas
   - Brown/gray-blue pigmented structures/pepper-like structures
   - Main linear vessels, or less commonly, irregularly distributed linear curved/branched vessels

   (b) Uncommon features
   - Shiny white streaks/crystalline structures
   - Purpuric spots/patches
   - Rosettes
   - Comedo-like openings, follicular keratotic plugs
2. The dermoscopic features of extragenital lichen sclerosus are as follows (Fig. 12.60):
   (a) White-yellow structureless areas
   (b) Comedo-like openings
   (c) Follicular keratotic plugs
   (d) Shiny white streaks

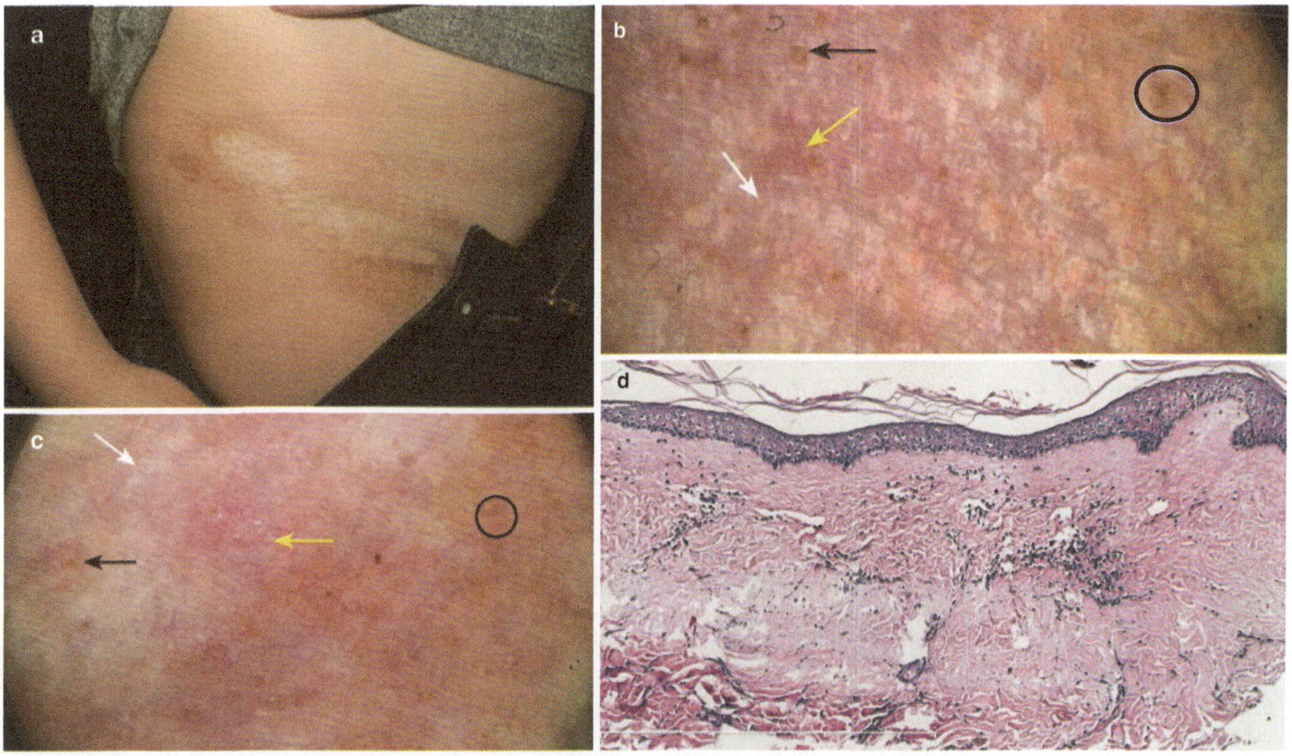

Fig. 12.58 Morphea. (**a**). Linear sclerotic atrophic plaque with hypopigmentation on the right groin. (**b**). White clouds (white arrow), branched vessels (yellow arrow), comedo-like openings (black arrow), and peripheral patchy brownish pigmentation (black circle) (×20). (**c**). White clouds (white arrow), branching vessels (yellow arrow), follicular keratotic plugs (black arrow), and brownish pigmentation (black circle) (×20). (**d**). Histopathological examination shows epidermal atrophy, basal cell vacuolar degeneration, collagen fiber thickening and sclerosis in the mid-dermis, a reduced number of adnexal structures, and the infiltration of sparse lymphocytes around the vessels and among collagen fibers (hematoxylin and eosin, ×40)

(e) Linear/dotted/branched vessels
(f) Brown/gray-blue pigmented structures

12.5 Cutaneous Vasculitis

Vasculitis encompasses a group of special conditions characterized by blood vessel wall inflammation. According to the size of the affected blood vessel, these conditions are divided into cutaneous small-vessel vasculitis (such as Henoch–Schonlein purpura, urticaria vasculitis, and erythema elevatum diutinum), small- to medium-vessel vasculitis (such as ANCA-associated small-vessel vasculitis), medium-vessel vasculitis (such as polyarteritis nodosa), and large-vessel vasculitis. Cutaneous small-vessel vasculitis mainly presents as palpable purpuric macules and papules and sometimes manifests as urticarial plaques, hemorrhagic vesicles/blisters, necrotic areas, or erythema-multiforme-like lesions. However, purpura is not a specific feature of vasculitis. Any disease that histologically causes blood vessel wall inflammation and extravasated erythrocytes can reveal purpura. The final diagnosis of cutaneous vasculitis requires histopathological examinations. Dermoscopy can help in the clinical diagnosis and differentiation and assist in biopsy positioning.

12.5.1 Dermoscopic Patterns of Purpuric Lesions

1. Homogeneous pattern

   The homogenous pattern presents as a diffuse homogenous structureless purpuric area, commonly seen in non-inflammatory purpuric disorders, such as those with a hemorrhagic tendency (warfarin overdosage) and an abnormal vascular wall or extravascular matrix (purpura senilis and steroid purpura).
2. Mottled/speckled pattern

   Violaceous blurred purpuric spots/blotches or well-demarcated purpuric globules on a purple or orange back-

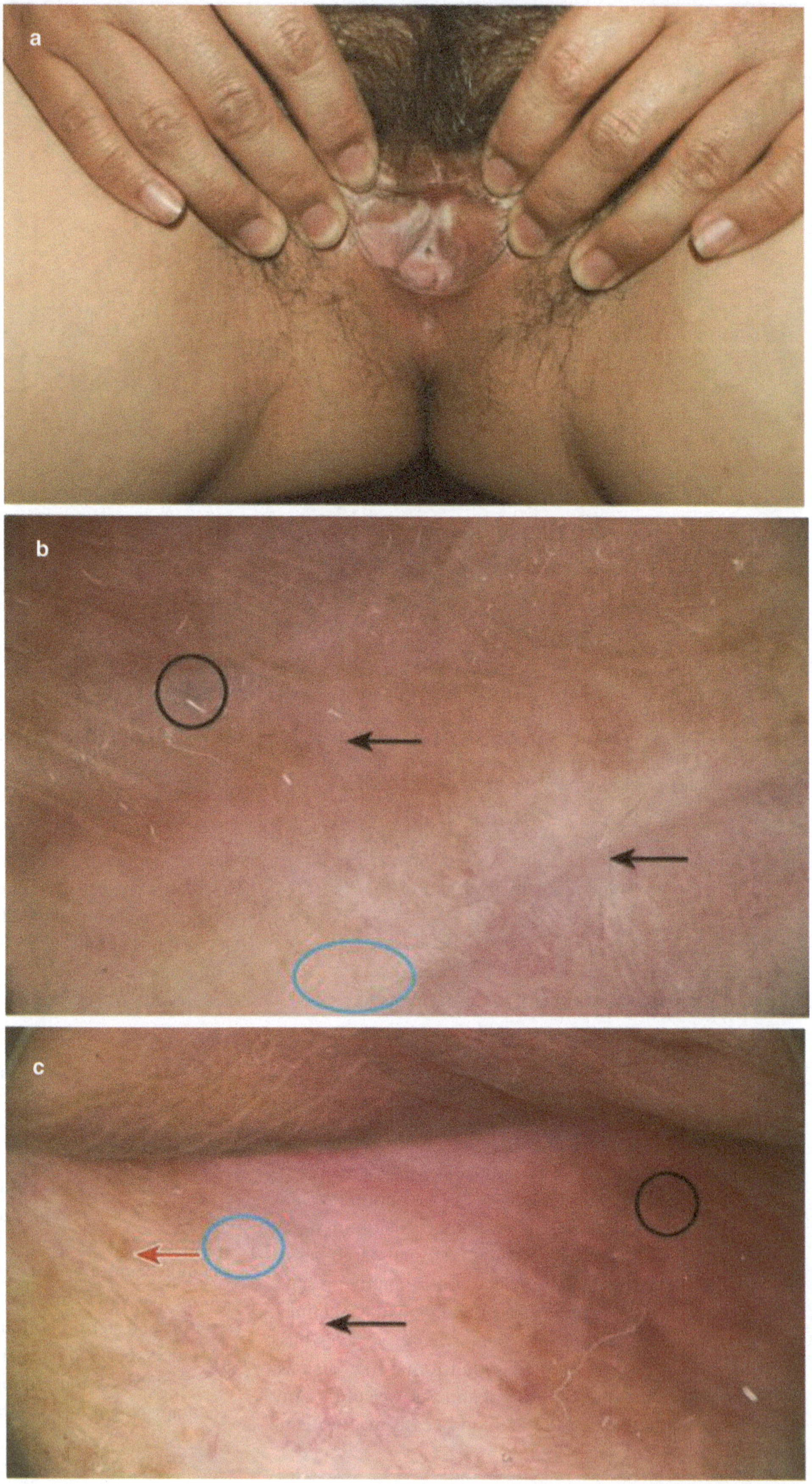

Fig. 12.59 Vulvar lichen sclerosus. (**a**). White sclerotic patches on the vulva with labia major and labia minor atrophy. (**b**). Irregularly distributed linear/dotted/linear curved vessels (black arrow), white-yellow structureless areas (blue circle), and purpuric spots/patches (black circle) (×20). (**c**). Irregularly distributed branched vessels (black arrow), white-yellow structureless areas (blue circle), blue-gray patchy pigmented structures (red arrow), and purpuric patches (black circle) (×20). (**d**). White-yellow structureless areas (blue circle), purpuric patches (black circle), and follicular keratotic plugs (yellow arrow) (×30). (**e**). Shiny white streaks (white arrow), brown patchy pigmented structures (red arrow), rosettes (white circle), and follicular keratotic plugs (yellow arrow) (×30). (**f**). Irregularly distributed dotted/branched vessels (black arrow), purpuric spots/patches (black circle), white-yellow structureless areas (blue circle), brown patchy pigmented structures (red arrow), and shiny white streaks (white arrow) (×20). (**g**). White-yellow structureless areas (blue circle), purpuric spots/patches (black circle), brown patchy pigmented structures (red arrow), rosettes (white circle), and shiny white streaks (white arrow) (×30). (**h**). White-yellow structureless areas (blue circle), purpuric spots/patches (black circle), shiny white streaks (white arrow), and comedo-like openings (yellow arrow) (×20). (**i**). Irregularly distributed dotted/branched vessels (black arrow), blue-gray/brown patchy pigmented structures (red arrow), and shiny white streaks (white arrow) (×20)

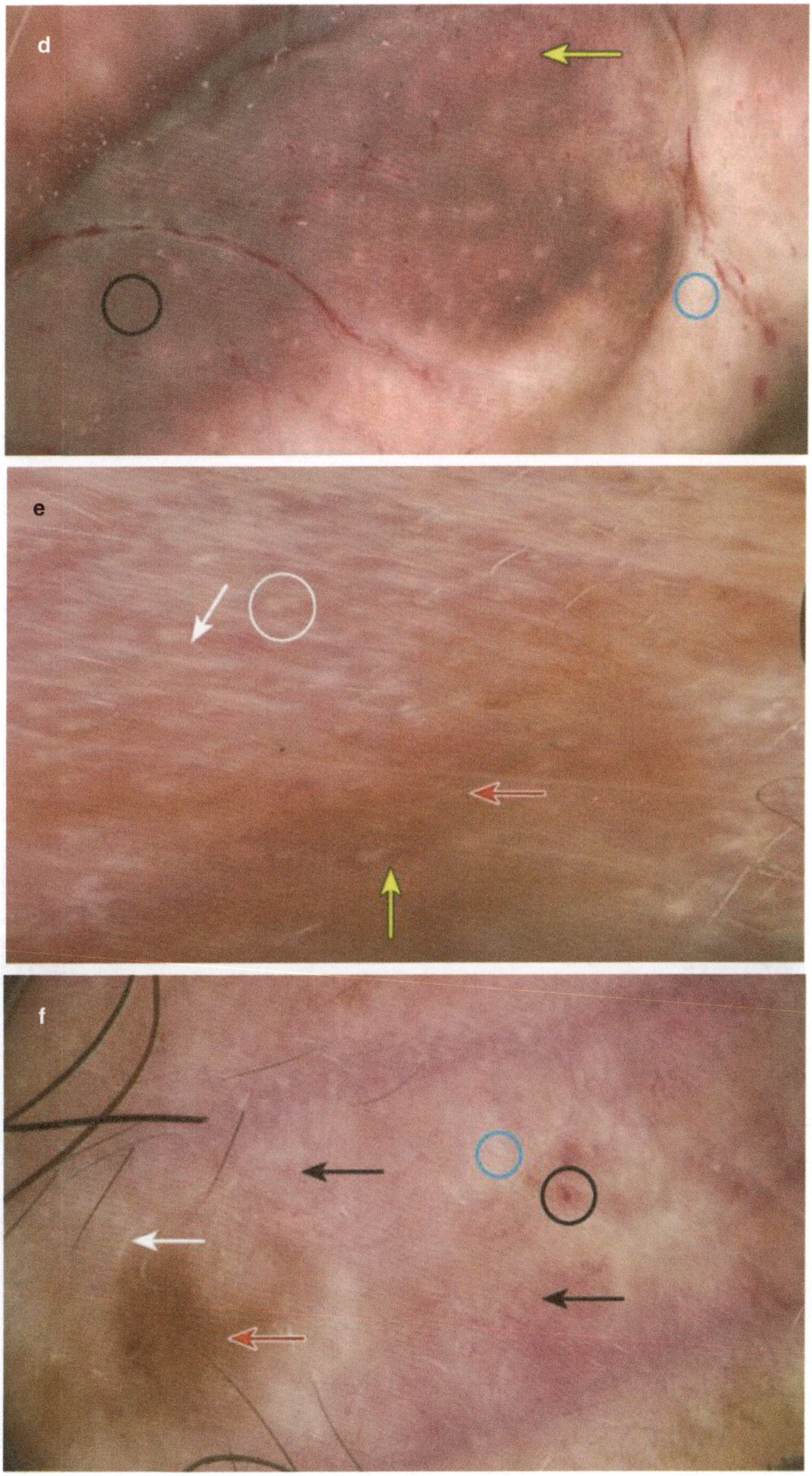

Fig. 12.59 (continued)

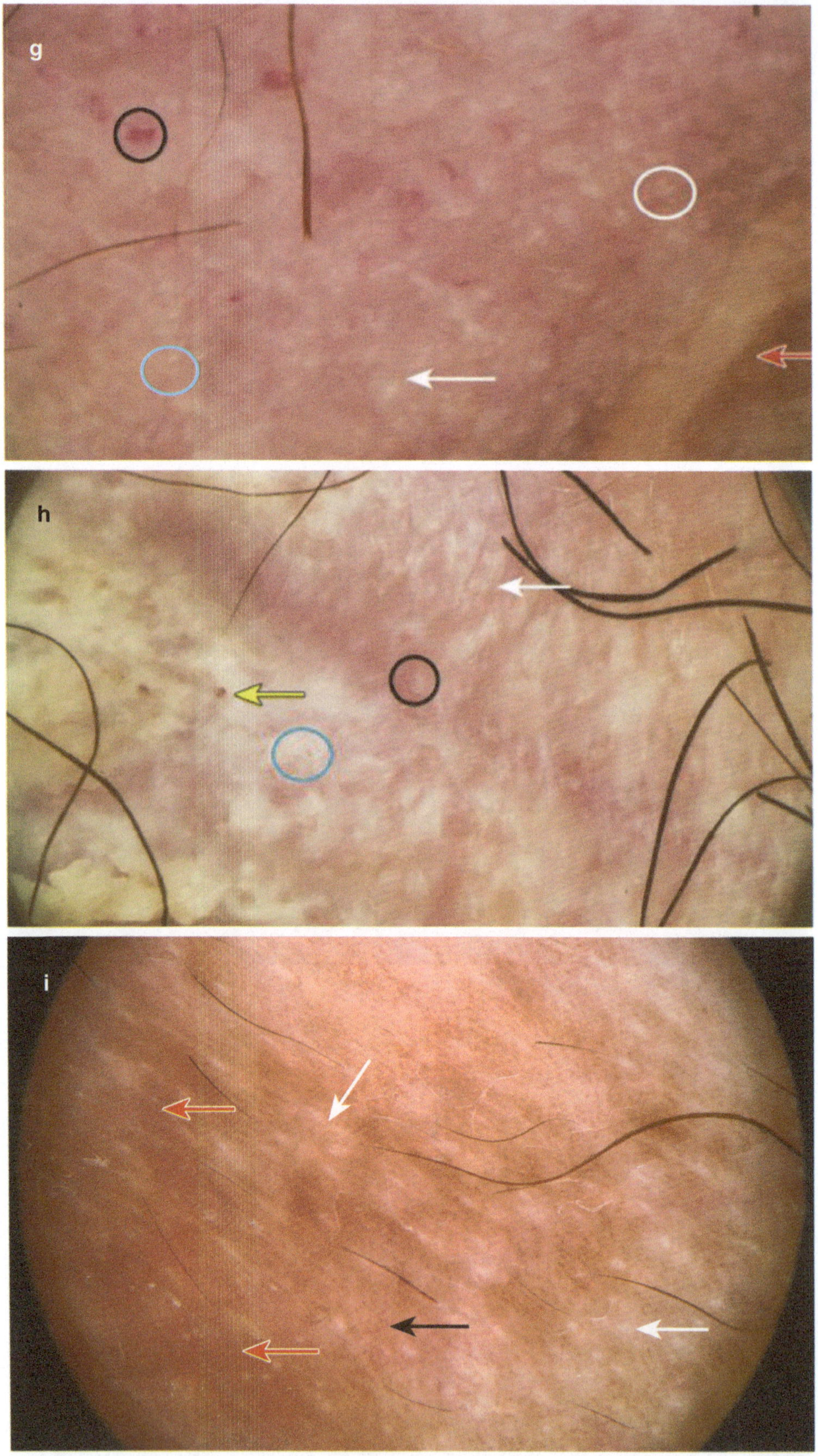

Fig. 12.59 (continued)

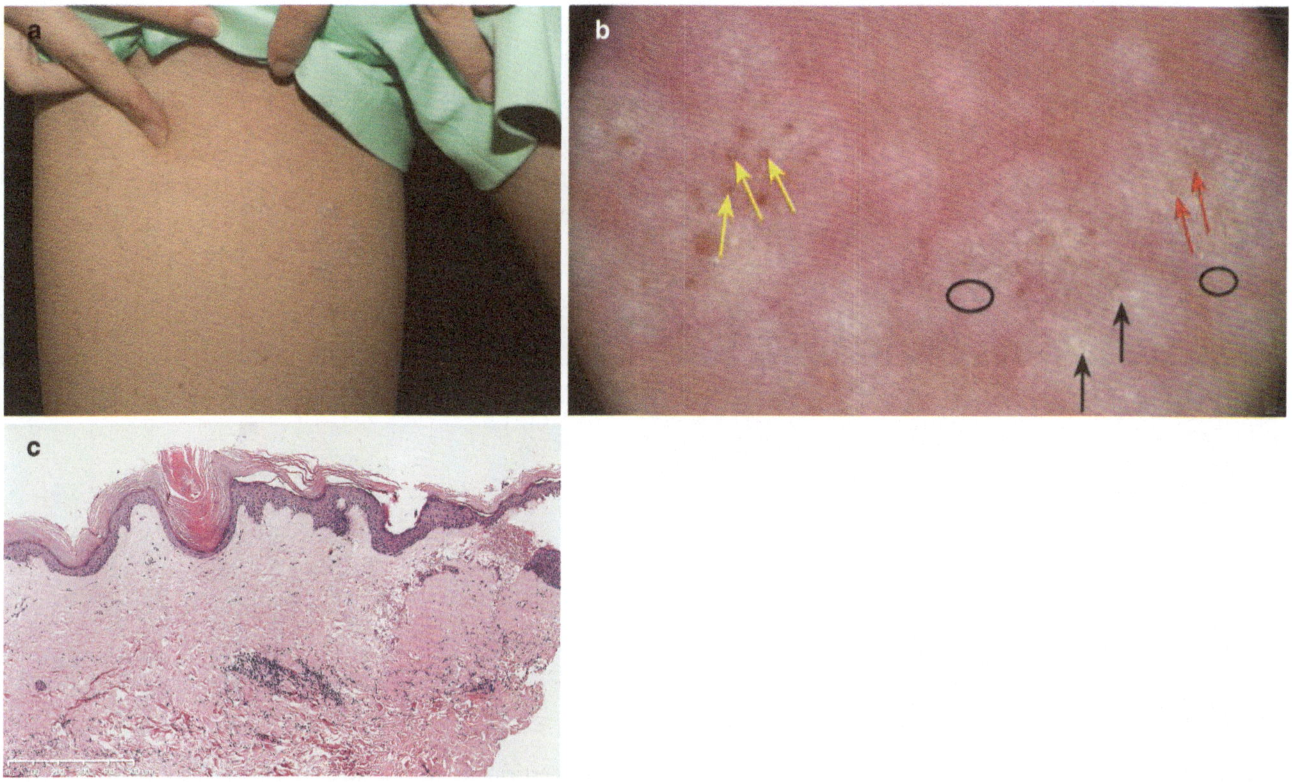

Fig. 12.60 Extragenital lichen sclerosus. (**a**). Multiple punctate atrophic white patches on the right leg. (**b**). White-yellow structureless areas (black circle), comedo-like openings (yellow arrow), follicular keratotic plugs (red arrow), shiny white streaks (circle), and sparse linear vessels (×20). (**c**). Histopathological examination shows hyperkeratosis, follicular plugs, and basal cell liquefaction degeneration. The homogenization of superficial dermis and sparse infiltration of lymphocytes among collagens can also be seen (hematoxylin and eosin, ×40)

ground*, commonly seen in leukocytoclastic vasculitis, such as Henoch–Schonlein purpura and pigmented purpuric dermatosis.

3. Perifollicular pattern

   The perifollicular pattern presents as a perifollicular purpuric halo, some concurring with spiral hair and follicular keratotic plugs, which can be seen in scurvy.

*A purple background reveals extravasated erythrocytes in the dermis, while an orange background is due to dermal hemosiderin deposition.

12.5.2 Henoch–Schonlein Purpura

The dermoscopic features of Henoch–Schonlein purpura are as follows (Fig. 12.61):

1. Reddish/purple background
2. Multiple purpuric dots
3. Purpuric globules
4. Dotted/linear/branched vessels

12.5.3 Pigmented Purpuric Dermatosis

12.5.3.1 All Subtypes of Pigmented Purpuric Dermatosis Are Dermoscopically Alike

The dermoscopic features of pigmented purpuric dermatosis are as follows (Figs. 12.62, 12.63, and 12.64):

1. Purpuric dots or globules
2. Dark-brown/coppery-red background
3. Other features, including dotted/linear/branched vessels, brown dots, and globules, a brown pigment network, and blue-gray dots.

12.5.3.2 Dermoscopy in the Differential Diagnosis of Lichen Aureus and Nummular Eczema (Fig. 12.65) (Table 12.8)

1. Lichen aureus presents as purpuric dots, blue-gray dots, and a brown pigment network on a copper-red background.
2. Nummular eczema presents as shiny yellow clods, scales, and blood crusts.

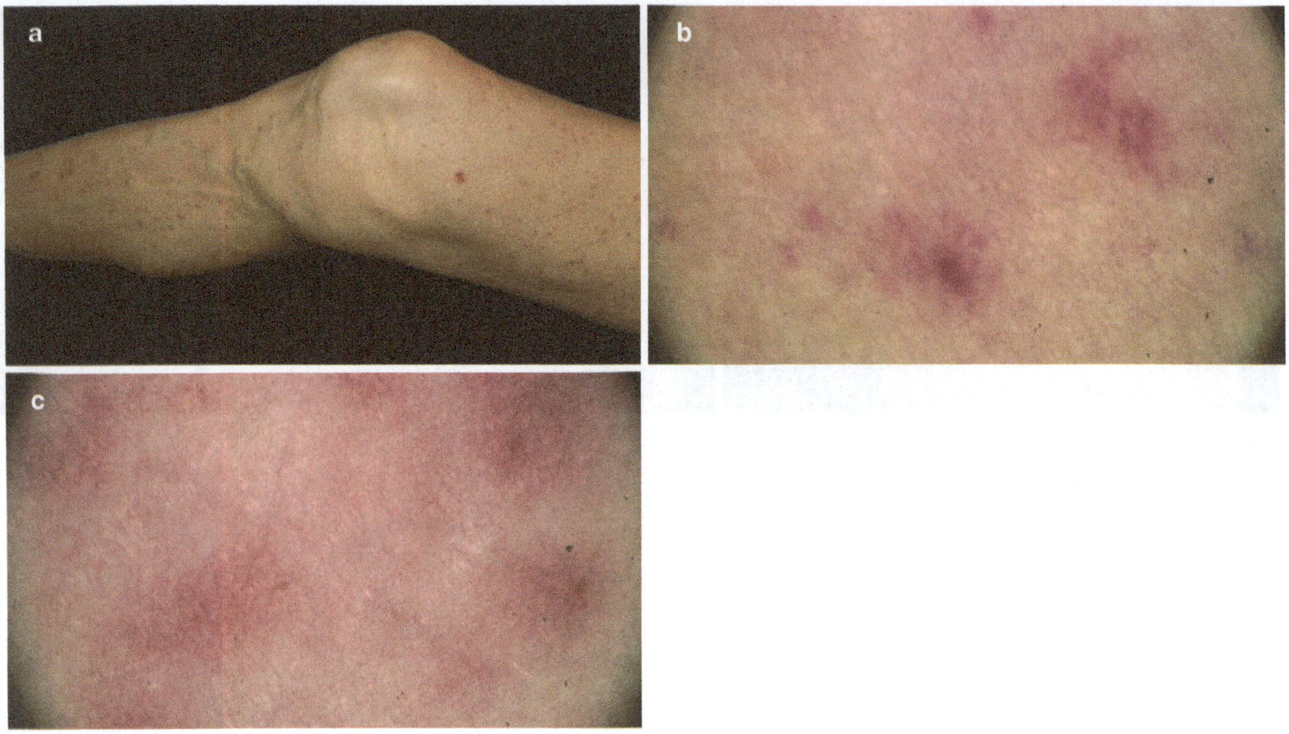

Fig. 12.61 Henoch–Schonlein purpura. (**a**). Sparse palpable purpura on the lower extremities. (**b**). Violaceous blurred purpuric spots on a purple-reddish background (×20). (**c**). Dotted/linear/branched vessels on a purple-reddish background (×20)

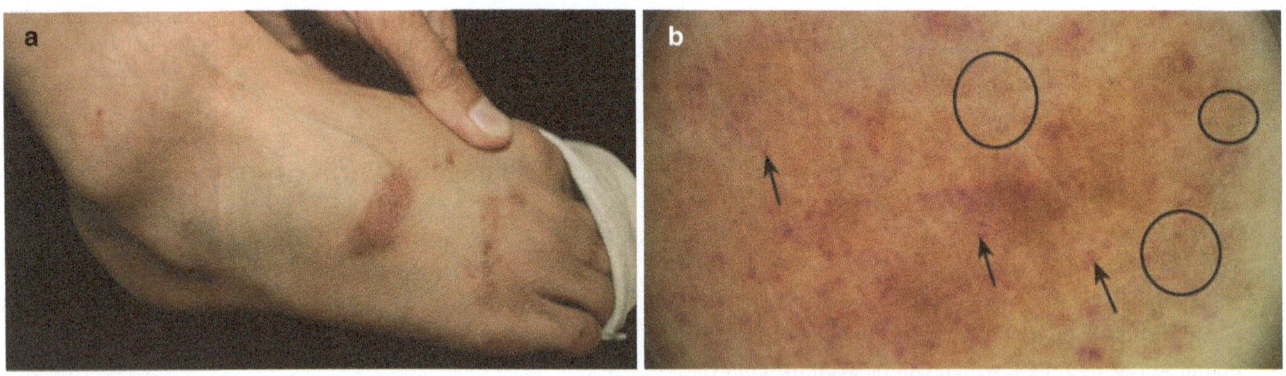

Fig. 12.62 Pigmented purpuric dermatosis. (**a**). Brown-red purpuric macules on the right dorsal foot and ankle. (**b**). Multiple purpuric dots (arrow), blurred linear vessels, and brown pigment networks (circle) on a copper-red/brown background (×20)

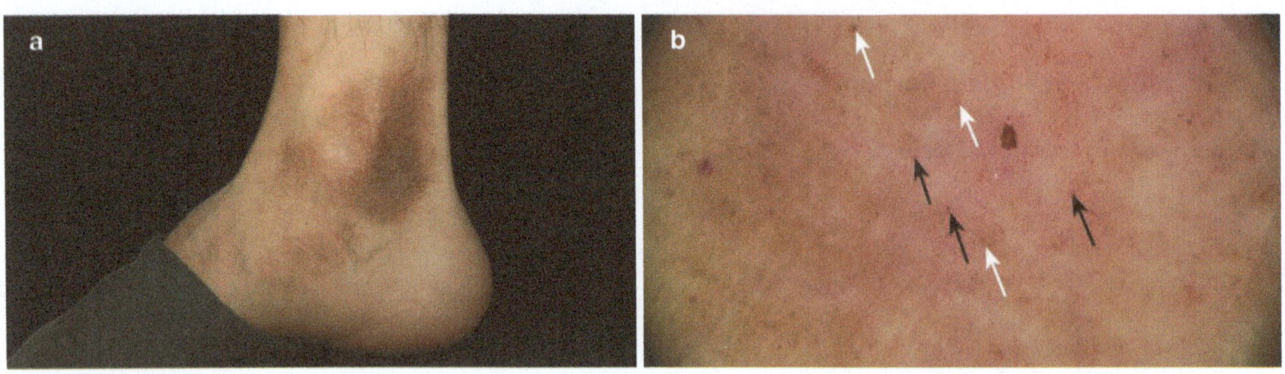

Fig. 12.63 Pigmented purpuric dermatosis. (**a**). Rusty lichenoid purpuric patches on the right ankle. (**b**). Multiple purpuric dots/globules (black arrow), dotted/short linear vessels, and brown dots/globules (white arrow) with hemorrhagic crusts on a brown background (×20)

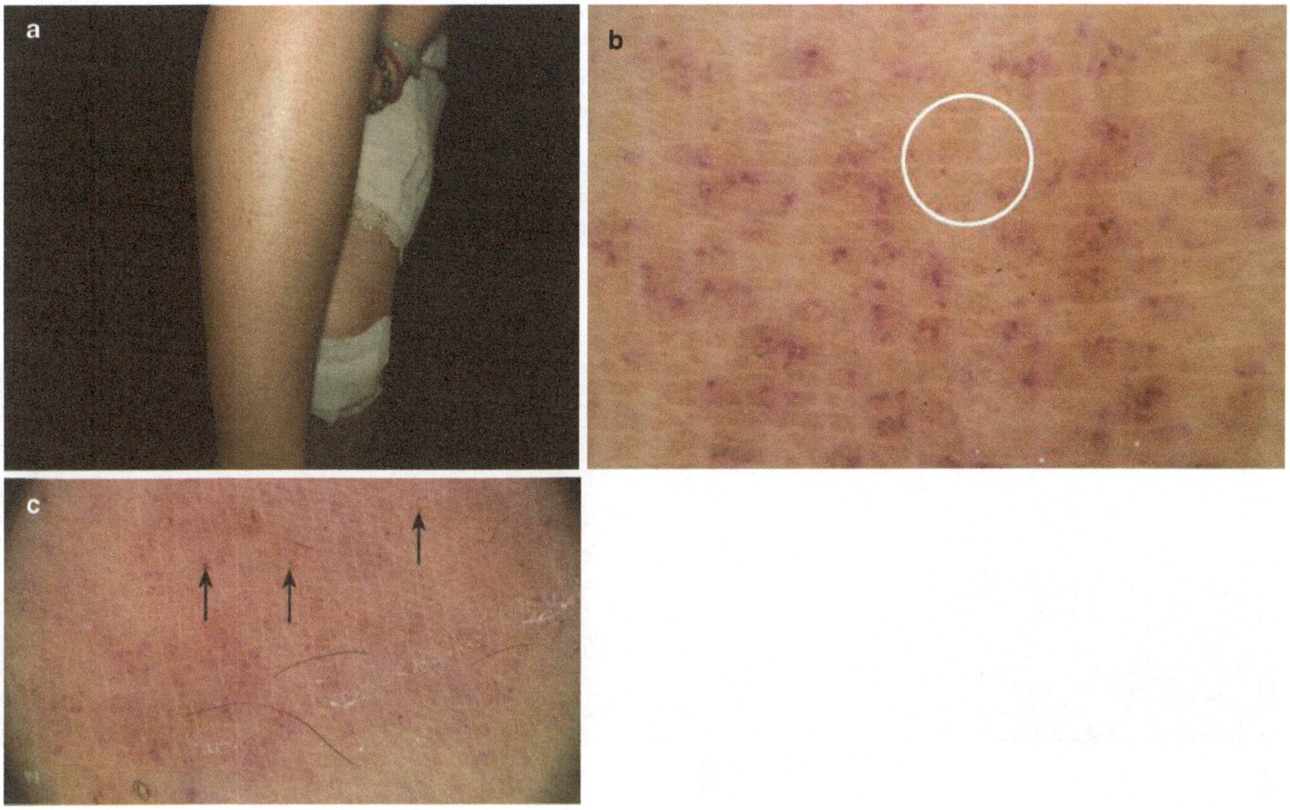

Fig. 12.64 Pigmented purpuric dermatosis. (**a**). Brown-red palpable purpuric papules on the lower extremities. (**b**). Purpuric dots/globules and prominent brown pigment networks (circle) on a brown background (×20). (**c**). Purpuric dots and many brown dots (arrow) on a brown background (×20)

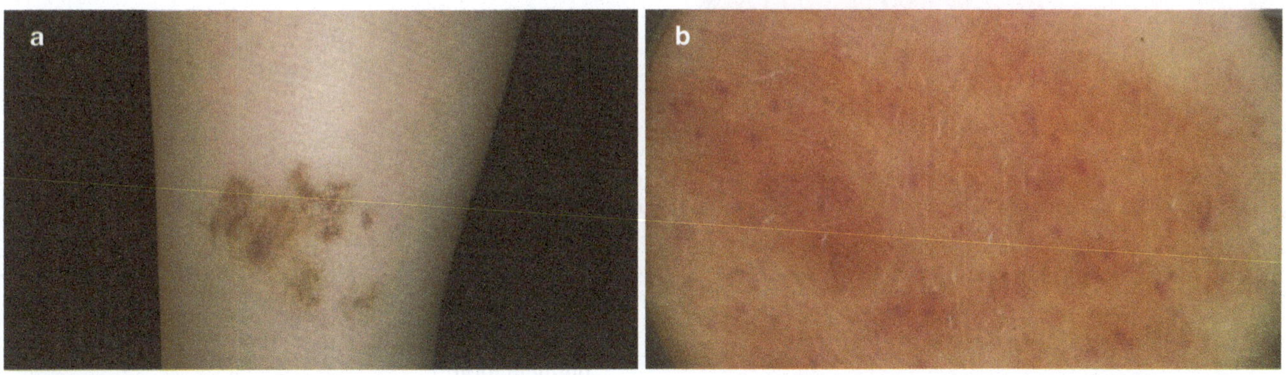

Fig. 12.65 Lichen aureus. (**a**). Yellow macules and brown-red purpuric papules on the right leg. (**b**). Purpuric dots/globules and a brown pigment network on a copper-red background (×20)

12.5.4 Urticarial Vasculitis

The dermoscopic features of urticarial vasculitis are as follows (Fig. 12.66):

1. Orange-brown background
2. Purpuric dots/globules
3. Blue-gray dots
4. Dotted/linear/branched vessels

Notably, purpuric dots or globules in urticarial vasculitis are less frequent in early lesions than in late lesions. Additionally, purpuric dots or globules are less frequent in urticarial vasculitis than in Henoch–Schonlein purpura and pigmented purpuric dermatosis. However, these features are highly indicative of urticarial vasculitis, enabling its discrimination from common urticaria, which lacks purpuric dots/globules and presents as linear vessels and reddish structureless avascular areas. Linear vessels are due to an ectatic subpapillary vascular plexus. Erythematous structureless areas are due to dermal edema. Notably, blue-gray blotches have been reported to be a helpful dermoscopic finding in aiding biopsy positioning for vasculitis.

Table 12.8 Comparison of dermoscopic features between lichen aureus and nummular eczema

Dermoscopic features	Lichen aureus	Nummular eczema
Dark-brown/copper-red background	+++	–
Purpuric dots	+++	–
Pigmented structures (gray dots/brown pigment network)	+++	–
Scales	–	+++
Shiny yellow clods	–	+++
Blood crusts	–	+++

Table 12.9 Comparison of dermoscopic features between lichenoid amyloidosis and macular amyloidosis

Dermoscopic features	Lichenoid amyloidosis	Macular amyloidosis
Central hub	+++	+++ no scarlike area
Pigmented structures	+++	+++
Shiny white streaks	+	–
Hemorrhagic spots	++	–

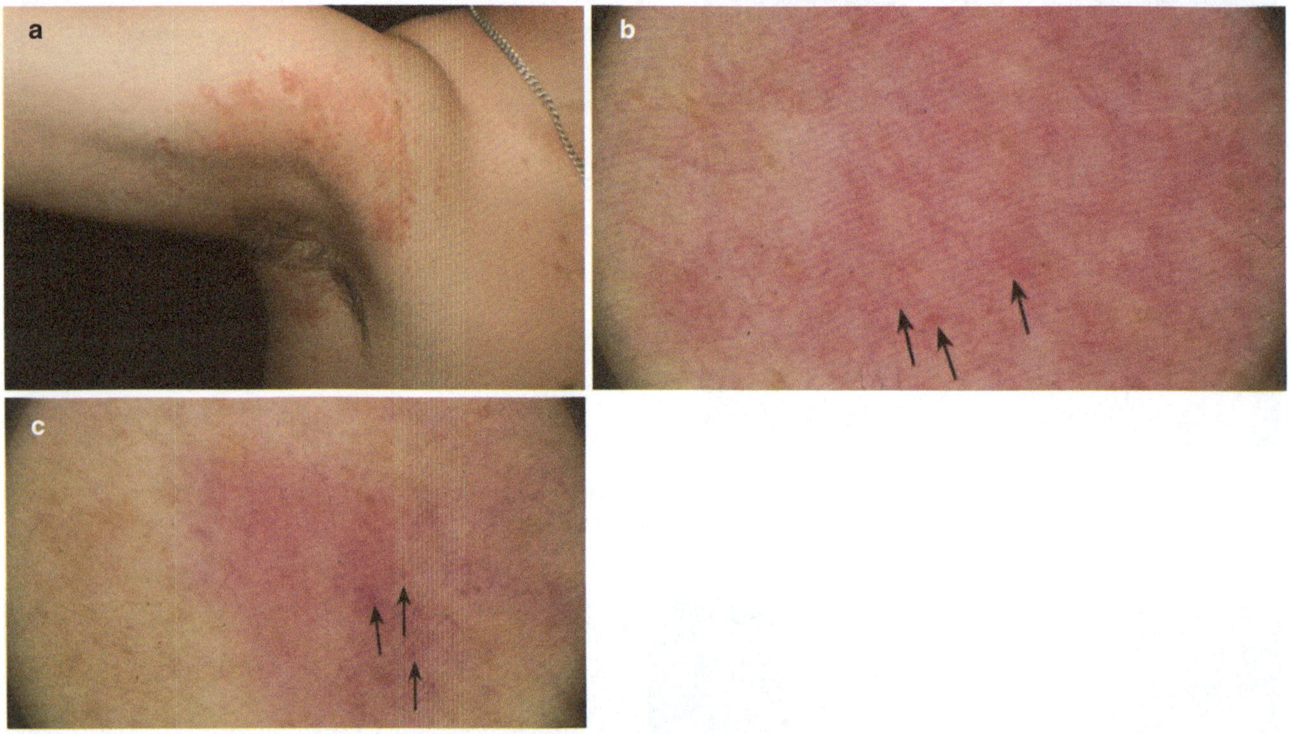

Fig. 12.66 Urticarial vasculitis. (**a**). Axilla wheals that last for more than 24 hours and are associated with a burning sensation and hyperpigmentation. (**b**). Linear and branched vessels as well as some purpuric dots (arrow) (×20). (**c**). Prominent purpuric globules (arrow) (×20)

12.6 Metabolic Dermatoses

12.6.1 Primary Cutaneous Amyloidosis

Primary cutaneous amyloidosis (PCA) is a common chronic disorder, with no systemic involvement, caused by amyloid deposition in the dermis. The most common subtypes of PCA are macular amyloidosis and lichen amyloidosis. The diagnosis of PCA mainly relies on the clinical manifestations. However, other inflammatory disorders, such as lichen simplex chronicus, postinflammatory pigmentation, and prurigo nodularis, may show similar symptoms. Dermoscopy can be useful in the differential diagnosis of PCA (Table 12.9).

12.6.1.1 Dermoscopic Features of Lichenoid Amyloidosis (Fig. 12.67)

1. Central hub
   (a) White and/or brown scarlike area
   (b) Corresponding to orthohyperkeratosis and/or acanthosis histologically
2. Surrounding various configurations of brown pigmentation
   (a) Corresponding to basal hyperpigmentation, pigmentary incontinence, and/or melanin granules appearing in amyloid deposits in the dermal papilla histologically
   (b) Shiny white streaks
   (c) Hemorrhagic spots

12.6.1.2 Dermoscopic Features of Macular Amyloidosis (Fig. 12.68)

1. Central hub
   (a) White and/or brown color, with no scarlike area.
   (b) The white central hub corresponds to the pathological change of orthohyperkeratosis and acanthosis. Brown central hubs are due to loosened, basket-weave orthokeratosis.

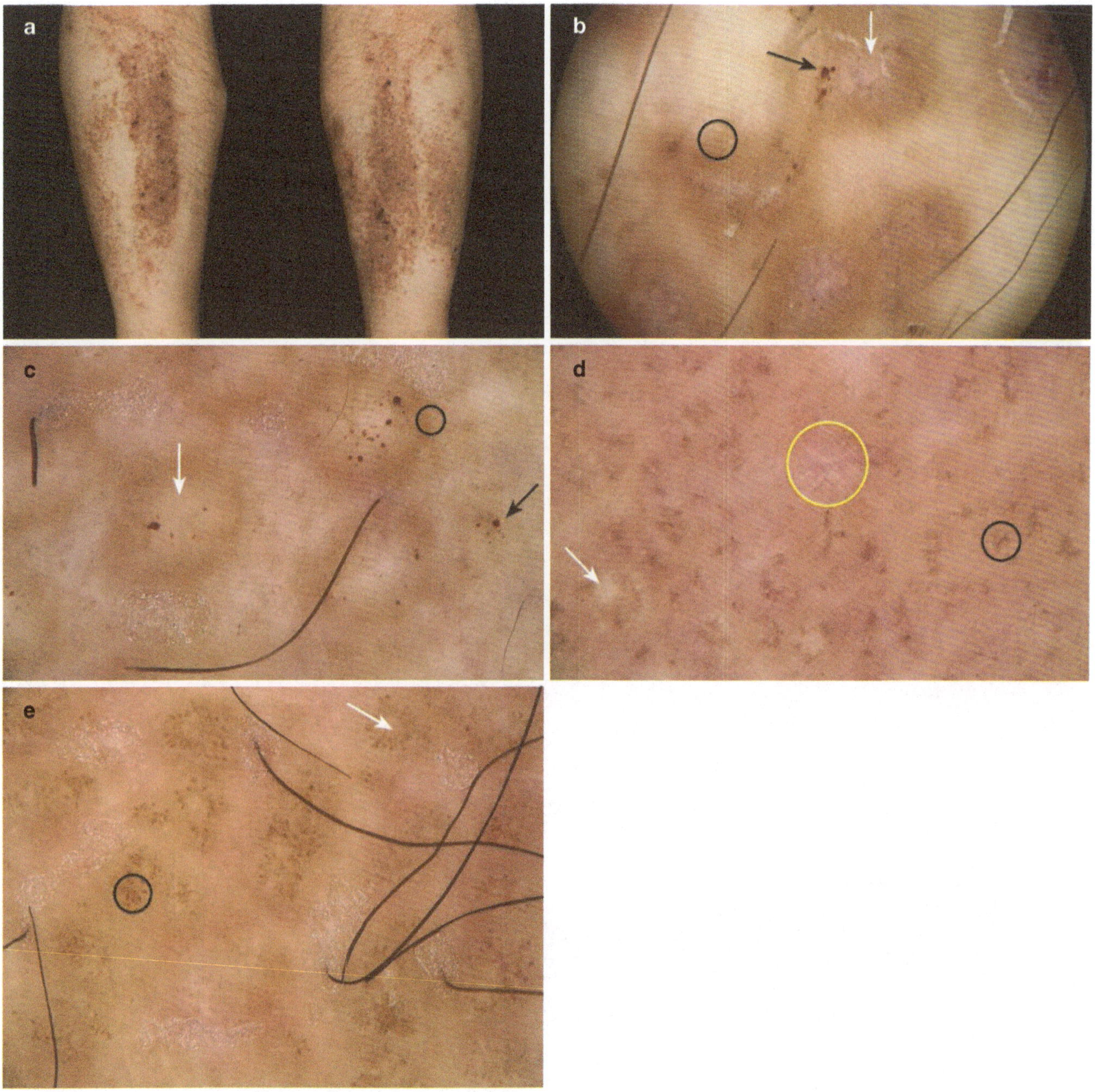

Fig. 12.67 Lichenoid amyloidosis. (**a**). Pretibial lichenoid papules, some coalescing into plaques. (**b**). Central hub (white arrow) surrounded by brown pigmented dots and patches (black circle), with sparse hemorrhagic spots (black arrow) (×20). (**c**). White central hub (white arrow) surrounded by brown pigmented patches (black circle), with sparse hemorrhagic spots (black arrow) (×40). (**d**). Shiny white streaks (yellow circle) and a brown and white central hub (white arrow) with brown pigmented globules, patches, and leaves (black circle) (×40). (**e**). White central hub (white arrow) surrounded by brown pigmented dots and globules, some distributed radially (black circle) (×40)

2. Various peripheral configurations of brown pigmentation correspond to basal hyperpigmentation, pigmentary incontinence, and/or melanin granules appearing in amyloid deposits in the dermal papilla histologically.

12.6.2 Acanthosis Nigricans

Acanthosis nigricans is characterized by the hyperpigmentation and papillary or velvet-like hyperplasia of the skin. There are many types of acanthosis nigricans, and their histological findings include mild to moderate hyperkeratosis and papillomatosis, irregular acanthosis, and basal hyperpigmentation.

The dermoscopic features of acanthosis nigricans are as follows (Fig. 12.69):

1. Ridge-groove pattern, presenting as deep and wide grooves and papillary ridges (some manifest as "sulci and gyri" patterns), with peripheral hyperpigmentation.
2. Chapped-land structures.

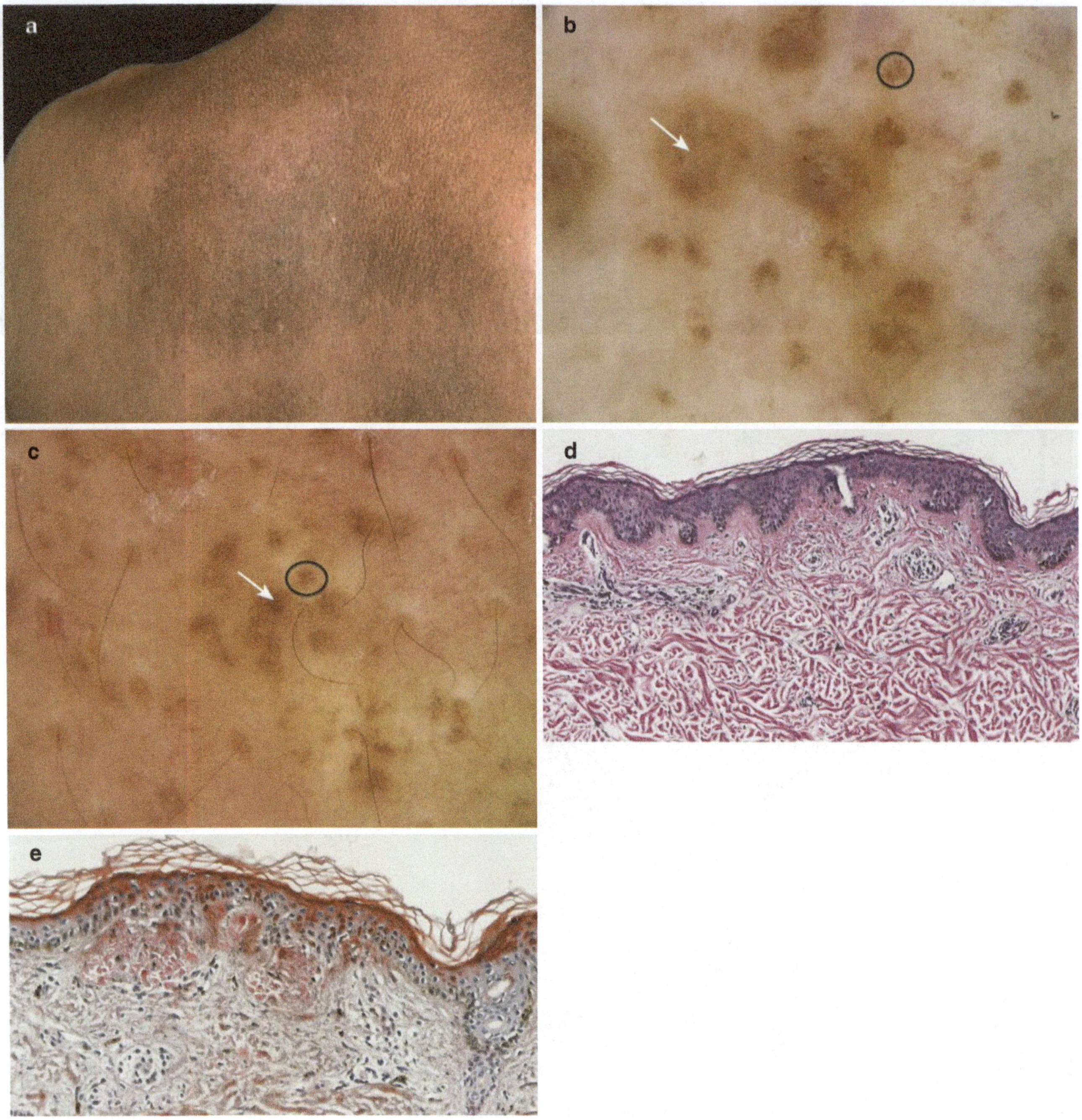

Fig. 12.68 Macular amyloidosis. (**a**). Rippled brown macules on the back. (**b**). Brown and white central hub (white arrow) surrounded by brown pigmented dots and patches (black circle) (×40). (**c**). Brown central hub (white arrow) surrounded by brown pigmented dots, globules, and lines (black circle) (×40). (**d**). Histopathological examination shows basket-weave orthokeratosis, basal hyperpigmentation, and amyloid deposits in the dermal papillae (hematoxylin and eosin, ×40). (**e**). Congo red staining was positive (×100)

12.7 Hyperpigmented/Hypopigmented and Other Inflammatory Diseases

12.7.1 Vitiligo

Vitiligo is an acquired hypopigmented dermatosis with unclear etiology, but it is probably related to inherited, autoimmune, and neuropsychiatric factors. Vitiligo is usually divided into generalized, segmental, and localized subtypes, among others. Unspecific manifestations of vitiligo may be misdiagnosed as other hypopigmented dermatoses, such as pityriasis alba, postinflammatory hypopigmentation, and amelanotic nevi. Dermoscopy can help in the differential diagnosis among these conditions.

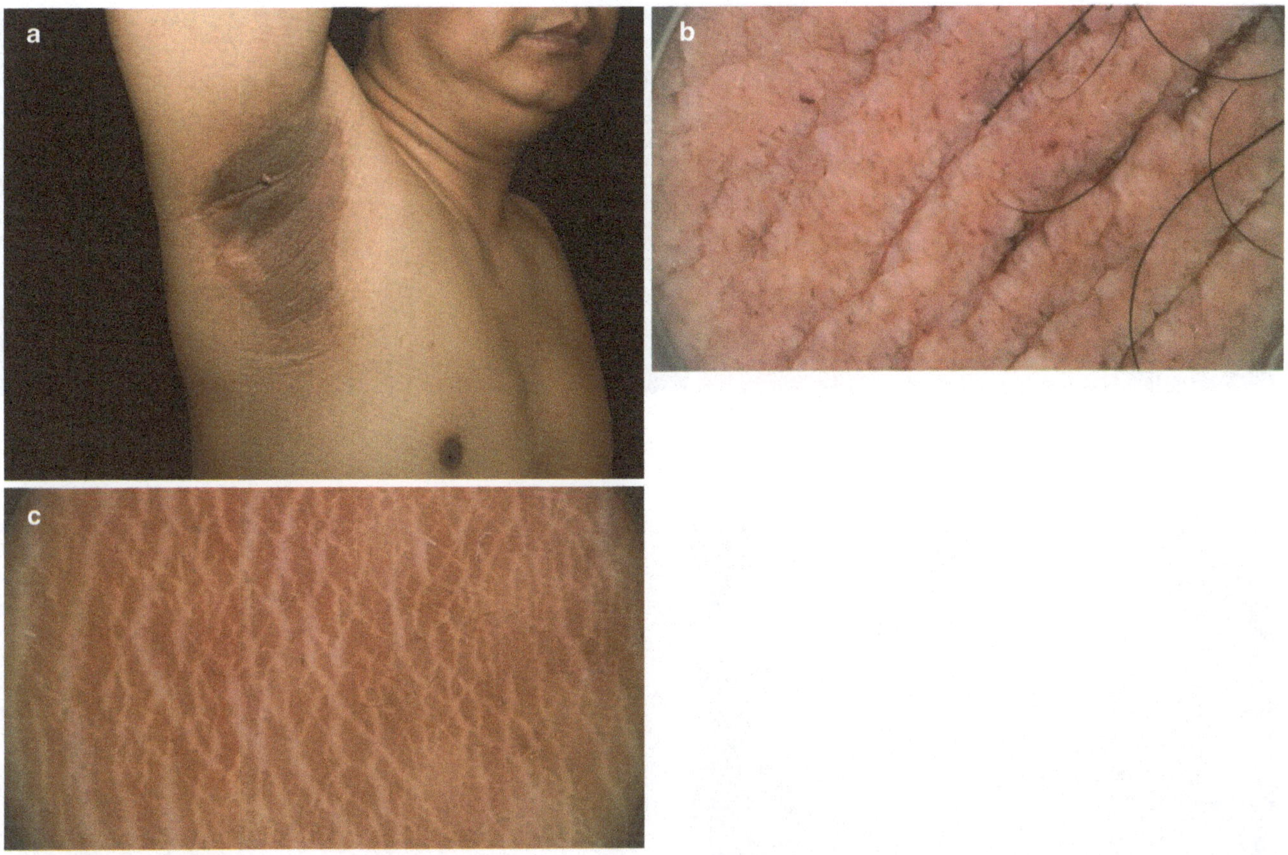

Fig. 12.69 Acanthosis nigricans. (**a**). Velvet-like thickening and hyperpigmentation of axilla. (**b**). Ridge-groove pattern, presenting as deep and wide grooves and papillary ridges, with peripheral hyperpigmentation (×20). (**c**). Chapped-land structures (×20)

Fig. 12.70 Vitiligo. (**a**). Ivory patches on the left arm. (**b**). Bright white areas, perifollicular pigmentation (circle), and sparse white vellus hair (×20)

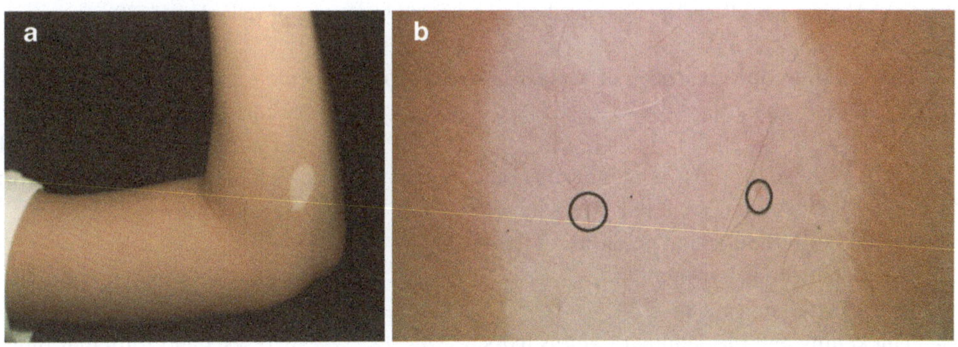

The dermoscopic features of vitiligo are as follows (Figs. 12.70 and 12.71):

1. Well-defined shiny white areas.
2. Perifollicular pigmentation (more frequent in repigmenting or progressing lesions).
3. Other features include white hair, perilesional pigmentation, reverse network-like pigmentation, network-like pigmentation, and telangiectasia.

Of note, well-defined bright white areas along with perifollicular pigmentation are specific features of vitiligo, which is of great value in the differential diagnosis of pityriasis alba, postinflammatory hypopigmentation, and amelanotic nevi.

12.7.2 Melasma

Melasma is a pigmentation disorder that presents as bilateral pigmented macules and occurs mainly in women. Melasma may result from increased estrogen levels. Dermoscopy can be utilized in the differential diagnosis and therapeutic effect evaluation of melasma.

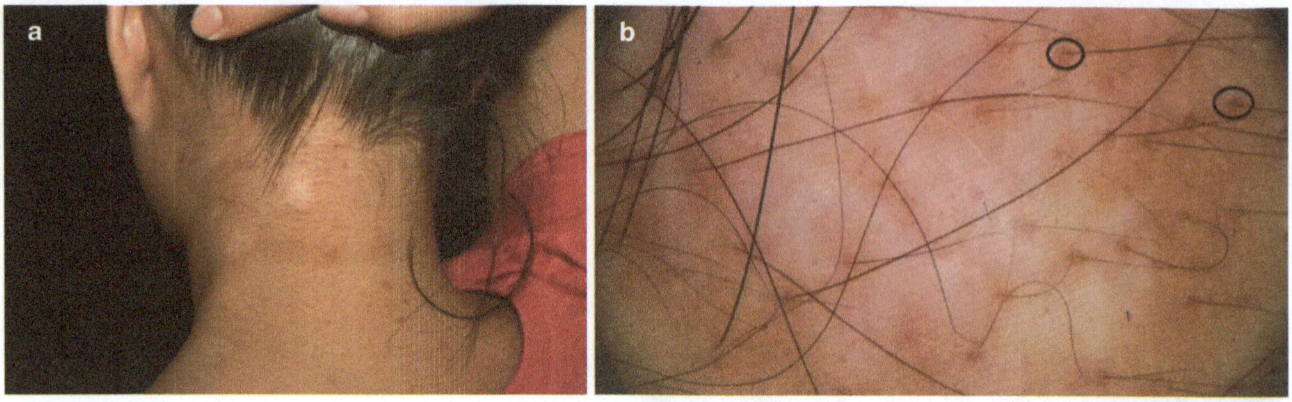

Fig. 12.71 Vitiligo. (**a**). Hypopigmented patches on the posterior neck. (**b**). Bright white areas, perifollicular pigmentation (circle), and perilesional pigmentation (×20)

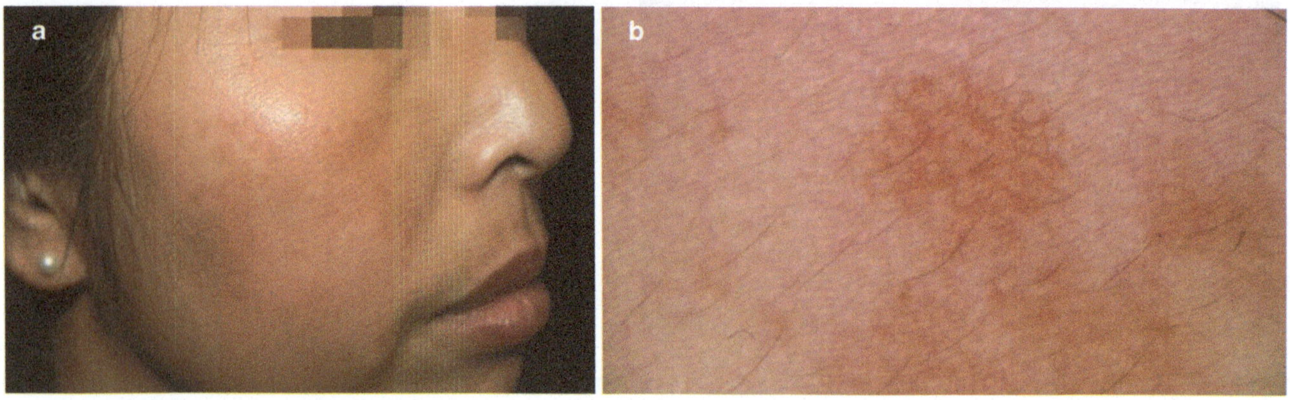

Fig. 12.72 Melasma. (**a**). Bilateral pigmented macules on the cheeks. (**b**). Light yellowish-brown homogeneous patches, pseudonetwork pigmentation, and brown curved/annular areas with the thickening and blackening of vellus hairs (×30)

The dermoscopic features of melasma are as follows (Fig. 12.72):

1. Light yellowish-brown homogeneous patches and dark-brown dots/globules/curved areas/annular areas, with spared perifollicular and periadnexal regions
2. Pseudonetwork pigmentation
3. Reticular telangiectasia
4. Thickening and blackening of vellus hairs

Dermoscopy has already been used in the differential diagnosis of melasma and other hyperpigmented disorders, such as Riehl's melanosis (presenting as diffused brownish hyperpigmentation and pseudonetwork pigmentation) and Ota's nevus (presenting as blue-gray linear pigmentation and hypopigmented dots).

12.7.3 Dowling–Degos Disease

Dowling–Degos disease is an autosomal-dominant inherited disease that is often sporadic clinically because of incomplete penetrance. Dowling–Degos disease commonly has an adult onset and is characterized by pigmentation involving large body folds and flexural areas.

The dermoscopic features of Dowling–Degos disease are as follows:

1. Brown to reddish-brown background
2. Central star-like pattern
3. Cysts and follicular plugs are sometimes seen

12.7.4 Confluent and Reticulated Papillomatosis

Confluent and reticulated papillomatosis, with a predilection for female patients aged 20–30, commonly presents as patchily or reticularly distributed brownish waxy papules on the scapular region, submammary region, and upper abdomen. The etiology of confluent and reticulated papillomatosis remains unknown but is probably related to obesity and diabetes. Confluent and reticulated papillomatosis is sometimes confused with or concurrent with acanthosis nigricans and

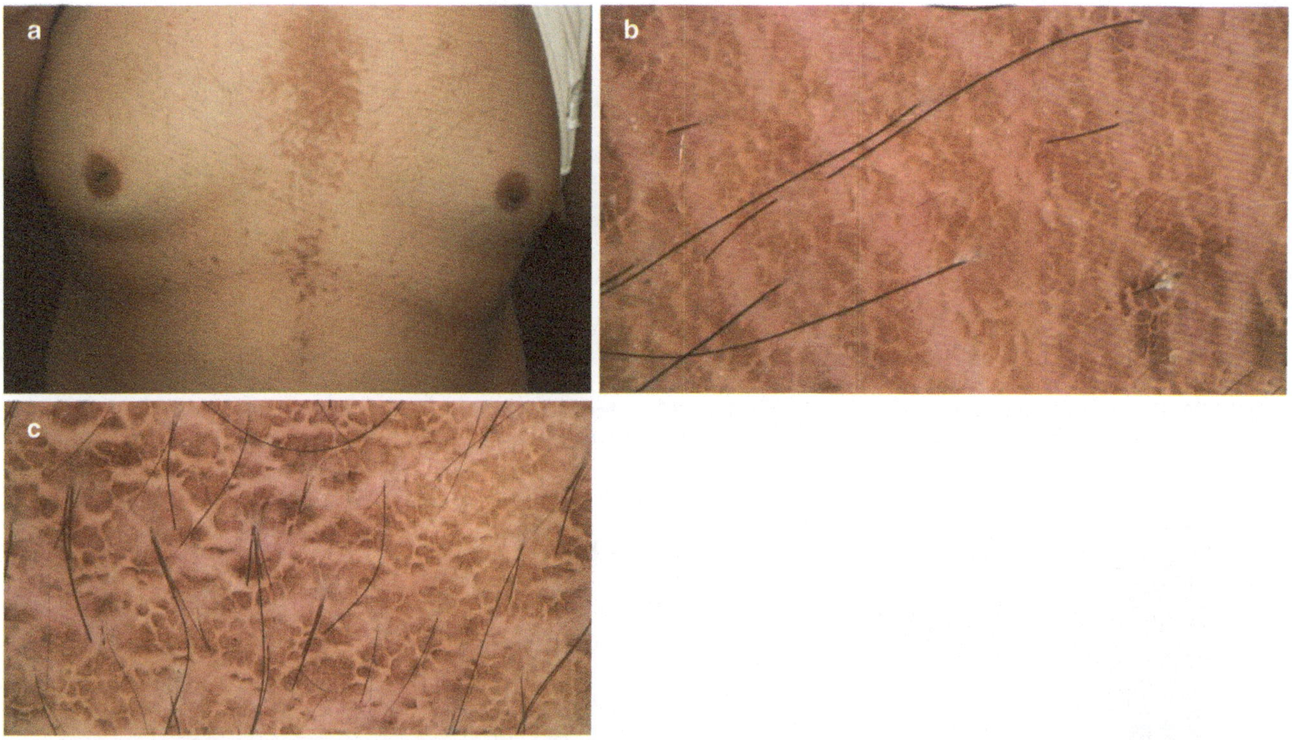

Fig. 12.73 Confluent and reticulated papillomatosis. (**a**). Brownish reticular papules and patches on the chest. (**b**). Dermoscopy shows well-demarcated homogeneous polygonal brownish pigmentation divided by white striae, which forms a sulcus appearance. White scales can also be seen. (**c**). Well-demarcated homogeneous polygonal brownish pigmentation divided by white or pale white striae, forming sulci and gyri patterns (×30)

tinea versicolor. Dermoscopy can assist in the diagnosis and differential diagnosis of these conditions.

The dermoscopic features of confluent and reticulated papillomatosis are as follows (Fig. 12.73):

1. Well-demarcated/ill-demarcated polygonal brownish pigmentation divided by white to pale white striae, forming cobblestone or sulci and gyri patterns
2. White scales

Histologically, brownish pigmentation and white scales correspond to the hyperpigmentation of the basal layer and the parakeratosis of the epidermis, respectively. The cobblestone or sulcus appearances correspond to epidermal papillomatous hyperplasia.

12.7.5 Porokeratosis

Porokeratosis is a heterogeneous group of entities that are characterized by abnormal keratinization. Except for porokeratosis of Mibelli, types of porokeratosis include disseminated porokeratosis, linear porokeratosis, disseminated actinic porokeratosis, and verrucous porokeratosis, among others. Different subtypes can occur in a single patient or family. The dermoscopic features of many types of porokeratosis have been reported previously.

The dermoscopic features of porokeratosis are as follows:

1. Peripheral keratotic rim with two free edges (also called a "white track" or "lines of volcanic crater"), corresponding to coronoid lamella histologically
2. Central white to brown homogeneous areas, red-brownish dots/granules, and multiple vascular patterns (dotted/linear)

The dermoscopic features of disseminated actinic porokeratosis are similar to those of porokeratosis of Mibelli. Pigmentation in the peripheral keratotic rim can also be seen in disseminated actinic porokeratosis, especially in the pigmented disseminated actinic porokeratosis subtype (Figs. 12.74 and 12.75). Additionally, rosettes are found in the verrucous porokeratosis subtype. Keratotic rims of porokeratosis are more prominently viewed with the furrow ink test or under ultraviolet dermoscopy. Ultraviolet dermoscopy shows a shiny "diamond necklace" appearance at the keratotic rim (Fig. 12.76). Dermoscopy can be useful in the differentiation between porokeratosis and psoriasis, since the latter shows no white keratotic rims.

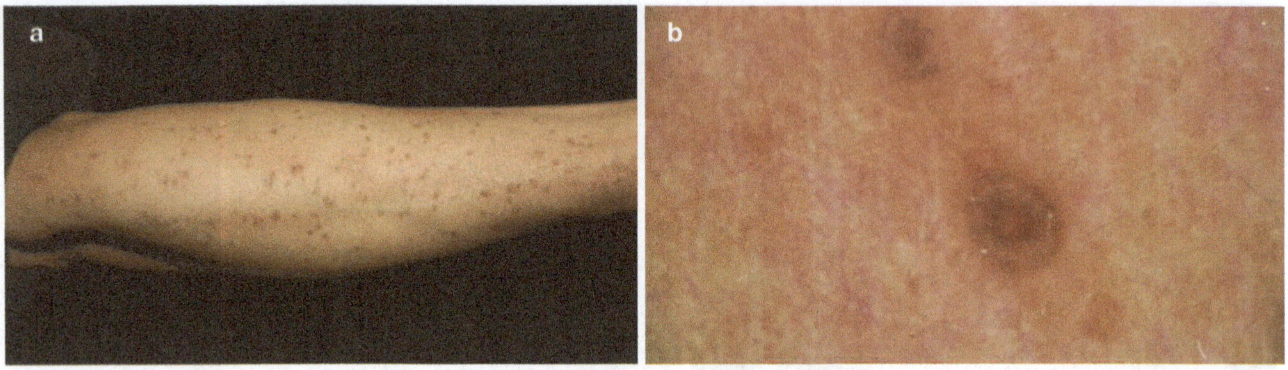

Fig. 12.74 Disseminated actinic porokeratosis. (**a**). Flat papules with peripheral keratotic rims. (**b**). Peripheral keratotic rim having two free edges (white track), a central brown homogeneous area, and peripheral pigmentation (×30)

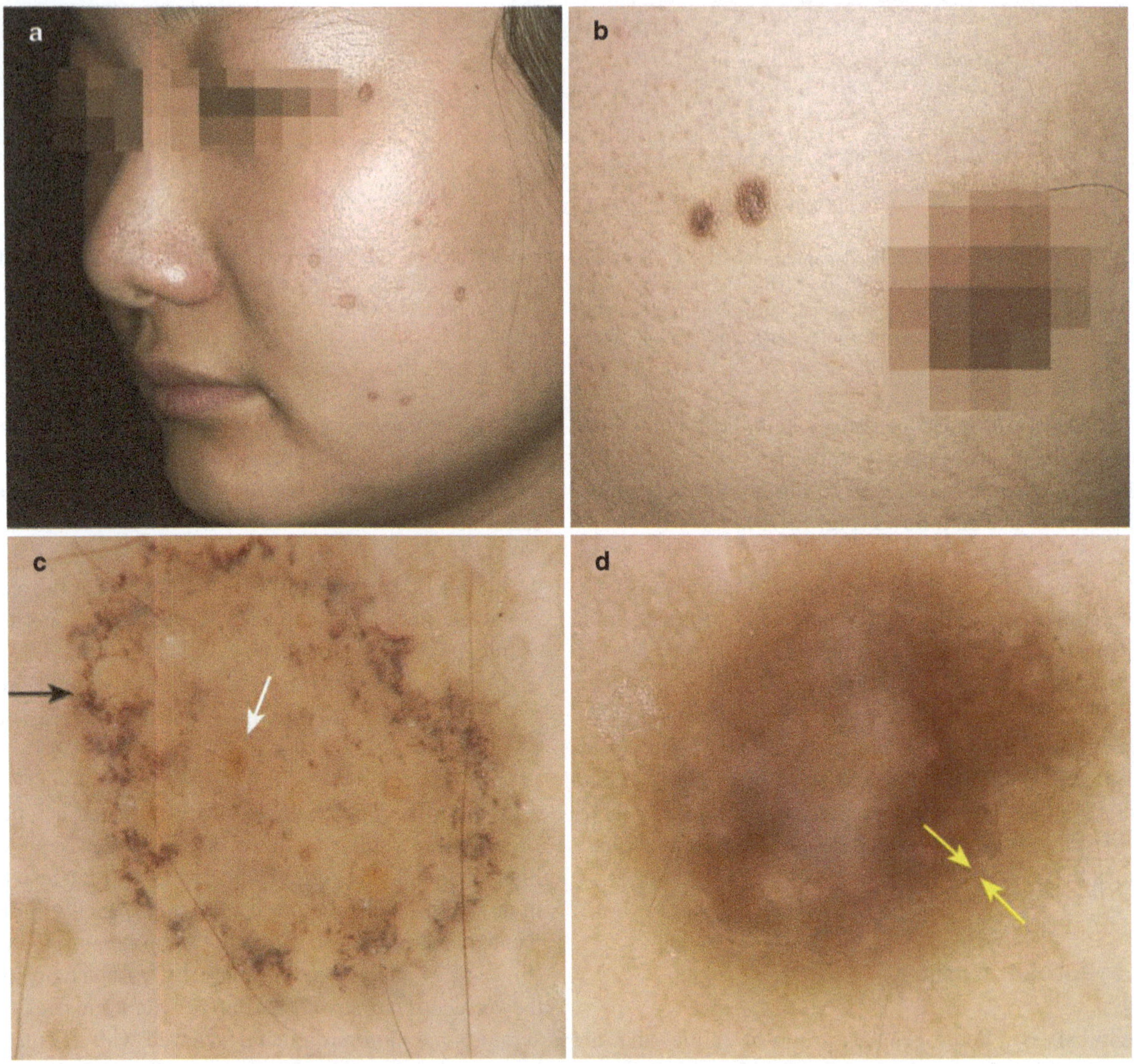

Fig. 12.75 Disseminated actinic porokeratosis. (**a** and **b**). Well-defined light-brown bean-sized round patches with peripheral elevated rims and central atrophy. (**c**). Peripheral brown pigmented dots and globules (black arrow), a few central dotted/patchy brown pigmented structures, and follicular keratotic plugs in the dilated follicles (white arrow). (**d**). Peripheral light-brown pigmentary structures, a white track (yellow arrow), and central white homogeneous area (×20)

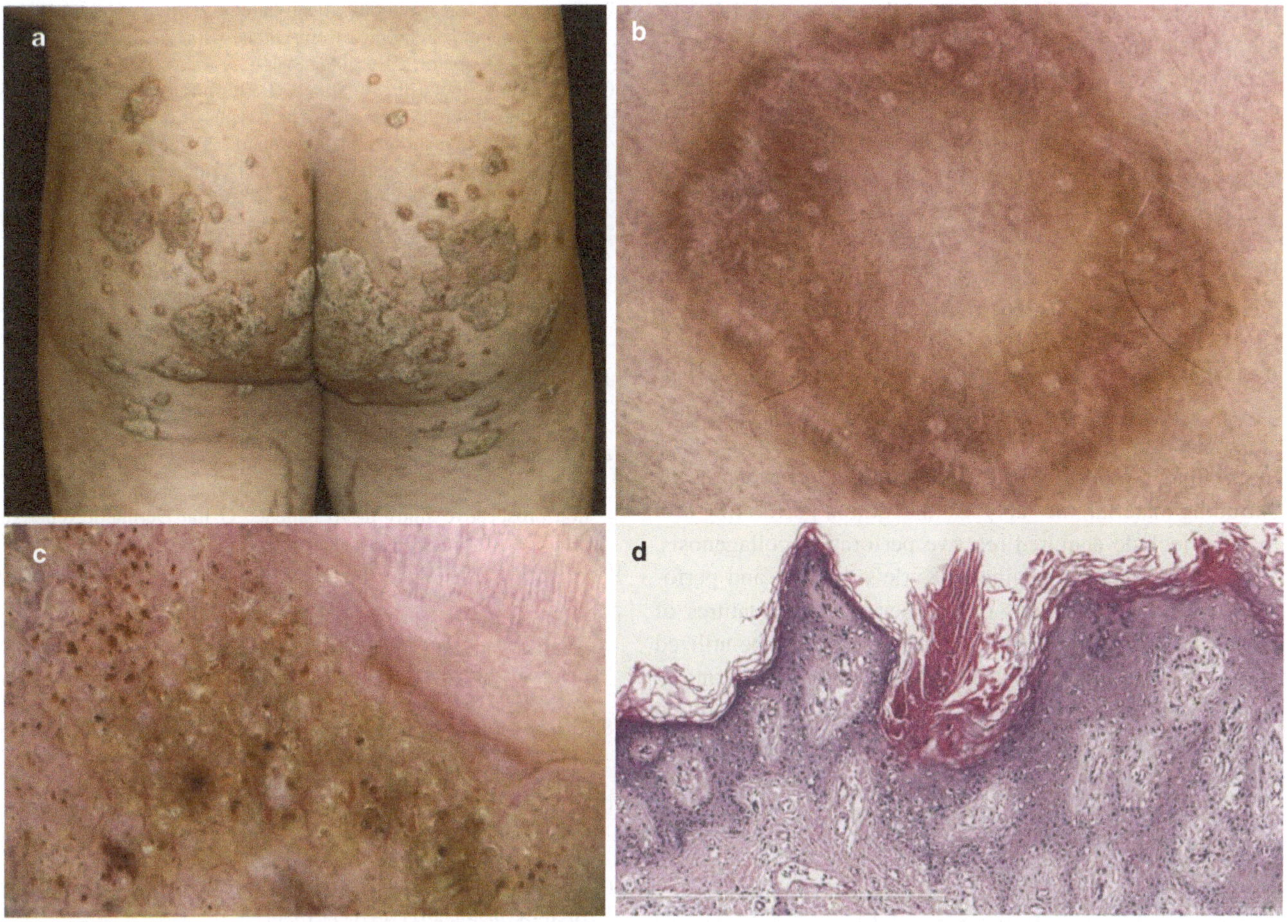

Fig. 12.76 Verrucous porokeratosis. (**a**). Well-demarcated brown verrucous keratotic plaques on the buttocks. (**b**). Peripheral keratotic rim with two free edges and central white homogeneous area with dotted vessels and rosettes (×20). (**c**). Papillomatous pattern with dotted vessels (×50). (**d**). Histopathological examination shows coronoid lamella, a diminished granular layer, and a number of dyskeratotic keratinocytes, corresponding to the diagnosis of porokeratosis (hematoxylin and eosin, ×100)

12.7.6 Darier's Disease

Darier's disease is an inherited acantholytic genodermatosis due to mutations in the ATP2A2 gene. The subtypes of Darier's disease include generalized and segmental Darier's disease. Darier's disease usually presents with generalized or localized hyperkeratotic, reddish-brown papules. Histological findings show acantholysis and cleft formation with dyskeratosis in the epidermis.

The dermoscopic features of Darier's disease are as follows:

1. Central yellowish to brownish areas having star-like/polygonal/round to oval shapes
2. Somewhat thin whitish halos
3. Pinkish background
4. With/without whitish scales
5. Dotted and/or linear vessels with/without peripheral halos

12.7.7 Grover's Disease

Grover's disease is an acquired disorder that typically presents as itchy, red-brownish papules and papulovesicles on the trunk. Histologically, Grover's disease presents as cleft formation in the epidermis. The histological patterns of Grover's disease are Darier-like, pemphigus-like, spongiotic, and Hailey–Hailey-like.

The dermoscopic features of Grover's disease are as follows:

1. The Darier-like histological pattern presents as central yellowish to brownish star-like/branched polygonal/round-oval shape and a peripheral white halo.
2. The spongiotic pattern presents as dotted/globular vessels with whitish scales over a red-yellowish background.

The dermoscopic features of diseases that are histologically characterized as acantholytic dyskeratosis, such as

Darier's disease, Darier-like Grover's disease, and BRAF inhibitor-induced acantholytic dyskeratosis, are similar because of the similar histological background. The central yellow-brownish area corresponds to compact hyperkeratosis and acanthosis, while the pinkish background and vascular patterns correspond to superficial dermic inflammation.

12.7.8 Acquired Perforating Dermatosis

Acquired perforating dermatosis is a group of disorders characterized by the invagination of the epidermis with the extrusion of dermal materials. Adults are susceptible to acquired perforating dermatosis. Based on the composition of the extruding material, the subtypes of acquired perforating dermatosis include acquired reactive perforating collagenosis, elastosis perforans serpiginosa, Kyrle's disease, and perforating folliculitis. Reports on the dermoscopic features of these entities are few. However, dermoscopy can be utilized in the differential diagnosis of acquired perforating dermatoses and nodular prurigo, which presents as a white starburst pattern surrounded by reddish/brown-yellowish crusts, erosions, and/or scales.

The dermoscopic features of acquired perforating dermatosis are as follows:

1. Reactive perforating collagenosis presents as a central yellowish-brown structureless area, surrounded by a white rim and an outer pink circle.
2. Perforating folliculitis presents as central bright white clods surrounded by a structureless gray area with outer brown reticular lines.

Further Reading

1. Sgouros D, Apalla Z, Ioannides D, et al. Dermoscopy of common inflammatory disorders. Dermatol Clin. 2018;36(4):359–68.
2. Xu C, Liu J, Liu Y. Application progress of dermoscopy in nonpigmented skin lesions. Chin Med J. 2014;94(46):3688–90.
3. Liu J, Zou X. Expert consensus on dermoscopic diagnosis of erythematous and Papulosquamous disorders. China J Leprosy Skin Diseases. 2016;32(2):65–9.
4. Errichetti E, Stinco G. Dermoscopy in general dermatology: a practical overview. Dermatol Ther. 2016;6(4):471–507.
5. Lallas A, Kyrgidis A, Tzellos TG, et al. Accuracy of dermoscopic criteria for the diagnosis of psoriasis, dermatitis, lichen planus and pityriasis rosea. Br J Dermatol. 2012;166(6):1198–205.
6. Xu C, Liu J, Chen D, et al. Significance of dermoscopy in the differential diagnosis of psoriasis vulgaris and eczema. Chin Med J. 2014;94(36):2833–7.
7. Errichetti E, Stinco G. Dermoscopy in differential diagnosis of palmar psoriasis and chronic hand eczema. J Dermatol. 2016;43(4):423–5.
8. Zalaudek I, Argenziano G. Dermoscopy subpatterns of inflammatory skin disorders. Arch Dermatol. 2006;142(6):808.
9. Errichetti E, Lacarrubba F, Micali G, et al. Differentiation of pityriasis lichenoides chronica from guttate psoriasis by dermoscopy. Clin Exp Dermatol. 2015;40(7):804–6.
10. Errichetti E, Piccirillo A, Stinco G. Dermoscopy as an auxiliary tool in the differentiation of the main types of erythroderma due to dermatological disorders. Int J Dermatol. 2016;55(12):e616–8.
11. Lallas A, Apalla Z, Argenziano G, et al. Dermoscopic pattern of psoriatic lesions on specific body sites. Dermatol. 2014;228(3):250–4.
12. Kim GW, Jung HJ, Ko HC, et al. Dermoscopy can be useful in differentiating scalp psoriasis from seborrhoeic dermatitis. Br J Dermatol. 2011;164(3):652–6.
13. Xu C, Chen D, Liu J. Application of dermoscopy in diagnosis and differential diagnosis of scalp psoriasis and seborrheic dermatitis. Chin Med J. 2014;94(44):3467–71.
14. Rossi A, Mandel VD, Garelli V, et al. Videodermoscopy scalp psoriasis severity index (VSCAPSI): a useful tool for evaluation of scalp psoriasis. Eur J Dermatol. 2011;21(4):546–51.
15. Rossi A, Pranteda G, Iorio A, et al. Efficacy of Iralfaris shampoo in the treatment of scalp psoriasis: a videodermoscopy evaluation prospective study in 70 patients. G Ital Dermatol Venereol. 2012;147(6):625–30.
16. Piraccini BM, Bruni F, Starace M. Dermoscopy of non-skin cancer nail disorders. Dermatol Ther. 2012;25(6):594–602.
17. Goncharova Y, Attia EA, Souid K, et al. Dermoscopic features of clinically inflammatory dermatoses and their correlation with histopathologic reaction patterns. Arch Dermatol Res. 2015;307(1):23–30.
18. Vazquez-Lopez F, Marghoob A. Dermoscopic assessment of long-term topical therapies with potent steroids in chronic psoriasis. J Am Acad Dermatol. 2004;51(5):811–3.
19. Lallas A, Argenziano G, Zalaudek I, et al. Dermoscopic hemorrhagic dots: an early predictor of response of psoriasis to biologic agents. Dermatol Pract Concept. 2016;6(4):7–12.
20. Navarini A, Feldmeyer L, Tondury B, et al. The yellow clod sign. Arch Dermatol. 2011;147(11):1350.
21. Thomas M, Yadav T, Khopkar U. The role of dermoscopy using a triple light source in the diagnosis of pityriasis rosea: an observational pilot study. Int J Dermatol. 2017;56(7):e147–8.
22. Lallas A, Apalla Z, Lefaki I, et al. Dermoscopy of early stage mycosis fungoides. J Eur Acad Dermatol Venereol. 2013;27(5):617–21.
23. Xu C, Liu J, Wang T, et al. Dermoscopic patterns of early-stage mycosis fungoides in a Chinese population. Clin Exp Dermatol. 2019;44(2):169–75.
24. Ping X, Cheng T. Dermoscopy of poikilodermatous mycosis fungoides (MF). J Am Acad Dermatol. 2016;74(3):e45–7.
25. Errichetti E, Stinco G. Dermoscopy as a supportive instrument in the differentiation of the main types of acquired keratoderma due to dermatological disorders. J Eur Acad Dermatol Venereol. 2016;30(12):e229–31.
26. Ankad BS, Beegouder SL. Pityriasis lichenoides et varioliformis acuta in skin of color: new observations by dermoscopy. Dermatol Pract Concept. 2017;7(1):27–34.
27. Luo Y, Chi C, Liu J, et al. Comparison of Dermoscopic features between classic and pigmented lichen planus. China J Leprosy Skin Diseases. 2016;32(9):533–6.
28. Pirmez R, Duque-Estrada B, Donati A, et al. Clinical and dermoscopic features of lichen planus pigmentosus in 37 patients with frontal fibrosing alopecia. Br J Dermatol. 2016;175(6):1387–90.
29. Baquero SE, Lorentelavirgen AI, Dominguez CJ, et al. Value of dermoscopy in the diagnosis and prognostic evaluation of linear pigmented lichen planus. Actas Dermosifiliogr. 2015;106(4):339–40.
30. Ankad BS, Beergouder SL. Hypertrophic lichen planus versus prurigo nodularis: a dermoscopic perspective. Dermatol Pract Concept. 2016;6(2):9–15.
31. Errichetti E, Piccirillo A, Stinco G. Dermoscopy of prurigo nodularis. J Dermatol. 2015;42:632–4.

32. Lallas A, Apalla Z, Karteridou A, et al. Dermoscopy for discriminating between pityriasis rubra pilaris and psoriasis. J Dermatol Case Rep. 2013;7(1):20–2.
33. Vazquez-Lopez F, Kreusch J, Marghoob A. Dermoscopic semiology: further insights into vascular features by screening a large spectrum of nontumoral skin lesions. Br J Dermatol. 2015;150(2):226–31.
34. Kaliyadan F. Dermoscopy of erythema multiforme. Indian Dermatol Online J. 2017;8(1):75.
35. Grazyna KW, Tomasz C, Tomasz K, et al. Dermoscopic follow-up of the skin towards acute graft-versus-host-disease in patients after allogeneic hematopoietic stem cell transplantation. Biomed Res Int. 2016;2016:4535717.
36. Lallas A, Argenziano G, Apalla Z, et al. Dermoscopic patterns of common facial inflammatory skin diseases. J Eur Acad Dermatol Venereol. 2014;28(5):609–14.
37. Lallas A, Sidiropoulos T, Lefaki I, et al. Photoletter to the editor: Dermoscopy of granuloma faciale. J Dermatol Case Rep. 2012;6(2):59–60.
38. Lallas A, Argenziano G, Longo C, et al. Polygonal vessels of rosacea are highlighted by dermoscopy. Int J Dermatol. 2014;53(5):e325–7.
39. Segal R, Mimouni D, Feuerman H, et al. Dermoscopy as a diagnostic tool in demodicidosis. Int J Dermatol. 2010;49(9):1018–23.
40. Kelati A, Mernissi FZ. Granulomatous rosacea: a case report. J Med Case Rep. 2017;11(1):230.
41. Micali G, Dall'oglio F, Verzi AE, et al. Treatment of erythematotelangiectatic rosacea with brimonidine alone or combined with vascular laser based on preliminary instrumental evaluation of the vascular component. Lasers Med Sci. 2018;33(6):1397–400.
42. Chi C, Luo Y, Liu J. Application of Dermoscopy in Discosmetic dermatosis. Chin J Dermatol. 2018;51(12):922.
43. Patricia AC, Silvia MR, Adriana VH, et al. Dermoscopy distinction of eruptive vellus hair cysts with molluscum contagiosum and acne lesions. Pediatr Dermatol. 2012;29(6):772–3.
44. Ayhan E, Alabalik U, Ayci Y. Dermoscopic evaluation of two patients with lupus miliaris disseminatus faciei. Clin Exp Dermatol. 2014;39(4):500–2.
45. Borgia F, Giuffrida R, Vaccaro M, et al. Photodynamic therapy in lupus miliaris disseminatus faciei's scars. Dermatol Ther. 2016;29(5):320–4.
46. Pellivano R, Tiodorovic-Zivkovic D, Gourhant JY, et al. Dermoscopy of cutaneous sarcoidosis. Dermatology. 2010;221(1):51–4.
47. Chauhan P, Meena D, Hazarika N. Dermoscopy of sarcoidosis: a useful clue to diagnosis. Indian Dermatol Online J. 2018;9(1):80–1.
48. Iman H, Fatima ZM. Dermoscopic features of sarcoidosis. Pan Afr Med J. 2014;18:111.
49. Errichetti E, Lallas A, Apalla Z, et al. Dermoscopy of granuloma annulare: a clinical and histological correlation study. Dermatology. 2017;233(1):74–9.
50. Bombonato C, Argenziano G, Lallas A, et al. Orange color: a dermoscopic clue for the diagnosis of granulomatous skin diseases. J Am Acad Dermatol. 2015;72(1 Suppl):S60–3.
51. Ramadan S, Hossam D, Saleh MA. Dermoscopy could be useful in differentiating sarcoidosis from necrobiotic granulomas even after treatment with systemic steroids. Dermatol Pract Concept. 2016;6(3):17–22.
52. Pellicano R, Caldarola G, Filabozzi P, et al. Dermoscopy of necrobiosis lipoidica and granuloma annulare. Dermatology. 2013;226(4):319–23.
53. Errichetti E, Stinco G. Dermatoscopy of granulomatous disorders. Dermatol Clin. 2018;36(4):369–75.
54. Lallas A, Zaballos P, Zalaudek I, et al. Dermoscopic patterns of granuloma annulare and necrobiosis lipoidica. Clin Exp Dermatol. 2013;38(4):425–7.
55. Navarrete-Dechent C, Puerto CD, Bajaj S, et al. Dermoscopy of elastosis perforans serpiginosa: a useful tool to distinguish it from granuloma annulare. J Am Acad Dermatol. 2015;73(1):e7–9.
56. Lallas A, Apalla Z, Lefaki I, et al. Dermoscopy of discoid lupus erythematosus. Br J Dermatol. 2013;168(2):284–8.
57. Jha AK, Sonthalia S, Sarkar R. Dermoscopy of discoid lupus erythematosus. Indian Dermatol Online J. 2016;7(5):458.
58. Inui S, Itami S, Murakami M, et al. Dermoscopy of discoid lupus erythematosus: report of two cases. J Dermatol. 2014;41(8):756–7.
59. Cervantes J, Hafeez F, Miteva M. Blue-white veil as novel dermatoscopic feature in discoid lupus erythematosus in 2 African-American patients. Skin Appendage Disord. 2017;3(4):211–4.
60. Lallas A, Apalla Z, Argenziano G, et al. Clues for differentiating discoid lupus erythematosus from actinic keratosis. J Am Acad Dermatol. 2013;69(1):e5–6.
61. Errichetti E, Piccirillo A, Viola L, et al. Dermoscopy of subacute cutaneous lupus erythematosus. Int J Dermatol. 2016;55(11):e605–7.
62. Errichetti E, Lallas A, Apalla Z, et al. Dermoscopy of Morphea and cutaneous lichen Sclerosus: clinicopathological correlation study and comparative analysis. Dermatology. 2017;233(6):462–70.
63. Shim WH, Jwa SW, Song M, et al. Diagnostic usefulness of dermatoscopy in differentiating lichen sclerous et atrophicus from morphea. J Am Acad Dermatol. 2012;66(4):690–1.
64. Borghi A, Corazza M, Minghetti S, et al. Clinical and dermoscopic changes of vulvar lichen sclerosus after topical corticosteroid treatment. J Dermatol. 2016;43(9):1078–82.
65. Borghi A, Corazza M, Minghetti S, et al. Dermoscopic features of vulvar lichen Sclerosus in the setting of a prospective cohort of patients: new observations. Dermatology. 2016;232(1):71–7.
66. Luo Y, Liu J, Chi C, et al. Analysis of Dermoscopic features of vulvar lichen Sclerosus. Chin J Dermatol. 2018;51(11):809–11.
67. Larre Borges A, Tiodorovic-Zivkovic D, Lallas A, et al. Clinical, dermoscopic and histopathologic features of genital and extragenital lichen sclerosus. J Eur Acad Dermatol Venereol. 2013;27(11):1433–9.
68. Vazquez-Lopez F, Garcia-Garcia B, Sanchez-Martin J, et al. Dermoscopic patterns of purpuric lesions. Arch Dermatol. 2010;146(8):938.
69. Ozkaya DB, Emiroglu N, Su O, et al. Dermatoscopic findings of pigmented purpuric dermatosis. An Bras Dermatol. 2016;91(5):584–7.
70. Suh KS, Park JB, Yang MH, et al. Diagnostic usefulness of dermoscopy in differentiating lichen aureus from nummular eczema. J Dermato. 2017;44(5):533–7.
71. Portela PS, Melo DF, Ormiga P, et al. Dermoscopy of lichen aureus. An Bras Dermatol. 2013;88(2):253–5.
72. Suh KS, Kang DY, Lee KH, et al. Evolution of urticarial vasculitis: a clinical, dermoscopic and histopathological study. J Eur Acad Dermatol Venereol. 2014;28(5):674–5.
73. Vazquez-Lopez F, Maldonado-Seral C, Solaer-Sanchez T, et al. Surface microscopy for discriminating between common urticaria and urticarial vasculitis. Rheumatology (Oxford). 2003;42(9):1079–82.
74. Vazquez-Lopez F, Fueyo A, Sanchez-Martin J, et al. Dermoscopy for the screening of common urticaria and urticaria vasculitis. Arch Dermatol. 2008;144(4):568.
75. Choo JY, Bae JM, Lee JH, et al. Blue-gray blotch: a helpful dermoscopic finding in optimal biopsy site selection for true vasculitis. J Am Acad Dermatol. 2016;75(4):836–8.
76. Chuang YY, Lee DD, Lin CS, et al. Characteristic dermoscopic features of primary cutaneous amyloidosis: a study of 35 cases. Br J Dermatol. 2012;167(3):548–54.
77. Luo Y, Liu J, Chi C, et al. Analysis of Dermoscopic features of primary cutaneous amyloidosis. Chin J Dermatol. 2017;50(7):478–81.
78. Chuh AT, Zawar V. Demonstration of residual perifollicular pigmentation in localized vitiligo—a reverse and novel application of digital epiluminescence dermoscopy. Compu Med Imaging Graph. 2004;28(4):213–7.
79. Li Y, Liu J, Sun QN. Dermoscopic features of melasma. Acta Academiae Medicinae Sinicae. 2015;37(2):226–9.

80. Sonthalia S, Jha AK, Langar S. Dermoscopy of melasma. Indian Dermatol Online J. 2017;8(6):525.
81. Manas C, Shekhar N. Dermoscopy of pigmentary disorders in Brown skin. Dermatol Clin. 2018;36(4):473–85.
82. Geibler S, Dyall-Smith D, Coras B, et al. Unique brown star shape on dermatoscopy of generalized Dowling-Degos disease. Australas J Dermatol. 2011;52(2):151–3.
83. Bernardes F, Quaresma MV, Rezende FC, et al. Confluent and reticulate papillomatosis of Gougerot-Carteaud and obesity: dermoscopic findings. An Bras Dermatol. 2014;89(3):507–9.
84. Nicola A, Magliano J. Dermoscopy of disseminated superficial actinic porokeratosis. Actas Dermosifiliogr. 2017;108(5):e33–7.
85. Jha AK, Sonthalia S, Lallas A. Dermoscopy of porokeratosis of Mibelli. Indian Dermatol Online J. 2017;8(4):304–5.
86. Sotoodian B, Mahmood MN, Salopek TG. Clinical and Dermoscopic features of pigmented disseminated superficial actinic porokeratosis: case report and literature review. J Cutan Med Surg. 2018;22(3):229–31.
87. Luo Y, Liu J. Image gallery: verrucous porokeratosis with characteristic histopathological and dermoscopic features. Br J Dermatol. 2017;176(4):e38.
88. Uhara H, Kamijo F, Okuyama R, et al. Open pores with plugs in porokeratosis clearly visualized with the dermoscopic furrow ink test: report of 3 cases. Arch Dermatol. 2011;147(7):866–8.
89. Thatte S, Kharkar VD, Khopkar US. "Diamond necklace" appearance in superficial porokeratosis. J Am Acad Dermatol. 2014;70(6):e125–6.
90. Chi C, Liu J. Image gallery: porokeratosis under the dermoscopic furrow ink test and ultraviolet light. Br J Dermatol. 2018;178(1):308.
91. Moscarella E, Longo C, Zalaudek I, et al. Dermoscopy and confocal microscopy clues in the diagnosis of psoriasis and porokeratosis. J Am Acad Dermatol. 2013;69(5):e231–3.
92. Enzo E, Vincenzo M, Enrico P, et al. Dermoscopy: a useful auxiliary tool in the diagnosis of type 1 segmental Darier's disease. Dermatol Pract Concept. 2016;6(2):53–5.
93. Errichetti E, Stinco G, Lacarrubba F, et al. Dermoscopy of Darier's disease. J Eur Acad Dermatol Venereol. 2016;30(8):1392–4.
94. Lacarrubba F, Boscaglia S, Nasca MR, et al. Grover's disease: dermoscopy, reflectance confocal microscopy and histopathological correlation. Dermatol Pract Concept. 2017;7(3):51–4.
95. Kittisak P, Tanaka M. Dermoscopic findings in a case of reactive perforating collagenosis. Dermatol Pract Concept. 2015;5(2):75.

13 Infectious and Parasitic Dermatoses

The diagnosis of infectious and parasitic dermatoses is based on pathogen detection, which often requires specialized laboratory physicians and expensive equipment and is time-consuming. However, dermoscopy, which is performed by dermatologists, is intuitive, convenient, and quick and can be used to obtain relatively accurate diagnostic information through observing dermoscopic features of lesions. It is especially suitable for primary care settings or telemedicine. In order to avoid cross-infection among patients, polarized noncontact dermoscopy can be applied since it does not require direct contact with the lesions. Disposable plastic wrap attached to surface of the contact plate with a coupling agent on it, or a disposable contact slide or microscope slide placed between dermoscope and the lesion can avoid direct contact.

As there is no large sample evidence-based studies on the dermoscopic features of infectious and parasitic dermatoses, clinicians still need to combine the medical history, clinical manifestations, necessary pathogen detection, and histopathological examinations to make a final diagnosis for skin lesions that cannot be confirmed via dermoscopy.

13.1 Condyloma Acuminatum

Condyloma acuminatum is a sexually transmitted disease caused by human papillomavirus (HPV) infection, with an average incubation period of three months, presenting as papules, keratotic plaques, and verrucous, papillary and cauliflower-like vegetations. Condyloma acuminatum mainly involves the coronal sulcus, glans, foreskin, frenula, urethra, penile body, perianal region, and scrotum in male patients, and cervical, vagina, vulva, anal canal, and perineum in female patients. Among these sites, urethral lesions are usually tiny, flat, and asymptomatic.

13.1.1 Dermoscopic Manifestations of Condyloma Acuminatum

Morphology: finger pattern, mosaic pattern (clustered dotted or glomerular vessels surrounded by a whitish network), papillary hyperplasia, verrucous hyperplasia, flat papules, and so on. There is often coexist of two patterns in each lesion.

Vessel morphology: dotted/glomerular vessels, curved (comma-shaped) vessels, circular vessels, and hairpin-like vessels (Fig. 13.1). Some keratinized skin lesions lack vascular manifestations and pigmentation can be seen.

During a acetowhite test, the wart turns white, and the vascular structures almost disappear under dermoscopy, due to the temporary degeneration of keratin on the surface, the contraction of vascular loop, and the decrease in blood flow caused by acetic acid. Therefore, dermoscopic examination should be done before a acetowhite test.

13.1.2 Significance of Dermoscopy in the Diagnosis and Treatment of Condyloma Acuminatum

Dermoscopy is especially important for the diagnosis of tiny condyloma acuminatum. It can not only confirm the diagnosis of condyloma acuminatum, but also help to identify tiny condyloma around the major lesion. The diagnosis of tiny condyloma acuminata mainly depends on the vascular structure, which is different from that of the surrounding tissue. In addition, the wart body is slightly raised, and the base of the wart in the mucosa is often milky white.

Condyloma acuminatum can be distinguished from pseudocondyloma, pearly penile papules, Bowenoid papulosis, and molluscum contagiosum under dermoscopy (Figs. 13.2, 13.3, 13.4, 13.5, 13.6, 13.7, 13.8, 13.9, 13.10, 13.11, 13.12, 13.13, 13.14, 13.15, and 13.16). Pseudocondyloma shows uniform finger-like protrusions,

J. Liu, X. Zou, *Practical Dermoscopy*, https://doi.org/10.1007/978-981-19-1460-7_13

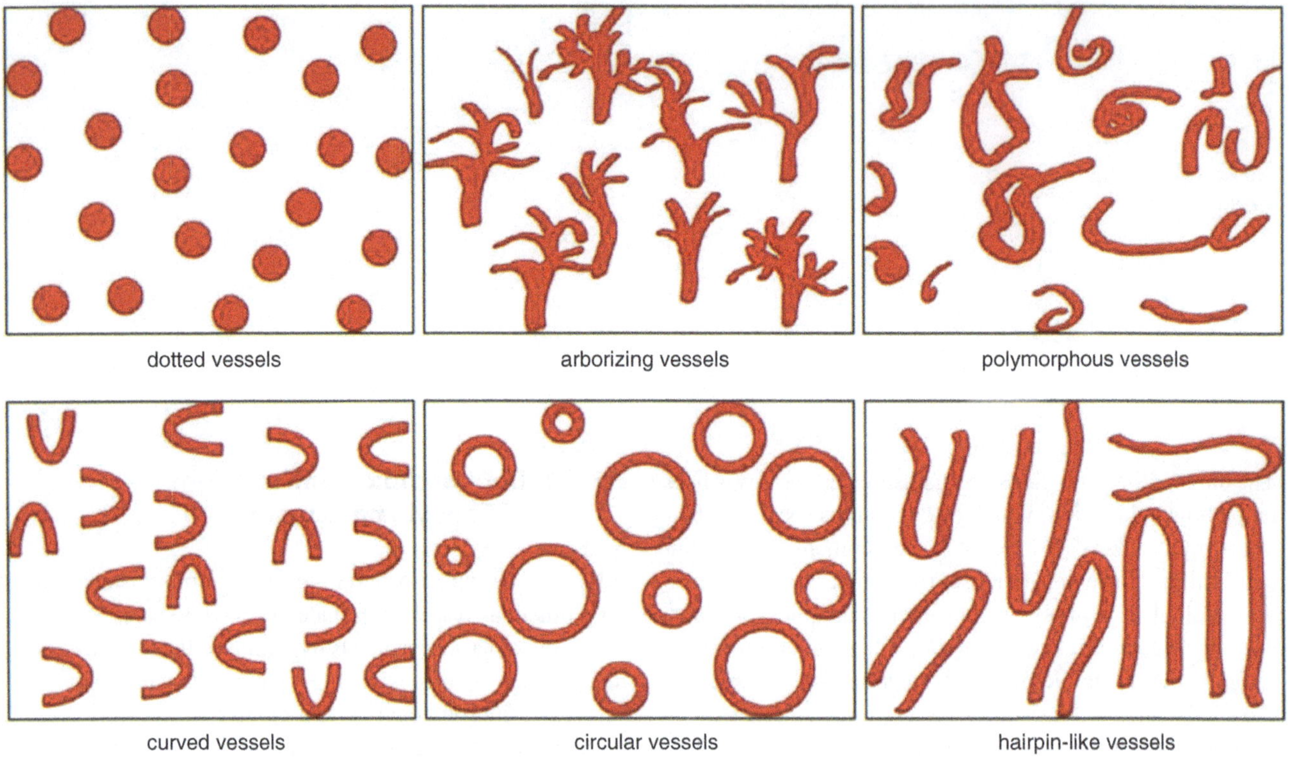

Fig. 13.1 Schematic diagram of vessel morphology

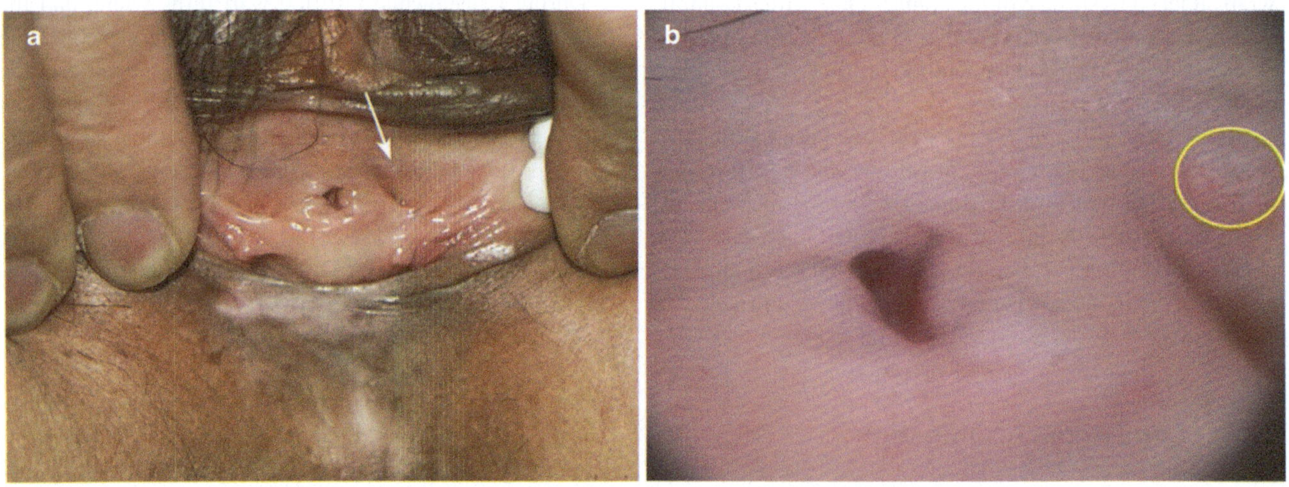

Fig. 13.2 Condyloma acuminatum (1). (**a**) Clinical appearance: a tiny skin lesion, whose diagnosis cannot be confirmed. (**b**) Dermoscopy: a flat papule with arborizing vessels (×10)

with dotted, glomerular, or comma-shaped vessels in the center. Pearly penile papules show uniform small papillary protrusions with dotted or globular vessels in the center. Bowenoid papulosis shows an unspecific pattern: light-brown to dark-brown papilloma or hyperkeratosis, brown-gray structureless areas, linear brown-gray dots, and dotted, globular, or hairpin-like vessels.

13.2 Verruca Plana

Verruca plana is an infectious dermatosis caused by HPV, and it mainly occurs in young adults, presenting as flat, round to oval, and rice- to soybean-sized papules with hazel or normal skin color and smooth surfaces that can be scattered or gathered in groups (Figs. 13.17, 13.18, and 13.19).

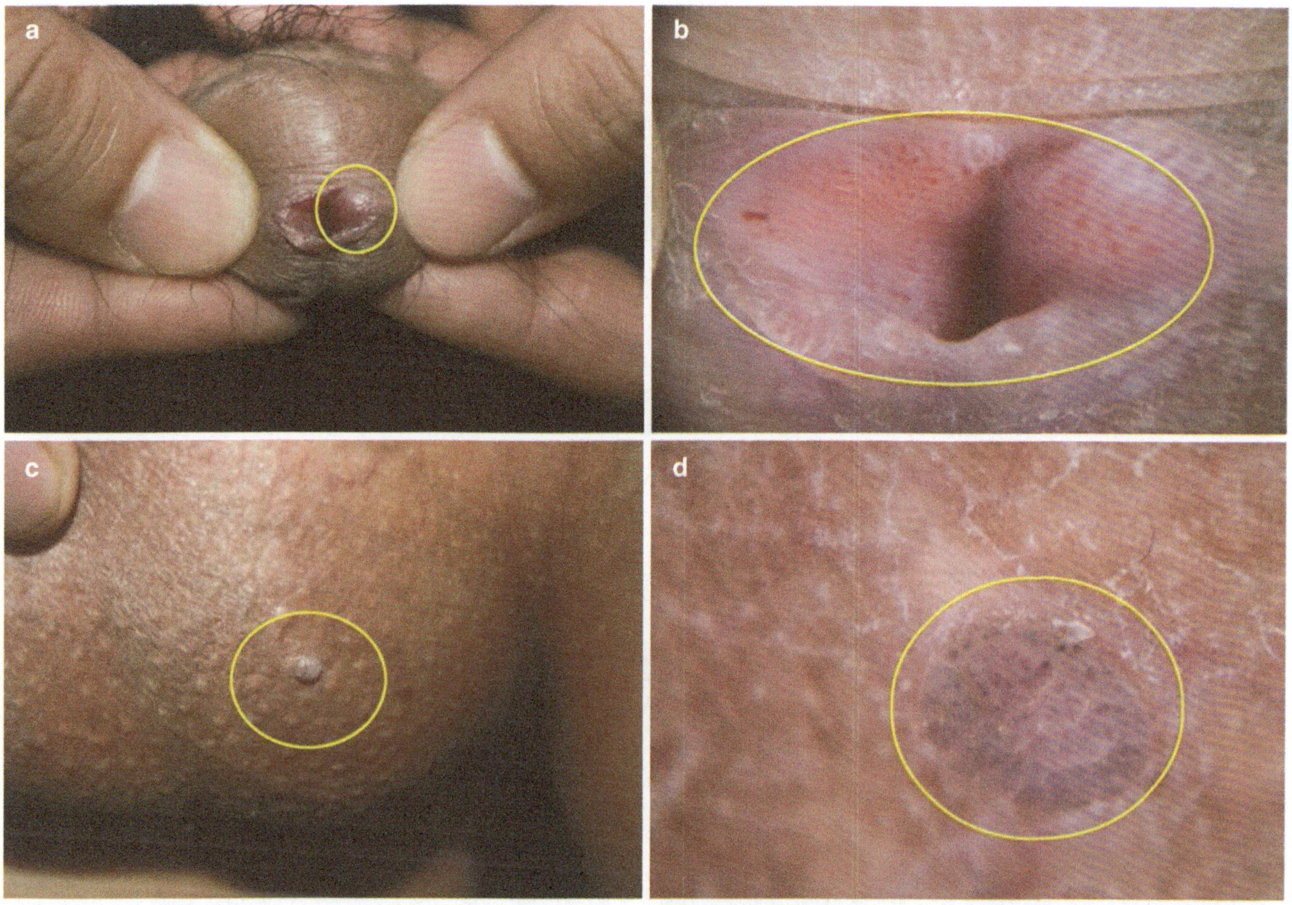

Fig. 13.3 Condyloma acuminatum (2). (**a**) Clinical appearance: a tiny skin lesion, whose diagnosis cannot be confirmed. (**b**) Dermoscopy: dotted, globular, or comma-like vessels (×10). (**c**) Clinical appearance of another lesion in the same patient: a flat, smooth, and brownish papule (×10). (**d**) Dermoscopy: papillary hyperplasia with dotted vessels and the mosaic pattern (×10)

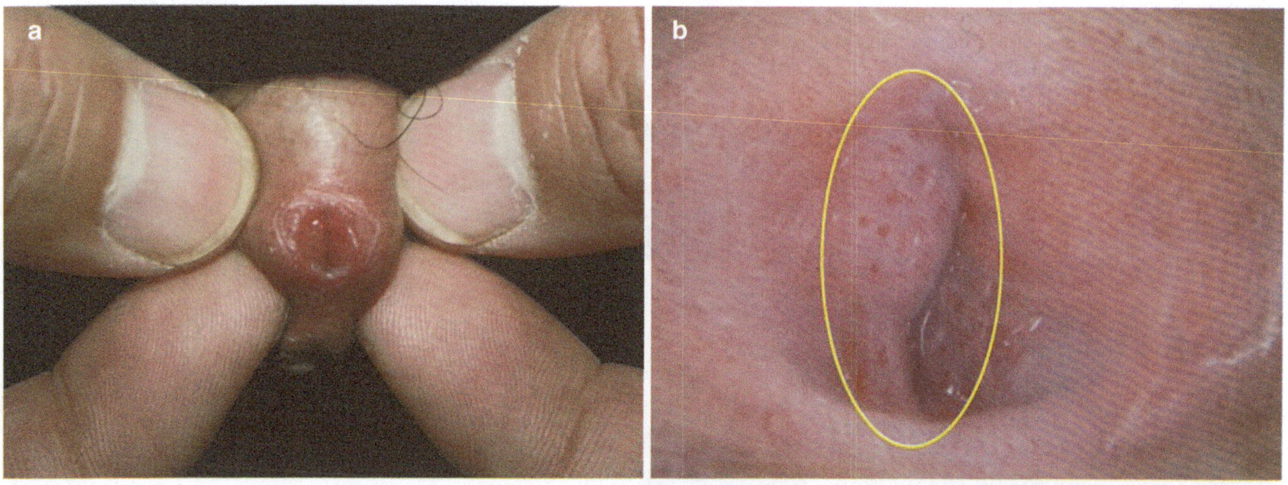

Fig. 13.4 Condyloma acuminatum (3). (**a**) Clinical appearance: no obvious warts. (**b**) Dermoscopy: a flat papule inside the urethra with dotted or globular vessels (×10)

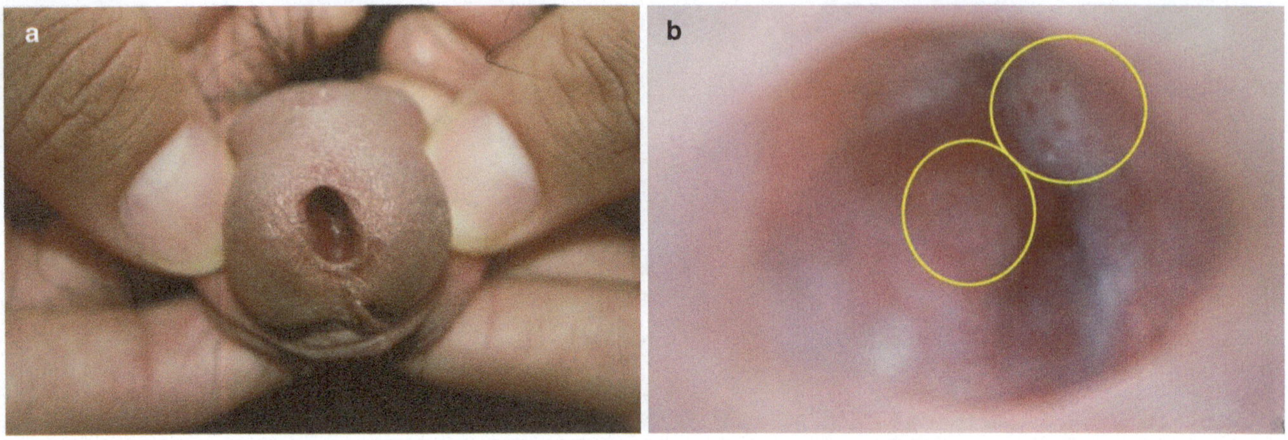

Fig. 13.5 Condyloma acuminatum (4). (**a**) Clinical appearance: no obvious warts. (**b**) Dermoscopy: multiple flat papules inside the urethra with dotted or globular vessels (×10)

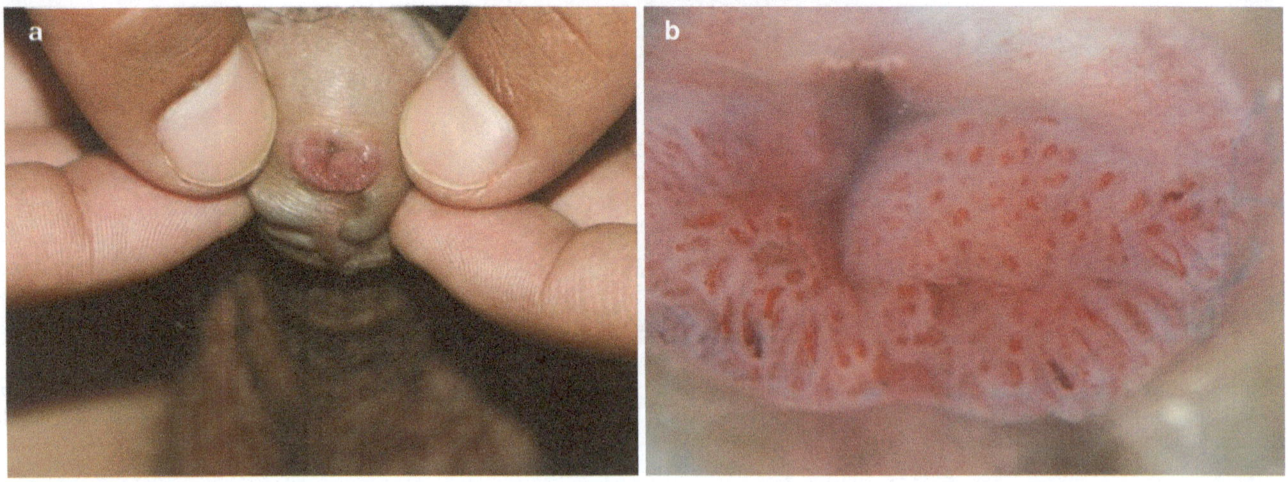

Fig. 13.6 Condyloma acuminatum (5). (**a**) Clinical appearance: wart body covers one-half of the urethral orifice. (**b**) Dermoscopy: papillary hyperplasia covers three-fourth of the urethral orifice with dotted, globular, or hairpin-like vessels (×10)

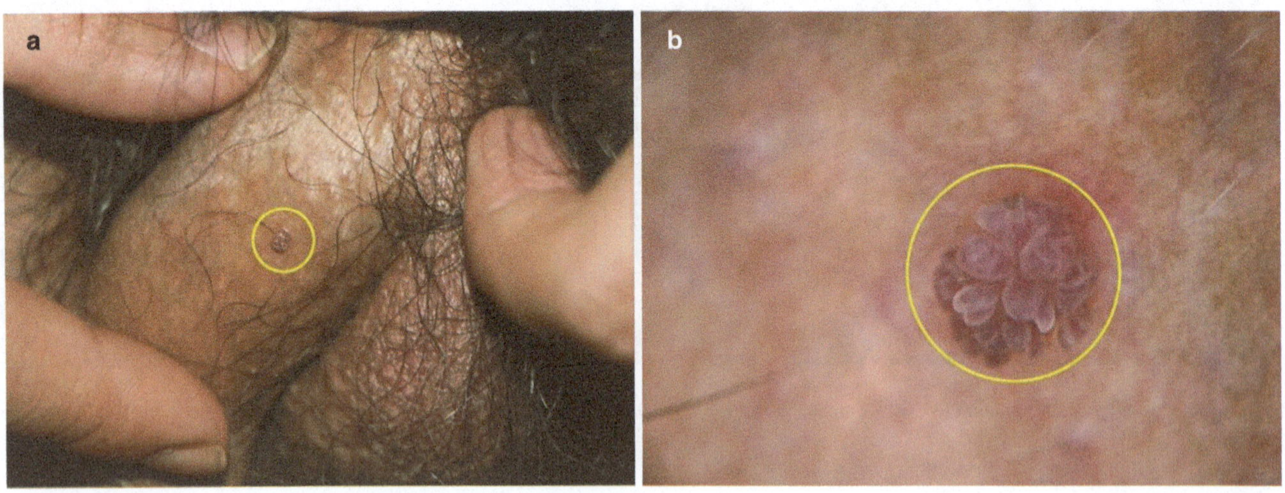

Fig. 13.7 Condyloma acuminatum (6). (**a**) Clinical appearance: flat, smooth, and brown papule. (**b**) Dermoscopy: clustered papillary hyperplasia with polymorphous vessels (×10)

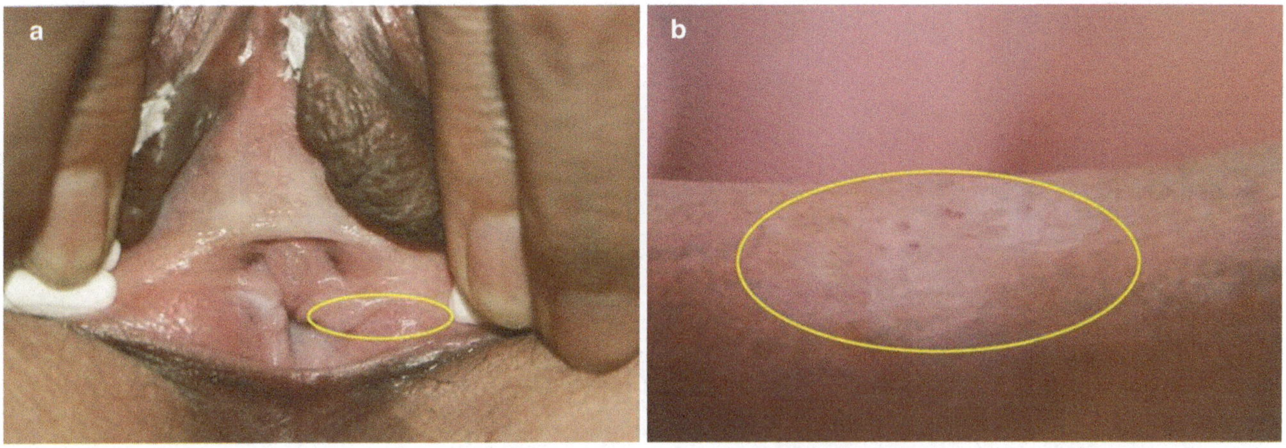

Fig. 13.8 Condyloma acuminatum (7). (**a**) Clinical appearance: generally normal. (**b**) Dermoscopy: flat papules with dotted or globular vessels (×10)

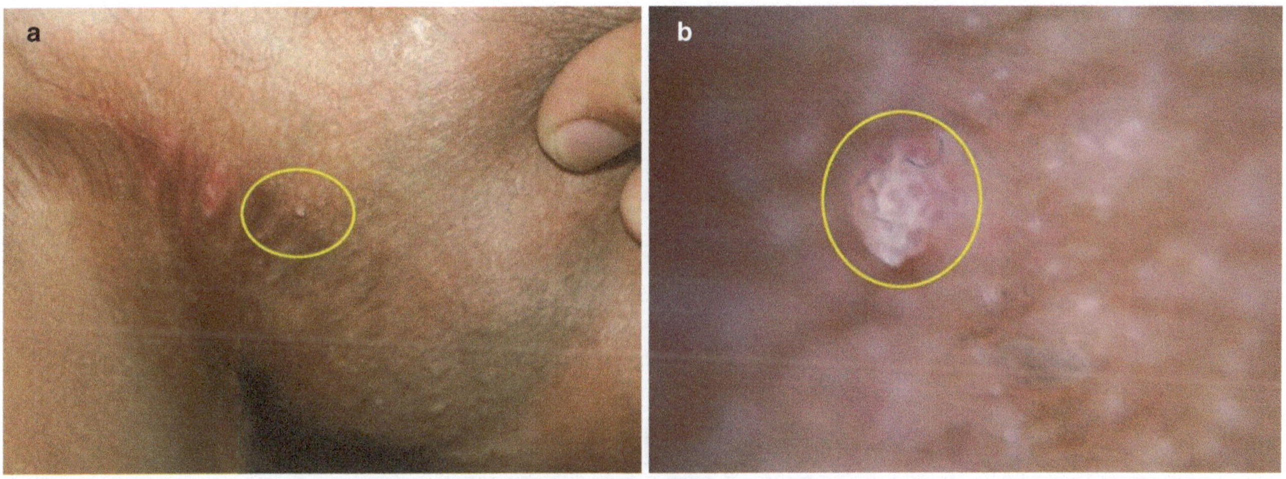

Fig. 13.9 Condyloma acuminatum (8). (**a**) Clinical appearance: a single skin-colored papule. (**b**) Dermoscopy: a single papillary papule with polymorphous vessels, surrounded by dotted white micro papules that are multiple tiny wart bodies (×10)

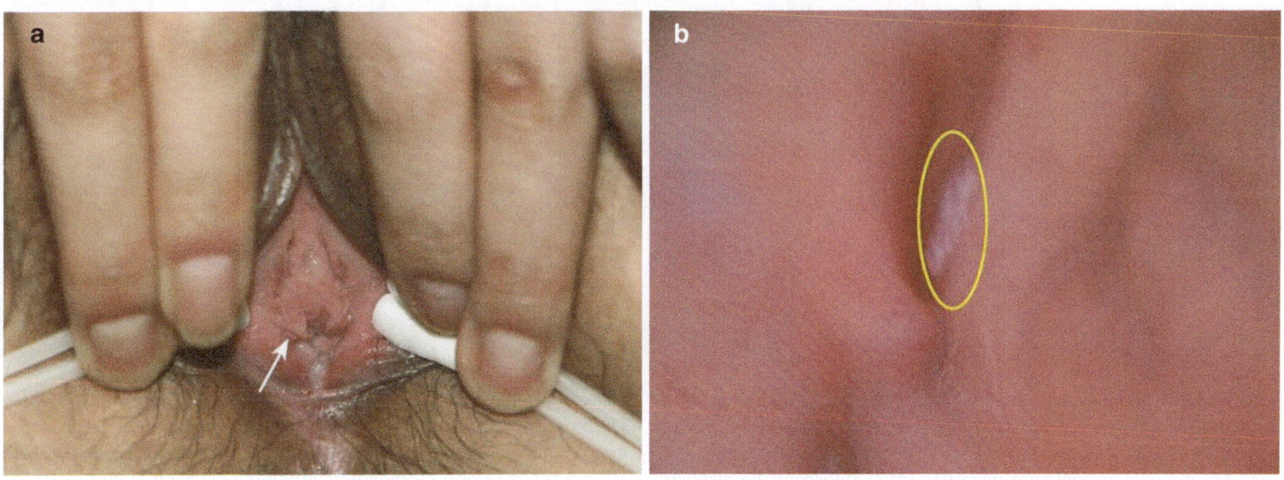

Fig. 13.10 Condyloma acuminatum (9). (**a**) Clinical appearance: single tiny skin-colored papule. (**b**) Dermoscopy: elongated milky white flat papule with polymorphous vessels (×10)

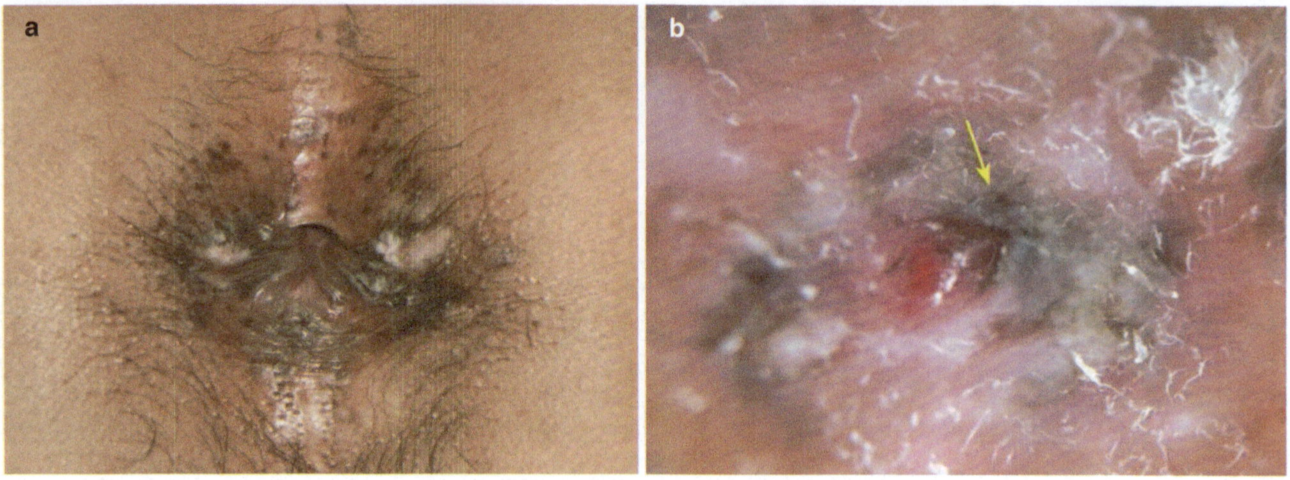

Fig. 13.11 Bowenoid papulosis. (**a**) Clinical appearance: multiple, perianal, brownish-black flat papules. (**b**) Dermoscopy: white- or brownish-gray structureless areas with no apparent vascular structure (×10)

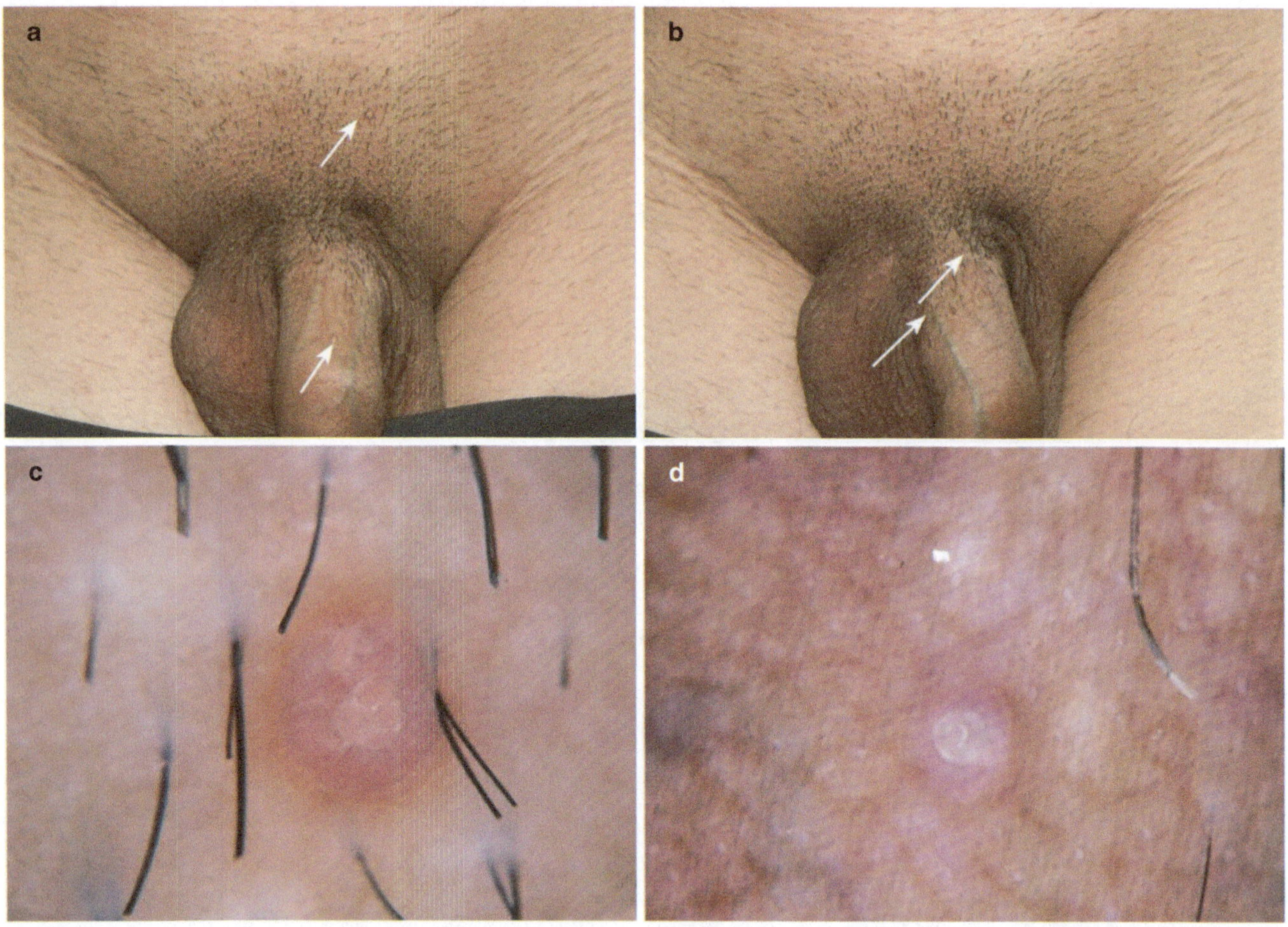

Fig. 13.12 Condyloma acuminatum and molluscum contagiosum. (**a**, **b**) Clinical appearance: four tiny lesions. (**c**) Dermoscopy: central clover-shaped amorphous structure with peripheral radial vessels, diagnosed as molluscum contagiosum (×10). (**d**) Dermoscopy: hemispherical warts with a central round yellow homogeneous area with peripheral crown-like vessels, diagnosed as molluscum contagiosum (×10). (**e**) Dermoscopy: papillary warts with polymorphous vessels, diagnosed as condyloma acuminatum (×10). (**f**) Dermoscopy: oval papules with polymorphous vessels, diagnosed as condyloma acuminatum (×10)

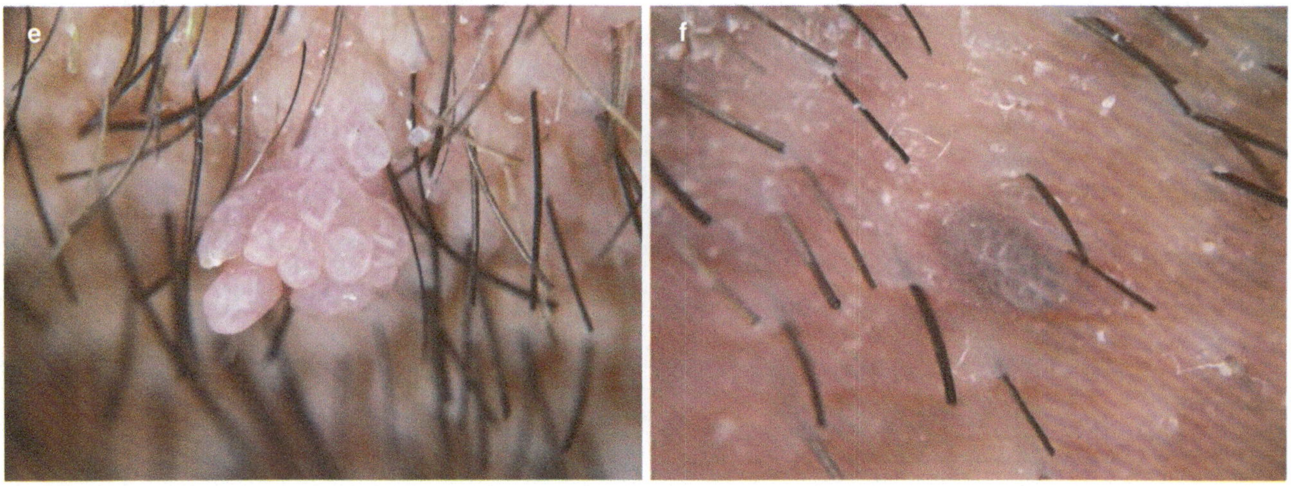

Fig. 13.12 (continued)

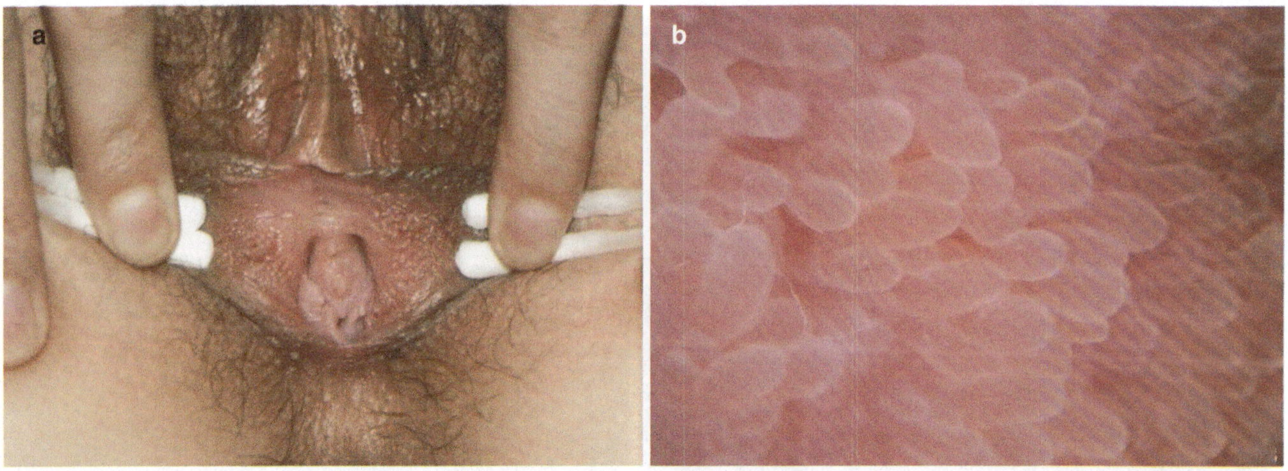

Fig. 13.13 Pseudocondyloma (1). (**a**) Clinical appearance: skin-colored papules clustered like fish roe. (**b**) Dermoscopy: uniform finger-like protrusions with smooth surfaces and dotted vessels (×10)

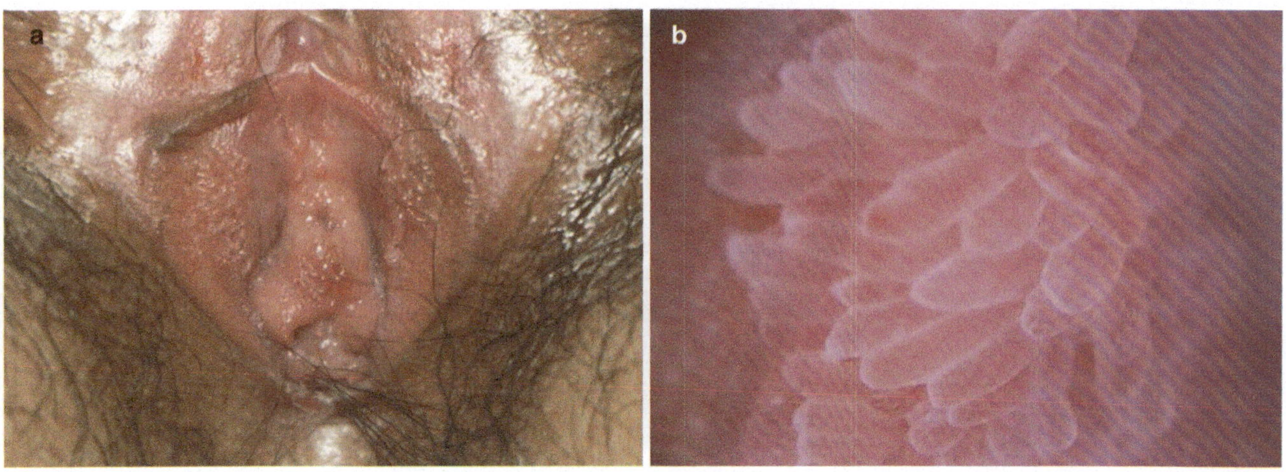

Fig. 13.14 Pseudocondyloma (2). (**a**) Clinical appearance: skin-colored papules clustered like fish roe. (**b**) Dermoscopy: uniform and consistent finger-like protrusions with smooth surfaces and dotted vessels inside (×10)

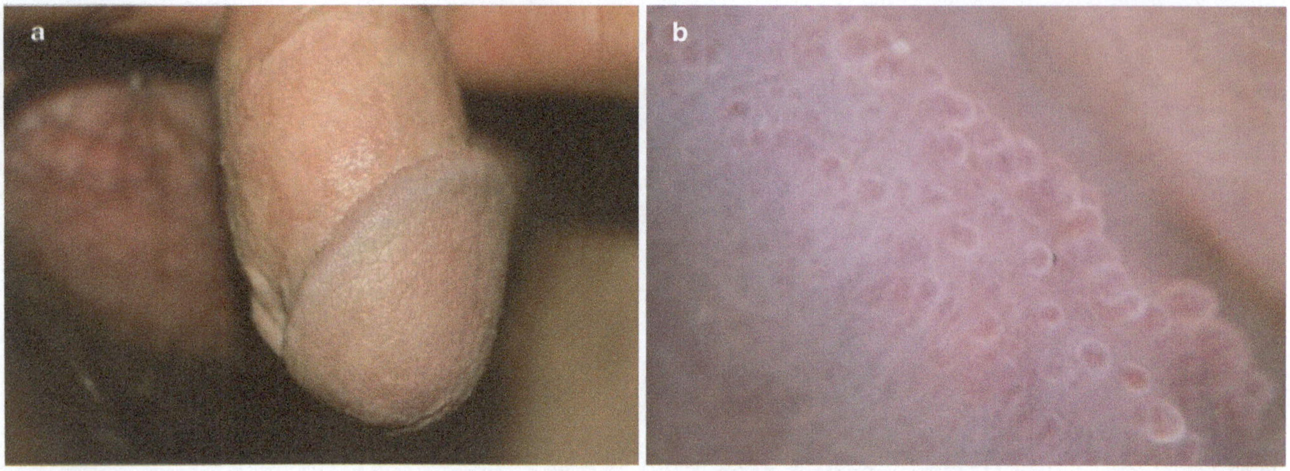

Fig. 13.15 Pearly penile papules (1). (**a**) Clinical appearance: small skin-colored papules of generally the same size encompass the coronal sulcus. (**b**) Dermoscopy: uniform papillary protrusions with dotted vessels and smooth surfaces (×10)

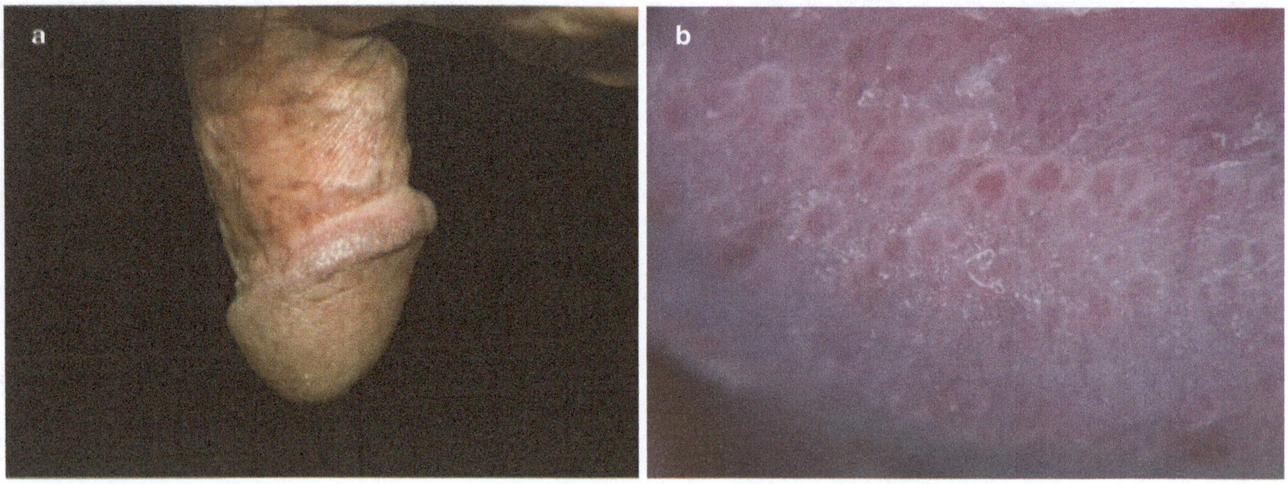

Fig. 13.16 Pearly penile papules (2). (**a**) Clinical appearance: small skin-colored papules, generally equal in size, located around the coronal sulcus. (**b**) Dermoscopy: uniform papillary protrusions with dotted vessels and smooth surfaces (×10)

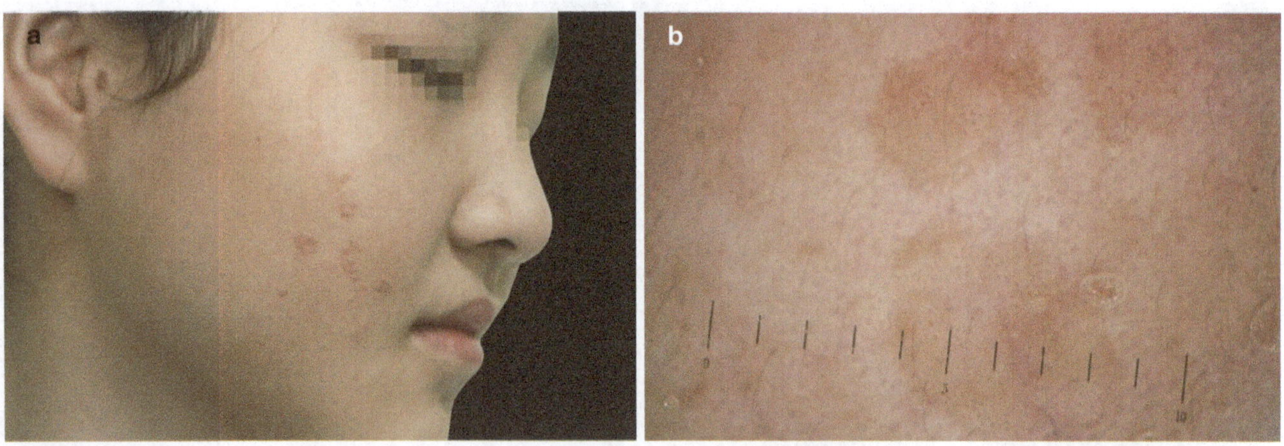

Fig. 13.17 Verruca plana (1). (**a**) Clinical appearance: skin-colored flat papules. (**b**) Dermoscopy: uniformly distributed dotted vessels and the mosaic pattern (×10)

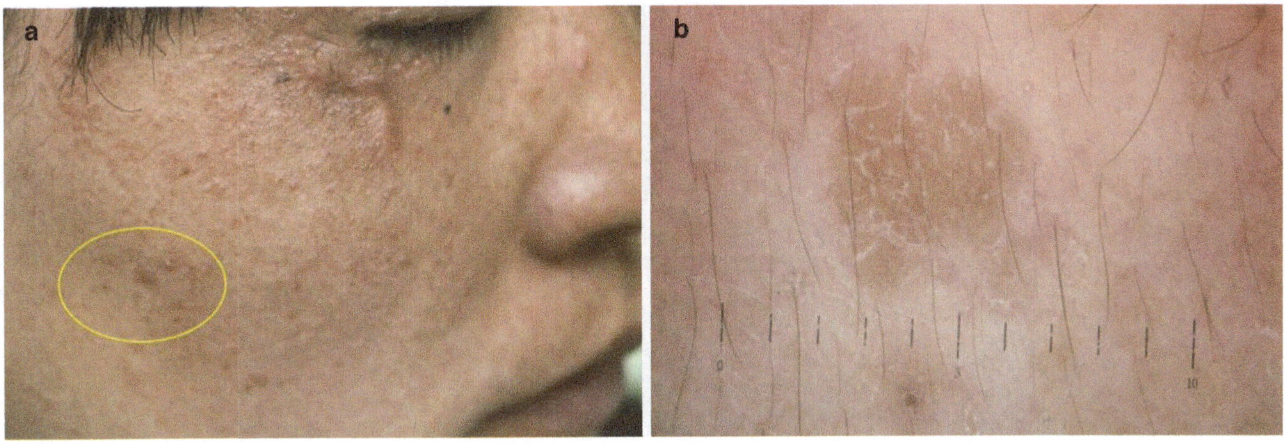

Fig. 13.18 Verruca plana (2). (**a**) Clinical appearance: skin-colored flat papules. (**b**) Dermoscopy: uniformly distributed dotted vessels and the mosaic pattern (×10)

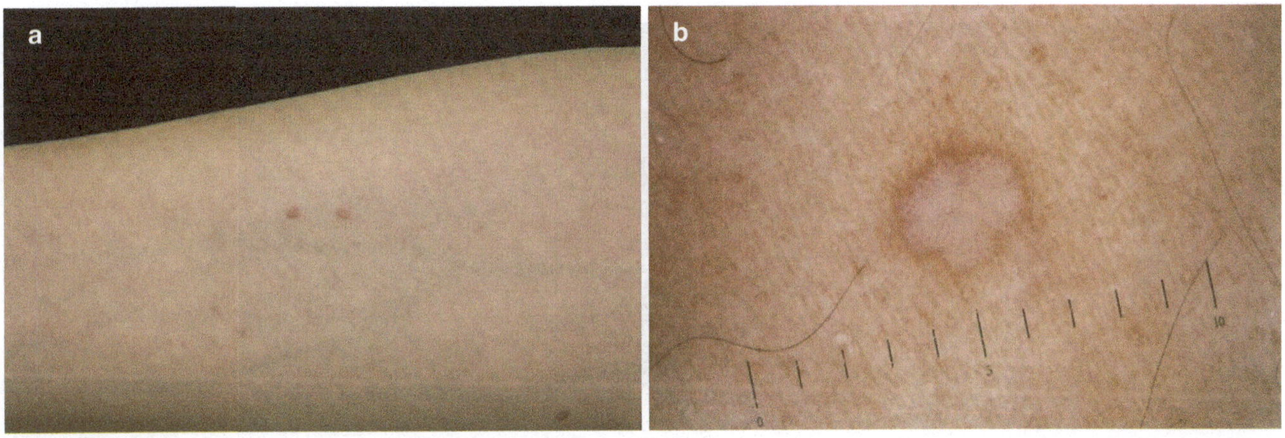

Fig. 13.19 Verruca plana (3). (**a**) Clinical appearance: skin-colored flat papules. (**b**) Dermoscopy: uniformly distributed dotted vessels and the mosaic pattern (×10)

13.2.1 Dermoscopic Manifestations of Verruca Plana

Dermoscopy shows regularly distributed dotted vessels on a light-brown, skin-colored to yellow background, histologically corresponding to the top of the capillaries in the dermal papillae.

13.2.2 Significance of Dermoscopy in the Diagnosis and Treatment of Verruca Plana

1. Differentiate it from solar lentigo and seborrheic keratosis.
2. Assess whether the disease is cured.

13.3 Verruca Vulgaris

Verruca vulgaris is an infectious dermatosis caused by HPV that mainly involves the fingers or dorsum of the hand in children and young adults, presenting as round to oval, light-yellow or dirty brown, single or multiple papillary lesions with rough surfaces (Figs. 13.20, 13.21, and 13.22).

13.3.1 Dermoscopic Manifestations of Verruca Vulgaris

Dermoscopy shows multiple papillary projections, with central red-dotted or looped vessels and peripheral white halos. These dotted vessels are slightly larger than those in verruca plana and are often accompanied by hemorrhage and capillary thrombosis.

13.3.2 Significance of Dermoscopy in the Diagnosis and Treatment of Verruca Vulgaris

1. Differentiate it from seborrheic keratosis.
2. Assess whether the disease is cured.

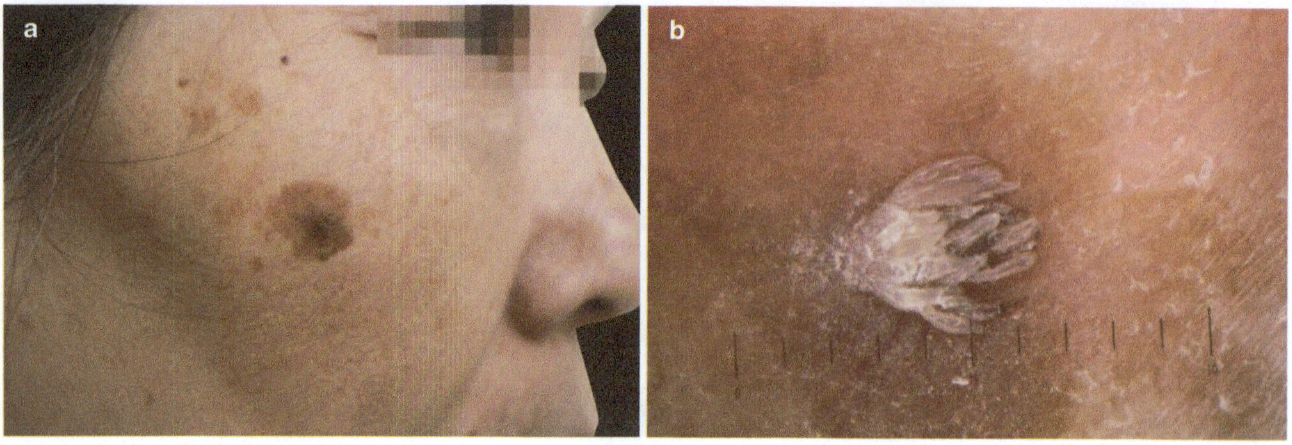

Fig. 13.20 Verruca vulgaris (1). (**a**) Clinical appearance: skin-colored papules on seborrheic keratosis. (**b**) Dermoscopy: finger-like protrusions with thrombus or hemorrhage (×10)

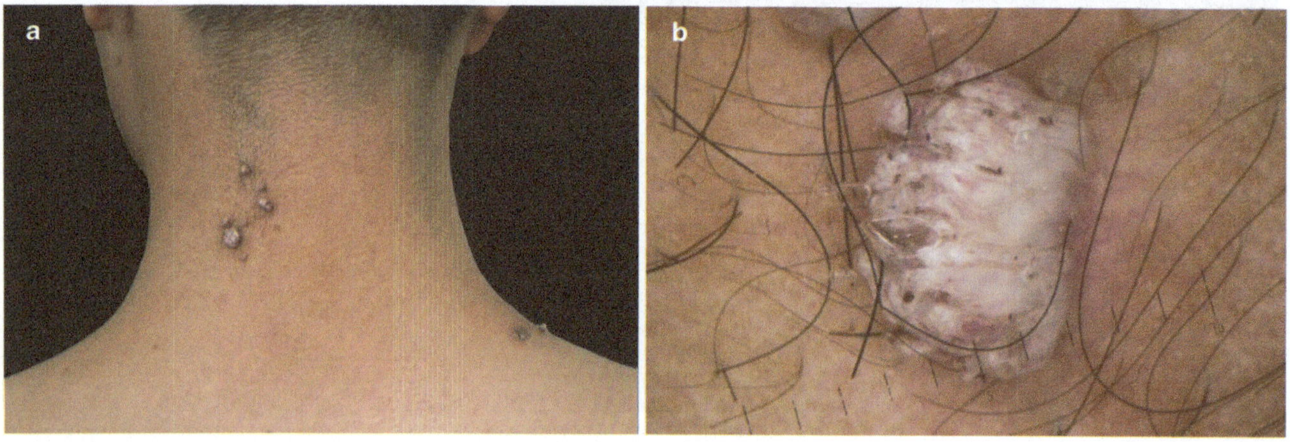

Fig. 13.21 Verruca vulgaris (2). (**a**) Clinical appearance: multiple verrucous hyperplastic keratotic skin lesions. (**b**) Dermoscopy: milky white verrucous hyperplasia with dotted, hairpin-like vessels and hemorrhages (×10)

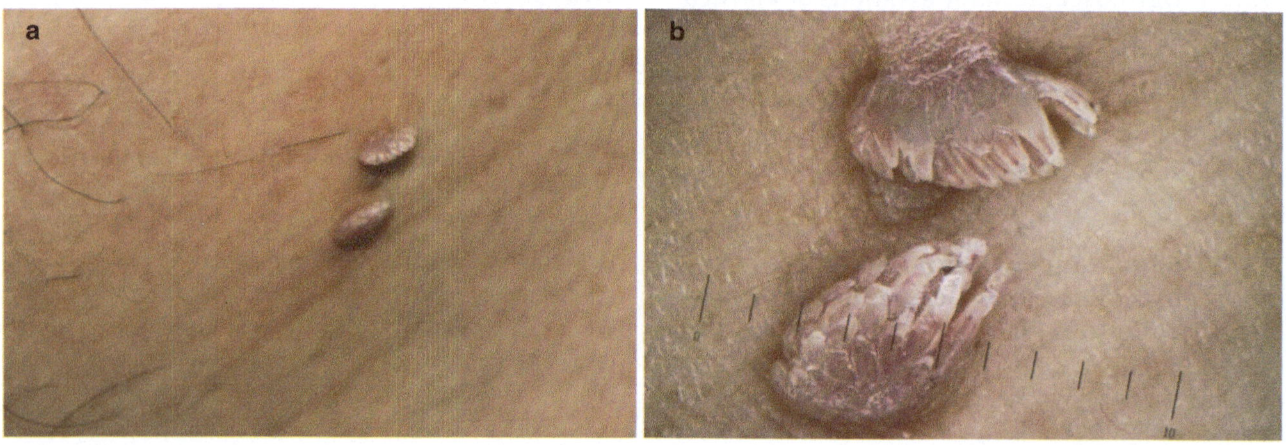

Fig. 13.22 Verruca vulgaris (3). (**a**) Clinical appearance: two verrucous hyperplastic keratotic skin lesions. (**b**) Dermoscopy: verrucous hyperplasia with dotted and hairpin-like vessels in the center (×10)

13.4 Periungual Warts

Periungual warts are verruca vulgaris that form around the nails. If a periungual wart spreads under the nail, it can cause damage to the nail plate, leading to fissures, pain, or secondary infection (Figs. 13.23 and 13.24).

13.4.1 Dermoscopic Manifestations of Periungual Warts

1. Verrucous hyperplasia with discontinuous dermatoglyphs and rough surface.
2. Dotted and globular vessels, hemorrhages, and thrombosis caused by pressure and friction.

13.4.2 Significance of Dermoscopy in the Diagnosis and Treatment of Periungual Warts

1. Differentiate it from onychomycosis.
2. Assess whether the disease is cured.

13.5 Verruca Plantaris

Verruca plantaris is a type of verruca vulgaris that occurs on the sole of the foot. Trauma or friction is the main inducement for it. It presents as a dirty-gray or gray-brown round keratotic lesion with a rough surface surrounded by a slightly thickened keratinized circle (Figs. 13.25 and 13.26).

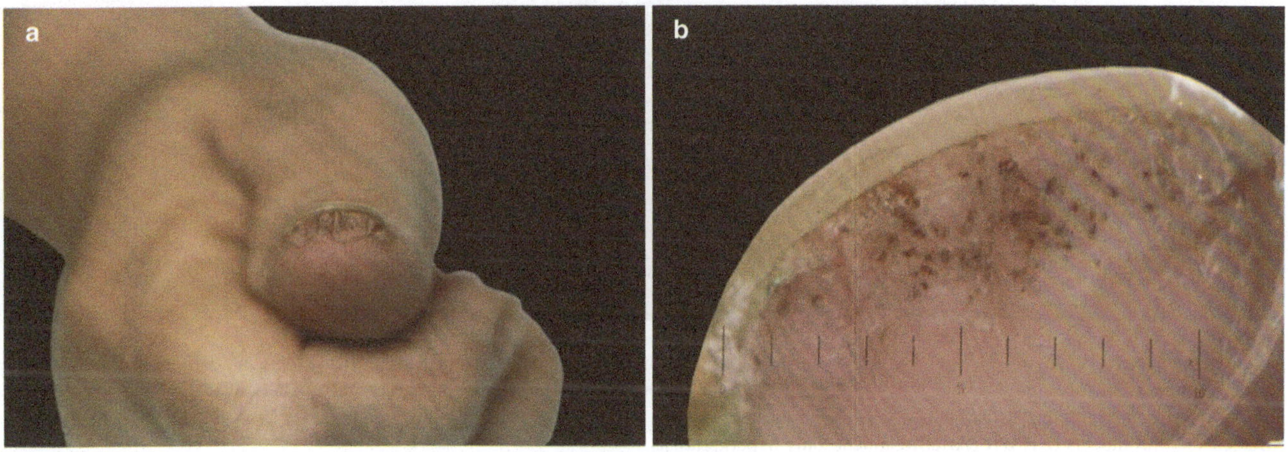

Fig. 13.23 Periungual wart (1). (**a**) Clinical appearance: verrucous hyperplastic lesion with a rough surface. (**b**) Dermoscopy: verrucous hyperplasia with rough keratotic surface and dotted vessels (×10)

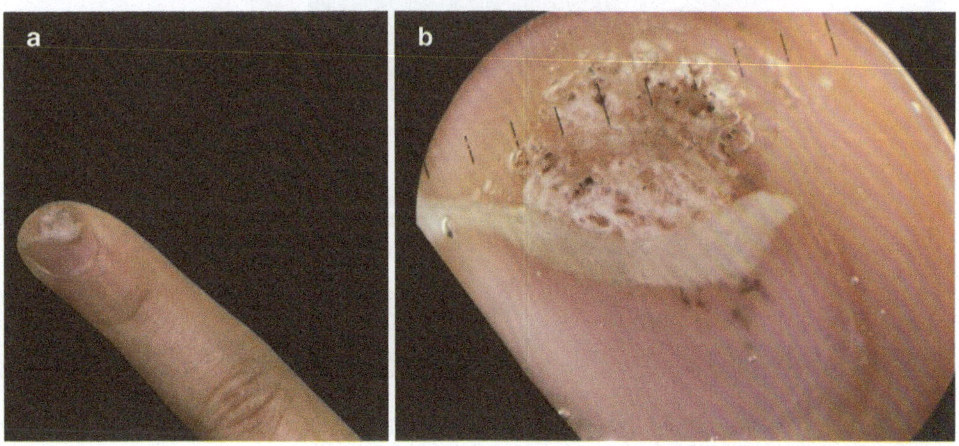

Fig. 13.24 Periungual wart (2). (**a**) Clinical appearance: verrucous hyperplastic lesion with a rough surface. (**b**) Dermoscopy: verrucous hyperplasia with a rough surface, dotted vessels, and subungual hemorrhages (×10)

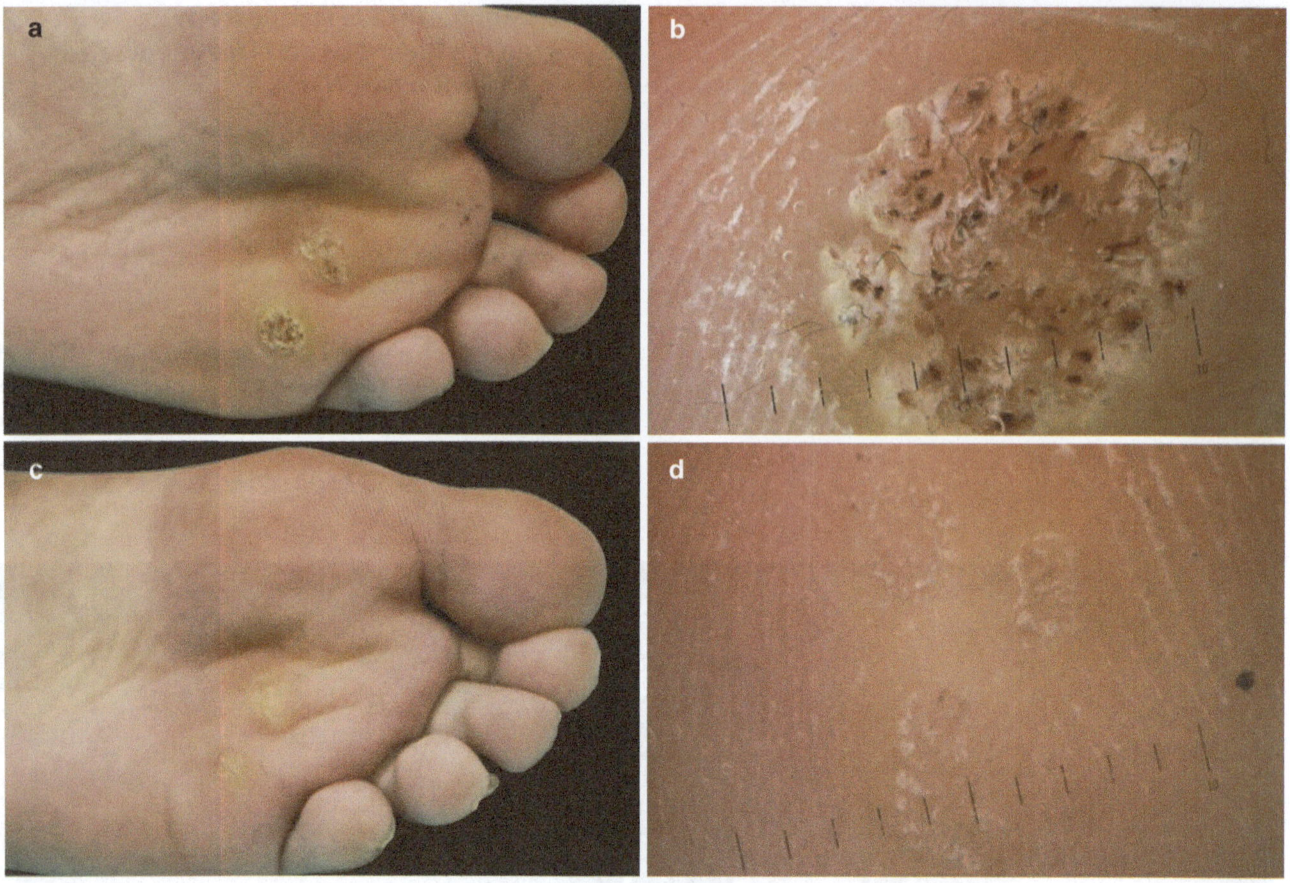

Fig. 13.25 Verruca plantaris (1). (**a**) Clinical appearance: keratotic hyperplastic lesion with a rough surface. (**b**) Dermoscopy: hyperkeratosis with a rough surface, discontinuous dermatoglyphs, spot hemorrhages, and thrombosis (×10). (**c**) After treatment, only hyperkeratosis is seen. (**d**) Dermoscopy: after treatment, hyperkeratosis and spot thrombosis can still be observed, which indicates that the lesion has not cured yet (×10)

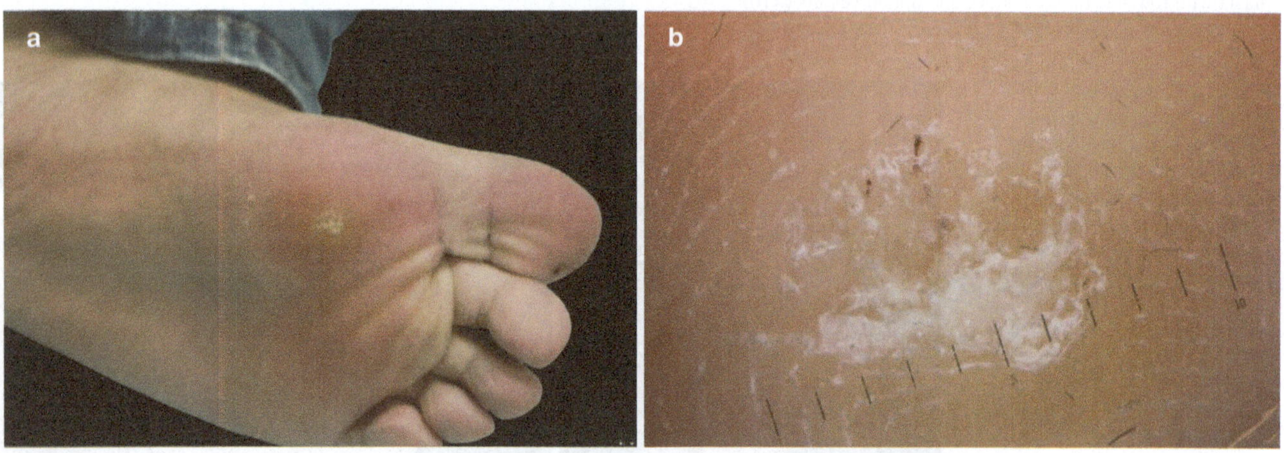

Fig. 13.26 Verruca plantaris (2). (**a**) Clinical appearance: hyperkeratotic lesion with a rough surface. (**b**) Dermoscopy: hyperkeratosis with a rough surface, discontinuous dermatoglyphs, and spot thrombosis (×10)

13.5.1 Dermoscopic Manifestations of Verruca Plantaris

1. Discontinuous dermatoglyphs with rough surface.
2. Light-brown or yellow structureless background, on which there are many irregular red-brown-black dots or linear streaks (hemorrhages) due to the long-term pressure or friction on the plantar foot.

13.5.2 Significance of Dermoscopy in the Diagnosis and Treatment of Verruca Plantaris

1. Differentiate it from a callus (Fig. 13.27), clavus (Figs. 13.28 and 13.29), and acral melanoma.
2. Assess whether the disease is cured.

13.6 Molluscum Contagiosum

Molluscum contagiosum is caused by a virus known as *Molluscum contagiosum* virus (MCV). Molluscum contagiosum may occur in any age, more frequent in children. The typical lesions are waxy, shiny, umbilicated, pearly papules with an average diameter of 2–4 mm (Figs. 13.30, 13.31, 13.32, 13.33, and 13.34).

13.6.1 Dermoscopic Manifestations of Molluscum Contagiosum

1. The typical feature is central orifice/umbilication with white or yellowish-white amorphous structures (including globular, polylobular, or clover-like aspects).
2. Surrounded by crown-like vessels (radial or branched).

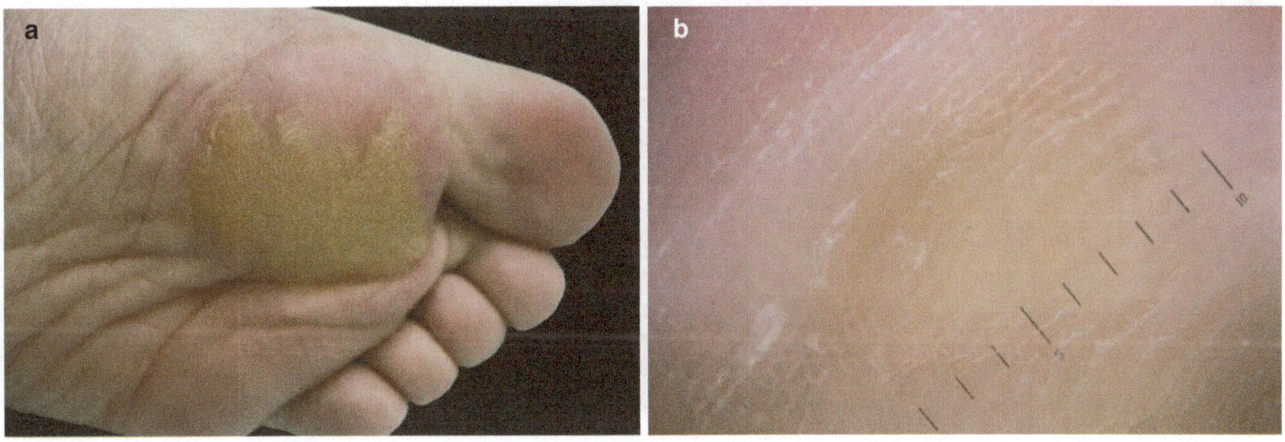

Fig. 13.27 Callus. (**a**) Clinical appearance: patchy hyperkeratotic lesion with a smooth surface. (**b**) Dermoscopy: hyperkeratosis with a smooth surface and continuous dermatoglyphs (×10)

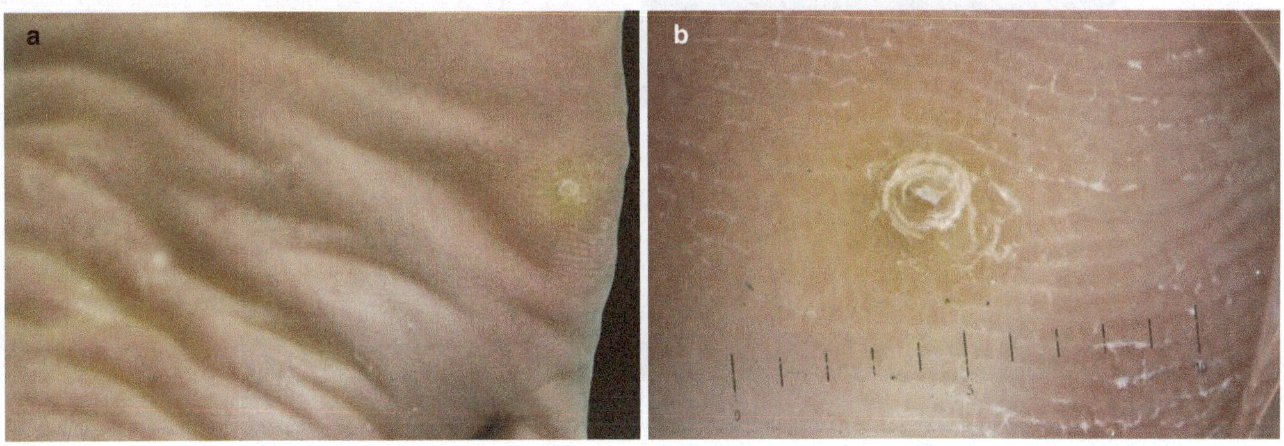

Fig. 13.28 Clavus (1). (**a**) Clinical appearance: a hyperkeratotic lesion with scales in the center. (**b**) Dermoscopy: hyperkeratosis on a light-yellow background, with central scales, discontinuous dermatoglyphs, and a peripheral light-brown halo (×10)

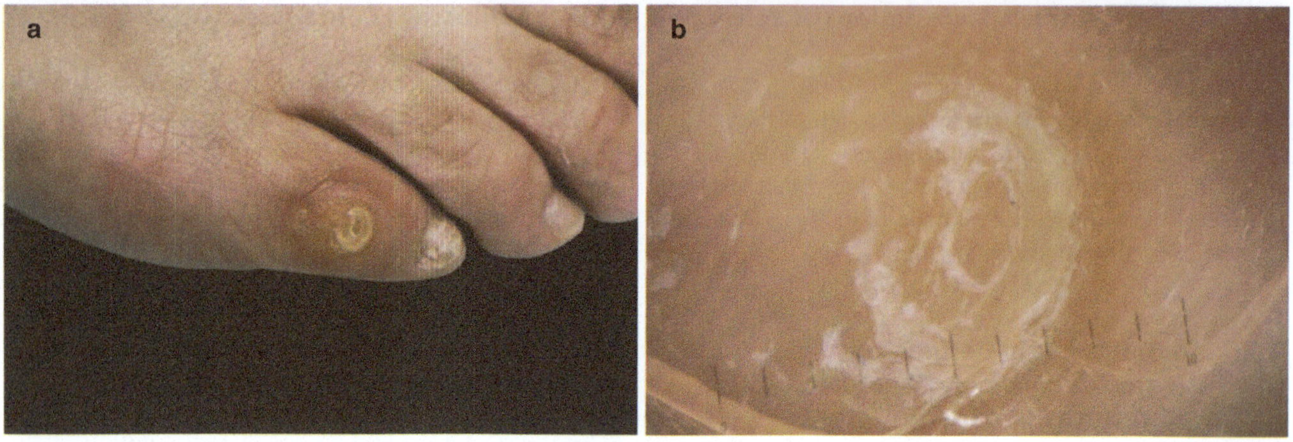

Fig. 13.29 Clavus (2). (**a**) Clinical appearance: a hyperkeratotic lesion with scales in the center. (**b**) Dermoscopy: hyperkeratosis on a light-yellow background, with central scales, discontinuous dermatoglyphs, and a peripheral light-brown halo (×10)

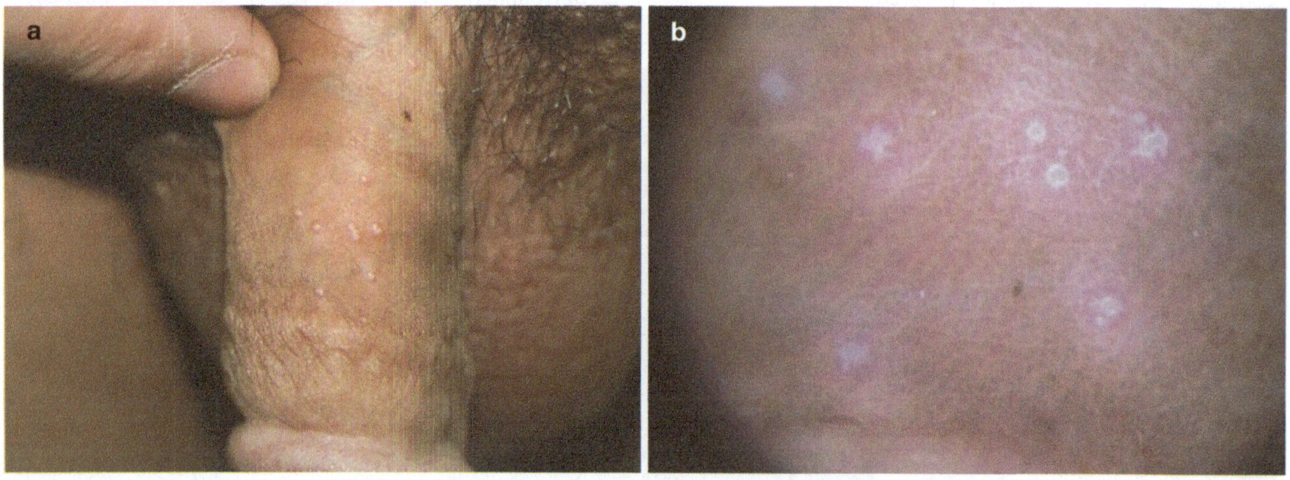

Fig. 13.30 Molluscum contagiosum (1). (**a**) Clinical appearance: multiple millet-sized papules. (**b**) Dermoscopy: white amorphous structures with peripheral erythematous halos (×10)

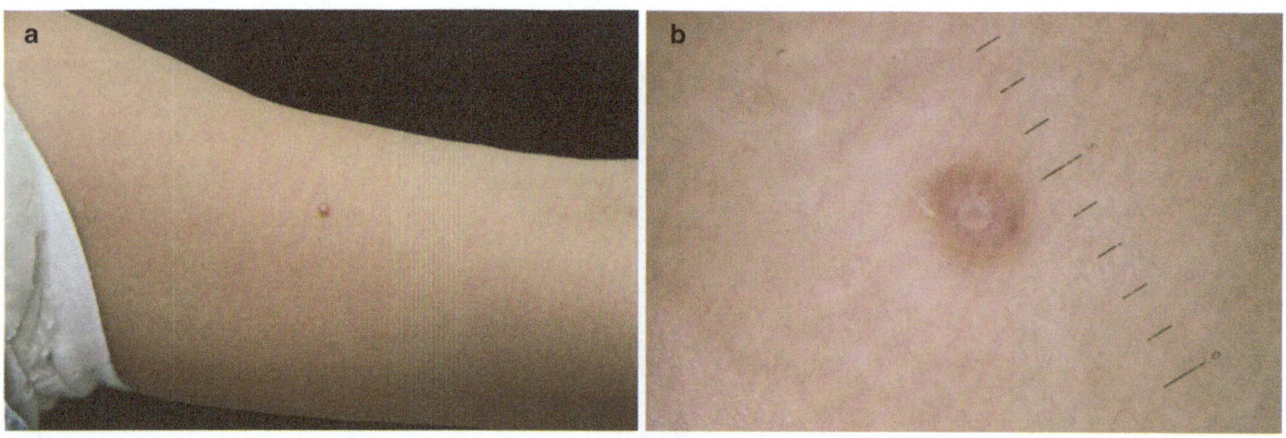

Fig. 13.31 Molluscum contagiosum (2). (**a**) Clinical appearance: a single skin-colored round papule. (**b**) Dermoscopy: central white amorphous structures with peripheral crown-like vessels, making up the halo-like pattern (×10)

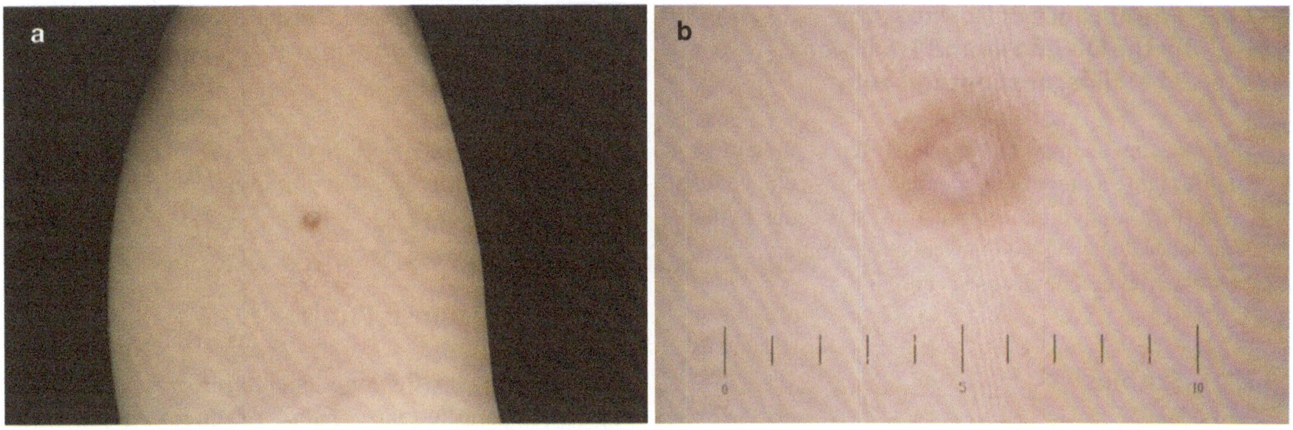

Fig. 13.32 Molluscum contagiosum (3). (**a**) Clinical appearance: a single skin-colored round papule. (**b**) Dermoscopy: white amorphous structures with central umbilication and peripheral crown-like vessels (×10)

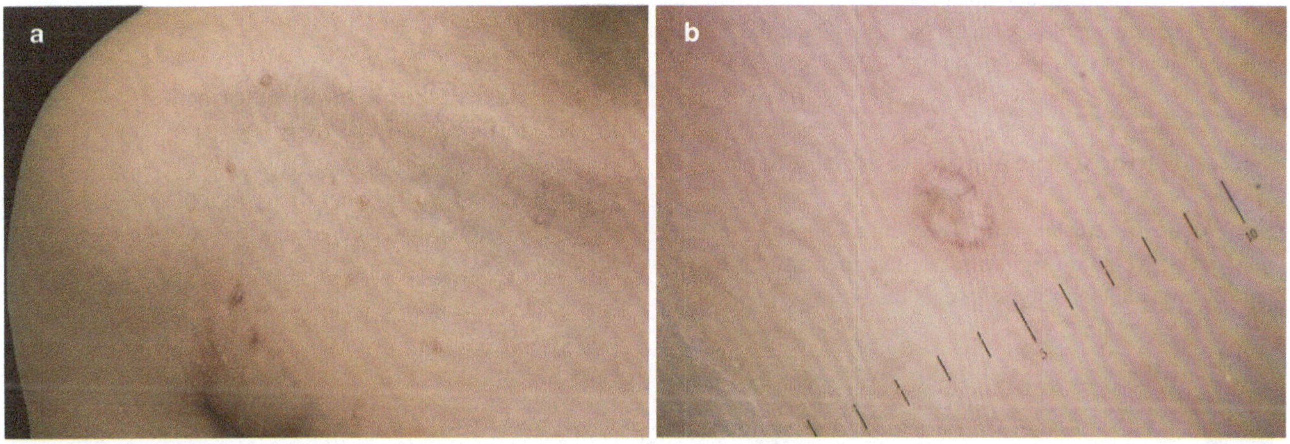

Fig. 13.33 Molluscum contagiosum (4). (**a**) Clinical appearance: multiple skin-colored papules. (**b**) Dermoscopy: central white amorphous structures with peripheral crown-like vessels (×10)

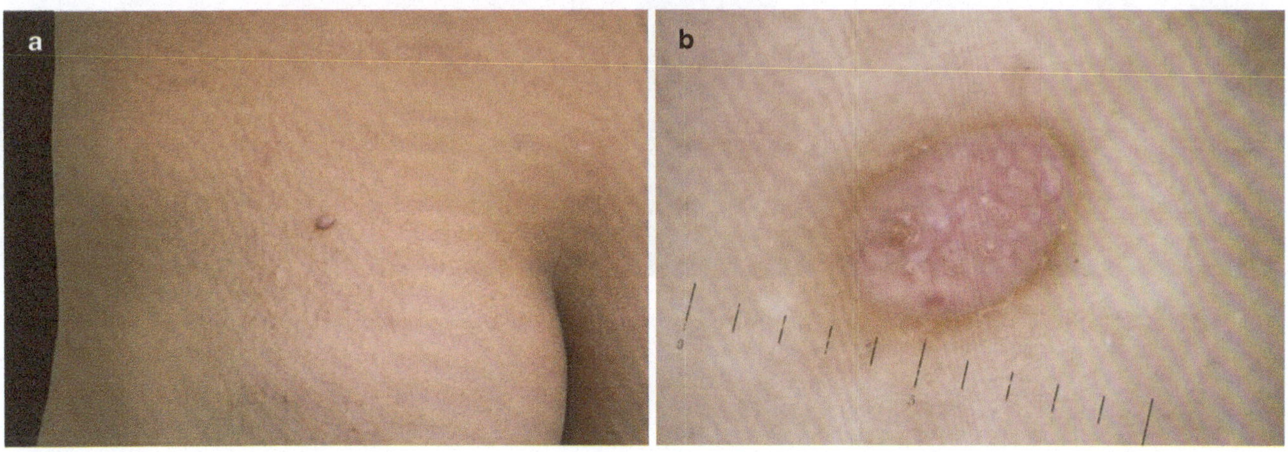

Fig. 13.34 Molluscum contagiosum (5). (**a**) Clinical appearance: a single skin-colored papule. (**b**) Dermoscopy: polylobular white amorphous structures with linear vessels (×10)

13.6.2 Significance of Dermoscopy in the Diagnosis and Treatment of Molluscum Contagiosum

1. Dermoscopy is important for the differentiation of single molluscum contagiosum, genital molluscum contagiosum, tiny condyloma acuminatum, sebaceous hyperplasia, sebaceous nevi, and sebaceous adenoma.
2. Assess whether the disease is cured.

13.7 Scabies

Scabies is a contagious skin disease caused by infestation with the mite *Sarcoptes scabiei var. hominis.* Skin lesions most commonly involve the interdigital spaces, flexor wrists, waist, lower abdomen, and inner thighs. Scabies is characterized by pruritic papules, vesicles or blisters, and the itch that is worse at night (Fig. 13.35).

13.7.1 Dermoscopic Manifestations of Scabies

Dermoscopy reveals the typical serpentine burrow and delta-wing jet with contrail sign where delta represents the anterior part of mite and contrail represents the burrow.

13.7.2 Significance of Dermoscopy in the Diagnosis and Treatment of Scabies

1. Conducive to noninvasive testing and diagnosis.
2. Helpful in differentiation of it from hand eczema.

13.8 Pediculosis Pubis

Pediculosis pubis is an infestation of the pubic area caused by the ectoparasite *Pthirus pubis*. The three stages in the life cycle of *Pthirus pubis* are egg, nymph, and adult. The parasite often attaches to pubic hair, where it bites and thus can cause severe itching (Fig. 13.36).

13.8.1 Dermoscopic Manifestations of Pediculosis Pubis

Polarized light can filter out the reflected light and enables three-dimensional and magnifying observation of the parasites or the eggs.

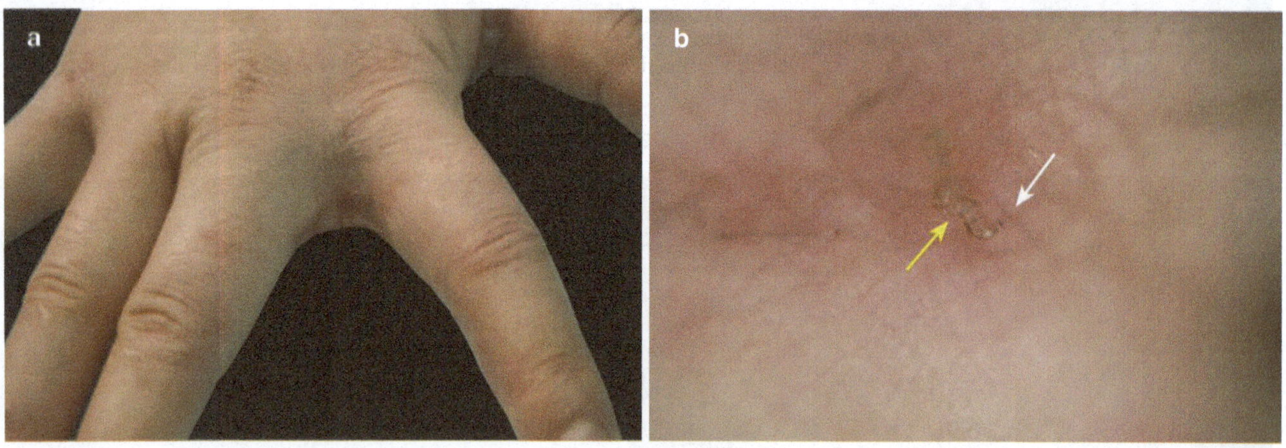

Fig. 13.35 Scabies. (**a**) Clinical appearance: small red papules between the fingers. (**b**) Dermoscopy: typical "serpentine burrow" (yellow arrow) and "delta-wing jet with contrail" sign (white arrow) (×10)

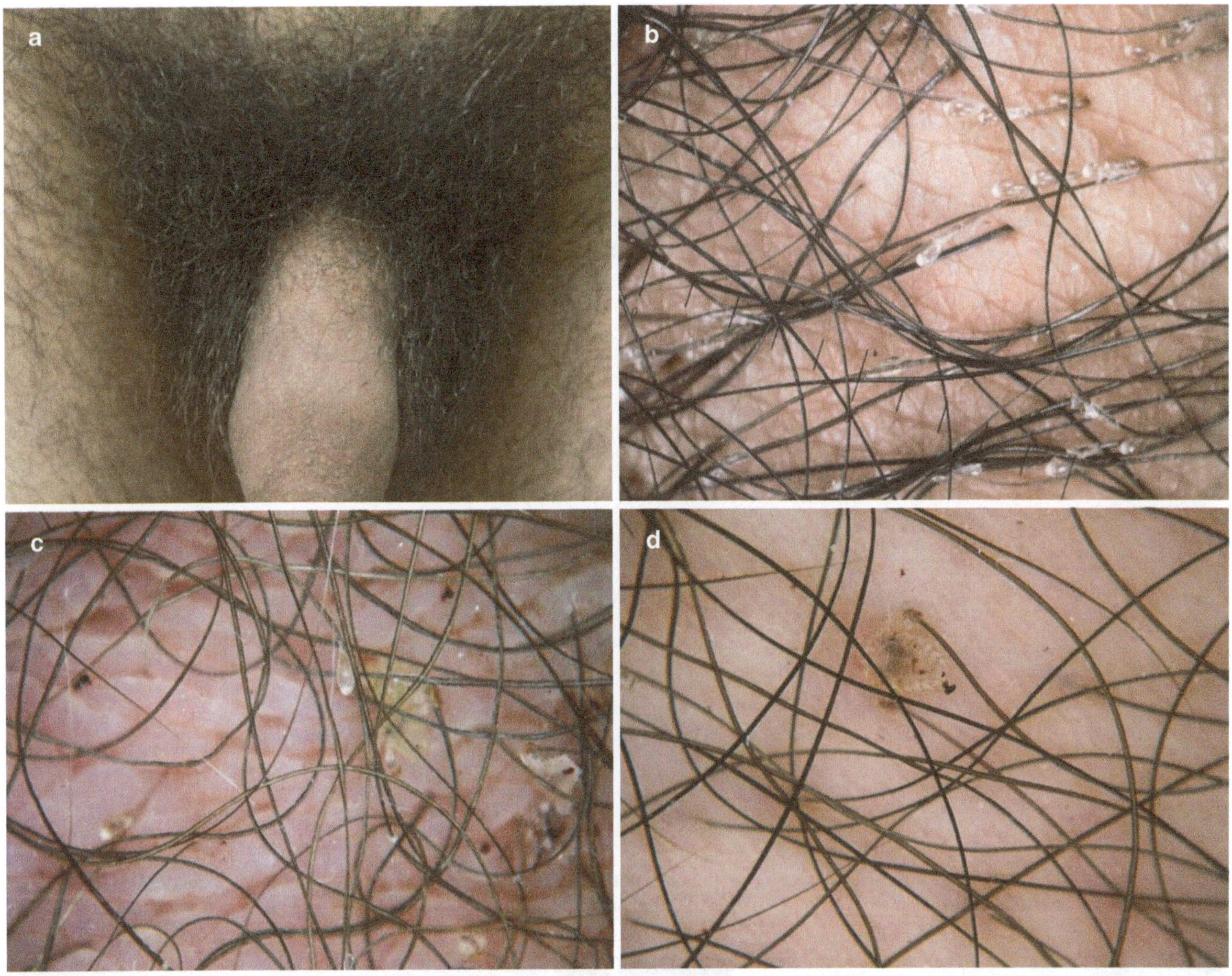

Fig. 13.36 Pediculosis pubis. (**a**) Clinical appearance: there seems to be white scales attached to the pubic hair. (**b**) Dermoscopy: Pthirus pubis eggs (×10). (**c**) Dermoscopy: *Pthirus pubis* eggs and adult (×10). (**d**) Dermoscopy: *Pthirus pubis* adult (×10)

13.8.2 Significance of Dermoscopy in the Diagnosis and Treatment of Pediculosis Pubis

Dermoscopy is helpful in the diagnosis of genital pruritus diseases.

13.9 Tick Bites

Tick bites can cause different degrees of local skin inflammation. A mild lesion presents as erythema with central ecchymosis, while a severe one may present with obvious edema, vesicles, and even persistent nodules and ulcers with tingling pain or itch (Fig. 13.37).

13.9.1 Dermoscopic Manifestations of Tick Bites

Dermoscopy shows the tick and the surrounding inflammation of the bite site.

13.9.2 Significance of Dermoscopy in the Diagnosis and Treatment of Tick Bites

Dermoscopy is helpful to confirm the diagnosis, and remove the tick.

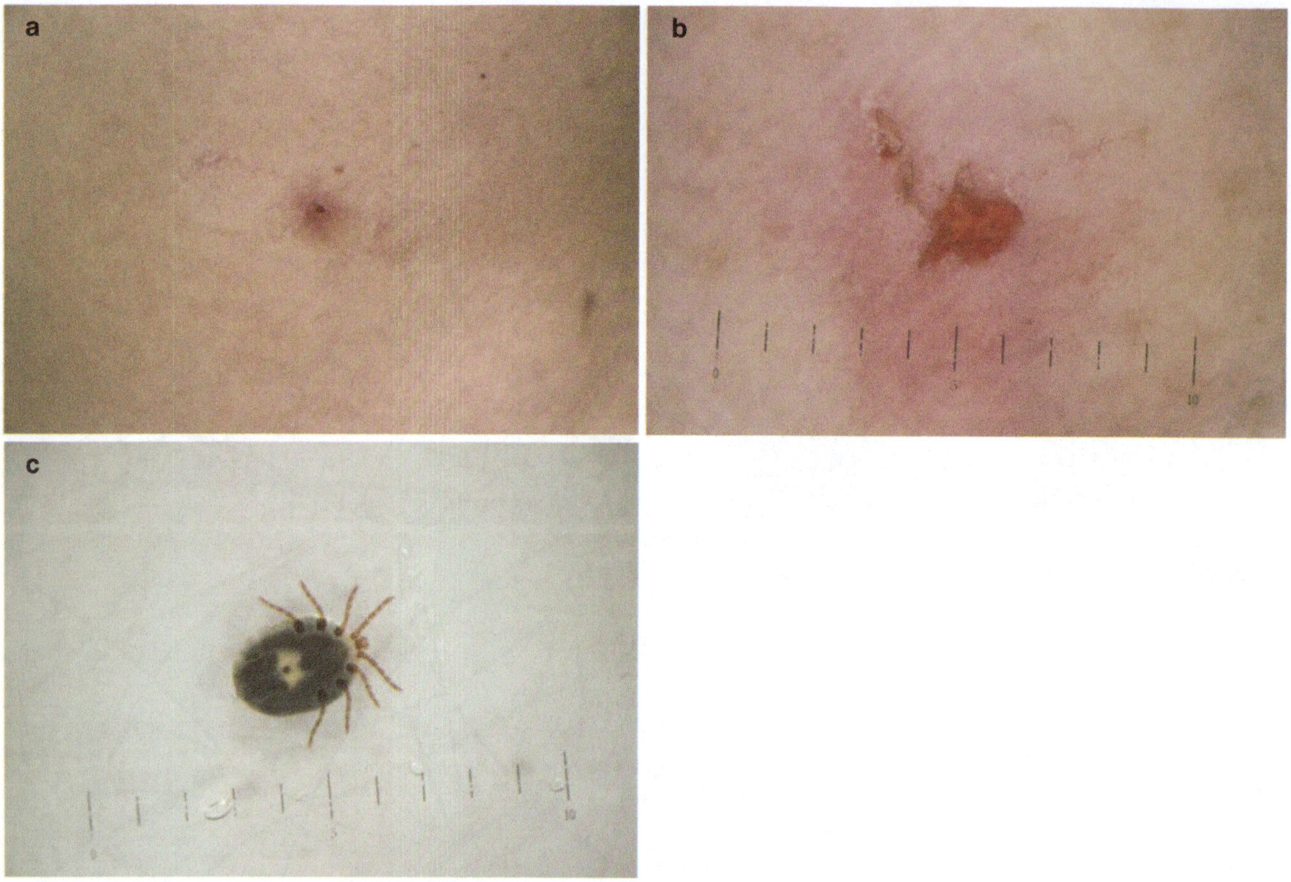

Fig. 13.37 Tick bite. (**a**) Clinical appearance: insect bite in the center of the inflammatory erythema. (**b**) Dermoscopy: congestion and erosion on the bite site with a surrounding erythematous halo (×10). (**c**) Adult tick under dermoscopy (×10)

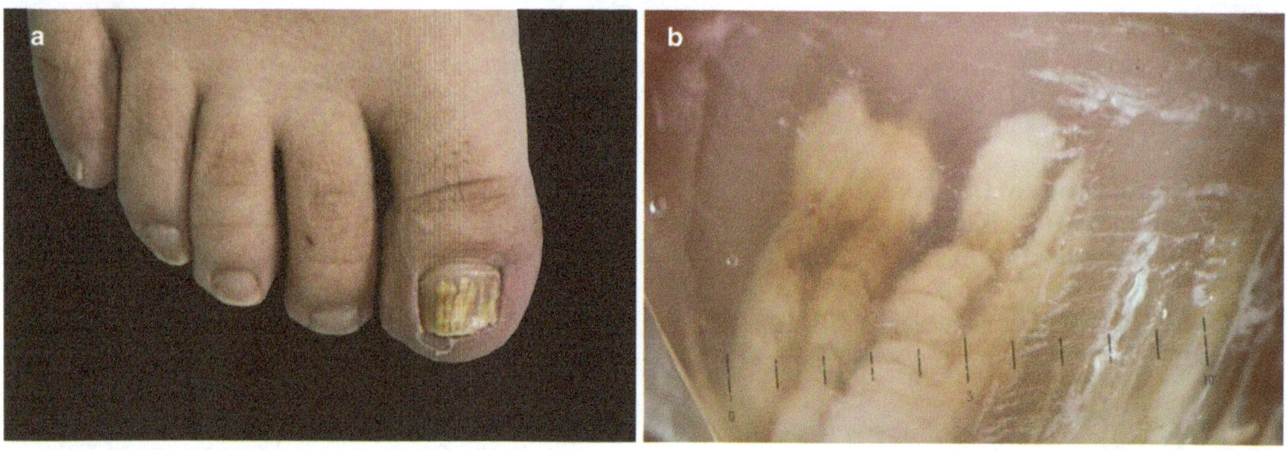

Fig. 13.38 Onychomycosis (1). (**a**) Clinical appearance: an irregular yellowish-brown nail. (**b**) Dermoscopy: irregular yellow or yellowish-white longitudinal streaks and a jagged proximal edge with an intermittent ascending pattern and irregular distal end (×10)

13.10 Onychomycosis

Onychomycosis is a fungal infection of the nail plate or nail bed caused by dermatophytes and other organisms like yeasts and molds, usually starting from a single nail and gradually involves other nails. The infection begins at the free edge, lateral edge, or lunula of the nail, showing dotted or irregular white or dirty-yellow localized turbid patches, and gradually extends to the whole nail plate, presenting as nail discoloration, thickening, tarnishing, and separation from the nail plate (Figs. 13.38 and 13.39).

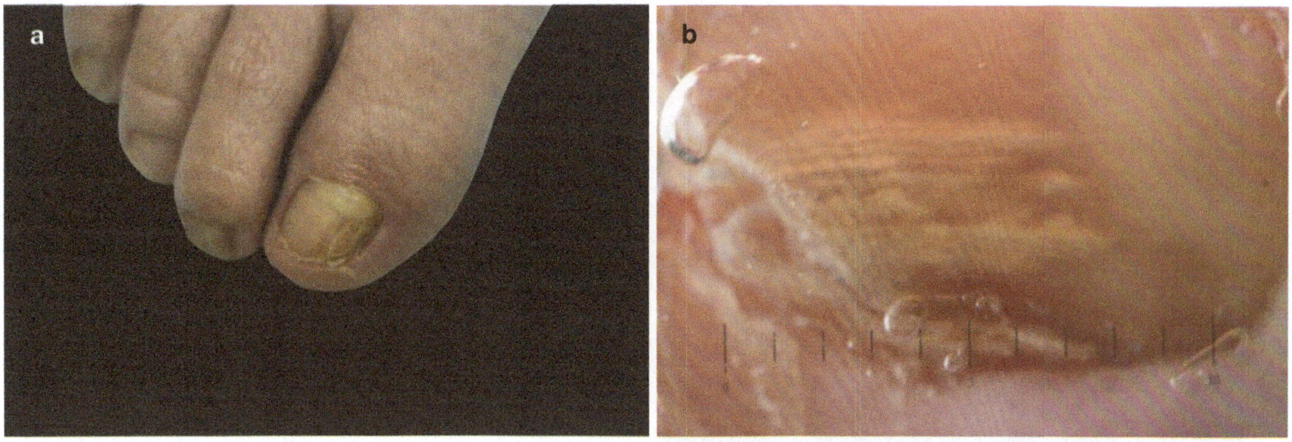

Fig. 13.39 Onychomycosis (2). (**a**) Clinical appearance: an irregular yellowish-brown nail. (**b**) Dermoscopy: irregular yellow or yellowish-white longitudinal streaks and a jagged proximal edge with an intermittent ascending pattern and irregular distal end (×10)

13.10.1 Dermoscopic Manifestations of Onychomycosis

The dermoscopic features of onychomycosis include pigmentation, onycholysis (distal and/or lateral edge), marbled-like turbid area, hemorrhagic debris, and longitudinal streaks on the nail plate; irregular yellow, white, brownish-black longitudinal streaks; and a jagged proximal edge with an intermittent ascending pattern and irregular distal end.

13.10.2 Significance of Dermoscopy in the Diagnosis and Treatment of Onychomycosis

1. Help in the differential diagnosis of it from nail lichen planus and nail psoriasis (see Chap. 12).
2. Assess the therapeutic effect in follow-up observation.

13.11 Tinea Versicolor

Tinea versicolor is a superficial fungal infection caused by *Malassezia furfur*. Tinea versicolor mainly occurs in summer and autumn in warm regions and involves the chest, back, and neck, presenting as well-demarcated, round to oval macules covered with thin chaff-like scales, which can be yellow, light-brown, or brown. Developed or nearly healed lesions can also manifest as hypopigmentation (Figs. 13.40, 13.41, and 13.42).

13.11.1 Dermoscopic Manifestations of Tinea Versicolor

1. Hyperpigmented: thin scales and a pigment network composed of brown streaks or diffuse brown pigmentation.
2. Hypopigmented: well-demarcated white patches with scales in the furrows.

13.11.2 Significance of Dermoscopy in the Diagnosis and Treatment of Tinea Versicolor

1. Assist in the differential diagnosis of it from vitiligo, nevus depigmentosus, guttate psoriasis, idiopathic guttate hypomelanosis, mycosis fungoides, and other hypopigmented skin diseases.
2. Assist in the differential diagnosis of it from pityriasis rosea, mycosis fungoides, and other hyperpigmented skin diseases.

13.12 Tinea Capitis

Tinea capitis, classified into tinea favosa, tinea blanca, and kerion, is a dermatophyte infection of the scalp and hair that can cause focal alopecia (Fig. 13.43).

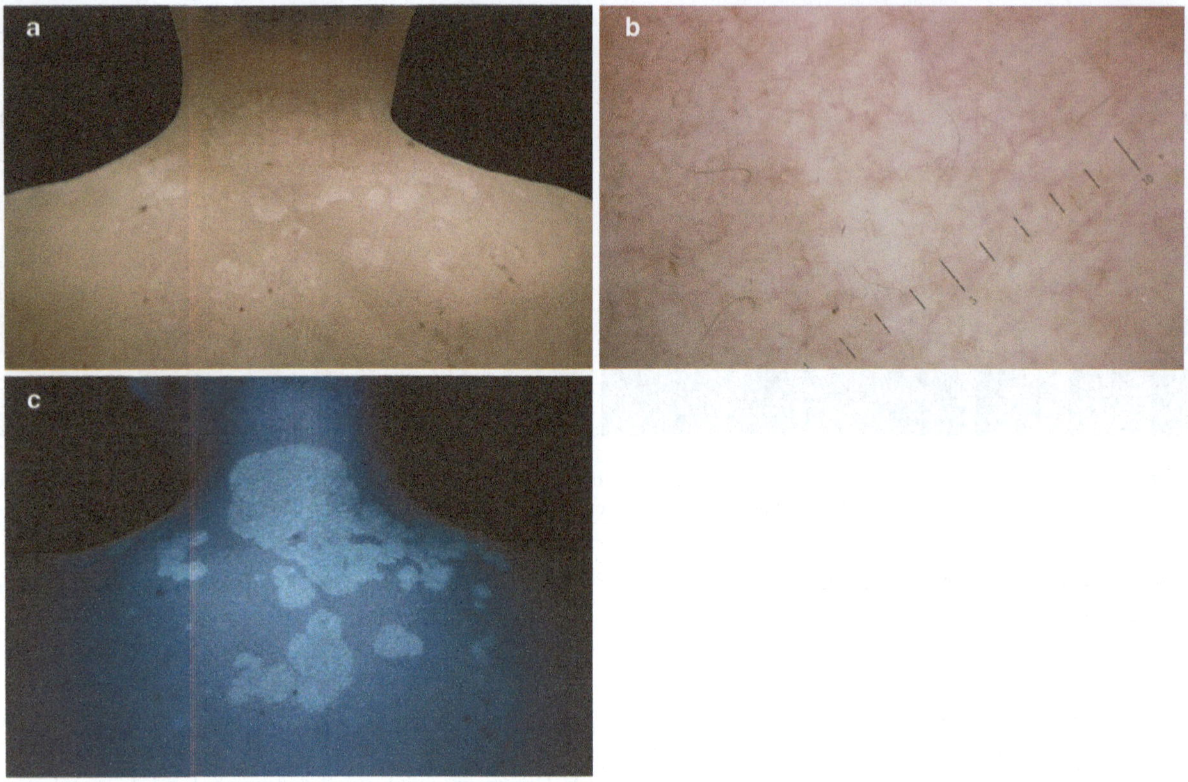

Fig. 13.40 Hypopigmented tinea versicolor (1). (**a**) Clinical appearance: well-demarcated pale-white patches. (**b**) Dermoscopy: well-demarcated white patches with scales in the furrows (×10). (**c**) Wood's lamp examination: well-demarcated white patches with fusion

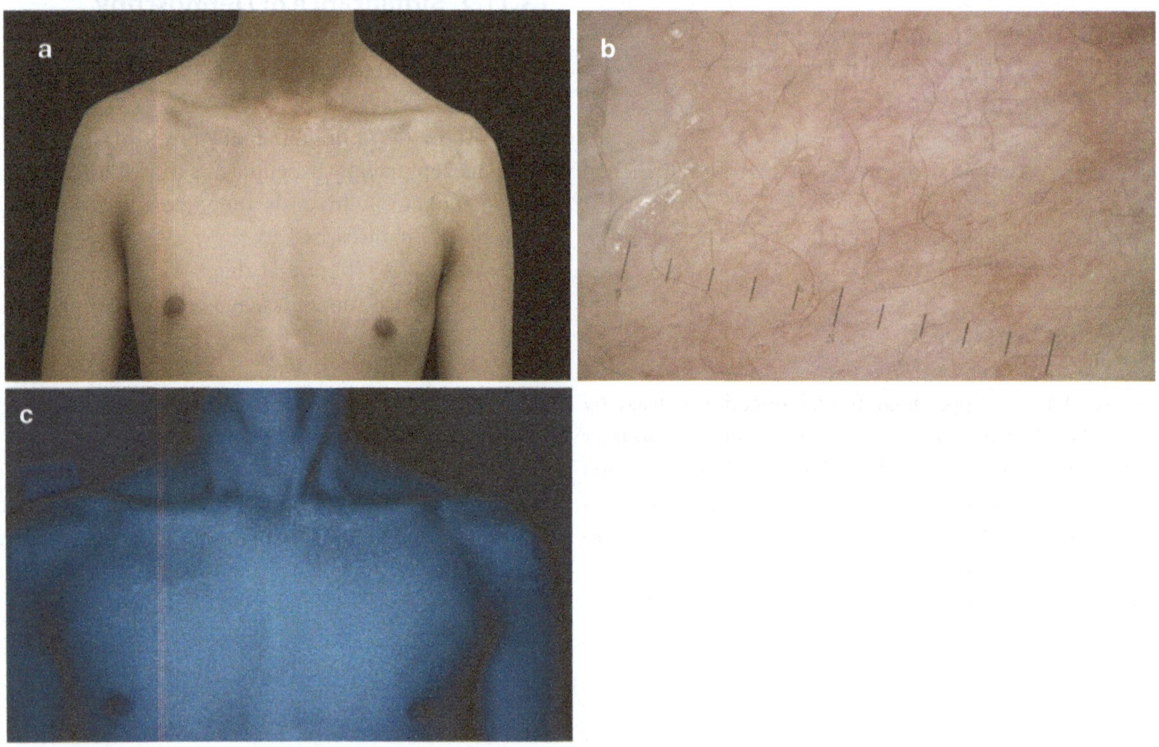

Fig. 13.41 Hypopigmented tinea versicolor (2). (**a**) Clinical appearance: well-demarcated patches with thin scales. (**b**) Dermoscopy: thin scales, white patches, and pigment network consisting of brown streaks (×10). (**c**) Wood's lamp examination: well-demarcated pale-white patches

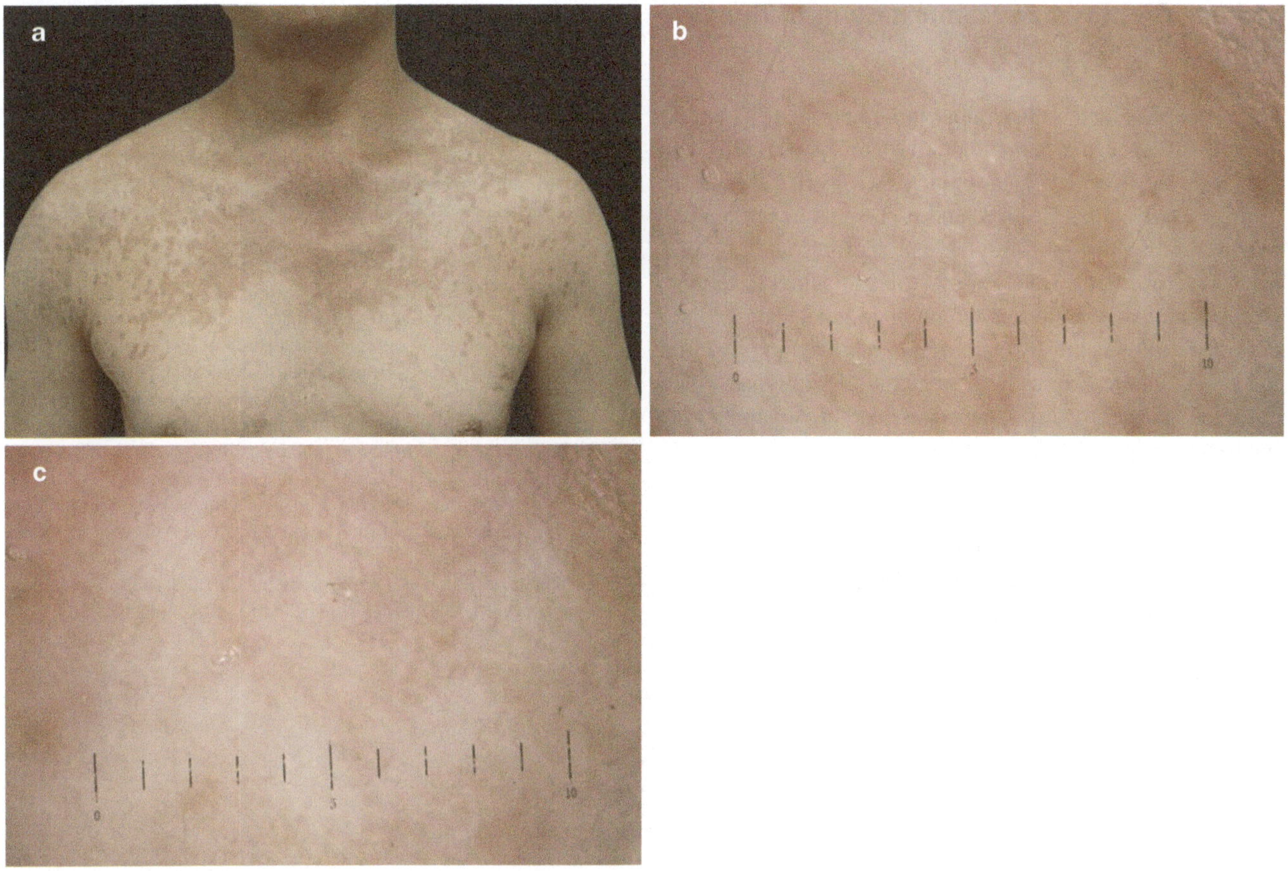

Fig. 13.42 Hyperpigmented tinea versicolor (1). (**a**) Clinical appearance: well-defined brown patches. (**b, c**) Dermoscopy: thin scales and a pigment network consisting of brown streaks or diffuse brown pigmentation (×10)

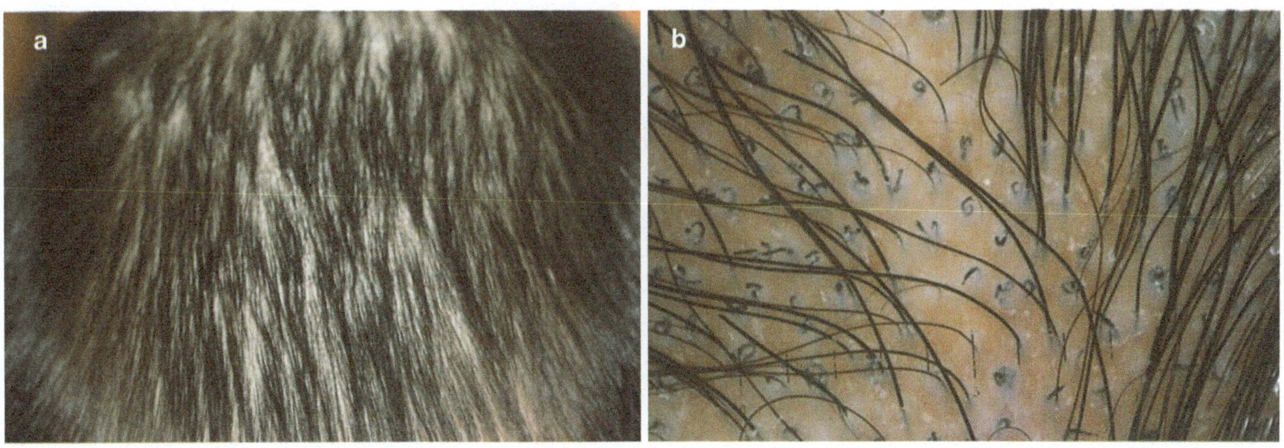

Fig. 13.43 Tinea capitis. (**a**) Clinical appearance: irregular patchy alopecia. (**b**) Dermoscopy: broken hair and "comma hair" (×10)

13.12.1 Dermoscopic Manifestations of Tinea Capitis

Dermoscopy shows broken hair, whose hair shaft looks like a comma, hence the name "comma hair." Dystrophic hair also can be found. Tinea blanca is mostly caused by *Microsporum canis* infection, and it presents as broken hair of different lengths and atrophic hair shafts, some of which are corkscrew, with white glossy scales attached to the hair shaft. Comma hair is not very common in tinea blanca. Black dot tinea capitis is mostly caused by *Trichophyton tonsurans* infection, manifesting as large amounts of "comma," "hairpin," and "question mark"-shaped hair and broken hair clinging to the scalp under dermoscopy.

13.12.2 Significance of Dermoscopy in the Diagnosis and Treatment of Tinea Capitis

Assist in the differential diagnosis of it from syphilitic alopecia, trichotillomania, alopecia areata, and other hair diseases.

Further Reading

1. Zhang Y, Jiang S, et al. Application of dermoscopy image analysis technique in diagnosing urethral condylomata acuminata. An Bras Dermatol. 2018;93(1):67–71.
2. Skin Imaging Group of Chinese Association of Integrative Medicine. Experts consensus on dermoscopic diagnosis of infectious and parasitic dermatoses. China J Leprosy Skin Disease. 2017;33(1):1–7.
3. Tschandl P, Argenziano G, Bakos R, et al. Dermoscopy and entomology (entomodermoscopy). J Dtsch Dermatol Ges. 2009;7(7):589–96.
4. Ianhez M, Cestari Sda C, Enokihara MY, et al. Dermoscopic patterns of molluscum contagiosum: a study of 211 lesions confirmed by histopathology. An Bras Dermatol. 2011;86(1):74–9.
5. Haliasos EC, Kerner M, Jaimes-Lopez N, et al. Dermoscopy for the pediatric dermatologist part I: Dermoscopy of Pediatric infectious and inflammatory skin lesions and hair disorders. Pediatr Dermatol. 2013;30(2):163–71.
6. Zhou H, Tang XH, De Han J, et al. Dermoscopy as an ancillary tool for the diagnosis of pityriasis versicolor. J Am Acad Dermatol. 2015;73:e205–6.
7. Errichetti E, Stinco G. Dermoscopy in general dermatology: a practical overview. Dermatol Ther (Heidelb). 2016;6(4):471–507.

14 Hair and Nail Diseases

14.1 Hair Diseases

Dermoscopy is also called trichoscopy when it is used to observe hair and scalp diseases. Trichoscopy is a convenient and effective imaging method that can be used to observe hair and scalp structures. Trichoscopy can provide information on hair shaft morphology, hair root morphology, skin surface microstructure, hair follicles, and capillaries. Trichoscopy can be used for the diagnosis and differential diagnosis of a variety of hair diseases, which is of great significance for the treatment and follow-up of hair diseases. For example, trichoscopy can be used as an objective means to monitor the hair growth cycle and reduce the number of unnecessary biopsies performed.

Many types of dermoscopy can be used to observe the scalp and hair. To observe scalp blood vessels, magnification needs to exceed 20 times. Polarized and nonpolarized dermoscopy can be used to observe the hair and scalp. Infiltrating dermoscopy often uses ethanol or water as a medium. Noninfiltrating polarized light dermoscopy is typically used to observe the scales around hair follicles.

Alopecia is a common hair disease that can be divided into acquired and congenital alopecia. Congenital alopecia is rare. Acquired alopecia can be divided into nonscarring alopecia or scarring alopecia on the basis of whether it causes permanent hair loss. Nonscarring alopecia is mainly caused by changes in the hair follicle cycle due to local immune and nonimmune factors. Nonscarring alopecia includes androgenic alopecia (AGA), alopecia areata, telogen alopecia, trichotillomania, and syphilitic alopecia. Scarring alopecia causes permanent alopecia, in which the hair follicles cannot regenerate after being damaged and are filled with hyperplastic collagen fibers. On the basis of whether hair follicles are targeted, scarring alopecia can be divided into primary and secondary alopecia. The pathogenic target of primary scarring alopecia is hair follicles, and the pathological changes of related diseases are mainly lymphocytic (such as discoid lupus erythematosus (DLE) and hair lichen planus), neutrophilic (such as alopecia folliculitis), mixed, and nonspecific. Secondary scarring alopecia involves hair follicle damage caused by local scalp diseases or physicochemical injuries, such as tinea capitis and burns.

Common hair diseases have specific dermoscopic signs corresponding to pathological changes. This chapter introduces only the dermoscopic manifestations of several typical alopecic diseases.

14.1.1 Androgenic Alopecia

AGA is a progressive hair loss disease that occurs in and after adolescence. AGA is mainly characterized by forehead hairline regression and/or a progressive reduction and thinning of hair on the top of head in men (Fig. 14.1), also known as male-pattern alopecia. In women, AGA is mainly characterized by a progressive reduction and thinning of hair on the top of head, with a small proportion of women with AGA experiencing diffuse thinning of the hair and usually no hairline regression.

The dermoscopic characteristics of early AGA are as follows (Fig. 14.2):

1. Hair diameter changes, with a difference in hair stem diameter of over 20%.
2. The proportion of vellus hair increases.
3. Brown peripilar sign: a brown ring with a diameter of approximately 1 mm can be seen around the hair follicle.
4. The proportion of hair follicles containing a single hair increases.
5. Yellow dot sign.

> **Tip**
> AGA should be differentiated from acute telogen alopecia, and the main feature of the latter is that the proportion of thinning hair stem in residual terminal hair is less than 20%.

J. Liu, X. Zou, *Practical Dermoscopy*, https://doi.org/10.1007/978-981-19-1460-7_14

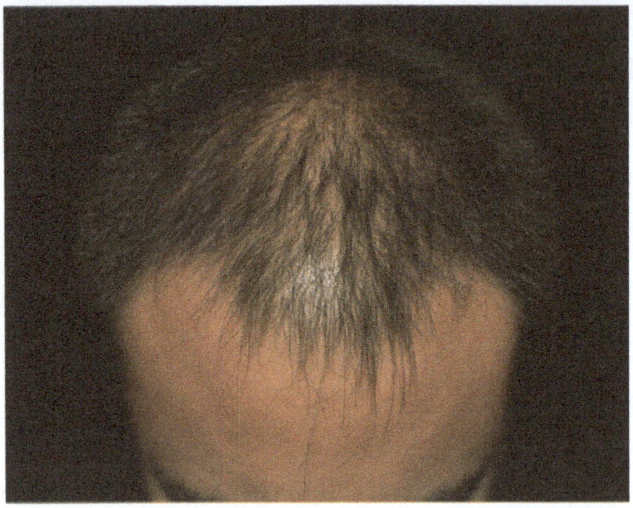

Fig. 14.1 Clinical manifestations of androgenic alopecia: the hair on the head of the patient is obviously sparse, and the hairline on the forehead has regressed, with an M-shape

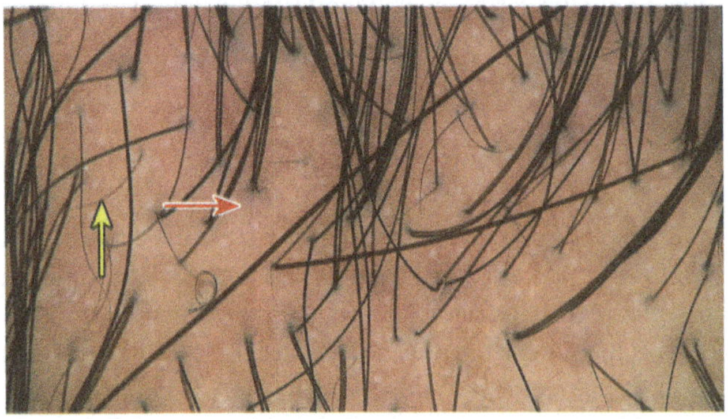

Fig. 14.2 Dermoscopic manifestations of androgenic alopecia: brown ring (red arrow) and thinning hair can be seen (yellow arrow, × 20)

The manifestations of AGA in female patients are similar to those in male patients, but the difference in hair stem diameter is not as obvious as in male patients. The number of hairs and the hair density in hair follicle units are mainly reduced. The yellow dot sign in female AGA patients indicates the progression of the disease.

> **Tip**
> A slightly sunken brown halo, that is, the brown peripilar sign, may be present around the hair follicle opening in the early stage of AGA, whereas the yellow dot sign is seen in the advanced stage of AGA.

The dermoscopic diagnostic criteria for AGA are as follows:

1. Major criteria.
   (a) More than 4 yellow dots can be seen in an image with a magnification of more than 70 times in the frontal area.
   (b) The average hair diameter of the frontal area is smaller than that of the occiput.
   (c) The proportion of thin hair (less than 0.03 mm) in the frontal area is more than 10%.
2. Minor criteria.
   (a) Increased frontal to occipital ratio of a single-hair pilosebaceous unit.
   (b) Vellus hair.
   (c) Frontal peripilar sign.

Two major criteria or 1 major criterion and 2 minor criteria must be met to make a diagnosis of AGA.

14.1.2 Alopecia Areata

Alopecia areata is an inflammatory and nonscarring alopecic disease with unknown etiology. Alopecia areata can occur in patients of any age. Some patients have mental stress or emotional fluctuations before the onset of alopecia areata, and most of them have no conscious symptoms. Some patients experience nail changes, such as nail white spots, nail pitting, and nail brittleness. Alopecia areata can be divided into three stages according to the development of the disease: the active stage, static stage, and recovery stage.

The dermoscopic characteristics of alopecia areata are as follows (Fig. 14.3):

1. Yellow dots
2. Black dots
3. Broken hairs
4. Short vellus hairs (length < 10 mm)
5. Exclamation mark hairs

The significance of the different dermoscopic manifestations is as follows:

1. The yellow dots and short vellus hairs are sensitive indicators, and the black dots, exclamation mark hairs, and broken hairs are specific indicators.
2. Exclamation mark hairs have diagnostic significance. These hairs mostly occur in the acute hair loss process of alopecia areata, which is related to hair follicle malnutrition.
3. The black dots, exclamation mark hairs, and short vellus hairs are related to disease activity.

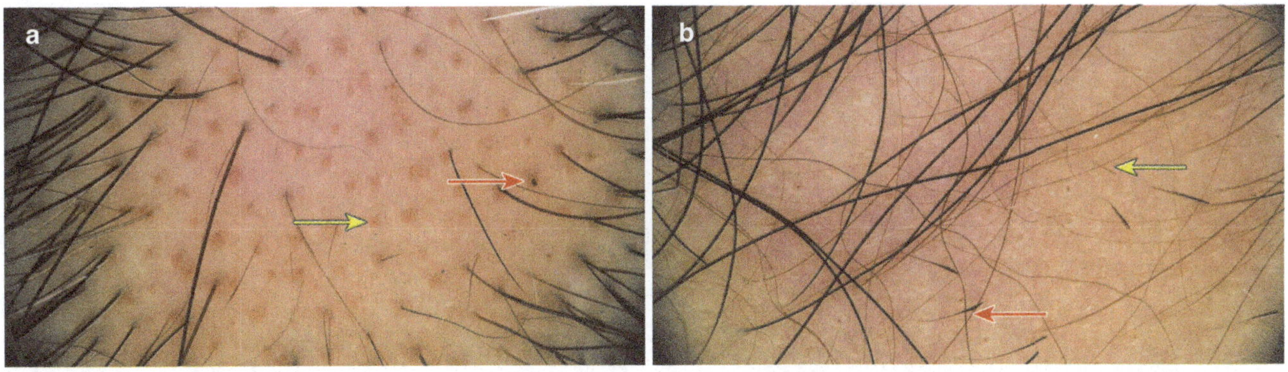

Fig. 14.3 (**a**) Dermoscopic manifestations of alopecia areata: black dots (red arrow) and yellow dots (yellow arrow, × 20). (**b**). Exclamation mark hairs (red arrow) and short vellus hairs (yellow arrow) can be seen, × 20)

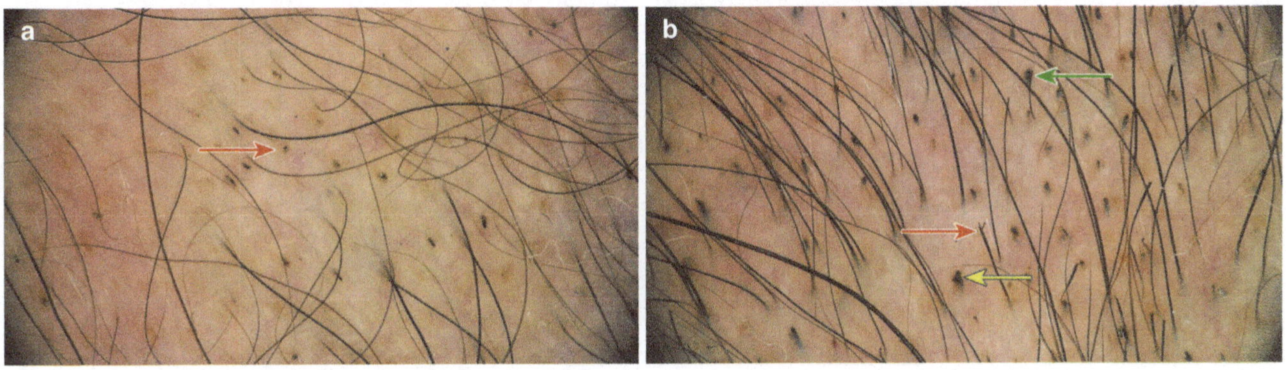

Fig. 14.4 Dermoscopic manifestations of trichotillomania: (**a**). The red arrow shows black dots (×20). (**b**). Broken hairs of different lengths and types, longitudinal fissuring at the end of hairs (red arrow), flame-like hair (yellow arrow), and tulip-like hair (green arrow, ×20)

14.1.3 Trichotillomania

Trichotillomania is an artificial type of traumatic hair loss. Patients with trichotillomania pull out their hair by themselves, resulting in patchy alopecia or total alopecia of the scalp. The onset of trichotillomania is related to abnormal moods, emotions, or environments and many other factors, as well as neurobiology. Clinically, trichotillomania needs to be differentiated from alopecia areata and tinea capitis.

The dermoscopic manifestations of trichotillomania are as follows (Fig. 14.4):

1. Broken hairs of different lengths
2. Black dots
3. Longitudinal fissuring at the end of hair
4. Various types of broken hairs, including curly hairs, flame-like hairs, the V-shaped sign, and tulip-like hairs
5. Hemorrhage spots and crusts

In the differential diagnosis of trichotillomania and alopecia areata, broken hairs of different lengths, longitudinal fissuring of hair, the V-shaped sign, and flame-like hairs under dermoscopy are more common in trichotillomania, while exclamation mark hairs, the thinning of hair tips, and yellow dots are more suggestive of alopecia areata.

14.1.4 Syphilitic Alopecia

Syphilitic alopecia is one of the clinical manifestations of secondary syphilis. Syphilitic alopecia occurs late (often 6 months) after being infected. Syphilitic alopecia is characterized by small and scattered patches of alopecia in the shape of insect bites, mainly distributed on the temporal and occipital areas (Fig. 14.5). Sometimes diffuse alopecia can occur, and eyelashes, the outer one-third of eyebrows, and body hair can also fall off.

The dermoscopic manifestations of syphilitic alopecia are as follows (Fig. 14.6):

1. Localized hairless areas.
2. Broken hairs of different lengths.
3. Brown rings can be seen around some hair follicles.
4. Black dots or yellow dots are occasionally seen.

Tip
Syphilitic alopecia is temporary. After syphilis is cured, the lost hair can regenerate.

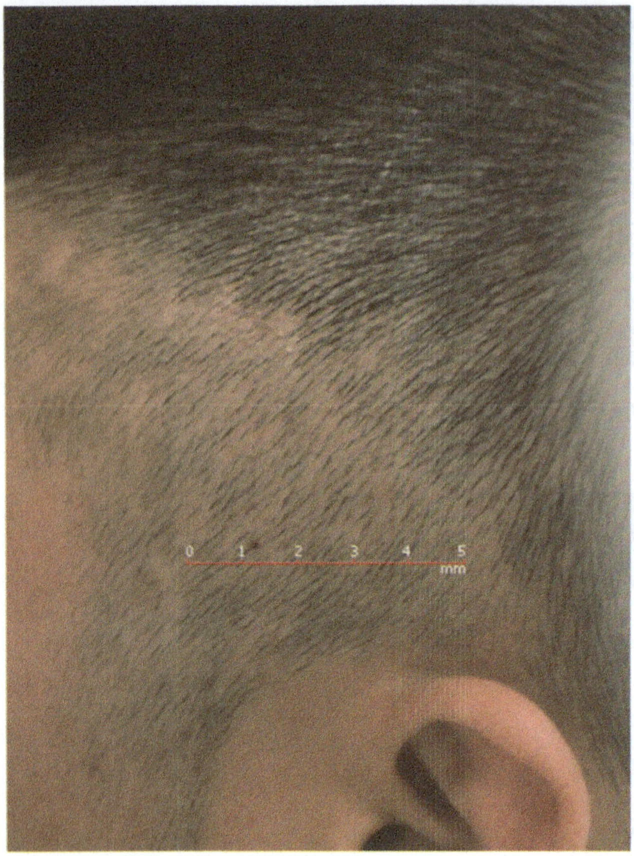

Fig. 14.5 Clinical manifestations of syphilitic alopecia: scattered insect-bite-like small alopecic spots can be seen on the temporal shaved area

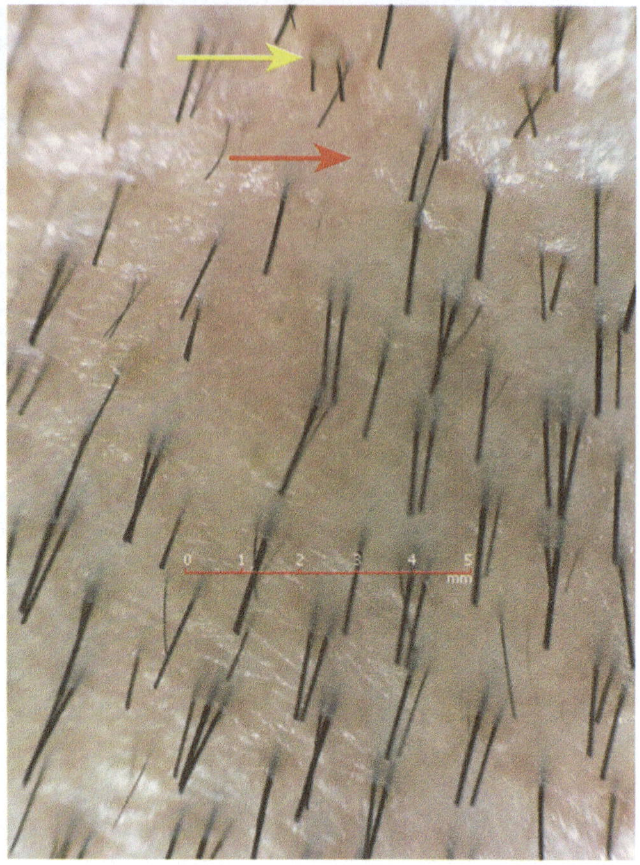

Fig. 14.6 Dermoscopic manifestations of patients with syphilitic alopecia: a localized hairless area (red arrow) and a brown ring around a hair follicle (yellow arrow) can be seen (× 20)

14.1.5 Discoid Lupus Erythematosus

Hair loss caused by DLE is a kind of scarring alopecia. Skin lesions are characterized by round or discoid erythema and plaques or papules with clear boundaries. Telangiectasia, scale attachment, hair follicle opening expansion, and hair follicular plugs are found on the surface. In the later stage, the center of the skin lesions shows atrophy and hypopigmentation with hair loss, as well as peripheral pigmentation (Fig. 14.7).

The dermoscopic manifestations of DLE are as follows (Fig. 14.8):

1. Red dots
2. White halo around hair follicles
3. Hair follicular plugs
4. Arborizing vessels

> **Tip**
> Red dots are areas of annular erythema and are mostly distributed around hair follicle openings. The presence of red dots is a specific indicator of the active stage of DLE and is related to a good prognosis.

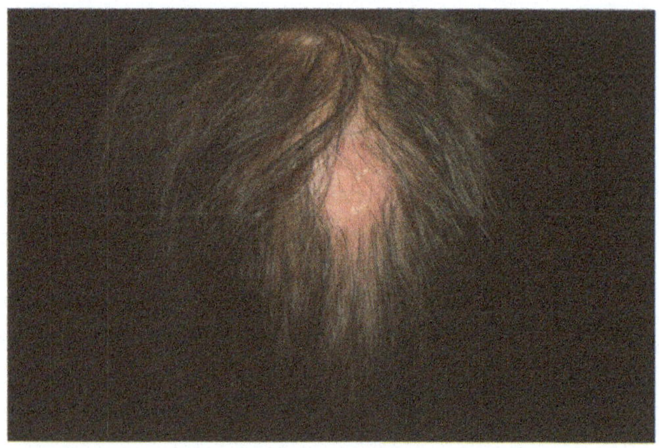

Fig. 14.7 Clinical manifestations of discoid lupus erythematosus: a round area of hair loss with central atrophic erythema, hypopigmentation, and sparse scales can be seen

14.1.6 Morphea

Scleroderma is a disease characterized by localized or diffuse fibrosis, sclerosis, and finally the atrophy of connective tissue of skin and internal organs. Scleroderma can be divided into two main forms: localized scleroderma (morphea) and systemic sclerosis (SSc).

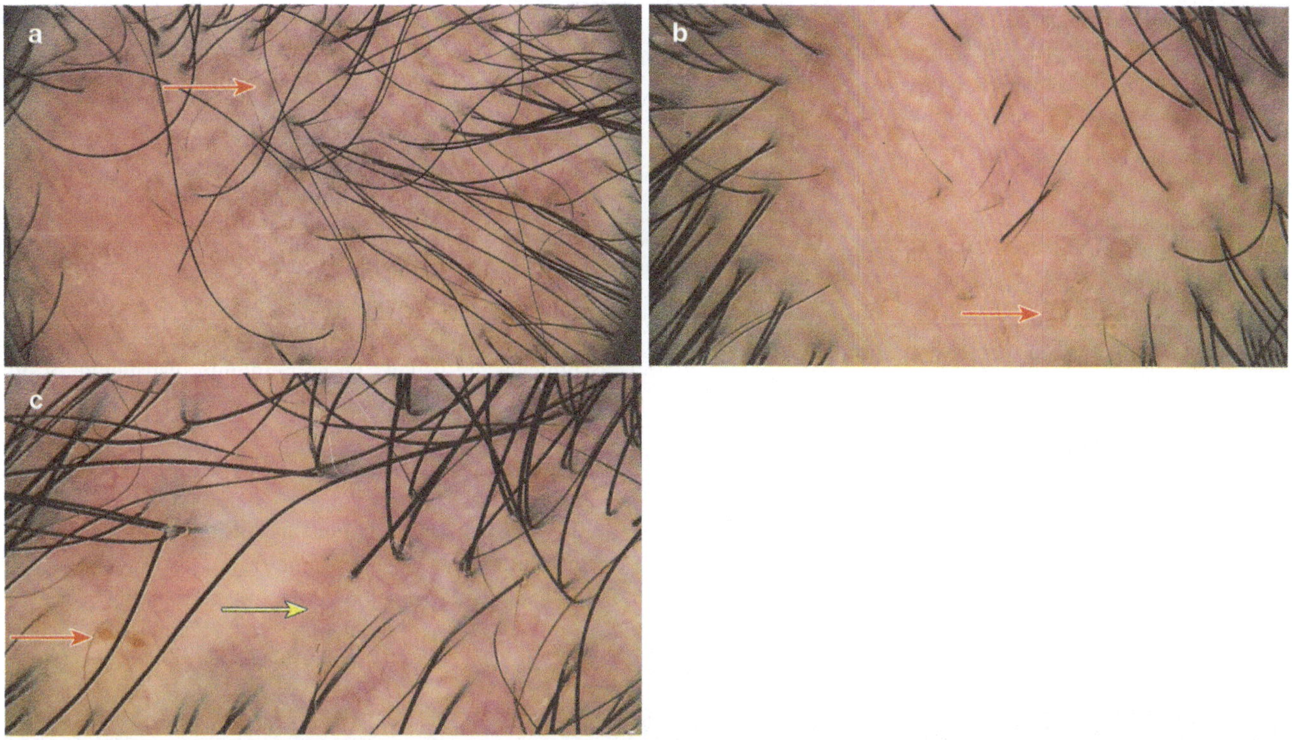

Fig. 14.8 Dermoscopic manifestations of discoid lupus erythematosus: (**a**). Red dots (red arrow) and brown pigment particles (×20). (**b**). Hair follicular plugs (red arrow), a white halo around a hair follicle, and arborizing vessels can be seen (× 20). (**c**). Hair follicular plugs (red arrow) and an arborizing blood vessel (yellow arrow) can be seen (× 20)

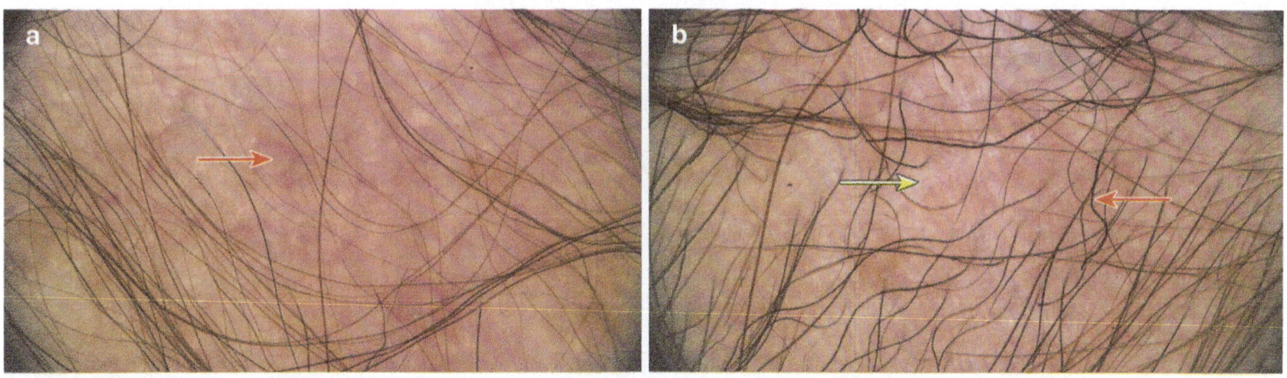

Fig. 14.9 Dermoscopic manifestations of morphea involving the scalp: (**a**). Hair follicle openings in the alopecic area disappear, and an irregular vascular shadow is seen (red arrow, ×20). (**b**). Broken and twisted hairs (red arrow) and a white area (yellow arrow) can be seen (× 20)

Morphea involving the scalp usually presents as sclerosing patchy alopecia, with obvious boundaries, dry and smooth surfaces, and peripheral mild erythema. Hair follicle openings can exist in the early stage but disappear in the late stage, accompanied by epidermal atrophy and sclerosis.

The dermoscopic manifestations of morphea involving the scalp are as follows (Fig. 14.9):

1. Skin atrophy and the absence of hair follicle openings
2. White areas
3. Black dots
4. Broken and twisted hairs
5. Irregular vascular shadow

14.1.7 Lichen Planopilaris

Lichen planopilaris (LPP), also known as lichen planus of hair follicles, is more common in women at the age of 30–70 but can also be seen in children. The clinical features of LPP are erythema around hair follicles, keratotic plugs surrounded by a narrow violaceous rim, and localized or generalized scarring alopecia. Cases of LPP occurring on the scalp are called scalp lichen planus, which needs to be differentially diagnosed from pseudopelade of Brocq.

The dermoscopic manifestations of hair lichen planus are as follows (Fig. 14.10):

1. Hair follicular plugs.
2. Scales and hair tubes around hair follicles.
3. Blue-purple patches caused by pigment incontinence.
4. White dots in late stage.
5. Hair follicle openings decrease or disappear.

14.1.8 Frontal Fibrosing Alopecia

Frontal fibrosing alopecia (FFA) refers to the regression of the hairline in the frontal and temporal areas and the eyebrow abscission of patients. FFA mostly occurs in postmenopausal women. Some scholars believe that FFA is a special subtype of LPP, but this is still controversial. Erythema around hair follicles can appear, especially at the hairline.

The dermoscopic findings of FFA are as follows (Fig. 14.11):

1. Erythema around hair.
2. Loss of vellus hair.
3. Scales around hair follicles.
4. Loss of hair follicle openings.
5. Scarring white splotch: a white irregular area without hair follicle openings. Unlike white spots, scarring white splotches are usually large, randomly distributed, of different sizes, and irregularly shaped.

Tip
FFA and hair lichen planus are difficult to distinguish under dermoscopy and pathology. The diagnosis of FFA mainly depends on clinical manifestations.

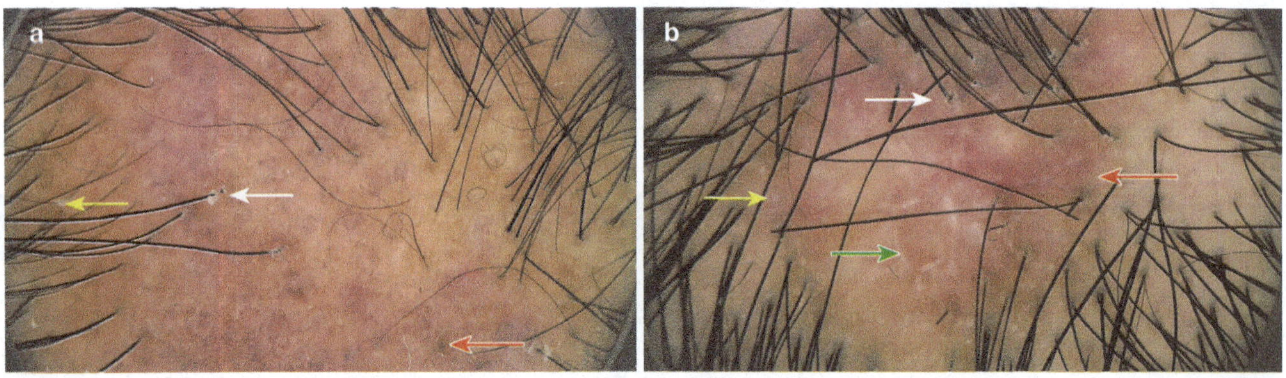

Fig. 14.10 Dermoscopic manifestations of hair lichen planus: (**a**). Scales around hair follicles (white arrow), hair tube type (yellow arrow), hair follicular plugs (red arrow), and blue-purple patches can be seen (×20). (**b**). Purple-red background (red arrow), Wickham striae (green arrow), white dots (yellow arrow), scales around hair follicles (white arrow), and reduced hair follicle openings can be seen (× 20)

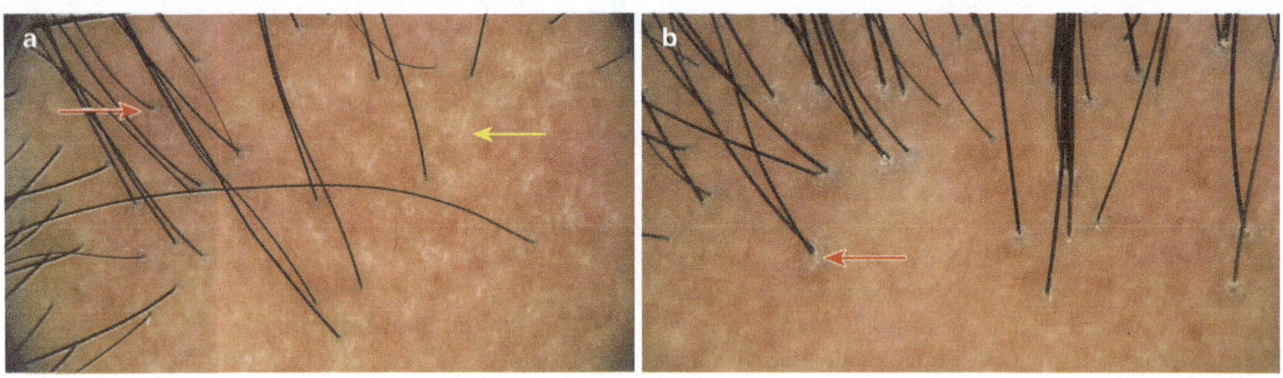

Fig. 14.11 Dermoscopic manifestations of frontal fibrosing alopecia: (**a**). Erythema around hair (red arrow) and a scarring white splotch (yellow arrow, × 20). (**b**). Scales around hair follicles can be seen (red arrow, × 20)

14.1.9 Folliculitis Decalvans

Folliculitis decalvans (FD) is a destructive folliculitis with permanent alopecia. The etiology of FD is unknown but may be related to an abnormal reaction to a bacterial infection (especially a *Staphylococcus aureus* infection). Most patients have a history of long-term seborrheic dermatitis. The common clinical manifestations are alopecic patches, inflammatory papules, pustules, and hair follicle hyperkeratosis. FD is always accompanied with pruritus or no obvious symptoms, mostly occurs in young adults.

The dermoscopic manifestations of FD are as follows (Fig. 14.12):

1. Clustered hair
2. Telangiectasia between hair follicles
3. Hair follicular plugs
4. Ulcers and blood crusts
5. Pustules around hair follicles
6. Hair follicle opening absence in the late stage

14.1.10 Folliculitis et Perifolliculitis Capitis Abscedens et Suffodiens

Folliculitis et perifolliculitis capitis abscedens et suffodiens is a rare chronic suppurative skin disease of the scalp. The etiology and pathogenesis of this disease are unclear but may be related to many factors, such as hair follicle atresia, bacterial infection, immune factors, sex hormones, smoking, and obesity. The main clinical manifestations of this disease are fluctuating nodules, interconnected sinuses, scarring alopecia, and red papules with abscesses on the scalp.

The dermoscopic manifestations of folliculitis et perifolliculitis capitis abscedens et suffodiens are as follows (Fig. 14.13):

1. Decreased or absent hair stem.
2. Yellow dots.
3. Black dots.
4. Broken hairs and short vellus hairs.
5. Hair follicular plugs.
6. Hair follicle openings exist in the early stage but are decreased or absent in the late stage.

14.2 Nail Diseases

In the diagnosis and treatment of nail diseases, dermoscopy can be used to magnify the subtle structures that are difficult to recognize with the naked eye. Dermoscopy can observe

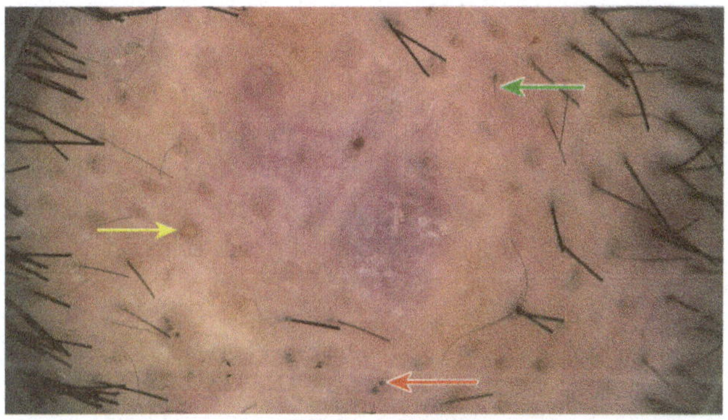

Fig. 14.13 Dermoscopic manifestations of folliculitis et perifolliculitis capitis abscedens et suffodiens: Hair follicle openings are partially absent, but black dots (red arrow), yellow dots (yellow arrow), short vellus hairs can be seen (green arrow, × 20)

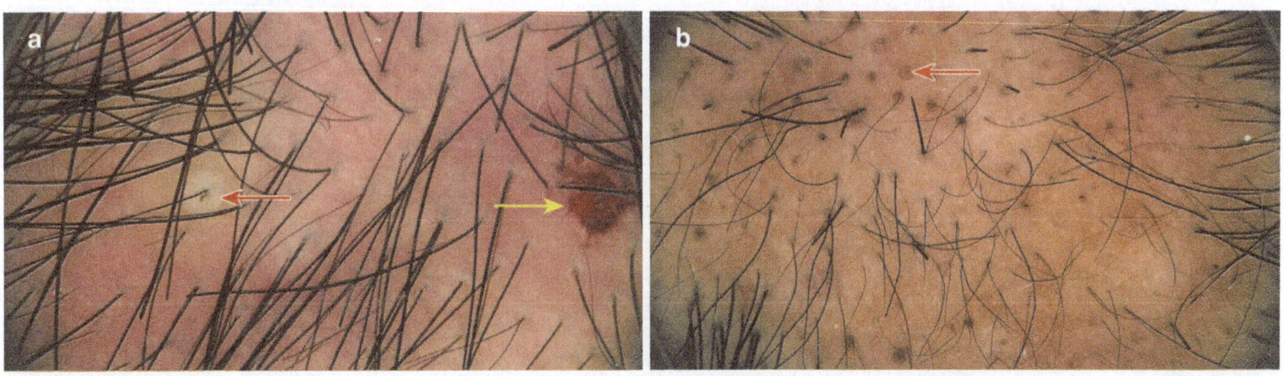

Fig. 14.12 Dermoscopic manifestations of alopecia folliculitis: (**a**). Telangiectasia between hair follicles, pustules around hair follicles (red arrow), and ulcers and blood crusts (yellow arrow) can be seen (× 20). (**b**). Part of the hair follicle openings are absent, and hair follicular plugs can be seen (red arrow, × 20)

not only the nail plate but also the microstructure and blood vessels of the proximal nail fold, nail matrix, nail bed, and nail free margin. Nail dermoscopy is also called onychoscopy.

The application of dermoscopy in nail diseases has expanded from pigmented diseases to various types of nail diseases, reducing the number of unnecessary biopsies of benign skin lesions performed. Onychoscopy has gradually become a powerful auxiliary diagnostic tool for nail disease. Studies have shown that dermoscopy can be used for the diagnosis of a variety of nail diseases, such as subungual hemorrhage, nail matrix nevus (NMN), nail melanoma, green nail syndrome, onychomycosis, nail lichen planus, nail psoriasis, nail changes in acrodermatitis continua, onychodystrophy, and nail squamous cell carcinoma. This section introduces the dermoscopic manifestations of common nail diseases.

14.2.1 Subungual Hemorrhage

Subungual hemorrhage, also known as subungual hematoma, refers to the accumulation of blood between nail matrix (or nail bed) and nail plate. Most subungual hemorrhages are caused by acute trauma or repeated chronic injury. The diagnosis of subungual hemorrhage caused by acute trauma combined with medical history is easy, but chronic hemorrhage caused by repeated injury needs to be differentiated from malignant melanoma. The clinical manifestation of subungual hemorrhage is brown to black dots or patches. As the nail grows, the haemorrhage spot gradually moves to the distal edge of nail plate.

According to the time of hemorrhage, the skin lesions can be red, purple, brown, and black under dermoscopy.

The dermoscopic manifestations of subungual hemorrhage are as follows (Fig. 14.14):

1. Homogeneous pigment pattern.
2. Globular pigment pattern.
3. Streak pattern.
4. Peripheral hypopigmentation.
5. Periungual hemorrhage.

> **Tip**
> Subungual hemorrhage is mostly characterized by the homogeneous or globular pigment pattern, generally without longitudinal full-length streaks on nail plate, which are more suggestive of nail melanocytic proliferative disease.

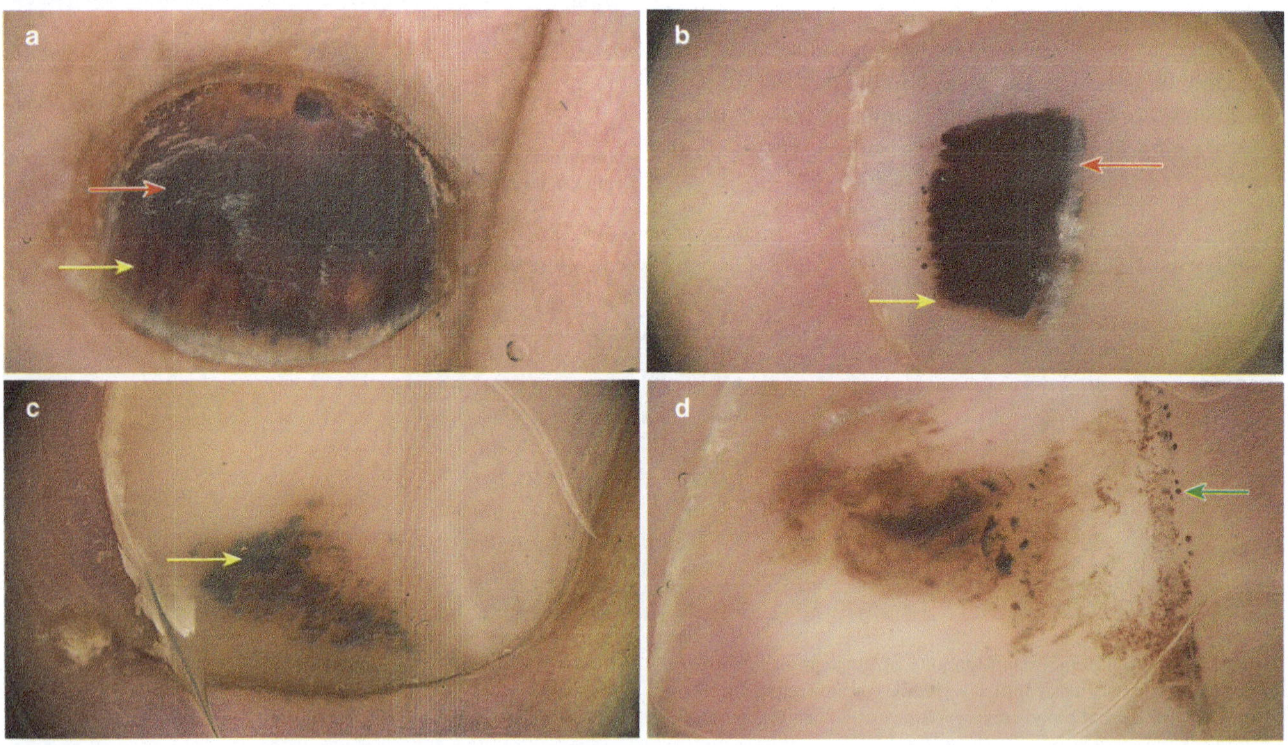

Fig. 14.14 Dermoscopic manifestations of subungual hemorrhage: (**a**). Diffuse brown to dark-red blotches are seen on nail plate, the color in the center is darker and peripheral color is lighter, and the homogeneous pattern (red arrow) and streak pattern (yellow arrow) can be seen (× 20). (**b**). Brown blotches with clear boundaries can be seen on the proximal plate; these blotches show the homogeneous pattern (red arrow) and peripheral hypopigmentation (yellow arrow, × 20). (**c**). Dark-red areas on the distal plate in a globular pattern (yellow arrow, × 20). (**d**). Irregular reddish brown blotches with clear boundaries on nail plate and hemorrhage spots around the nail can be seen (green arrow, × 20)

The significance of specific signs under dermoscopy is as follows:

1. The homogeneous pattern, which is characterized by diffuse blotches with uniform color, representing the color of dried bloodstains, is the most common pattern.
2. The globular pattern and streak pattern represent aggregated blood.
3. Peripheral hypopigmentation shows that the color gradually fades when the pigment expands from the center to the outside.
4. Periungual hemorrhage indicates that subungual hemorrhage is related to nail trauma.

14.2.2 Nail Matrix Nevus

An NMN is caused by the proliferation of melanocytes and is one of the causes of longitudinal melanonychia striata. Skin lesions usually occur in childhood, often involving fingers (especially the thumb). The most common clinical manifestations of NMN are nail striped pigmentation.

The dermoscopic manifestations of NMN are as follows (Fig. 14.15):

1. Brown background
2. Longitudinal streaks with regular thickness, spacing, color, and parallelism

Tip
Regular brown pigmentation in the nail is mostly the manifestation of a benign nevus.

Studies have shown that compared with adult NMN, childhood NMN often show more melanoma-like characteristics, such as wide and irregular streaks, multiple colors, and the Hutchinson sign.

14.2.3 Nail Melanoma

Nail melanoma is caused by abnormal proliferation of melanocytes, which is a malignant tumor and the 5-year survival rate is only 15%. Clinically, nail melanoma often manifests as a dark-brown to black longitudinal pigment band, accompanied by ulceration, hemorrhage, nail peeling, nail loss, and nail destruction.

The dermoscopic manifestations of nail melanoma are as follows (Fig. 14.16):

1. Brown background.
2. Brown to black longitudinal streaks with irregular thickness, spacing, color, and parallelism. The lesions may be wide at the proximal end and narrow at the distal end.
3. Hutchinson sign (the pigmentation of the periungual area).
4. Micro-Hutchinson sign (invisible to the naked eye but visible under dermoscopy).
5. Damage to and distal cracking of the nail plate.

Tip
When high-risk signs are observed under dermoscopy, biopsy is recommended to identify skin lesions.

Studies have shown that the Hutchinson sign is positive in all nail melanomas without a brown background or irregular streaks. When considering brown background, irregular

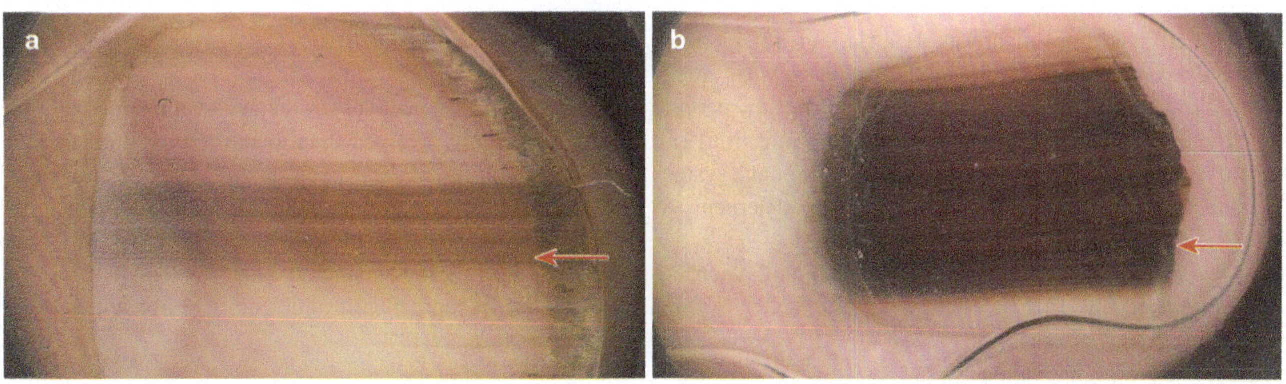

Fig. 14.15 Dermoscopic manifestations of a nail matrix nevus: (**a**). The longitudinal brown pigment band (red arrow) can be seen on the nail plate, with uniform color, and presents as regular straight lines (× 20). (**b**). The longitudinal red brown streaks (red arrow) on the nail plate can be seen, of which the spacing, color, and parallelism are regular (× 20)

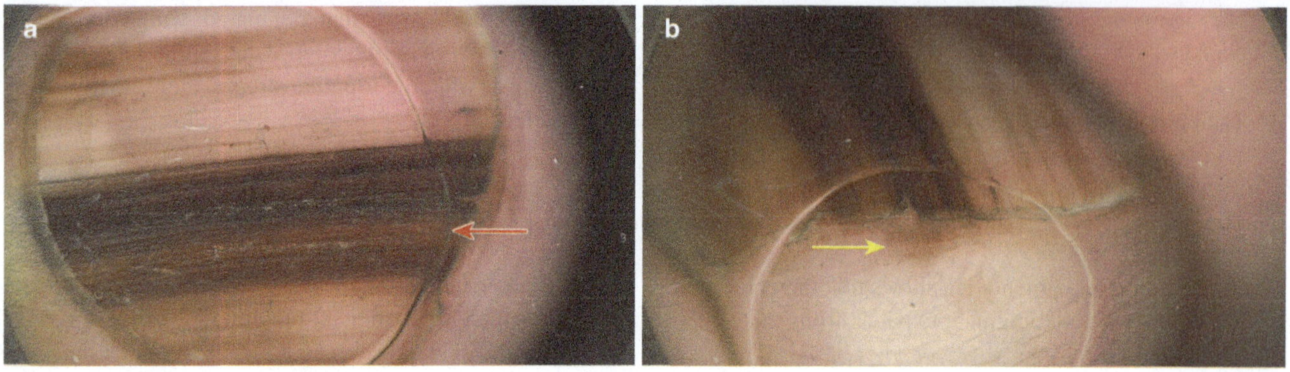

Fig. 14.16 Dermoscopic manifestations of nail melanoma: (**a**). Longitudinal brown pigment bands (red arrows) of different colors and widths. The lesion is confirmed as a nail melanoma by histopathology (× 20). (**b**). Uneven brown pigment streaks along the nail plate, brown pigmentation extending onto the hyponychium (Hutchinson sign, yellow arrow), and nail plate fissure (× 20)

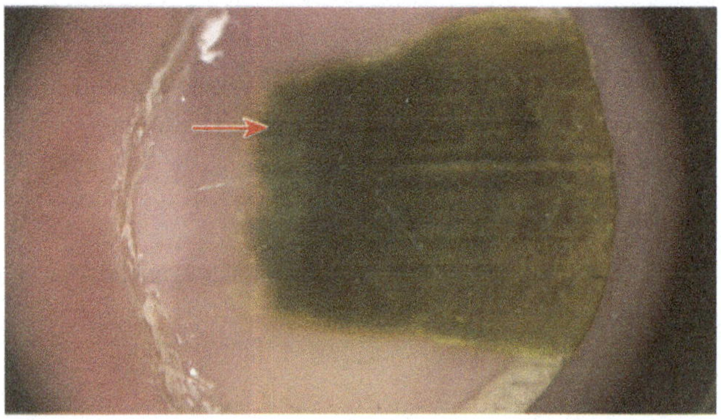

Fig. 14.17 Dermoscopic manifestations of green nail syndrome: dark-green pigmentation with clear boundaries (red arrow) can be seen at the distal end of the nail plate, and green color fades to yellow at the margin of the nail plate (× 20)

streaks, and Hutchinson sign together, the diagnostic accuracy of nail melanoma reaches almost 100%.

14.2.4 Green Nail Syndrome

Green nail syndrome manifests as a dark-green- or blue-green-dyed nail caused by *Pseudomonas aeruginosa* infection. Bacterial infection of nails rarely affects healthy people, but bacterial infection (such as *P. aeruginosa* infection) can occur in patients with onycholysis caused by immune system dysfunction, long-term exposure to water or detergent, or nail trauma.

The dermoscopic manifestations of green nail syndrome are as follows (Fig. 14.17):

1. Dark-green pigmentation.
2. Green color fades to yellow at the periphery of the discoloration.

14.2.5 Onychomycosis

Onychomycosis can be divided into the distal subungual type, white superficial type, and proximal subungual type, among which the distal subungual type is the most common. The clinical manifestations are nail bed hyperkeratosis, a yellowing and thickening of the distal nail plate, and nail peeling. In severe cases, the whole nail bed and nail plate are involved.

The dermoscopic manifestations of onychomycosis are as follows (Fig. 14.18):

1. Serrated edge at the junction of the normal nail and the lesion, and the serrated peak faces the proximal nail plate.
2. Yellow and white longitudinal streaks on the nail plate.
3. Distal irregular termination.

Tip
A serrated edge is important to distinguish onychomycosis and nail psoriasis.

14.2.6 Nail Lichen Planus

Lichen planus often involves the nail, and fingernails are more commonly involved than toenails. Longitudinal ridging and fissuring of the nail plate with thinning and distal splitting are the most common clinical manifestations of nail lichen planus. Nail bed involvement is also possible, with mild onycholysis and subungual hyperkeratosis.

The dermoscopic manifestations of nail lichen planus are as follows (Fig. 14.19):

1. On the nail matrix, longitudinal streaks, pitting, paronychia, a pterygium, red patches, and rough nails.

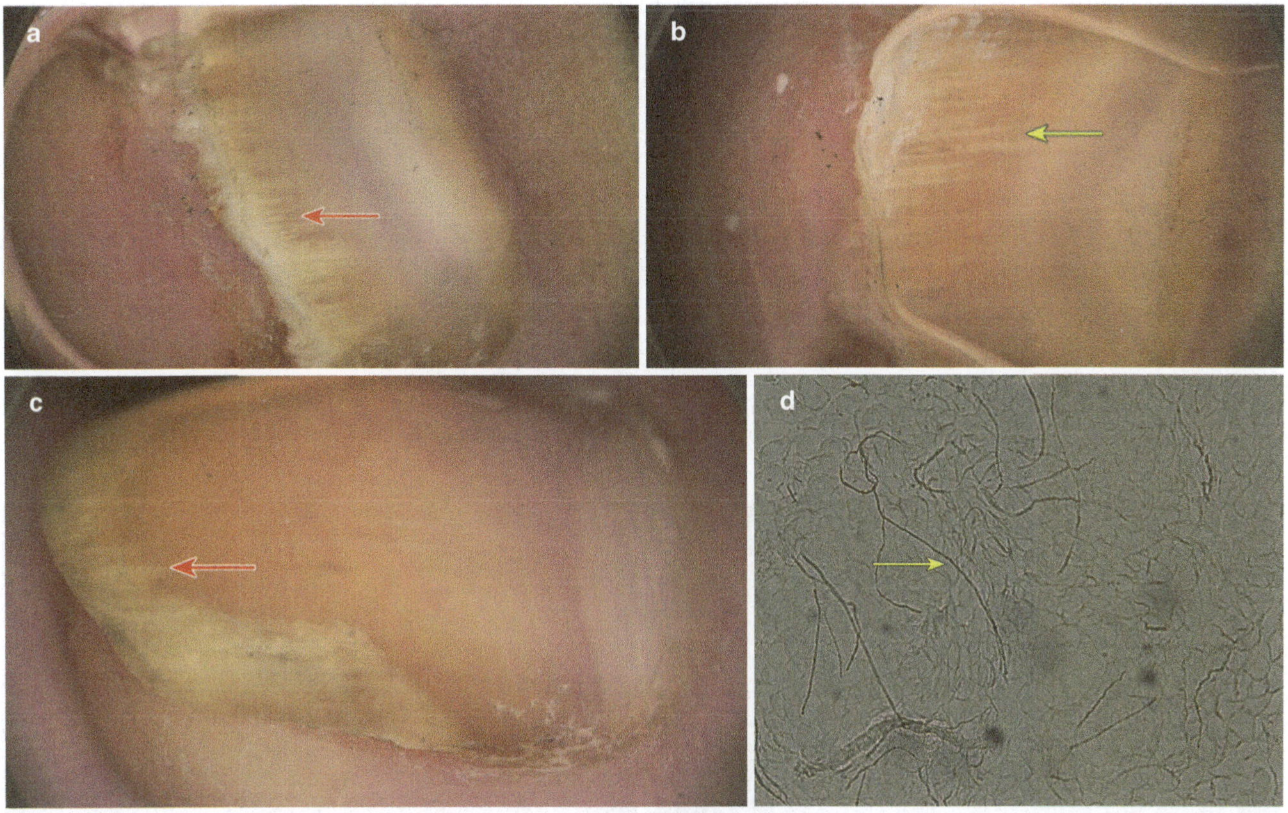

Fig. 14.18 Dermoscopic manifestations of onychomycosis (distal subungual type). (a). The distal nail plate is damaged, and a serrated edge can be seen (red arrow, × 20). (b). The distal nail plate is damaged, and yellow-white longitudinal streaks (yellow arrows) can be seen (× 20). (c). At the junction of the normal nail and the lesion, a sharp peak of the serrated edge toward the proximal nail (red arrow) can be seen (× 20). (d). The KOH preparation of the patient in c, which shows a great quantity of hyphae (yellow arrow)

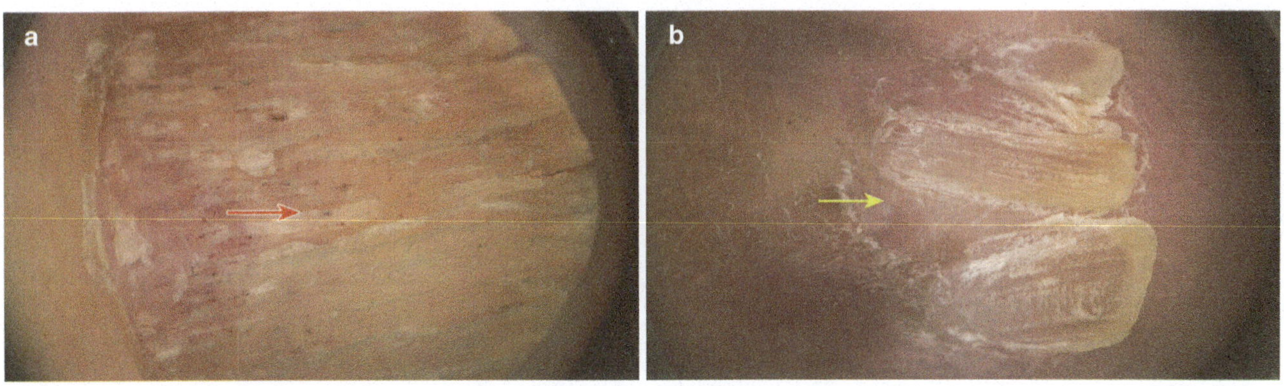

Fig. 14.19 Dermoscopic manifestations of nail lichen planus: (a). Nail plate fragmentation (red arrow), longitudinal streaks, and fragmented hemorrhage (× 20) n. (b). Nail splitting, nail plate atrophy, and a pterygium (yellow arrow, × 20)

2. On the nail bed, nail fragmentation, nail discoloration, onycholysis, hyperkeratosis under nails, and fragmented hemorrhage.
3. As the disease develops, the nail matrix, nail bed, and periungual skin can be affected at the same time, which manifests as a longitudinal ridge bulge and nail plate atrophy gathered at the center of the nail bed and even onychomadesis in severe cases.

14.2.7 Nail Psoriasis

Up to 50% of psoriasis patients have nail changes, and nail changes can be the only manifestation of psoriasis. The typical clinical manifestations of nail psoriasis include irregular pitting, the oil-drop sign on the nail bed, and nail peeling with erythema on the boundary. In addition, there are some nonspecific nail abnormalities, including nail bed

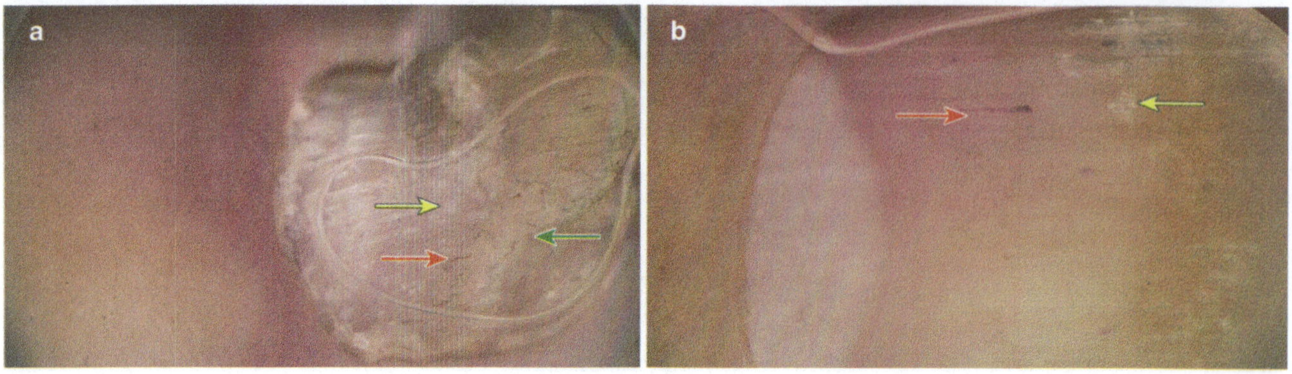

Fig. 14.20 Dermoscopic manifestations of nail psoriasis: (**a**). Fragmented hemorrhage under the nail (red arrow), nail pitting (yellow arrow), and a distal nail defect (green arrow, × 20). (**b**). Pitting (yellow arrow) and longitudinal subungual hemorrhage (red arrow) (× 20)

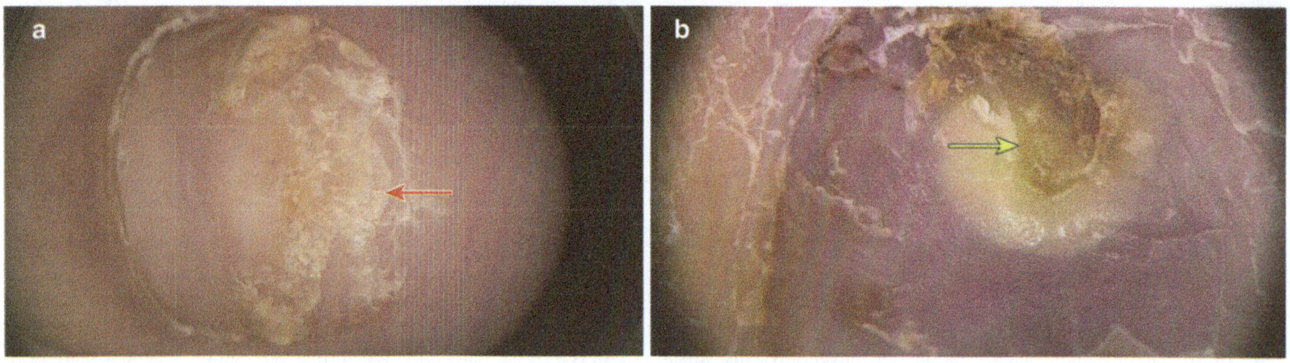

Fig. 14.21 Dermoscopic manifestations of nail changes in acrodermatitis continua: (**a**). Partial absence of the nail, with yellowish white scales at the distal end (red arrow, × 20). (**b**). The nail plate is exfoliated, and yellow pustules (yellow arrow) and scales can be seen on the nail bed (× 20)

hyperkeratosis, nail plate thickening, nail exfoliation, and paronychia.

The dermoscopic manifestations of nail psoriasis are as follows (Fig. 14.20):

1. Fragmented hemorrhage.
2. Nail pitting.
3. Distal nail dissection.
4. Subungual telangiectasia.

Subungual telangiectasia, nail stria, paronychia, and nail pitting under dermoscopy are positively correlated with the severity of the disease.

14.2.8 Nail Changes in Acrodermatitis Continua

Nail acrodermatitis is one of the typical clinical features of acrodermatitis continua, which often manifests as recurrent pustules around the nail and under nail plate. Other symptoms include nail peeling, nail removal, and periungual scales.

The dermoscopic manifestations of nail changes in acrodermatitis continua are as follows (Fig. 14.21):

1. Yellowish white hyperkeratosis/scales.
2. Pustules.

> **Tip**
> Pustules on the nail bed are characteristic of nail changes in acrodermatitis continua.

14.2.9 Onychodystrophy

Onychodystrophy refers to the abnormal shape and structure of nails caused by various factors. The clinical manifestations of onychodystrophy are nail thinning, turbidity, and deformation. The etiology of nail dystrophy is complex and can be related to other skin diseases, such as psoriasis, eczema, and systemic diseases. In addition, drugs and local factors can also cause onychodystrophy. Some patients have no obvious inducement, which is called idiopathic onychodystrophy.

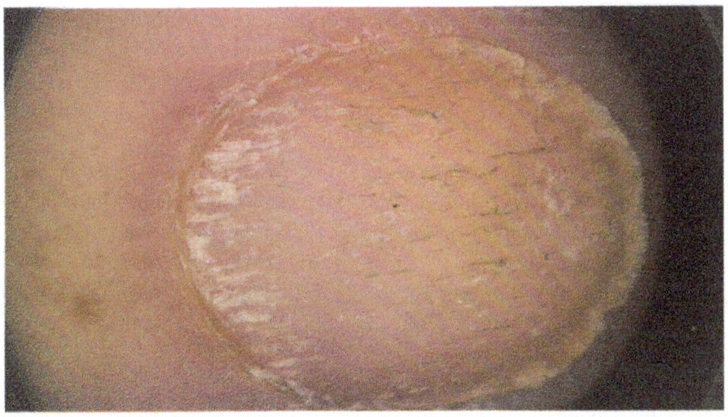

Fig. 14.22 Dermoscopic manifestations of nail dystrophy: regular patches and cracks can be seen on the nail plate (× 20)

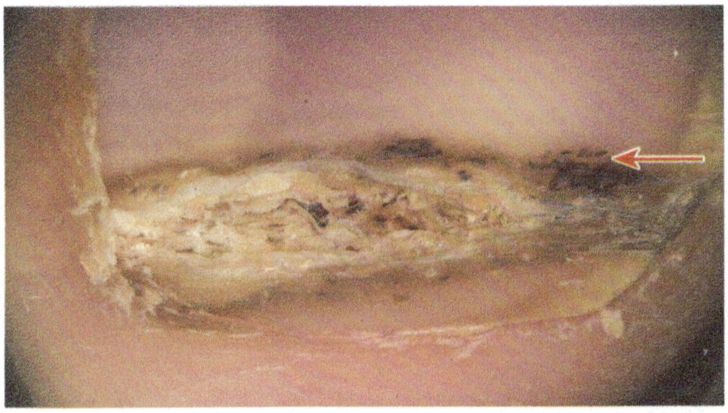

Fig. 14.23 Dermoscopic manifestations of nail squamous cell carcinoma: longitudinal red line on the nail plate, in which yellow and white scales, tumors, and patchy hemorrhages can be seen (red arrow, × 20)

The dermoscopic manifestations of onychodystrophy are as follows (Fig. 14.22):

1. Regular patches.
2. Partially or completely homogeneous background.

14.2.10 Nail Squamous Cell Carcinoma

Squamous cell carcinoma of the nail is the most common malignant tumor of the nails. Nail squamous cell carcinoma mostly involves the fingernails of middle-aged men. Clinically, there are chronic periungual or subungual tumors, which may form ulcerations and hemorrhages, as well as periungual swelling and inflammation.

The dermoscopic manifestations of nail squamous cell carcinoma are as follows (Fig. 14.23):

1. Longitudinal nail black line or red line
2. Irregular blood vessels
3. Patchy hemorrhages

Further Reading

Section 14.1: Hair Diseases

1. Trueb RM, Rezende HD, Diaz MFRG. Dynamic trichoscopy. JAMA Dermatol. 2018;154(8):877–8.
2. Pirmez R, Tosti A. Trichoscopy tips. Dermatol Clin. 2018;36(4):413–20.
3. Karadagkose O, Gulec AT. Clinical evaluation of alopecias using a handheld dermatoscope. J Am Acad Dermatol. 2012;67(2):206–14.
4. Mahmoudi H, Salehi M, Moghadas S, et al. Dermoscopic findings in 126 patients with alopecia areata: a cross-sectional study. Int J Trichology. 2018;10(3):118–23.
5. Tawfik SS, Sorour OA, Alariny AF, et al. White and yellow dots as new trichoscopic signs of severe female androgenetic alopecia in dark skin phototypes. Int J Dermatol. 2018;57(10):1221–8.
6. Rakowska A, Slowinska M, Kowalska-Oledzka E, et al. Dermoscopy in female androgenic alopecia: method standardization and diagnostic criteria. Int J Trichology. 2009;1(2):123–30.
7. Waskiel A, Rakowska A, Sikora M, et al. Trichoscopy of alopecia areata: an update. J Dermatol. 2018;45(6):692–700.
8. Lacarrubba F, Micali G, Tosti A. Scalp dermoscopy or trichoscopy. Curr Probl Dermatol. 2015;47:21–32.
9. Khunkhet S, Vachiramon V, Suchonwanit P. Trichoscopic clues for diagnosis of alopecia areata and trichotillomania in Asians. Int J Dermatol. 2017;56(2):161–5.
10. Piraccini BM, Broccoli A, Starace M, et al. Hair and scalp manifestations in secondary syphilis: epidemiology, clinical features and trichoscopy. Dermatology. 2015;231(2):171–6.
11. Doche I, Hordinsky MK, Valente NY, et al. Syphilitic alopecia: case reports and trichoscopic findings. Skin Appendage Disord. 2017;3(4):222–4.
12. Lallas A, Apalla Z, Lefaki I, et al. Dermoscopy of discoid lupus erythematosus. Br J Dermatol. 2013;168:284–8.
13. Saceda-Corralo D, Tosti A. Trichoscopic features of linear morphea on the scalp. Skin Appendage Disord. 2018;4(1):31–3.
14. Saceda-Corralo D, Fernandez-Crehuet P, et al. Clinical description of frontal fibrosing alopecia with concomitant lichen planopilaris. Skin Appendage Disord. 2018;4(2):105–7.
15. Nascimento L, Enokihara M, Vasconcellos M. Coexistence of chronic cutaneous lupus erythematosus and frontal fibrosing alopecia. An Bras Dermatol. 2018;93(2):274–6.

Section 14.2: Nail Diseases

16. Alessandrini A, Starace M, Piraccini BM. Dermoscopy in the evaluation of nail disorders. Skin Appendage Disord. 2017;3(2):70–82.
17. Mun JH, Kim GW, Jwa SW, et al. Dermoscopy of subungual haemorrhage: its usefulness in differential diagnosis from nail-unit melanoma. Br J Dermatol. 2013;1138(13):1224–9.
18. Ohn J, Choe YS, Mun JH. Dermoscopic features of nail matrix nevus (NMN) in adults and children: a comparative analysis. J Am Acad Dermatol. 2013;75(3):535–40.
19. Ohn J, Jo G, Cho Y, et al. Assessment of a predictive scoring model for dermoscopy of subungual melanoma in situ. JAMA Dermatol. 2018;154(8):890–8913.
20. Inoue Y, Menzies SW, Fukushima S, et al. Dots/globules on dermoscopy in nail-apparatus melanoma.Int. J Dermatol. 2014;53(1):88–92.
21. Romaszkiewjcz A, Slawinska M, Sobjanek M, et al. Nail dermoscopy (onychoscopy) is useful in diagnosis and treatment follow-up

of the nail mixed infection caused by *Pseudomonas aeruginosa* and *Candida albicans*. Postepy Dermatol Alergol. 2018;35(3):327–9.
22. Bhat YJ, Mir MA, Keen A, et al. Onychoscopy: an observational study in 237 patients from the Kashmir Valley of North India. Dermatol Pract Concept. 2018;8(4):283–91.
23. Nakamura R, Broce AA, Palencia DP, et al. Dermatoscopy of nail lichen planus. International J Dermatol. 2013;52(13):1384–7.
24. Golinska J, Sar-Pomian M, Rudnicka L. Dermoscopic features of psoriasis of the skin, scalp and nails – a systematic review. J Eur Acad Dermatol Venereol. 2019;33:648–60.
25. Yorulmaz A, Artuz F. A study of dermoscopic features of nail psoriasis. Postepy Dermatol Alergol. 2017;34(1):28–35.
26. Errichetti E, Stinco G. Dermoscopy in facilitating the recognition of acrodermatitis continua of Hallopeau. J Dermatol. 2017;44(11):e286–7.
27. Ramos Pinheiro R, Domingues TD, Sousa V, et al. A comparative study of onychomycosis and traumatic toenail onychodystrophy dermoscopic patterns. J Eur Acad Dermatol Venereol. 2019;33:786–92.

Computer-Aided Diagnosis of Dermoscopic Images

15

Although dermoscopy helps doctors diagnose skin lesions, the diagnosis of skin lesions with the naked eye is subjective, and there can be significant differences among even trained experts' diagnoses. Computer-aided diagnosis of dermoscopic images is an effective way to solve this problem. The system can intelligently extract and identify diseased tissues and has the function of quantitative measurements and analysis, making the diagnosis more accurate and objective.

Computer-aided diagnosis of dermoscopic images includes four steps: preprocessing, image segmentation, feature extraction, and disease recognition, as shown in Fig. 15.1. Preprocessing is mainly used to remove blur, uneven lighting, hair noise, etc. to improve the quality of the image; image segmentation is used to extract the skin lesion target from the normal skin background; feature extraction is used to transform the skin lesion target description in a way that can be calculated mathematically; and disease recognition is used to identify the target based on the data obtained by feature extraction, thereby determining the type of the lesion.

Many technical methods are used to accomplish computer-aided diagnosis. These methods can be roughly divided into traditional machine learning methods and deep learning methods. The diagnostic method based on traditional machine learning strictly follows the steps above to process and obtain the diagnostic result. The diagnostic method based on deep learning uses a convolutional neural network (CNN) for end-to-end processing, which can directly generate segmentation results without preprocessing or directly recognize the type of skin lesion after inputting images into the network. This chapter will introduce the technology of computer-aided diagnosis of dermoscopic images from two aspects: traditional machine learning and deep learning.

15.1 Computer-Aided Diagnosis Based on Traditional Machine Learning

Traditional machine learning methods regard each step of the computer-aided diagnostic system as an independent part, with each part processed separately and each result connected in series to obtain the final diagnosis. Each process has different image processing methods. For example, in the image segmentation step, methods based on Otsu's thresholding, region growth, statistical region fusion, etc. are commonly used to extract skin lesions from the image. In the disease recognition step, skin lesions can be recognized by a back-propagation (BP) neural network or support vector machine (SVM). Considering that this book is intended for medical professionals, and this chapter mainly focuses on the understanding of computer-aided diagnostic systems, this chapter will introduce relatively simple methods of image processing for each step and will not go deeper into the complex techniques.

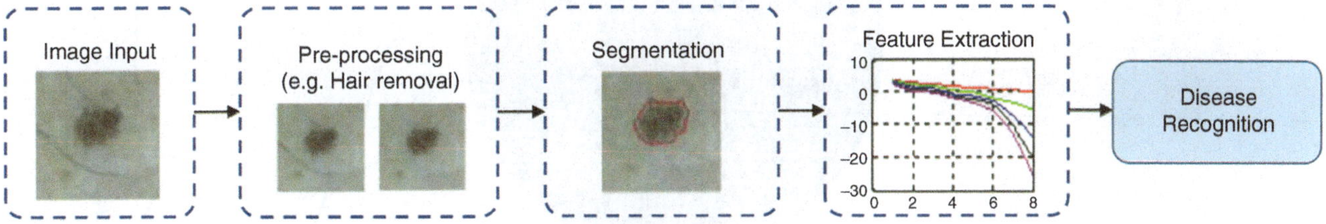

Fig. 15.1 Flowchart of computer-aided diagnosis of dermoscopic images

J. Liu, X. Zou, *Practical Dermoscopy*, https://doi.org/10.1007/978-981-19-1460-7_15

15.1.1 Preprocessing

Preprocessing is used to improve the quality of dermoscopic images. Here, we take hair denoising as an example to illustrate image preprocessing.

15.1.1.1 Hair Extraction Based on the Black Top-Hat Transform

The black top-hat transform is a commonly used morphological filter that can detect structures darker than the surrounding background in an image. Assume that f is the input image, g is the structuring element, and $f{\cdot}g$ represents a closing operation, which is defined as

$$f{\cdot}g = [f \oplus (-g)\ominus(-g) \quad (15.1)$$

where $-g$ is the symmetric set of g about the origin point, which is obtained by rotating g relative to the origin point at 180 degrees. That is, the closing operation dilates f with $-g$ and then erodes the result with $-g$. The black top-hat transform is defined as

$$\mathrm{Valley}(f) = (f \cdot g) - f \quad (15.2)$$

The black top-hat operator detects the valley structure in the image; therefore, it is also called the valley detector. In the dermoscopic image, the hair can be seen as a valley signal because its brightness value is darker than that of the surrounding pixels. Figure 15.2 (b) gives the result of the valley detection of Fig. 15.2 (a). We can see that weak hairs and strong hairs are highlighted together, and the contrast between hair pixels and other nonhair pixels is greatly improved. Then, the hair target is extracted by binarizing Fig. 15.2 (b), as shown in Fig. 15.2 (c).

15.1.1.2 Hair Removal Based on a Partial Differential Equation

Assuming that the initial image to be recovered is $I_0(i,j)$, image recovery is a process of gradually obtaining improved versions, and a series of intermediate results obtained in this process is regarded as an iterative image series $I_n(i,j)$. The process is mathematically described as follows:

$$I^{n+1}(i,j) = I^n(i,j) + \frac{\lambda}{s}\sum_{p \in D} c\left(\nabla^t I(i,j)\right)\nabla I^t(i,j) \quad (15.3)$$

where (i, j) represents the coordinates of pixel points; D represents the neighborhood of pixel (i, j), usually four adjacent points (up, down, left, and right); s represents the number of neighborhood points; the constant λ is a positive number, and it reflects the weight of the distribution coefficient, i.e., the degree of smoothness; n represents the current step, i.e., the number of iterations; $\nabla I(i,j)$ represents the Laplace gradient of pixel (i, j); c is the diffusion coefficient; and t is the order of the gradient, usually set to 1–2, and an overlarge t may destroy the information of the nonhair area.

For the color image of skin melanoma, the hair area obtained in Fig. 15.2 (c) is used as the mask, and the pixels at the mask are calculated in the three domains of R, G, and B by formula (15.3). Figure 15.3 shows an example of hair occlusion information recovery, where λ is taken as 0.8; neighborhood D is the upper, lower, left, and right pixels; and the number of iterations is 30. The recovery result is consistent with the understanding of skin lesion textures by the human eye.

15.1.2 Image Segmentation

Otsu's thresholding, also known as the maximum interclass variance thresholding, was proposed by Otsu from Japan in 1980. The method is derived based on the principle of discrimination and least squares, with which good results can be obtained.

Let the gray value of an image be level 1~m, and the number of pixels of the gray value i be n_i, and then divide it into

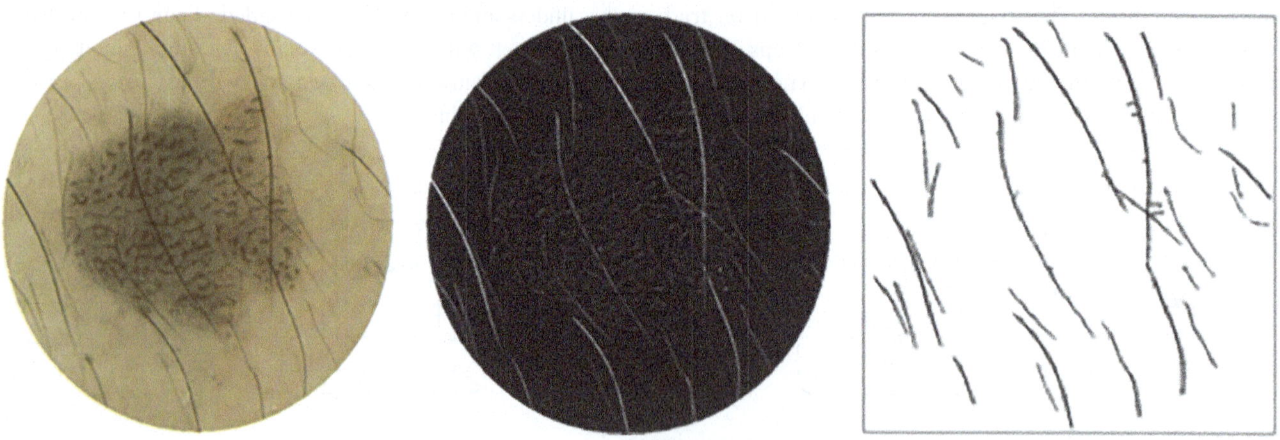

Fig. 15.2 An example of hair enhancement and binarization based on the black top-hat transform

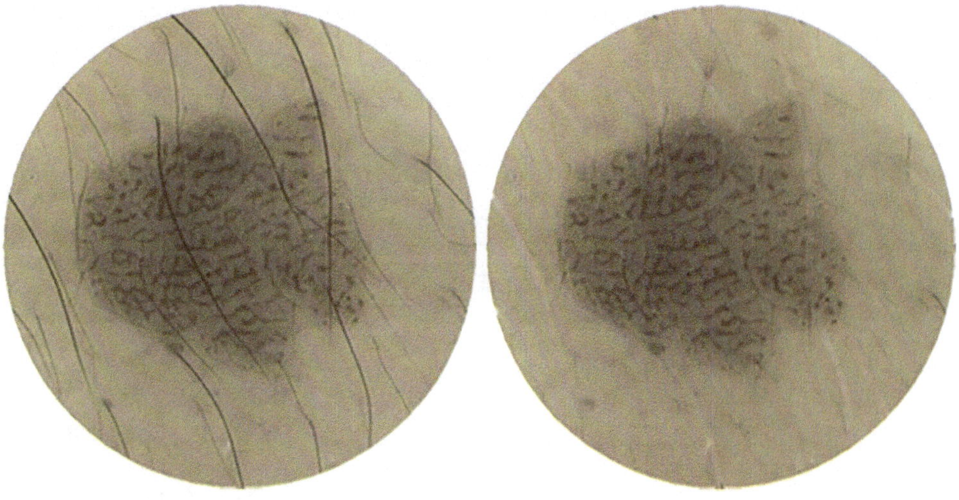

Fig. 15.3 An example of hair occlusion information recovery using the partial differential equation method

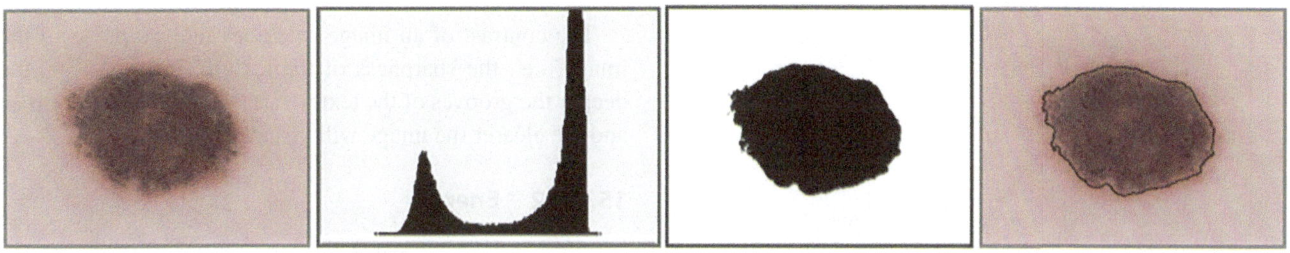

Fig. 15.4 An example of Otsu's thresholding segmentation

two groups, $C_0 = \{1\sim t\}$ and $C_1 = \{t + 1\sim m\}$ with t, then the variance between the two groups is calculated as follows:

$$\delta^2(t) = w_0 w_1 (\mu_1 - \mu_0)^2 \tag{15.4}$$

where μ_0 and μ_1 are the mean values of the two groups, and w_0 and w_1 are the probabilities of the two groups.

By changing t from 1 to m, we find the value of t when the above formula reaches a maximum value. That is, find the value of t^* when $\max\delta^2(t)$ is reached; then, t^* is the expected threshold. Figure 15.4 is an example of how Otsu's thresholding performs segmentation on a dermoscopic image, where (a) is the image to be segmented, and (b) is its histogram. The target and background of the image correspond to two peaks, and the best threshold falls between the two peaks. This threshold can be used to perform binarization to obtain the result shown in (c). Finally, (d) shows the result of covering the boundary line in (c) onto the original image, and the target is successfully segmented.

15.1.3 Feature Extraction

After image segmentation, the target area is obtained. For the computer to recognize the diseases, the color, texture, shape, and boundary of the target must be described with more concise and clearer values and variables. These values and variables generated from the original image reflect the main information of the target area. Here, we take texture features as an example to introduce the feature extraction process of dermoscopic images.

Generally, texture refers to repeated local patterns and their arrangement rules in the image; it is a regular change in the gray level or color of image pixels, which is related to spatial statistics, as shown in Fig. 15.5. The gray-level co-occurrence matrix is one of the most commonly used texture statistical analysis methods. This method reflects the comprehensive information of the image in direction, interval, change amplitude and speed by calculating the probability of transition from one gray level to another between two pixels in a specific direction and distance in the image. Let $f(x, y)$ be a gray image of $N \times N$ and $d = (dx, dy)$ be a displacement vector, where dx is the displacement in the row direction, dy is the displacement in the column direction, and L is the maximum grayscale of the image. The gray-level co-occurrence matrix is defined as the probability $p(i, j| d, \theta)$ of the simultaneous occurrence of pixels with distance $\delta = \left(dx^2 + dy^2\right)^{\frac{1}{2}}$ and gray level j, starting from the pixels with gray level i of $f(x, y)$, as shown in Fig. 15.6. The formula is as follows:

$$p(i,|j,|d,|\theta) = \{(x,y)|f(x|y) = i|f(x+dx|,y+dy) = j\} \tag{15.5}$$

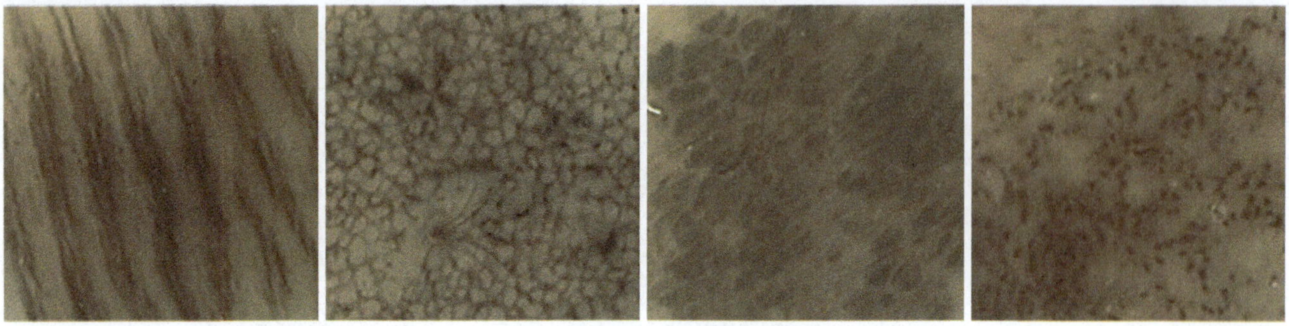

Fig. 15.5 Several kinds of textures in dermoscopic images

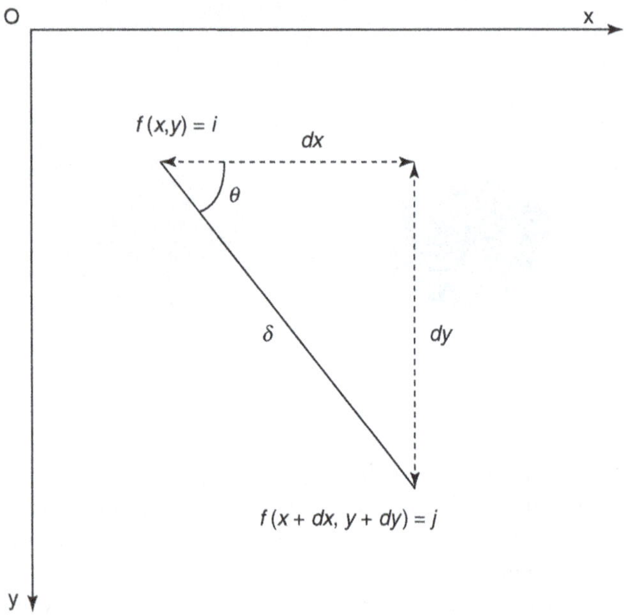

Fig. 15.6 Pixel pairs of the gray-level co-occurrence matrix

then we obtain probability by normalizing it,

$$\hat{p}(i,|j,|,d,|,\theta) = \frac{p(i,|j,|,d,|,\theta)}{S} \tag{15.6}$$

where S is the sum of the elements.

The gray-level co-occurrence matrix reflects the comprehensive information of the image gray-level distribution about direction, neighborhood and change amplitude, but it cannot directly provide the characteristics of distinguishing texture. Therefore, it is necessary to further extract the features describing the image texture from the gray-level co-occurrence matrix to quantitatively describe the texture characteristics. In the following subsections, we introduce the five most commonly used characteristics.

15.1.3.1 Contrast

$$\text{CON} = \sum_i \sum_j (i-j)^2 \hat{p}(i,|j,|,d,|,\theta) \tag{15.7}$$

The contrast of an image describes the sharpness of the image, i.e., the sharpness of the texture. In the image, the deeper the grooves of the texture are, the greater the contrast and the clearer the image will visually be.

15.1.3.2 Energy

$$\text{ASM} = \sum_i \sum_j \hat{p}(i,|j,|,d,|,\theta)^2 \tag{15.8}$$

Energy, or angular second moment (ASM), is a measure of the uniformity of the image gray distribution. When the element distribution of the gray-level co-occurrence matrix is more concentrated on the main diagonal, it means that the gray-level distribution of the image is more uniform from local areas. From the perspective of the whole image, the texture is coarser and the ASM is larger, which means that the coarse texture contains more energy; in contrast, the fine texture has a smaller ASM and contains less energy.

15.1.3.3 Correlation

Correlation measures the similarity of the elements of the gray-level co-occurrence matrix in the direction of rows or columns.

$$C(d,\theta) = \frac{\sum_i \sum_j ij\,\hat{p}(i,j|d,\theta) - \mu_1\mu_2}{\sigma_1^2\sigma_2^2} \tag{15.9}$$

where $\mu_1 = \sum_i i \sum_j \hat{p}(i,j|d,\theta)$, $\mu_2 = \sum_j j \sum_i \hat{p}(i,j|d,\theta)$

$$\sigma_1^2 = \sum_i (i-\mu_1)^2 \sum_j \hat{p}(i,j|d,\theta), \quad \sigma_2^2 = \sum_j (j-\mu_2)^2 \sum_i \hat{p}(i,j|d,\theta)$$

15.1.3.4 Entropy

$$\text{ENT} = -\sum_i \sum_j \hat{p}(i,|j,|d,|,\theta)\log_2 \hat{p}(i,|j,|d,|,\theta) \quad (15.10)$$

Entropy is a measure of the amount of information an image has, and texture information also belongs to image information. If the image has no texture, the gray-level co-occurrence matrix is almost zero, and the entropy is close to zero. If the image has more fine textures, the values in the gray-level co-occurrence matrix are approximately equal, and the entropy of the image reaches a maximum. If fewer textures are distributed in the image, the entropy of the image is small.

15.1.3.5 Inverse Different Moment

$$\text{Hom} = \sum_i \sum_j \frac{\hat{p}(i,j|d,\theta)}{1+(i-j)^2} \quad (15.11)$$

The inverse difference moment is a measure of the local change in image texture, which reflects the regularity of texture. The more regular the texture is, the greater the inverse different moment will be, and vice versa.

The five texture features above are extracted by a gray-level co-occurrence matrix. For the description of texture features, there are also other methods, such as Gabor features and local binary pattern (LBP) features. In fact, for the feature extraction of skin lesions, including color, boundary, shape, and other aspects, there are many description methods. Therefore, in computer-aided diagnostic systems, the feature extraction of skin lesions can usually reach dozens or even thousands of data points. These data will be input into the classifier to recognize the skin lesions.

15.1.4 Disease Recognition

After the image is enhanced, restored or segmented, the target area can be separated from the background and moved to the lesion classification stage. There are many classification methods, but each has its advantages and disadvantages. Therefore, it is necessary to select the appropriate method according to the actual needs. The BP neural network is a feedforward multilayer neural network that is used by many researchers to classify skin lesions. The structure of the BP network serves as a basis for the deep learning network. Therefore, we take the BP network as an example to illustrate the process of disease recognition.

15.1.4.1 Principle of a BP Neural Network

The basic component in a neural network is the neuron. In a biological neural network, each neuron is connected to other neurons. When a neuron is "excited," it will send chemicals

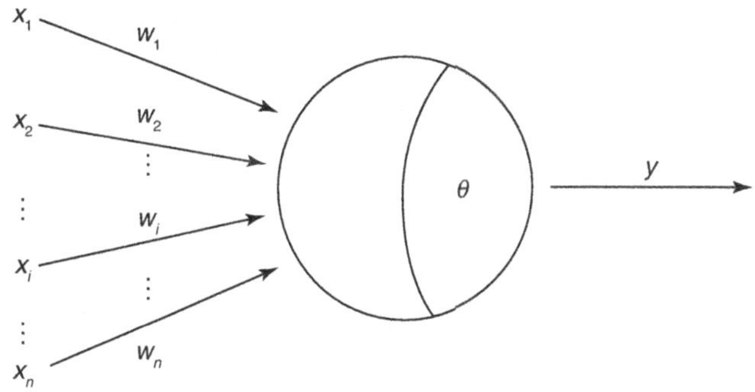

Fig. 15.7 The M-P neural model

to the connected neurons, thereby changing the potential in those neurons; if the potential of a certain neuron exceeds a threshold value, then it will be activated.

In 1943, McCulloch and Pitts abstracted the above situation as a simple model shown in Fig. 15.7, which is the "M-P neuron model" that is commonly used today. In this model, a single neuron receives input signals from n other neurons, passes them through a weighted connection, and processes the "activation function" to generate the output of the neuron. In Fig. 15.7, x_i represents the input from the i-th neuron, w_i represents the connection weight of the i-th neuron, θ represents the threshold, and y represents the output value of the neuron.

The ideal activation function is the step function shown in Fig. 15.8 (a), which maps the input value to the output value "0" or "1." "1" corresponds to neuron excitement, and "0" corresponds to neuron suppression. However, the step function has undesirable properties such as discontinuity and nonsmoothness. Therefore, the sigmoid function is commonly used as the activation function. The formula is as follows:

$$f(x) = \frac{1}{1+e^{-x}} \quad (15.12)$$

The classic sigmoid function, shown in Fig. 15.8 (b), squeezes the input value from a large range to the range of (0, 1); therefore, it is also called the "squeeze function."

A BP neural network includes an input layer, an output layer, and several hidden layers between them. The coupling relationship is formed in a single feedforward manner, and there is no interconnection between neurons in the same layer. Figure 15.9 gives a simple BP network model with a hidden layer. According to the BP learning algorithm, an input mode of the network is sent from the input layer to the hidden layer and is then sent to the output layer through hidden layers in between. After processing by the output layer unit, an output mode is obtained. Therefore, a BP neural network is called a feedforward structure. If there is an error between the output response and the expected output mode and it does not meet the requirements, the correction and

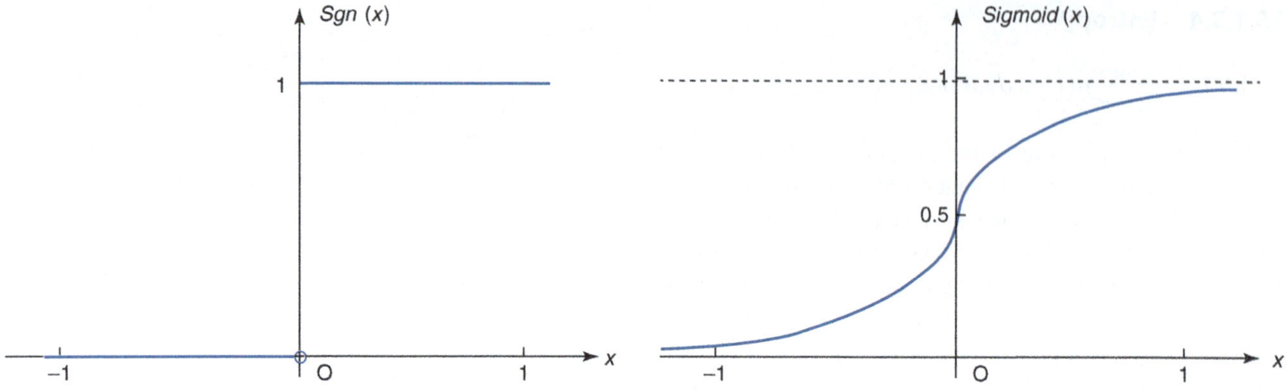

Fig. 15.8 Classic neuron activation function

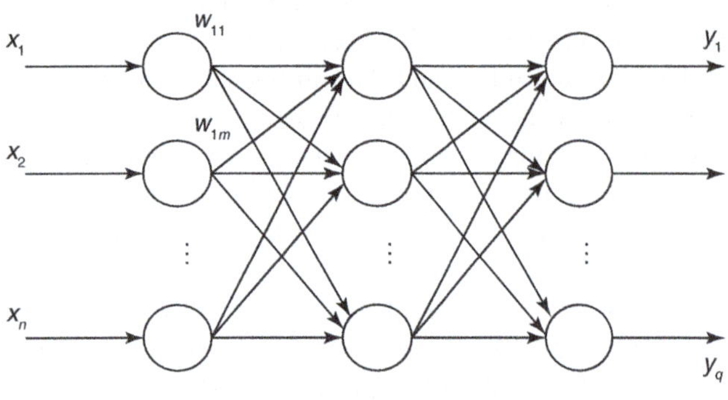

Fig. 15.9 Three-layer back-propagation network model

optimization of the weight can be achieved through the back-propagation of the error.

A BP neural network learning adopts the gradient descent method, which includes two steps: the forward propagation of the input mode and the backward propagation of the input error. First, it is necessary to use the input mode to find the actual output corresponding to it, as shown in Eq. (15.13),

$$y_k = f\left(s_k\right) = \frac{1}{1+\exp\left(-\sum_{j=1}^{p} v_{kj} b_j + \theta_k\right)}, \quad k = 1,2,\cdots,q \tag{15.13}$$

where y_k is the value of the k-th unit in the output layer, s_j is the activation value of each neuron in the hidden layer, v_{kj} is the weight from the hidden layer to the output layer, b_j is the output value of the hidden layer j unit, and θ_k is the output layer unit threshold.

In the forward propagation step, we obtain the actual output value of the network. When the error between the actual output value and the expected output value is greater than the limited value, the network must be corrected. The correction here is carried out from back to front; therefore, it is called error back-propagation, which is calculated from the output layer to the hidden layer and then from the hidden layer to the input layer.

We first calculate the correction error of the output layer, as shown in Eq. (15.14),

$$d_k = \left(o_k - y_k\right) y_k \left(1 - y_k\right), \quad k = 1,2,\cdots,q \tag{15.14}$$

where y_k is the actual output and o_k is the expected output.

Then, the correction error of each unit of the hidden layer is calculated as

$$e_j = \left[\sum_{k=1}^{q} v_{kj} d_k\right] b_j \left(1 - b_j\right), \quad j = 1,2,\cdots,p \tag{15.15}$$

The connection weight of the output layer to the hidden layer and the correction value of the output layer threshold are shown in Eqs. (15.16, 15.17),

$$\Delta v_{kj} = \alpha \cdot d_k \cdot b_j \tag{15.16}$$

$$\Delta \theta_k = \alpha \cdot d_k \tag{15.17}$$

where b_j is the output of the hidden layer j unit, d_k is the correction error of the output layer, and α is a learning coefficient greater than 0 and less than 1.

The correction value from the hidden layer to the input layer is shown in Eqs. (15.18, 15.19),

$$\Delta w_{ji} = \beta \cdot e_j \cdot x_i \tag{15.18}$$

$$\Delta \theta_j = \beta \cdot e_j \tag{15.19}$$

where e_j is the correction error of the hidden layer j unit, and β is the learning coefficient greater than 0 and less than 1.

To minimize the output error of a network, for each set of training inputs of the BP neural network, the network usually remembers the mode through hundreds of thousands of training iterations. Each training iteration actually repeats the input pattern described above. The learning result must be examined at the end of each iteration. The purpose of this examination is mainly to check whether the output error has been slight enough. If so, the entire learning process is ended; otherwise, the cyclic training is continued.

15.1.4.2 Classification of Benign and Malignant Melanocytic Tumors Based on a BP Network

Dermoscopic image classification based on traditional machine learning methods can be used for the benign and malignant classification of skin melanocytic tumors. We collected 240 images of melanocytic tumors for classification experiments, including 80 malignant samples and 160 benign samples. Out of the 240 images, 50% were used for the training set and 50% were used for the test set. According to the characteristics of skin melanocytic tumor images, we extracted features such as color, texture, and shape in the RGB color space and obtained 57 features in total. These 57 features were used as the input for the BP network, namely, $x_1, x_2 \ldots, x_n$ in Fig. 15.7, where n is 57. Our BP network structure was N-N-1, the learning rate was 0.7, the maximum training round was 1000, the expected error rate was 0.03, and the activation function was the sigmoid function. We trained the BP network using the above steps. After the training was completed, the trained BP model was evaluated on the test set. The model finally achieved 80.0% sensitivity and 93.75% specificity, and the final classification accuracy was 89.17%.

15.2 Computer-Aided Diagnosis Based on Deep Learning

Traditional methods require complicated preprocessing of the original images and require experienced engineers to manually design feature extractors and select appropriate classifiers for classification. Therefore, the generalization ability is not strong, and it is difficult to implement complex multiclassification tasks. With the advent of the era of big data and the development of computer hardware, deep learning technology has gradually exerted its advantages in the field of medical imaging. The computer-aided diagnostic method based on deep learning mainly uses the CNN for end-to-end processing, which omits the preprocessing process and outputs the segmentation result or directly classifies and recognizes the skin damage target input to the network. This section first briefly introduces the basic components of CNNs and then discusses the application of deep learning methods in skin lesion segmentation and classification.

15.2.1 Principle of Convolutional Neural Networks

CNNs, as a kind of deep learning method, are deep feedforward artificial neural networks. The input layer and hidden layer of ordinary neural networks are generally fully connected, which leads to a large number of parameters, and the extracted features do not have spatial information. A CNN features the local receptive field for extracting effective spatial information through a convolution layer. The local receptive field and weight sharing can greatly reduce the number of parameters.

15.2.1.1 Components of Convolutional Neural Networks

Generally, the structure of a CNN includes an input layer, convolution layer, pooling layer, full connection layer, activation function layer, output layer, and loss function layer.

A. Input layer

The input layer inputs an image. The size of the color image input is M × N × 3. M × N is the resolution of the image, and 3 is the number of channels, namely, the R, G, and B channels.

B. Convolutional layer

The convolutional layer is the core of a CNN, and most of the calculations are generated by convolutional layers. The most important idea of the convolution layer is the local receptive field and weight sharing. The local receptive field makes the extracted features contain local information. The number of convolution kernels in the convolutional layer determines the number of feature maps obtained after the input data pass through the layer. The size of a convolution kernel determines the size of the local receptive field; that is, each neuron is connected with only some input neurons, and the depth of this local area is the same as that of the input data, as shown in Fig. 15.10.

The convolution operation uses the convolution kernel to slide on the input two-dimensional data for calculation and obtain the result, i.e., the feature map, through the activation function. The value of the convolution kernel is the weight coefficient. Each convolution calculation performs a weighted summation on each channel of the input image and the corresponding position of the convolution kernel and then adds a bias term. The formula is as follows:

$$x_j^l = \sum_{i \in M_j} x_j^{l-1} * k_{ij}^l + b_j^l \tag{15.20}$$

where l refers to the l-th layer of the network, x_j^l is the j-th feature map output by this layer, M_j is the set of pixels

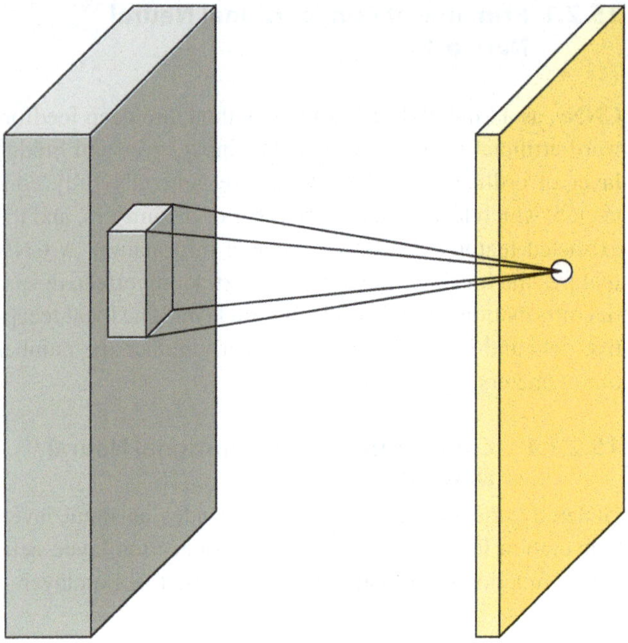

Fig. 15.10 Local receptive field of the convolution kernel

corresponding to the convolution kernel, k_{ij}^{l} is the i-th parameter in the convolution kernel, and b_j^l is the bias item.

Weight sharing is also used to further reduce the number of parameters; that is, the convolution kernel parameters corresponding to each neuron are consistent.

C. Pooling layer

The pooling layer is also called the downsampling layer and is usually located after the convolutional layer. The pooling operation downsamples the input data to reduce parameters and the number of calculations and to prevent overfitting. Additionally, the feature map also introduces invariance to a certain extent. The pooling filter replaces the entire window with one value so that the key of the feature can be highlighted without paying much attention to the position or direction information. The formula for pooling calculation is as follows:

$$x_j^l = \mathrm{down}\left(x_j^{l-1}\right) \tag{15.21}$$

where down(x) is the downsampling function, and the commonly used downsampling functions include taking the average value, intermediate value, maximum value, etc.

D. Full connection layer

The fully connected layer is usually located in the last layers of a CNN, including the output layer. Fully connected means that each output neuron of this layer is connected to all the input neurons. Figure 15.11 shows how neurons are fully connected. This layer maps the feature information to the sample label space of the final output layer and finally outputs the probability that the sample is in each category for classifying the features. However, since the fully connected layer is connected to every neuron of the input data without weight sharing, there are many parameters in the fully connected layer. To reduce the parameters of the network, global average pooling can sometimes be used to replace the fully connected layer.

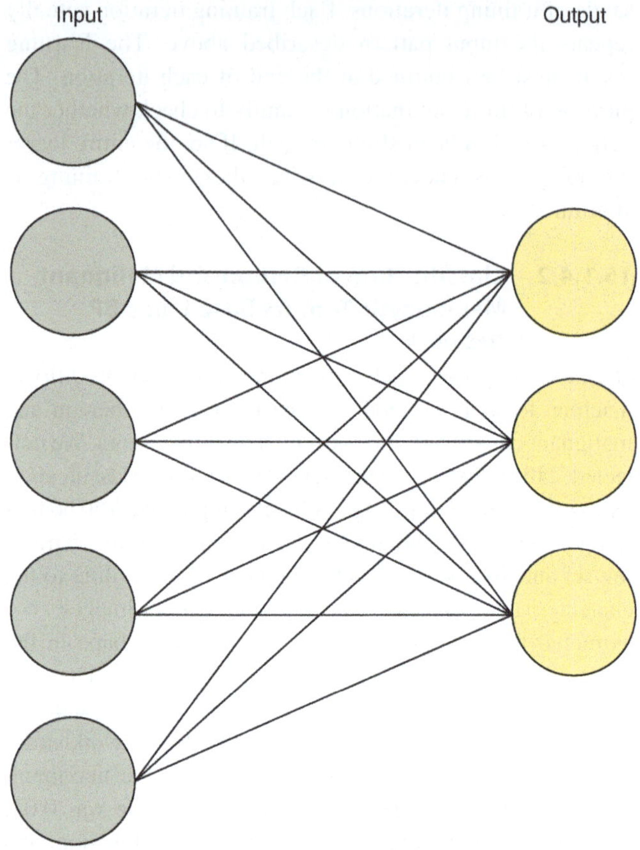

Fig. 15.11 Fully connected structure

E. Activation function layer

The activation function layer is used to introduce nonlinear factors since the description of a nonlinear network is much denser than that of a linear network. The activation function features nonlinearity, differentiability, monotonicity, and a finite output range. The earliest activation function used is the sigmoid function, as shown in formula (15.12). However, the sigmoid function has the disadvantage that the derivative value is small, especially when it is far from 0 and the derivative is close to 0, which easily leads to the disappearance of the gradient in the training process. Therefore, the rectified linear unit (ReLU) was proposed for solving the problem, and the formula is as follows:

$$\text{ReLU}(x)=\begin{cases} x & x>0 \\ 0 & x\le 0 \end{cases} \quad (15.22)$$

As shown in Fig. 15.12, when the input is greater than 0, the output of the function is equal to the input, and when the input is less than or equal to 0, the output of the function is 0, which is more similar to the activation mechanism of neurons. Moreover, compared with the sigmoid function, the convergence speed of the network becomes faster, and the accuracy is improved.

F. Softmax output layer

The Softmax function, also the normalized exponential function, is actually the logarithmic normalization of the gradient of the finite-term discrete probability distribution. The range of neuron parameters passing through the fully connected layer is often difficult to determine, which troubles the back-propagation calculation in the training process. Therefore, in practice, the Softmax function is often used as the final output layer of neural networks in multiclassification tasks.

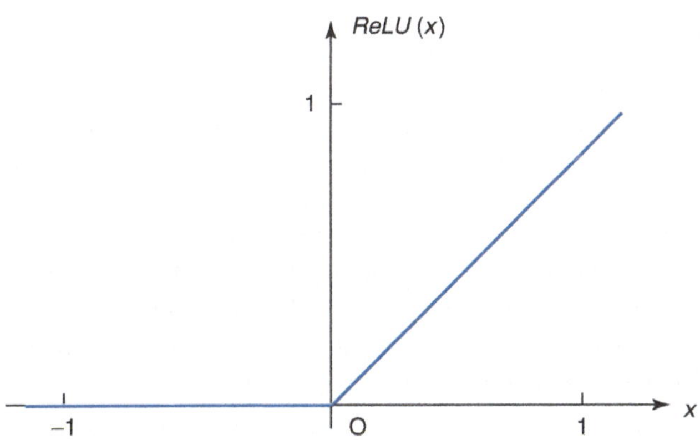

Fig. 15.12 The rectified linear unit (ReLU)

The Softmax function is shown in Fig. 15.13. The first step of the function transforms the prediction result of the model into an exponential function to ensure the nonnegativity of the output probability. To ensure that the sum of the probabilities of each prediction is equal to 1, the converted result needs to be normalized by e^z. Subsequently, the converted result is divided by the sum of all index results, which is the percentage of the converted result to the total, thereby converting the multicategory output into a probability value. The final probability value has two properties: (1) the predicted probability is a nonnegative number, and (2) the sum of the probabilities of various prediction results is equal to 1.

G. Loss function

The loss function is a key part of a CNN. Since CNNs are basically supervised learning, a loss function is needed to calculate the disparity between the expected output result and the real output result to evaluate the performance of the model. The key of the CNN training process is the back-propagation algorithm, that is, back-propagating according to the current loss, changing the value of each layer of parameters, and then iterating repeatedly so that the loss is continuously reduced until the final convergence.

The segmentation task uses the Dice coefficient loss function. This method is inspired by binary classification. The essential idea is to calculate the degree of overlap between the test result and the true value. The output range is from 0 to 1, indicating that the process goes from a complete noncoincidence to a complete coincidence. During the training process, the network proceeds to the reduced range of the loss function; therefore, the actual loss function is the complement of the Dice coefficient. The calculation formula is

$$\text{loss}=1-\text{DC}=1-\frac{2(A\cap G)}{A+G} \quad (15.23)$$

where DC represents the Dice coefficient, A represents the actual segmentation result, and G represents the true value of

Fig. 15.13 Softmax function

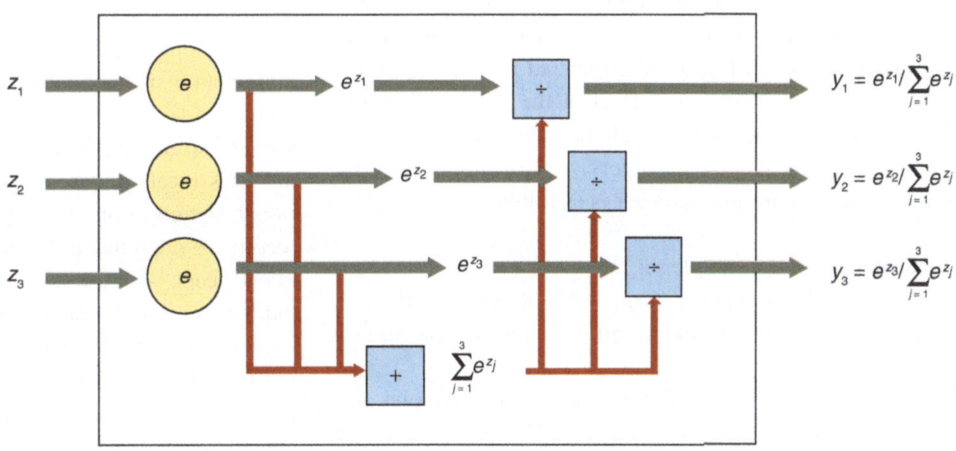

the segmentation. In the process of training, the network parameters are updated according to the reduced direction of loss so that the consistency between the segmentation result and the true value increases.

The classification task uses the cross-entropy loss function. Cross-entropy was first applied to information theory to describe the distance between the test vector and the truth vector. In practical problems, when we obtain a set of prediction vectors, we calculate the cross-entropy between the vector and the truth binary vector. The smaller the cross-entropy is, the closer their probability distributions and the better the prediction effect will be. By continuously reducing the cross-entropy, the neural network obtains more suitable parameters. The loss function is as follows:

$$\text{loss} = \frac{1}{n}\sum_{i=1}^{n}\left[y_i \log\left(\widehat{y_i}\right) + \left(1 - y_i\right)\log\left(1 - \widehat{y_i}\right)\right] \quad (15.24)$$

where n represents the number of images in each batch and y_i represents the category truth label. If the original image is melanoma, $y_i = 1$; otherwise, $y_i = 0$. $\widehat{y_i}$ represents the actual predicted probability, ranging from 0 to 1. In the training process, the network parameters are updated according to the decreasing direction to continuously improve the probability of correct prediction.

The general CNN network structure connects the convolution layer, pooling layer, and nonlinear activation function layer as a whole. This structure extracts the local features of the network, maps the extracted features to the final classification probability, and finally obtains the required results.

15.2.1.2 Training Process of Convolutional Neural Network

The training process of a CNN is similar to that of a BP network. After the predicted value is obtained through forward propagation, a back-propagation algorithm is used to calculate the partial derivative of the loss function to each weight, and then the weight is updated by the gradient descent method. The selection of hyperparameters in the training of CNNs is important, and the convergence results of neural networks largely depend on the initialization of these parameters. An ideal parameter initialization scheme makes training more effective, while a bad initialization scheme will not only affect the convergence effect of the network but also cause gradient dispersion or gradient explosion.

Generally, a CNN uses a supervised learning method for training, and the training process is as follows:

1. Select a training sample set.
2. Initialize the weights and thresholds of the network.
3. Select a vector from the training sample set and input it into the network.
4. Calculate the output value of the selected samples and compare it with the ideal output value; then, obtain the error value.
5. Use the obtained error value to back-propagate and adjust the weights and thresholds in the network according to the method of minimizing the error.
6. Finally, compare the total error E and the given error threshold ε . If $E \le \varepsilon$, go to the next step; If $E > \varepsilon$, the network has not reached the expected goal, and a return to step (3) is necessary to continue training.
7. After the training, a well-learned CNN is obtained.

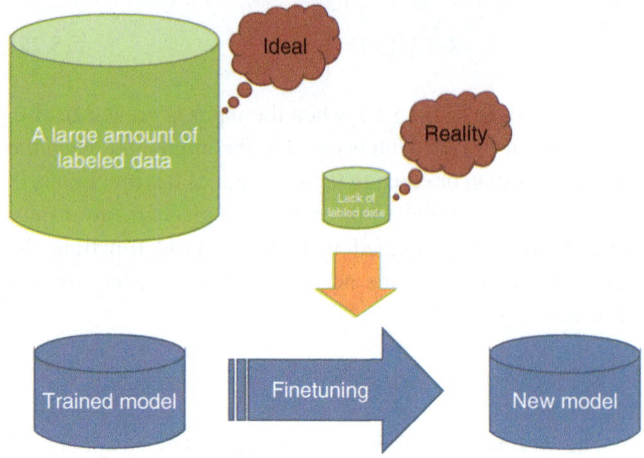

Fig. 15.14 Transfer learning in network training

However, there is often a lack of labeled data in practical scenarios due to various conditions. The network trained from scratch requires a large amount of labeled image data, which will consume considerable material, manpower, and time costs. In view of the limited resources in the actual scenario, researchers have proposed a transfer learning method to train the network. Considering that most data or tasks are relevant, transfer learning uses the learned model parameters to accelerate and optimize the learning efficiency of the model. The principle is shown in Fig. 15.14.

15.2.2 Typical Convolutional Neural Network Model

CNNs are one of the pioneering research results inspired by the combination of neurobiology and artificial neural networks. Compared with traditional methods, CNNs have the characteristics of strong applicability, simultaneous feature extraction and classification, strong generalization ability and fewer global optimization training parameters. This method has become an important milestone in the field of deep learning. In recent years, with the improvements in computational power and hardware performance, the depth of CNNs has increased, resulting in many typical network structures, including AlexNet and GoogLeNet. These networks have good performance in the segmentation and classification of dermoscopic images. This section will introduce these common networks.

15.2.2.1 AlexNet

In 2012, Alex designed an 8-layer CNN structure with a convolution kernel size of 11 × 11. He used the ReLU as the activation function and dual parallel GPU to realize network training. AlexNet won the championship in the ImageNet competition (1000 classes, approximately 1.28 million images), far exceeding second place by 10 percentage points. The network structure is shown in Fig. 15.15.

The operation of the first layer of the network is shown in Fig. 15.16. The left square is the input layer with a 3-channel image with a size of 224 × 224. The small square on the right is the convolution kernel with a size of 11 × 11 and a depth of 3. Each time a convolution kernel is used to perform a convolution operation in the input layer, we obtain a feature map with a depth of 1.

Therefore, in AlexNet, the length and width pixels of the input images are both 224, and the depth is 3. After five convolutional layers' calculations, the fully connected layer of the last three layers maps the two-dimensional feature information to the sample label space of the final output layer and finally outputs the probability in each category to classify the disease.

15.2.2.2 VGG-Nets

VGG-Nets was proposed by the Visual Geometry Group (VGG) of Oxford University. This network won first place in

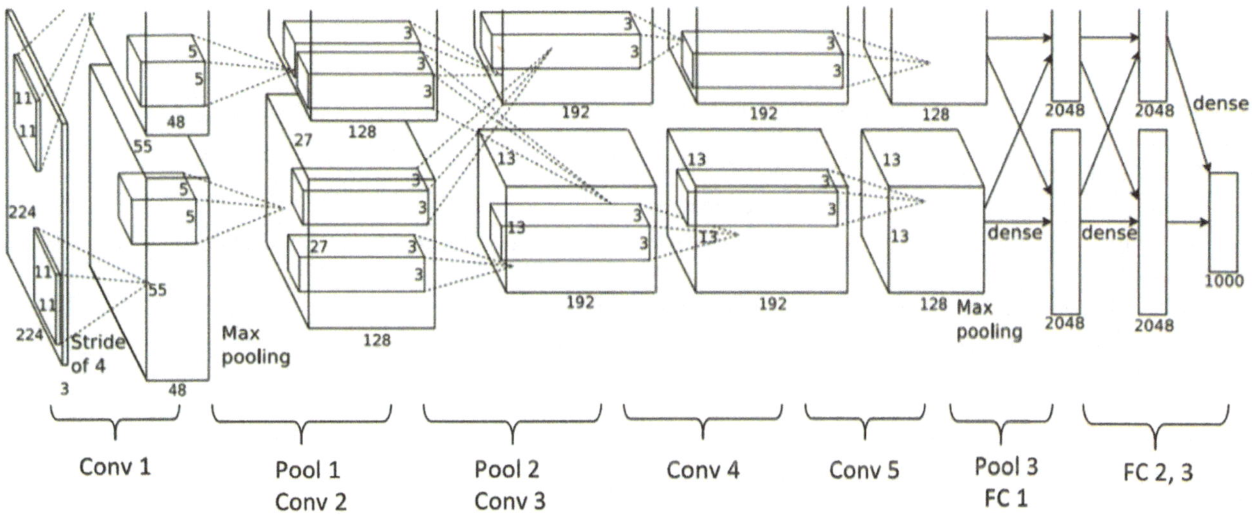

Fig. 15.15 AlexNet structure

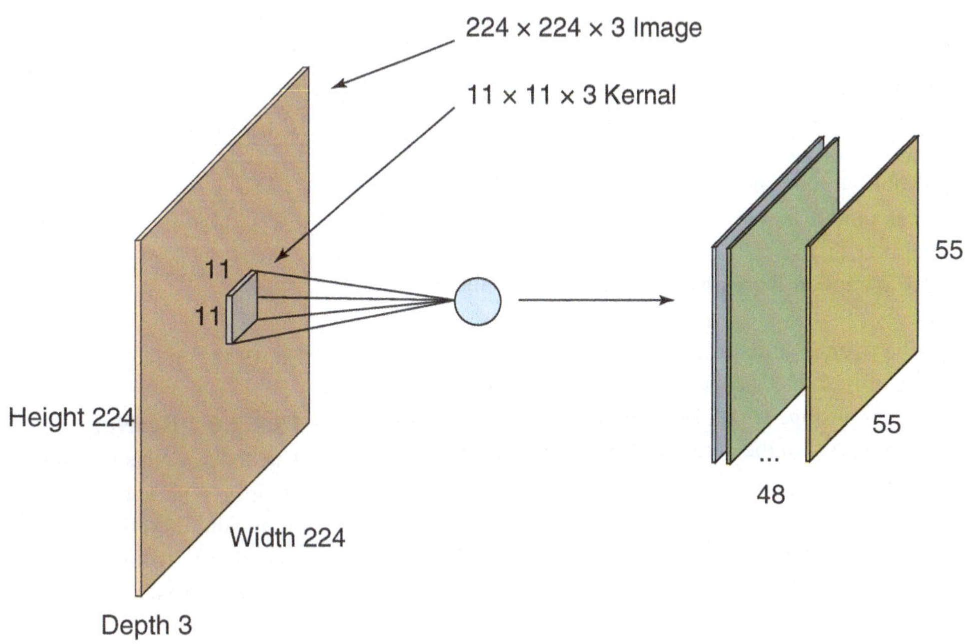

Fig. 15.16 First layer operation of AlexNet

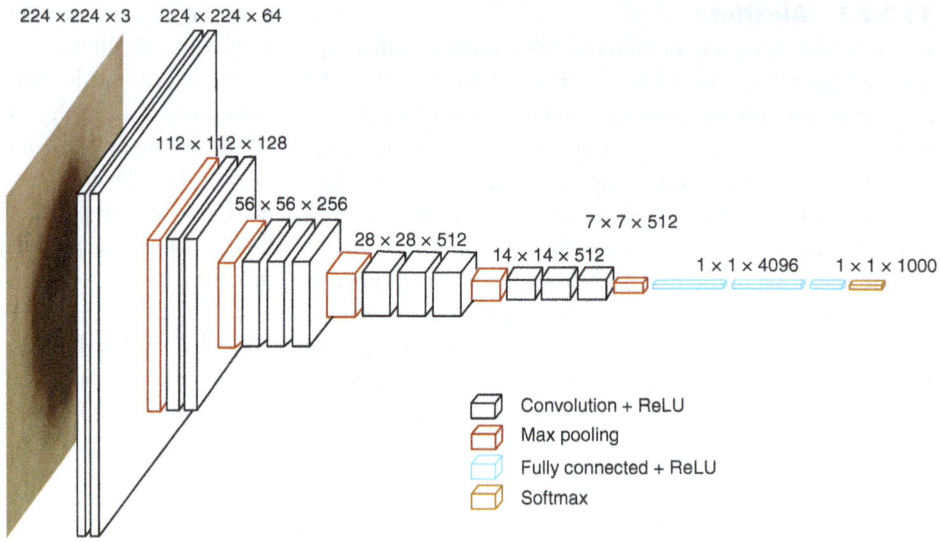

Fig. 15.17 VGG16-Nets structure

the 2014 ImageNet competition for positioning tasks and second place for classification tasks. VGG-Nets can be regarded as the deepened version of AlexNet, which adopts the structure of a convolution layer and a fully connected layer. According to the different network depths, VGG-Nets can be divided into VGG16 and VGG19. Figure 15.17 shows the structure of VGG16-Nets. Compared with the structure of AlexNet, VGG-Nets adopts several consecutive convolution kernels with a size of 3 × 3 to replace the larger convolution kernels in AlexNet, which improves the depth of the network and enhances the ability of the network, learning more complex patterns and ensuring the same perception field.

15.2.2.3 GoogLeNet

GoogLeNet defeated VGG-Nets in the 2014 ImageNet competition for classification tasks and won the championship. The network introduces the concept structure instead of the traditional operation of simple convolution activation. Inception is a network in network structure, and Fig. 15.18 shows the V1 and V3 versions. The Inception structure stacks convolution and pooling operations together and finally splices output features of the same size. On the one hand, Inception increases the width of the network; on the other hand, Inception increases the adaptability of the network to scale.

The overall structure of the original GoogLeNet is composed of multiple Inception-v1 modules connected in series, as shown in Fig. 15.19. With the further exploration of and improvements in the network structure, Inception has undergone multiple version upgrades to form a more complex network structure suitable for practical problems, further improving the expression ability of the network without increasing the number of calculations.

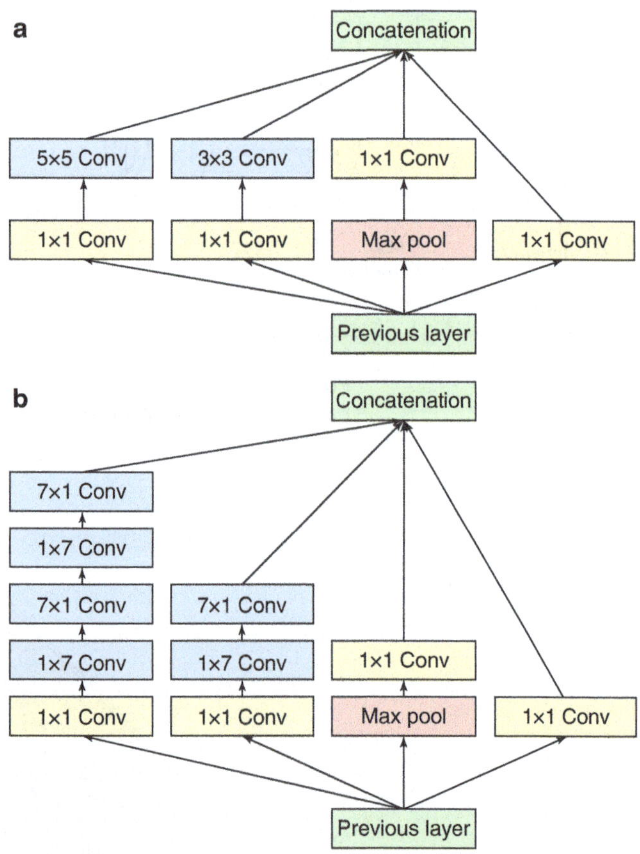

Fig. 15.18 (**a**) Inception-v1. (**b**) Inception-v3

15.2.2.4 ResNet

The above CNNs lose information during information transmission and lead to gradient disappearance or gradient explosion; therefore, deep networks are usually hard to train well. ResNet directly detours the input information to the output to protect the integrity of the information. The entire

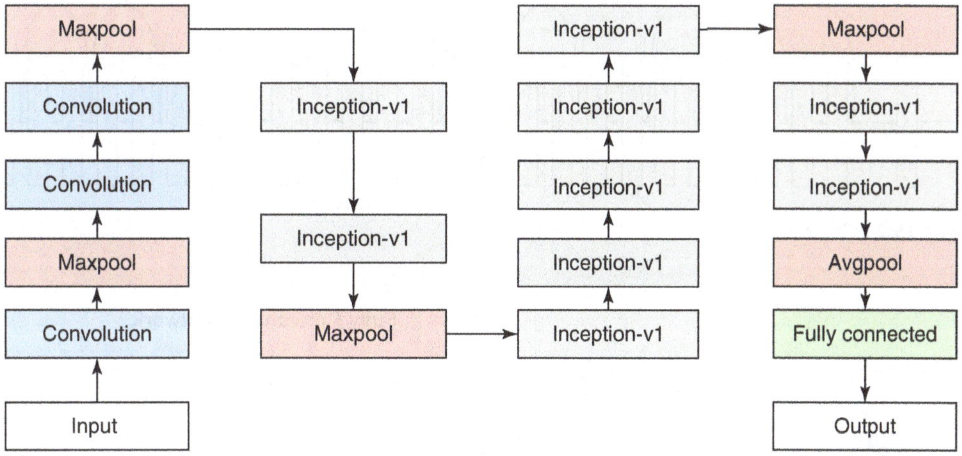

Fig. 15.19 GoogLeNet structure

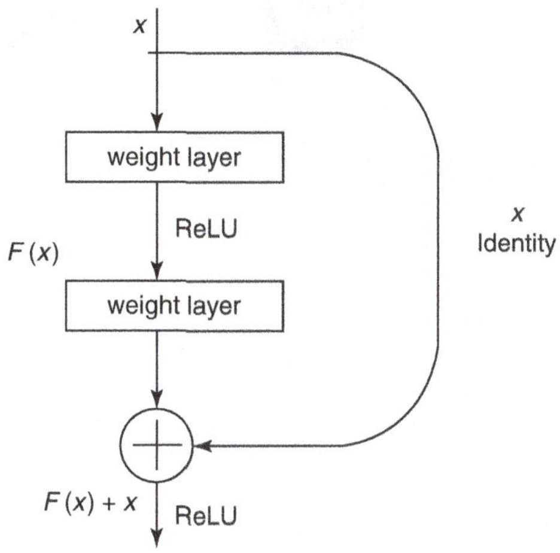

Fig. 15.20 A residual unit structure

network needs to learn only the part of the difference between input and output, simplifying the learning objectives and difficulties. Figure 15.20 shows the structure of a residual unit. Assuming that the input of a neural network is x and the expected output is $H(x)$, if we directly pass the input x to the output as the initial result, then the object we need to learn is $F(x) = H(x) - x$. In this way, ResNet changes the learning object, no longer learning a complete output $H(x)$ but only the difference between output and input, i.e., the residual to simplify the learning difficulty.

Based on this unique residual unit, Fig. 15.21 shows a 34-layer residual network. In practical problems, the number of layers can reach as high as 100, which greatly improves the generalization ability of the network.

15.2.3 Dermoscopic Image Segmentation Based on a Multiscale Fully Convolutional Neural Network

In the computer-aided diagnosis process for skin lesions, image segmentation is of great significance. Accurate skin lesion boundaries can provide a reliable basis for the subsequent analysis of skin lesions. However, the skin lesion area often has complex and diverse colors, blurred borders, and serious hair occlusion, all of which make the segmentation of dermoscopic images very challenging.

To solve the problem of image segmentation, a commonly used method is a fully convolutional network (FCN). Different from CNNs, FCNs do not use the full connection layer in the back part of the network but replace the full connection layer with a convolution layer, which is the reason why they are called FCNs. After the input image of an FCN is convolved and pooled, a smaller heatmap is obtained, upsampling is used to restore the heatmap to the same size as the input image, and the heatmap is then output as the result of segmentation. This process is visually represented in Fig. 15.22.

In practical problems, the skin lesion area is sometimes a small target. When this occurs, a multiscale FCN can be used to segment the dermoscopic image. Figure 15.23 shows a multiscale FCN designed by our research group. The network consists of a backbone and two branches with different scales of receptive fields. The backbone is obtained by fine-tuning the first ten layers of the VGG16 network to map features to high-dimensional space. The global branch is fine-tuned from the 11th to 15th layers of the VGG16 network. To obtain global features, this branch uses a hole algorithm to expand the receptive field. The local branch is composed of four convolutional layers with a convolution kernel size of 3×3, and the convolution kernel parameters are obtained by random initialization. Compared with the global branch, the local branch has a smaller receptive field and pays more attention to targets with small lesions. We cascade global features and local features to generate a prediction probability map and use bilinear interpolation to enlarge the prediction probability map to the original image size. The final segmentation result is classified by the Softmax classifier pixel by pixel.

Figure 15.24 shows the classification results generated by different branches of multiscale networks. The global branch ensures that the larger skin lesions are segmented, and the local branch segments the small targets that may have skin

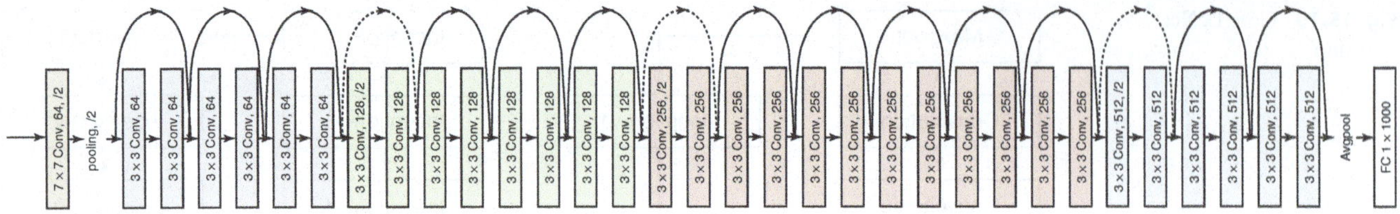

Fig. 15.21 ResNet structure

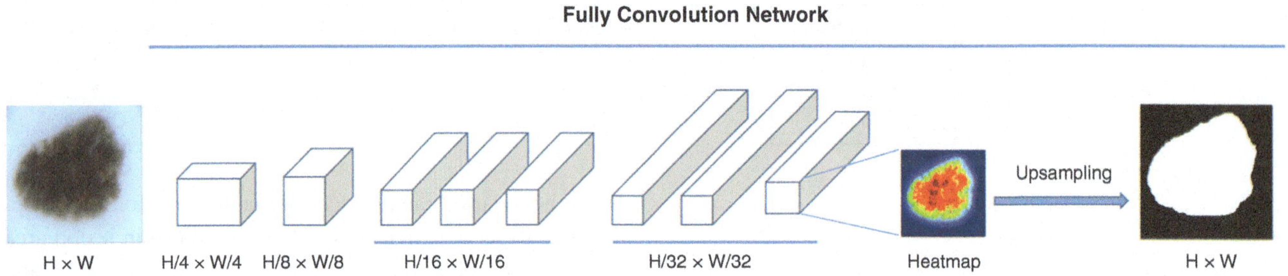

Fig. 15.22 Fully convolutional network structure

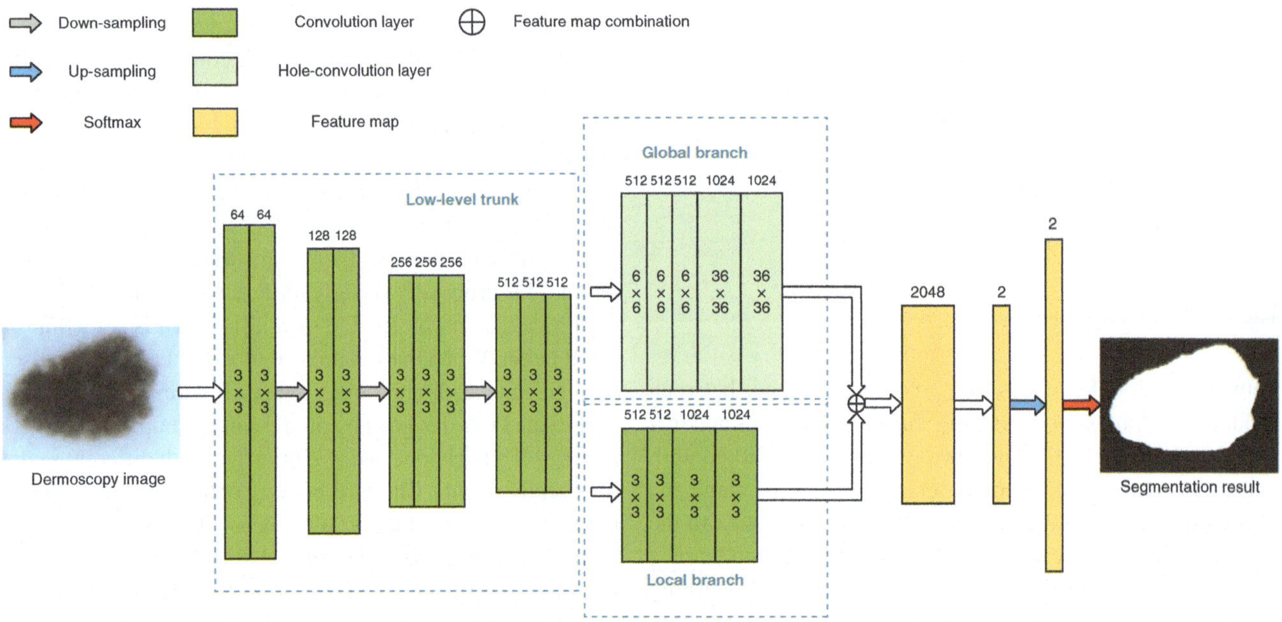

Fig. 15.23 Multiscale fully convolutional network structure

lesions. Through the integration of the two branches, we finally obtain a segmentation result suitable for large and small targets.

15.2.4 Skin Lesion Recognition Based on a Convolutional Neural Network

With powerful classification networks, a large number of training samples and appropriate training strategies, deep learning plays a great advantage in computer-aided diagnosis. In January 2017, Stanford University Artificial Intelligence Laboratory, in cooperation with Stanford School of Medicine, proposed a method that automatically classifies dermoscopic and clinical skin lesion images using deep learning and published the research results in an article in the journal *Nature*, which received widespread attention.

In computer-aided diagnosis, CNNs need a sufficient amount of training data as well as neural networks with strong classification performance; otherwise, it is difficult for CNN to learn appropriate features, and overfitting is a dilemma. The Stanford team has built a very large skin image

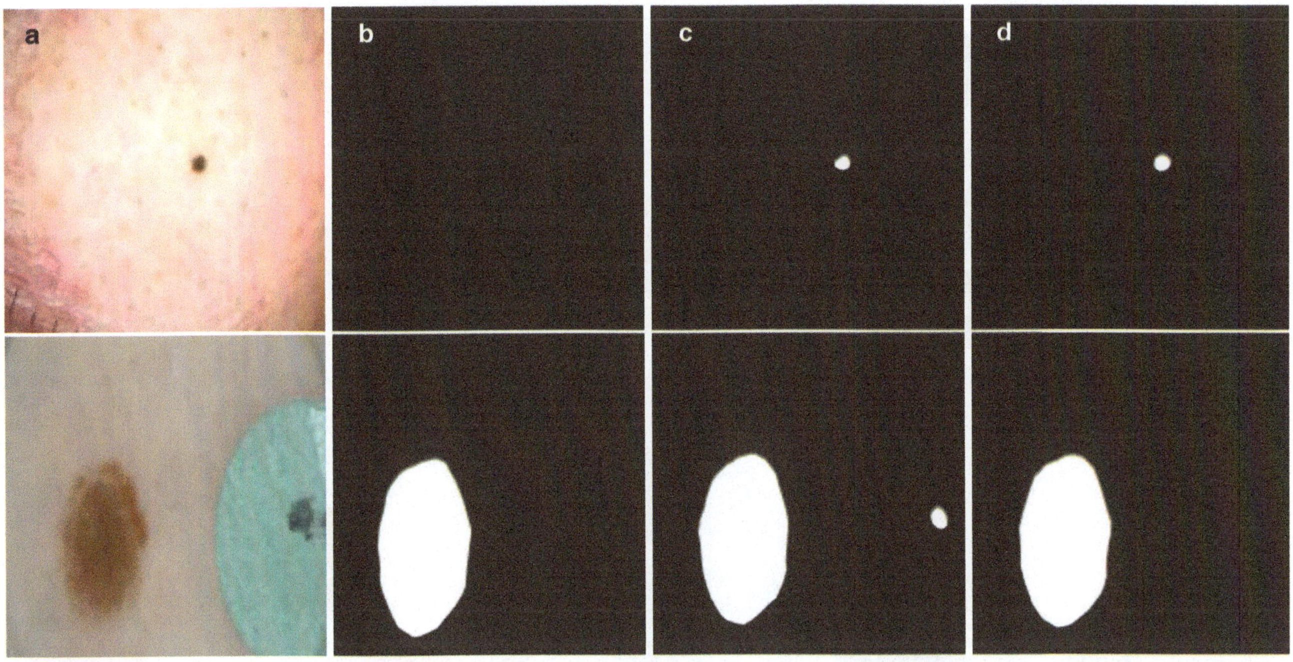

Fig. 15.24 (**a**) Original image. (**b**) Segmentation result by global branch. (**c**) Segmentation result by local branch. (**d**) Final segmentation result

database of up to 129,450 images, including 2032 different diseases, which provides a powerful boost for the training of CNNs. In the data preparation stage, the team proposed an automatic recursive algorithm called PA (disease partitioning algorithm) to aggregate 2032 skin diseases into 757 classes (training classes) with a more uniform distribution according to the skin disease classification tree structure shown in Fig. 15.25 so as to ensure microgranularity classification and sufficient training data for each class.

The team chose GoogLeNet Inception-v3 as its classification network and applied transfer learning technology to its own database. The network structure is shown in Fig. 15.26. GoogLeNet Inception-v3 is one of the CNN models with the strongest classification performance. Pretrained with nearly 1.3 million images in the ImageNet database, GoogLeNet has strong data abstraction capabilities, feature extraction capabilities, and image classification capabilities. The team used the image database to fine-tune the parameters of the trained GoogLeNet Inception-v3 and obtained the CNN model used for skin lesion classification. The team carried out classification experiments on the dataset with 3 or 9 coarse-grained labels and compared the results of CNN with the diagnostic results of two professional doctors. The classification accuracy of the model on the 3-classification and 9-classification tasks reached 72.1% and 55.4%, respectively, while that of the two professional doctors was 65.6% and 53.3% and 66.0% and 55.0%, respectively. Therefore, classification algorithms based on deep learning have the potential to reach or even exceed the diagnostic accuracy of professional doctors.

At present, scholars from various countries have explored the application of deep learning in computer-aided diagnosis by constructing different skin disease datasets, using different CNN networks and evaluation methods, and have achieved good classification results. However, there are still many problems to be solved in using CNNs. ① There is still a lack of a unified database and a unified evaluation method to train and evaluate CNNs, which makes it impossible to compare the experimental results of different teams. In the future, more databases and CNN evaluation methods need to be standardized. ② At present, deep learning is mostly single-center and single-race research, and there is no artificial intelligence model suitable for all races in the world. ③ There is still a lack of information about the patient's medical history (age, sex, the time of onset, the duration of disease, etc.), the clinical characteristics of skin lesions (inspection, palpation, etc.), and the method of combining the results of examination and multidimensional skin imaging. ④ Current research involves a few disease types, which is different from the many disease types encountered in clinical practice, and the types of diseases need to be expanded in deep learning research. Current deep learning applications are mostly limited to the multiclass diagnosis of skin imaging. However, the diagnosis of tumor malignancy and the choice of treatment are equally important to dermatologists. Therefore, we look forward to more research on the application of deep learning in other aspects of dermatology diagnosis and treatment and multicentre cooperation to further leverage deep learning methods in dermatology.

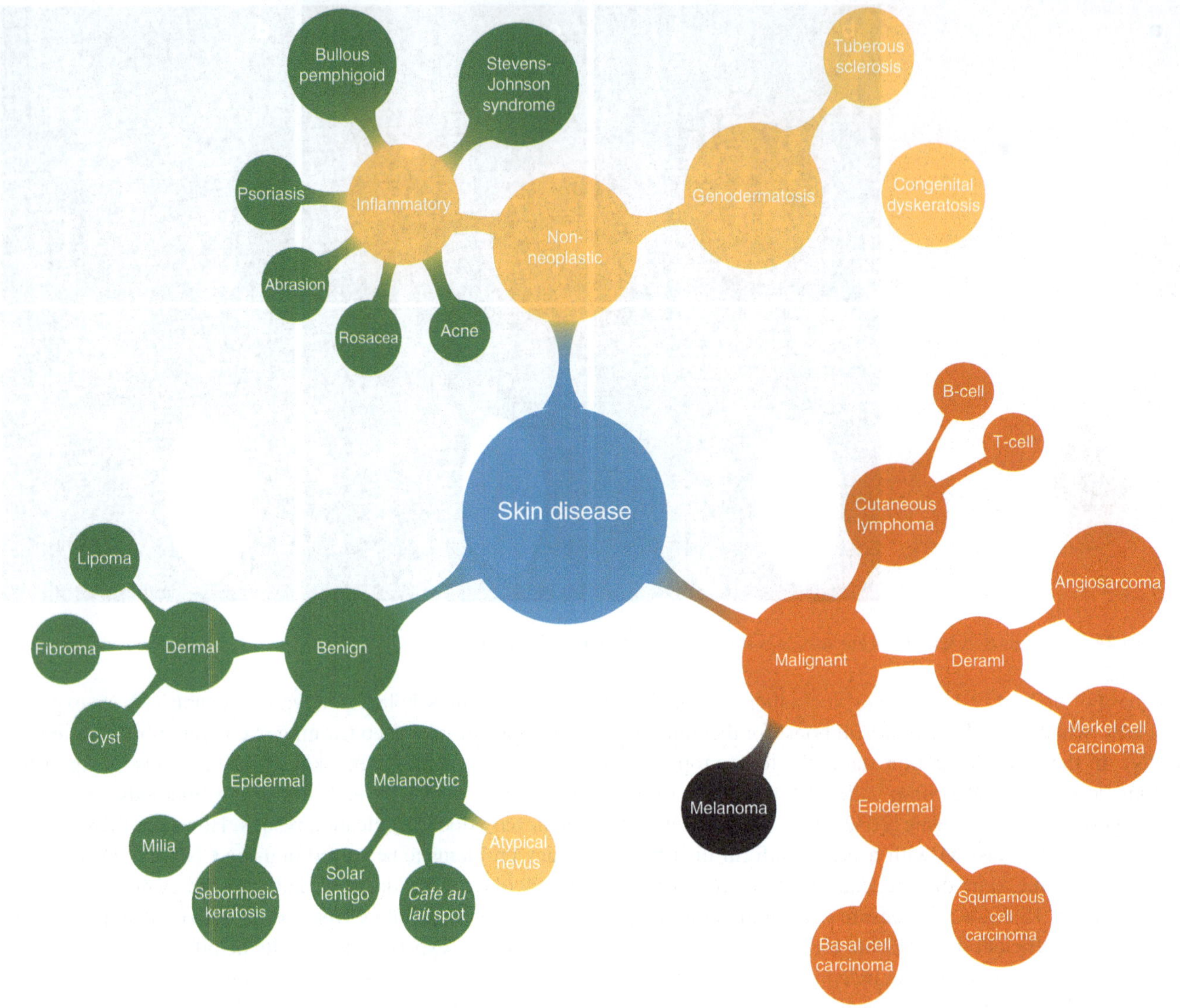

Fig. 15.25 Tree structure of skin disease classification

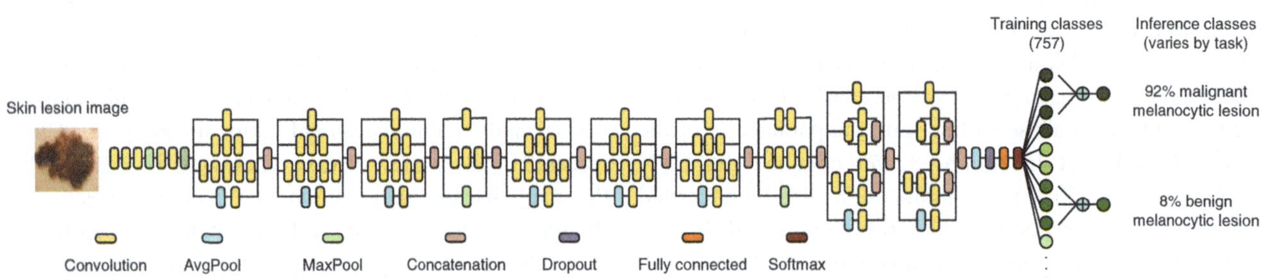

Fig. 15.26 Skin lesion classification model based on GoogLeNet Inception-v3

Further Reading

1. Krizhevsky A, Sutskever I, Hinton G. ImageNet classification with deep convolutional neural networks. Adv Neural Inf Proces Syst. 2012;25(2):1097–105.
2. Simonyan K, Zisserman A. Very deep convolutional networks for large-scale image recognition. Comput Sci. 2014;1 https://doi.org/10.48550/arXiv.1409.1556.
3. Szegedy C, Liu W, Jia Y, et al. Going deeper with convolutions. Comput Sci. 2014; https://doi.org/10.48550/arXiv.1409.4842.
4. He K, Zhang X, Ren S, et al. Deep residual learning for image recognition [C]//2016 IEEE conference on computer vision and pattern recognition (CVPR). IEEE Computer Society; 2016.
5. Long J, Shelhamer E, Darrell T. Fully convolutional networks for semantic segmentation. IEEE Trans Pattern Anal Mach Intell. 2014;39(4):640–51.
6. Esteva A, Kuprel B, Novoa RA, et al. Dermatologist-level classification of skin cancer with deep neural networks. Nature. 2017;542(7639):115–8.
7. Wang S, Liu J, Zhu C, et al. Comparison of dermatologists and deep convolution neural network in the diagnosis of pigmented nevus and seborrheic keratosis. Chin J Dermatol. 2018;51(7):486–9.
8. Zhang XY, Wang SQ, Liu J, et al. Towards improving diagnosis of skin diseases by combining deep neural network and human knowledge. BMC Med Inform Decis Mak. 2018;18(S2):69–76.
9. Wang S, Liu J. Research progress of deep learning assisted automatic classification of skin images. Chin J Dermatol. 2020;53(12):1037–40.

The manufacturer's authorised representative in the EU is Springer
Nature Customer Service Centre GmbH, Europaplatz 3, 69115 Heidelberg,
Germany. If you have any concerns regarding our products, please
contact ProductSafety@springernature.com

Printed and bound by CPI Group (UK) Ltd, Croydon, CR0 4YY
02/10/2026
02226756-0001